Complementary, Integrative and Alternative Medicine

Complementary, Integrative and Alternative Medicine

Editor: Nicolas Mooney

AMERICAN
MEDICAL PUBLISHERS
www.americanmedicalpublishers.com

AMERICAN
MEDICAL PUBLISHERS
www.americanmedicalpublishers.com

Cataloging-in-Publication Data

Complementary, integrative and alternative medicine / edited by Nicolas Mooney.
p. cm.
Includes bibliographical references and index.
ISBN 978-1-63927-048-4
1. Alternative medicine. 2. Integrative medicine. 3. Medicine. I. Mooney, Nicolas.
R733 .C66 2022
615.5--dc23

American Medical Publishers,
41 Flatbush Avenue,
1st Floor, New York,
NY 11217, USA

ISBN 978-1-63927-048-4 (Hardback)

Contents

Preface

The purpose of the book is to provide a glimpse into the dynamics and to present opinions and studies of some of the scientists engaged in the development of new ideas in the field from very different standpoints. This book will prove useful to students and researchers owing to its high content quality.

The medical treatments which are used instead of traditional therapies fall under the umbrella of alternative medicine. This includes a wide range of health care products and therapies such as acupuncture, chiropractic, magnetic field therapy, etc. Integrative medicine is an approach to care that puts the patient at the center and addresses the full range of physical, emotional, mental, social, spiritual and environmental influences that affect a person's health. The diagnostic and therapeutic disciplines that are used in conjunction with conventional medicine are known as complementary medicine. Complementary, integrative and alternative medicine often use natural substances such as foods, herbs, animal and fungal products, minerals, non-vitamin supplements and megavitamins. This book outlines the concepts and applications of complementary, integrative and alternative medicine in detail. It is compiled in such a manner, that it will provide an in-depth knowledge about the theory and practice of this subject. This book will serve as a reference to a broad spectrum of readers.

At the end, I would like to appreciate all the efforts made by the authors in completing their chapters professionally. I express my deepest gratitude to all of them for contributing to this book by sharing their valuable works. A special thanks to my family and friends for their constant support in this journey.

Editor

1

Prevalence and Factors Associated with Parental Traditional Medicine Use for Children in Motta Town, Amhara Regional State, Ethiopia, 2014

Tenaw Gualu Melesse[*1], **Yohannes Ayalew**[2], **Girma Alem Getie**[1], **Haymanot Zeleke Mitiku**[1] **and Girmay Tsegaye**[1]

[1]*Department of Nursing, College of Health Sciences, Debremarkos University,Debremarkos, Ethiopia*

[2]*Departments of Nursing and Midwifery, School of Allied Health Sciences, College of Health Science, Addis Ababa University, Addis Ababa, Ethiopia*

[*]**Corresponding author**: Tenaw Gualu Melesse, Department of Nursing, College of Health Sciences, Debremarkos University Debremarkos, Ethiopia, E-mail: tenawgualu@yahoo.com

Abstract

Background: Traditional medicine is the ancient and culture bound medical practice which existed in human societies before the application of modern science to health. Around 80% of Ethiopians relies on traditional medicines. Although some traditional medical practices in children are useful and contributing positively and need to be strengthen, some are harmful from the perspective of health. In Ethiopia, studies conducted so far are very limited and focused on adults. As a result, this study was conducted to assess the prevalence and factors associated with parental traditional medicine practice for children.

Objective: The aim of this study was to assess prevalence and factors associated with parental traditional medicine use for children in Motta Town.

Methods: Community based cross-sectional study design was used. Data was collected using structured interviewer administered questionnaire. The study was conducted among 381 households selected using systematic random sampling method. Both descriptive and inferential statistics were used to present the data. Odds ratio, binary and multiple logistic regression were used to assess the association between dependent and independent variables.

Result: It was found that 88.2% of parents had used either forms of traditional medicine for their children. The top therapies used were herbs (66.9%), religious therapies (52.8%), massage (22.8%), bone settler (21.8%) and traditional birth attendants (13.1%). Female parents, low educational level, accessibility of traditional medicine, low price and perceived effectiveness were significantly associated with parental traditional medicine use for children.

Conclusion and recommendation: There was high parental traditional medicine practice for children in this study. Female parents, low educational status, easily accessibility, cheap in price and perceived effectiveness were significant predictors. The integration of traditional medicine as part of modern medicine and controlling mechanism should be strengthen. Community education and further research on its efficacy and safety should also be done.

Keywords: Traditional medicine; Parent; Children; Motta; Ethiopia

Abbreviations:

AOR: Adjusted Odds Ratio; ASD: Autism Spectrum Disorder; CAM: Complementary and Alternative Medicine; CI: Confidence Interval; COR: Crude Odds Ratio; HEW's: Health Extension Workers; MDG: Millennium Development Goal; SPSS: Statistical Package for Social science; TM: Traditional Medicine; USA: United States of America; WHO: World Health Organization.

Introduction

World Health Organization (WHO) defines traditional medicine as diverse health practices, approaches, knowledge and beliefs incorporating plant, animal, and/or mineral based medicines, spiritual therapies, manual techniques and exercises applied singularly or in combination to maintain well-being, prevent illness as well as to diagnose and treat illness [1].

In Asia and Latin America, for example, population continues to use traditional medicine. In China, traditional medicine accounts for around 40% of all health care delivered. On the other hand, up to 80% of people in Africa use traditional medicine to meet their health care needs [1]. Ethiopian people have been using traditional medicine since time immemorial. Around 80% of its population relies on traditional medicines [2].

There are many factors that push people to rely on traditional, complementary and alternative medicine all over the world in recent times. Because it is easily accessible, more affordable, closely corresponds to the patients ideology and less paternalistic than modern medicine, the appeal of traditional, complementary and alternative medicine increases [3].

Irrational use of medicine is a major problem worldwide. It is estimated that more than half of all medicines are prescribed, dispensed or sold inappropriately and that half of all patients fail to take them correctly. This contributes to enormous health and economic impacts both at a personal and national level [4]. As a result, pediatric use of complementary and alternative medicine (CAM) therapies raises legal as well as clinical concerns [5].

Children are dependent on their parents. They cannot fight for their health rights. And some traditional practices like harmful traditional health practices were found to be killing practices for children. These practices are violating the children's health rights and hindering the country from achieving millennium development goal (MDG 4) [6].

Even though the use of traditional complementary and alternative therapies in children has recently shown explosive growth, there is little scientific evidence of benefit, a need for better regulatory oversight, and continuing gaps in the knowledge and attitudes of pediatric health professionals [7].

In Ethiopia, studies conducted so far are very limited and focused on adult traditional medical practices. The use of traditional medicine has not been widely studied among children. Therefore, this cross-sectional study was conducted to assess prevalence and predictors of parental traditional medicine use for children. So determining the rational of increased childhood traditional medicine utilization has paramount importance and it will fill the gaps in this regard.

Objectives

General objective: To assess the prevalence and factors associated with parental traditional medicine use for children in Motta town, Amhara Regional State, Ethiopia, 2014.

Specific objective: To determine the prevalence of parental traditional medicine use for children for the last twelve months. To identify factors associated with parental traditional medicine use for children

Methods and Materials

Study area: The study was conducted in Motta town which is found in East Gojjam Zone, Amhara region of Ethiopia.

Study design: Community based cross-sectional study design was used.

Study period: The data was collected from March to April/2014.

Source population: All parents having under eighteen years of age children who live in Motta Town.

Study population: All randomly selected parents having under eighteen years of old children who fulfill the inclusion criteria were included.

Inclusion criteria: Parents who were permanent residents at least for six months have under eighteen years old children who live with them at least for six months. Available at the time of data collection were included.

Exclusion criteria: Parents who were seriously ill or unable to give the required information during data collection period were excluded.

Sample size: A total of 381 households were included in this study.

Sampling procedure: Study populations (parents having under eighteen years old children) were selected using systematic sampling technique.

Instrument and measurement

The data collection tool was a structured interviewer administered questionnaires. Either the father or mother of the children was interviewed. But priority was given for the mother because mothers are close to their children than fathers. Structured interviewer administered questionnaires adapted and modified from previous researches done on similar topics [8-11] and was translated in to the local language (Amharic). The questionnaire consists of five parts. The first part consisted of predisposing factors. Under this part, the questionnaire dealt about parental socio demographic characteristics and value - believe systems. The second part comprised of prevalence of utilization of TM. The third part of the questionnaire comprised enabling factors. The fourth part of the questionnaire was about need factors and the last section was regarding health care experience.

Personnel

Eight health extension workers (HEWs) were involved in the data collection.

Data quality control

Data collectors (HEWs) were trained on how to interview and record and assigned out of their respective kebeles to minimize information bias. In order to assess the validity and reliability of the instrument, clarity of the questions and respondent reaction to the question and interviewer, pre-test was done in another kebeles at 5% of actual respondents. After the pre-test unclear questions were collected and interviewers adjusted themselves as required. But the data from the pre-test was not included in the analysis. When the head of household (mother/father) was unavailable during data collection period, repeated trials until three times were done. During the data collection time, regular monitoring and supervision of the overall activity was done by the supervisors and principal investigator to ensure the quality of data.

Data processing and analysis

The data was cleaned, coded and entered in Epi data version 3.1 and transferred to SPSS version 20.0 for analysis. Finally, descriptive and inferential statistics were used to summarize the data.

Variables

Dependent variable: Parental traditional medicine use for children

Independent variables: Predisposing Factors such as socio demographic characteristics of parents (age, sex, religion, marital status, economic level, education, family size and resident). Enabling Factors (cost, accessibility and source of referral). Need Factors (conditions such as promotion, prevention and treatment, type of illness, perception of illness and parental rating of child health). Health Care Experience (parental CAM use, dissatisfaction with modern medicine, efficacy of CAM, fear of side effect of modern medicine and cost of modern medicine) (Table 1).

Ethical consideration

Ethical approval and clearance to conduct this research were obtained from Research and Ethical Review Committee of Department of Nursing and Midwifery, School of Allied Health Sciences, College of Health Science, Addis Ababa University. Permission to conduct the study was also requested from Motta Town Administration. Voluntariness was asked and signed on the consent form. The aim of the study was explained and participants were informed about confidentiality of the data.

Result

Prevalence of traditional medicine utilization for children

Among the total 381 participants of this study, 336(88.2%) had used at least one form of traditional medicine for their children in the last 12 months. Among this 79.8% were females and 8.4 were males. Herbal medicine were most commonly practiced 255(66.9%) followed by religious/prayer practice 201(52.8%), massage 87(22.8%), bone settler 83(21.8%), tooth extractors 38(10.8%) and 16(4.2%) have mentioned as they used other forms of traditional medicine named: Yehareg ressa, Salehu dress and Yebuda medhanit in their culture

Variable		Frequency(N)	Percentage(%)
Sex	Male	41	10.8
	Female	340	89.2
Age (years)	≤25	63	16.5
	26-35	179	47
	36-45	108	28.3
	>45	31	8.1
Religious affiliation	Orthodox	228	59.8
	Muslim	145	38.1
	Others*	8	2.1
Marital status	Single	18	4.7
	Married	233	61.2
	Divorced	86	22.6
	Widowed	44	11.5
Educational status	Unable to read and write	192	50.4
	Read and write	103	27
	Primary school (1-8)	28	7.3
	High school (9-12)	32	8.4
Residence	Urban	252	66.1
	Sub urban	129	33.9
Number of children (<18 years)	Less than three	271	71.1
	Three- four	104	27.3
	Greater than four	6	1.6
Monthly income (Ethiopian birr)	<500	180	47.2
	500-850	114	29.9
	851-1500	56	14.7
	>1500	31	8.1

*Catholic and Protestant

Factors associated with traditional medicine practice

Respondents were asked to list what their reasons were to use traditional medicine for their child/children. Among these (47.5%) mentioned accessibility, (34.4%) cheap in price, (31.5%) having low income, (15%) referred by someone else and 4.7% mentioned lack of time for emergency problems and cultural acceptability of traditional medicines. Study participants have used traditional medicine to treat different health problems (Figure 1).

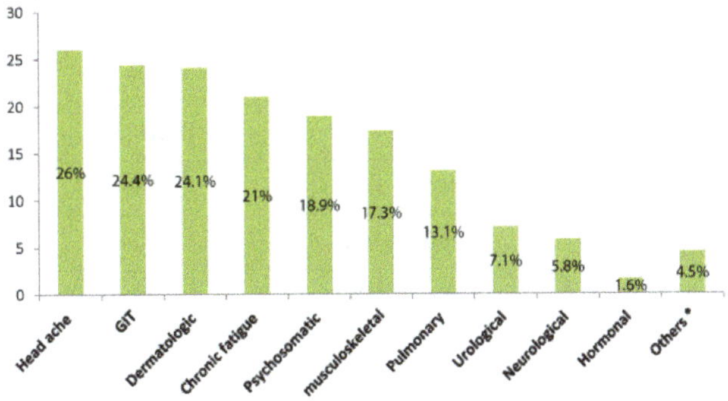

Figure 1: Frequency of children symptoms treated by parental traditional medicine in Motta town, Amhara region, North West Ethiopia, April 2014. (In the last 12 months) Note: *Eye problems, Ear problems.

Study participants were asked about their reasons for applying traditional than modern medicine. From this, nearly half of respondents (47.2%) used because as it was effective when selected correctly, (37.8%) difficulty in accessing health care facility (20.2%) fear of using drugs and side effect, (11.3%) satisfaction with traditional medicine, (6%) dissatisfaction with modern medicine, (3.9%) less efficacy of modern medicine and (4.5%) mentioned non-curable diseases with modern medicine and cultural acceptability (Table 2).

Variables		**Frequency (N)**	**Percentage (%)**
Have you ever used TM for yourself in the last 12 months?	Yes	316	82.9
	No	65	17.1
Who had used CAM?	Mother only	169	44.4
	Father only	95	24,9
	Both	117	30.7
How do you indicate the level of TM efficacy?	Very poor	6	1.6
	Poor	87	22.8
	Fair	52	13.6
	Very good	170	44.6

	Excellent	66	17.3
How do you indicate your level of satisfaction after TM use?	Completely dissatisfied	9	2.4
	Somewhat dissatisfied	79	20.7
	Neither satisfied nor dissatisfied	15	3.9
	Somewhat satisfied	154	40.4
	Completely satisfied	124	32.5

Over all how do you rank the quality of your experience with modern healthcare systems?	Very bad	5	1.3
	Bad	15	3.9
	Good	82	21.5
	Very good	111	29.1
	Extremely good	168	44.1

Table 2: Health care experience of participants in Motta town, Amhara region, North West Ethiopia, April 2014 (In the last 12 months, N=381).

Variables		**Parental TM use for children**			
		Yes	**No**	**COR (95%CI)**	**AOR (95%CI)**
Sex	Male	32(8.4)	9(2.4)	1	1
	Female	304(79.8)	36(9.4)	2.38(1.05-5.37)	2.66(1.11- 6.40)*
Educational status	Illiterate	174(45.7)	18(4.7)	3.56(1.32-9.62)	3.10(1.10-8.84)*
	Read and write	92(24.1)	11(2.9)	3.08(1.06-8.97)	3.45(1.12-0.61)*
	Primary(1-8)	25(6.6)	3(0.8)	3.07(0.70-3.46)	4.80(1.02-2.67)*
	High school	26(6.8)	6(1.6)	1.6(0.46-5.52)	0.97(0.26-3.66)
	Above high school	19(5.0)	7(1.8)	1	1
Monthly income	<500 birr	162(42.5)	18(4.7)	3.68(1.47-9.20)	
	500-850 birr	102(26.8)	12(3.4)	3.48(1.31-9.26)	
	851-1500 birr	50(13.1)	6(1.6)	3.41(1.08-0.75)	
	>1500 birr	22(5.8)	9(2.4)	1	
Accessibility of TM	Yes	168(44.1)	13(3.4)	2.46(1.25-4.86)	2.97(1.42-6.18)*
	No	168(44.1)	32(8.4)	1	1
Cheap in price	Yes	122(32.0)	9(2.4)	2.28(1.06-4.89)	2.41(1.10-5.43)*
	No	214(56.2)	36(9.4)	1	1
Parental TM use	Yes	284(74.5)	32(8.4)	2.22(1.10-4.51)	
	No	52(13.6)	13(3.4)	1	
Effectiveness of TM	Yes	167(43.8)	13(3.4)	2.43(1.23-4.80)	2.48(1.21-5.08)*
	No	169(44.4)	32(8.4)	1	1
Difficulty in accessing modern medicine and cost	Yes	135(35.4)	9(2.4)	2.69(1.25-5.76)	
	No	201(55.1)	36(9.4)	1	
1=Reference *p-value<0.05(significant)					

Table 3: Bivariate and multivariate logistic regression analysis of factors associated Parental TM use for children in Motta Town, Amhara Region, North West Ethiopia, April 2014 (N=381).

Discussion

In this cross-sectional study, the prevalence of parental traditional medicine use for children was 88.2%. It was higher when compared to a research done in Kuala Lumpur, Malaysia, 84.5% [12] and Southern Arizona, 64% [13]. The difference might be from methodological and cultural differences between the studies. The previous studies were conducted at health care setting and this study was community based.

In a health care setting study, people could be said that they have experience with modern health care system, so the prevalence of traditional medicine use for children might be decreased (Table 3).

In this study, the most commonly used TM therapies were herbal medicine (66.9%), religious therapy (52.8%), massage (22.8%) and bone settler (21.8%). This study is in line with a research done in Southern Arizona where spiritual therapies were most commonly used [13]. This might be due to in Ethiopia also most of the people are religious and religious therapies are given priority. However, the study was in contrary in most cases with the study conducted in Eastern-Harargie district of Oromya region, Ethiopia, where uvulectomy, tonsillectomy, cauterization, milk tooth extraction, spiritual healing and herbal medicine were the most commonly used therapies [6]. The difference could be from the study population; in this study, participants were parents having under eighteen years old children and in previous study participants were parents having under five years old children. And uvulectomy, tonsillectomy, cauterization, milk tooth extraction are commonly practiced among under five children not for older children. In addition, because these are invasive procedures now a days the practices are somewhat decreased.

Some of the socio-demographic characteristics were significantly associated with parental traditional medicine use for children. Adjusting for other factors, sex of the parent was significantly associated with parental traditional medicine practice. Females were 2.66 times more likely to use traditional for their children than males. This was in congruent with studies done in India, Ireland and USA where female gender was an independent predictive factor of CAM use [14-16]. This might be; because female parents spent most of their time with their children than male parents and they are near to their children. But a study done in Addis Ababa, showed there is no significance difference between sexes [2]. The difference might be from the methodology of the study. In a study done at Addis Ababa, the study participants were traditional healers and patients who attend traditional clinic for themselves.

Another factor that affects parental traditional medicine practice was educational level. Parental educational status was significantly associated with parental TM use for children in this study. Illiterate parents were 3.10 times more likely to practice traditional medicine for their children than parents above high school educated. This is not in line with previous studies done in Calabria and Finland where parents who use traditional medicine for their children were more educated [17-20]. This could because; this study was community based and most of the participants were illiterate.

Resources found within the family and the communities were another pushing factors for traditional medicine practice [21]. In this study, accessibility of traditional medicine was significantly associated with parental use for children. Those parents who perceived traditional medicine as it is being easily accessible were 2.97 times more likely to use traditional medicine for their children when compared to those who perceived as it isn't accessible. This is in line with another study, where accessibility and acceptance of treatments were predictive of parental CAM use for ASD [19].

From the total participants 131(34.4%) perceived traditional medicine as it is cheap. Adjusting for other factors, parents who recognized traditional medicine as it is being cheap enough were 2.4 times more likely to practice for their children than those who didn't perceive as it is cheap. It was lower than a study done in Ghana where 58.6% users of traditional health care services claimed that traditional medical services are "cheap" [22]. This may be due to the socio-economic and market differences between participants in Ghana and Ethiopia.

Perceived effectiveness of traditional medicine was another factor significantly related with parental traditional medicine utilization. In this study, 167 (43.8%) of participants perceived traditional medicine as effective when selected correctly and had used for their children. Adjusting for other factors, those who perceived traditional medicine as effective were 2.48 times to use for their children than those who perceived as it is not accessible. This was in agreement with a study done among Calabrian children, where perception of the efficacy of traditional medicine was high in all interviewed [17].

Although parental use of traditional medicine for themselves was significantly associated with childhood traditional medicine practice in previous studies [13,16,19,22]. In this study, there wasn't significant difference between parents who had used for themselves and those who hadn't used it previously. Probably this could be because child and maternal health service have received government attention currently and health education has been given at large to the parents regarding children's health.

Conclusion

There was high parental traditional medicine practice for children in this study (88.2%). This indicates the contribution of traditional medicines to the public health is significant. The study showed that for the majority of parents traditional medicines were among the options to promote, prevent and treat their children's health/health problems. The most commonly used traditional medicine therapies were herbal medicines, religious practice, massage, bone settlers, and tooth extraction in order. Female parents, low educational status of parents, easily accessibility of traditional medicines, being cheap in price and perceived effectiveness of traditional medicines were predictors for parents to use traditional medicine for their children.

Recommendation

1. Since perceived efficacy is predictor for traditional medicine use, safety and efficacy of traditional medicine should be studied further.
2. Controlling mechanism should be set regarding traditional healers and traditional medicine accessibility.
3. Education, support and counseling should be given to community at large and particularly to the women regarding traditional medicines.
4. Further national wide research (quantitative and qualitative) including children's characteristics should be conducted.

Acknowledgement

First and for most thanks to the Almighty GOD who is our power and strength. Our gratitude extends to Motta town administration, data collectors and study participants. It is our admiration to Addis Ababa University and Debre Markos University for their financial support to conduct this study

Authors contribution

The authors have contributed their unreserved effort throughout this study in data collection, preparation of the manuscript and approval of the final manuscript.

Conflict of interest

We declare that we have no competing interests

References

1. WHO (2002) WHO traditional medicine strategy 2002-2005. World Health Organization Geneva
2. Birhan W, Giday M, Teklehaymanot T (2011) The contribution of traditional healers' clinics to public health care system in Addis Ababa, Ethiopia: a cross-sectional study. J Ethnobiol Ethnomed 7: 39.
3. Santé Omdl (2001) Legal Status of Traditional Medicine and Complementary-alternative Medicine: A Worldwide Review: Worlds health organization WHO WHO Medicines Strategy
4. Cohen MH, Kemper KJ (2005) Complementary therapies in pediatrics: a legal perspective. Pediatrics 115: 774-780.
5. Sadik EA GT, Mengistu B (2013) Aspects of Common Traditional Medical Practices Applied for Under Five Children in Ethiopia, Oromia Region, Eastern-Harargie District, Dadar Woreda, 2011 G.C. J Community Med Health Educ. 3: 237.
6. Woolf AD, Gardiner P (2010) Use of complementary and alternative therapies in children. Clin Pharmacol Ther 87: 155-157.
7. Ellison CG, Bradshaw M, Roberts CA (2012) Spiritual and religious identities predict the use of complementary and alternative medicine among US adults. Prev Med 54: 9-12.
8. Oshikoya KA, Senbanjo IO, Njokanma OF, Soipe A (2008) Use of complementary and alternative medicines for children with chronic health conditions in Lagos, Nigeria. BMC Complement Altern Med 8: 66.
9. Curlin FA, Rasinski KA, Kaptchuk TJ, Emanuel EJ, Miller FG, et al. (2009) Religion, clinicians, and the integration of complementary and alternative medicines. J Altern Complement Med 15: 987-994.
10. Kim JH, Nam CM, Kim MY, Lee DC (2012) The use of complementary and alternative medicine (CAM) in children: a telephone-based survey in Korea. BMC Complement Altern Med 12: 46.
11. Hamidah A, Rustam ZA, Tamil AM, Zarina LA, Zulkifli ZS, et al. (2009) Jamal R. Prevalence and parental perceptions of complementary and alternative medicine use by children with cancer in a multi-ethnic Southeast Asian population. Pediatric blood & cancer 52: 70-74.
12. Sanders H, Davis MF, Duncan B, Meaney FJ, Haynes J, et al. (2003) Use of complementary and alternative medical therapies among children with special health care needs in southern Arizona. Pediatrics 111: 584-587.
13. Pankaj G, Prateek S, Saurabh R (2011) Determinants of self-medication practices in an urban slum community. Asian J Pharm Clin Res 4: 54-57.
14. Chang KH, Brodie R, Choong MA, Sweeney KJ, Kerin MJ (2011) Complementary and alternative medicine use in oncology: a questionnaire survey of patients and health care professionals. BMC Cancer 11: 196.
15. Yussman SM, Ryan SA, Auinger P, Weitzman M (2004) Visits to complementary and alternative medicine providers by children and adolescents in the United States. Ambul Pediatr 4: 429-435.
16. Dolceamore TR, Altomare F, Zurlo F, Miniero R (2012) Use of alternative-complementary-medicine (CAM) in Calabrian children. Ital J Pediatr 38: 70.
17. Vlieger AM, van de Putte EM, Hoeksma H (2006) [The use of complementary and alternative medicine in children at a general paediatric clinic and parental reasons for use]. Ned Tijdschr Geneeskd 150: 625-630.
18. Hall SE (2013) Factors Affecting Parents' Decisions to Treat Their Children with Autism Spectrum Disorder with Complementary and Alternative Treatments
19. Hämeen-Anttila KP, Niskala UR, Siponen SM, Ahonen RS (2011) The use of complementary and alternative medicine products in preceding two days among Finnish parents - a population survey. BMC Complement Altern Med 11: 107.
20. Gyasi RM, Mensah CM, Adjei PO-W, Agyemang S (2011) Public perceptions of the role of traditional medicine in the health care delivery system in Ghana. Global Journal of Health Science 3: 40.
21. Hurvitz EA, Leonard C, Ayyangar R, Nelson VS (2003) Complementary and alternative medicine use in families of children with cerebral palsy. Dev Med Child Neurol 45: 364-370.
22. Adams D, Dagenais S, Clifford T, Baydala L, King WJ, et al. (2013) Complementary and alternative medicine use by pediatric specialty outpatients. Pediatrics 131: 225-232.

2

Hahnemann's Theory of Psora in the Light of Modern Science

Ghosh AK*

The Jagaddal Noapara Homoeopathic Medical Association, West Bengal, India

***Corresponding author**: Ghosh AK, Secretary, The Jagaddal Noapara Homoeopathic Medical Association, West Bengal, India, E-mail: mail.dr.ajoy@gmail.com

Abstract

Hahnemann observed that the non-venereal chronic diseases originate from a diseased condition or disposition to disease transferring from generation to generation for thousands of years. He named the diseased condition as Psora behaving as the fostering soil for almost all possible disease. According to Hahnemann Psora developed from suppression of itch disease by external application in ancient times. Hahnemann considered the peculiar cutaneous eruption was the outward manifestation of internal itch disease, the Psora. Therefore, any external treatment to remove the skin manifestation is detrimental to the patient and should be avoided. Some eminent dermatologist's perspicacious observation reveals that suppression of some kinds of skin diseases result in virulent internal disorder. It is again justified by another instance that under proper homoeopathic treatment of a chronic disease having history of suppressed skin manifestation in the past, the old eruption definitely reappear satisfying Dr. Hering's law of cure. Health is the result of the dynamic equilibrium among the disease agent, human host and the environment. Human host possessing hereditary factors have an immense role in the production of large number of diseases. Thus to bring cure to any disease especially chronic disease, one should focus one's attention towards the patient [host] to find out the fundamental cause without ignoring the disease agents and the environmental factors acting as exciting or maintaining cause. Hahnemann's 'Theory of Chronic Disease' serves as a pioneer to the key of ideal cure of innumerable chronic diseases. Until and unless, Miasm [the fundamental cause of all natural diseases] is done away with by dint of antimiasmatic treatment, the permanent cure of chronic disease is not possible.

Keywords: Non-venereal chronic diseases; Hahnemann's theory; Psora; Miasm.

Introduction

In the homoeopathic world "miasm" has raised a lot of controversy. Some stalwarts look upon it as a mere fantasy of Hahnemann and find no practical value of it in homoeopathic treatment. But others regard the theory of chronic miasm as the key to the achievement of homoeopathy in curing chronic disease. Treating natural diseases during thirty years by the homoeopathic method of treatment, Hahnemann perceived, the chronic diseases could not be perfectly cured by the simple similar medicines selected on the present symptoms associated with dietetic and hygienic measures and not even by vigorous, robust constitution. With passage of time the disease grew worse in addition to other more serious symptoms until the organism is fully destroyed. After thorough research to find out the cause behind the failure of similar remedies to cure the chronic diseases, Hahnemann noticed ,--though the medicine prescribed, could subside the chronic disease for the time-being, yet the disease came back in a rather varied form with new symptoms. This led him to the conclusion that the presenting symptoms of a chronic disease represent merely the tip of a floating ice-berg. Hence, the original disease being deep-seated, the whole history of chronic disease associated with accessory circumstances should be taken into consideration. Hahnemann also observed interestingly, the origin of most of the non-venereal chronic diseases lying in a peculiar type of skin eruption, frequently suppressed by a faulty practice. In spite of corroboration on his observation by some of the physicians of his time, most of them failed to accept any relation persisting between skin diseases and other diseases. However, Hahnemann considered, the peculiar cutaneous eruption sometimes only of a few vesicles accompanied by intolerable voluptuous tickling itching was the outward manifestation of internal itch disease, the psora [1].

The word Psora originates from Hebrew word 'tsorat' meaning a groove or fault [2]. Hahnemann explained Psora as a diseased condition or disposition to disease transferring from generation to generation for thousands of years behaving as a fostering soil for almost every possible diseased condition. Psora, like other general diseases manifest outwardly only when, the whole economy has been completely affected. As the human skin does not evolve itself, without the co-operation of the rest of the living whole, it is irrational and thoughtless to consider any skin disease as merely the disease of the skin alone in which the internal portion of the organism takes no part. Therefore, any external treatment to remove the skin manifestation is detrimental to the patient and should be avoided [1]. With the progress of modern science, the skin disease thoroughly studied in association with other diseases, establishing the fact that the skin diseases are to be closely related to the other internal disorders.

Controversy on Hahnemann's theory of chronic disease

Publication of Hahnemann's book on chronic disease in 1828 brings forth a violent stir in the whole medical world. Very few books in the history of medicine produced so much controversy among the physicians. Even Barron Erust George Brunnow to whom Hahnemann had dedicated his work, was antagonistic to the view of Hahnemann regarding chronic diseases [3]. Hufeland [contemporary to Hahnemann] quoted, "At last the physician discovers that there is underlying, a hidden scabies or syphilis" [4]. In 1838, the Central

Congress of homoeopath in Frankfurt passed a resolution condemning the doctrine [5].

On the other hand many homoeopaths recognized the theory of chronic diseases as the most important discovery of Hahnemann. Stapf highly appreciated the book on chronic diseases as for its surprising explanations on the nature and treatment of chronic illness and emphasized to follow the doctrine strictly [6]. Boenninghausen and Hering, the staunch supporter of 'Psora theory' took it granted heartily [6].

After Hahnemann's expiry a number of homoeopathic stalwarts like Clarke [7], Stuart Close [8], Robert [9], Kent [10], O. Lesser [11], Von Grauvogl and others averred 'the doctrine of Psora is irrevocable' [12]. But a considerable number of homoeopathic physicians like Hering and Hughes are against Hahnemann's view regarding undue generalization in tracing all diseases to one primary disease-process [5].

Opinion of modern researchers: To keep pace with the progress of modern science various scientists carried on researches to unmask the mystery of 'Psora'. Stuart Close identified psoric miasm and Koch's tubercle bacilli were to be synonymous [8]. Mackenzie [13] has made an interesting attempt to substitute 'focal infection' for Psora, implying thereby the identification of the psoric miasms with strepto-staphylo and other pyogenic micro-organism. During researches in the Immunity School at University College Hospital, Dr. Edward Bach found that 'chronic intestinal organism lower general resistance, consequently local bacterial infections are almost certain to occur' [14]. This ultimately makes a person susceptible to various diseases. He concluded that poisoning from certain organisms in the intestinal tract was the cause of chronic diseases and that on the removal of theses toxins the so-called chronic complaints disappear. Thus in his opinion, Psora and intestinal toxaemia were identical. Dr. Wheeler and Dr. Dishington also supported to Dr. Bach [14]. In 1926 Bach published his book 'Chronic Disease—A Working Hypothesis', written in collaboration with Dr. C.E.Wheeler of London, who had assisted him in his researches at London Homoeopathic Hospital. Dr. Paterson [15] of Glasgow, the well-known bacteriologist and homoeopath conducted a research work on bowel flora in the same line of Dr. Bach and demonstrated that the non-lactose fermenting organisms of the bowel are related to disease on the one hand, to the homoeopathic remedies on the other. His careful research revealed the same truth as Dr. Bach observed i.e. the patient's clinical condition and susceptibility depend on the change of his bowel flora. He declared, "In the treatment of chronic disease, it is near impossible to get successful results without a full knowledge of Hahnemannian doctrine of miasms." K. C. Chandran tried to analyze the concept of Miasms and Chronic disease in the light of scientific understanding of molecular biology [16]. Among others who have attempted to explain Hahnemann's theory of chronic disease, Bodman [17], Clignett [18], Eardley [19], Gordon Ross [20], Ross [21], Twentyman [22], Zissu [23], Ian Watson [24], Vithoulkas [25] are worth-mentioning.

Reflection of emotion upon the skin

The skin is the visible reflector of emotion and psychological disorder being just like a sensitive photographic plate on which emotional states such as anger by flushing, embarrassment by blushing and fear by paleness etc. are reflected.

Obermayer [26], on the basis of few clinical clues concludes that emotional problems are playing an important role in the genesis of any dermatitis. For example, pruritus is often utilized as a tension outlet. In atopic dermatitis, feeling of anger or guilt may be released through scratching. Urticaria can be an outlet for suppressed anger about unjust life situations. Rosacea may be a sign of the individual's feeling of inferiority and guilt in relation to handling problems arising at work. In hand dermatitis [dyshidrosis], vesiculation frequently follows anxiety situation within 24-28 hours. Psychiatric investigation of the more common dermatologic condition by Wittkower and Russel also coincides with Obermayer's view. Effective treatment may be obtained only by psychotherapy.

Emotional difficulties early in life lead to 'alopecia areata' of severe form where the scalp, beard and body hairs are involved. A 2-week time interval is apparently required for the development of alopecia areata following documentable trauma; this observation has been made in over 300 consecutive cases of alopecia areata, 20 of which have been reported in detail. Relief of emotional stress arrests further hair loss and within several months re-growth may occur. In case emotional problem persisting the disease progresses to alopecia totalis [entire head] or to alopecia universalis [entire body]. "In a 26 year old man alopecia areata developed four times during world war-II. The hair loss occurred each time within two weeks after he had participated in an island invasion in the south pacific. The hair regrew each time his unit was moved to a rest area between operations with permanent re-growth of all the hair at the end of the war" [27].

Griesmer [28] in his survey regarding the incidence of emotionally triggered dermatosis on 4,576 patients found that the eruption of about 34 percent was apparently precipitated by stress. The eczemas and acne clearly were not only very frequently seen, but also their exacerbation seemed to have occurred after stressful situations in over half the patients; atopic eczema and hand eczema seemed to have been emotionally triggered in three quarters of the cases. After the pioneer work of Alexander [29], a number of psychosomaticians tried to explain the pathogenesis of psychocutaneous diseases but still now the matters remain unsolved.

Dermatosis due to internal diseases

Numerous type of skin diseases are discussed, though the aetiology of most of them remains obscure. Genetic predisposition or morbid susceptibility for skin diseases plays an important role in its development like acne vulgaris, atopic dermatitis, psoriasis alopecia, vitiligo and many other conditions. Hahnemann concluded that Psora being manifested primarily as disease, any skin manifestation should not be taken into consideration with the skin only. This truth is focused in the light of modern science. In fact, skin as a mirror of health of a person, reflecting numerous internal disorders upon it. The manifestation of same type of skin disease may differ according to age and diathetic tendencies. A number of genetic and developmental abnormalities have both neurological and cutaneous manifestations most probably due to the common origin of the nervous system and the epidermis from the ectoderm. The skin is affected by malnutrition, whether caused by insufficiency, excessive demands, dietetic imbalance or mal absorption. It is also affected by endocrine and metabolic disturbances, including disordered activities of the pituitary, thyroid and para-thyroids, pancreas, suprarenal and gonads. Pruritus may occur in liver diseases, with or without jaundice, particularly in billiary cirrhosis. Chronic renal disease with uraemia may cause general pruritus and a light brown diffuse pigmentation of the skin. Diabetes mellitus may be associated with infection include boils, carbuncles, ulcers, gangrene, tinea of the feet and the groin and infectious eczematous dermatitis. Asthma may alternate with attacks of Urticaria or may co-exist with it.

Therefore modern medical science unveils Hahnemann's idea that no external application but internal medicine essentially requires to cure skin manifestation due to internal diseases.

Adverse effects of suppression of skin disease by external application

In confirming with his own view Hahnemann in his book 'Chronic Diseases', gave an account of a cases of experiences of the writers in all centuries regarding the injurious effects[sever bodily or mental sufferings] of suppressed eruption [30].

Some eminent dermatologist's perspicacious observation reveals that suppression of some kinds of skin diseases result in virulent internal disorder and occasional death ultimately.

According to Brocq [31] the rapid disappearance of an eczematous eruption in a young child may be followed by pulmonary congestions of the most dangerous kind (Atopic march). He observed also that it is especially in middle life that alternations between eczematous lesions on the skin and visceral manifestations of greater or less gravity [pulmonary, renal, intestinal, cardiac, cerebral etc.] are most likely to show themselves.

Sir Morris [32] observed eczema which appears at puberty alternates with neurotic conditions, more especially with asthma and commencing osteoarthritis. He noted that the irritation of the skin may, as pointed out by Kaposi, set up reflex irritation in the intestine, preventing the proper digestion of food. The irregularities of the bowels react in turn on the skin, and thus a vicious cycle is established. The most common intestinal complication of skin diseases is dyspepsia. Gout is also a frequent complication.

A too rapid cure of eczema in children or its spontaneous disappearance may produce grave metastasis like bronchitis, dysenteric enteritis or pulmonary congestion, sometimes followed by death. In adults especially in old people, the disappearance of generalized eczema may be followed by the same accidents or by other manifestations such as asthma, rheumatism etc. These metastasis also occur in other dermatitis than eczema; prurigo may alternates with bronchitis; psoriasis with rheumatism, dyspnoea etc. [33].

Chronic suffering from rosacea may produce eye lesions, such as keratitis, conjunctivitis and blepharitis. Atopic eczema is one manifestation of a triad of atopic conditions the other two being bronchial asthma and hay fever [34].

Application of corticosteroids, topically and systematically in atopic dermatitis causes severe complication such as cataracts causing blindness [35].

In sub-acute and chronic eczema success often depends more on the dermatologist's understanding of the patient's personality, social domestic conditions and ability to carry out the treatment satisfactorily than on the choice of topical application. For contact dermatitis all hand creams or lotions should be forbidden [36].

Substances which are poorly absorbed through intact skin may penetrate diseased skin freely. So any substance used for topical application in skin disease produces serious systemic effects [37].

It is observed by the physicians that there is a relationship between eczema and asthma. According to BBC NEWS, scientists believe that they have found what triggers many children with eczema to go on to develop asthma. The US team at the Washington University School of Medicine showed that a substance made by the damaged skin triggered asthma symptoms in mice. The same substance, thymic stromal lymphopoietin [TSLP] is also produced in the lungs of asthma patients. Early treatment of the skin rash and blocking TSLP production might stop asthma developing in young patients with eczema, they hope. Drugs that act on TSLP might also protect against asthma developing even in cases that are not linked to eczema [38]. It is estimated that more than six million Australians have suffered from eczema at some stage of their lives – and more than 90% developed this condition before their fifth birthday. Medical experts have long been mystified by way so many eczema sufferers also develop asthma and allergies – what they call the atopic march. Studies show that 50-60% of children with severe eczema go on to develop childhood asthma. It has shown that a substance secreted by damaged and broken skin (caused by the itchy eczema) moves through the body and can trigger asthmatic symptoms. These findings suggest that the early treatment and control of skin rashes caused by eczema may stop asthma developing [39].

Eczema and asthma are closely related by the reason that both may have similar pathogenic mechanism underlying their manifestations. Both are due to the effect of hypersensitivity reactions which are mediated by IgE Antibody affixed to the surface of mast cells and basophiles, and both can be triggered by exposure to allergens [40-42].

Hahnemann's theory is again justified by another instance that under proper homoeopathic treatment of a chronic disease having history of suppressed skin manifestation in the past, the old eruption definitely reappear satisfying Herring's law of cure. This incidence comes to be every day phenomenon found in any homoeopathic clinic, hospital or health centre. The distinguished homoeopathic physicians mentioned their own cases in their books. If we go through the case records from the respective books, we can see that in a considerable number of cases, the Hering's Law of Cure can be verified. For quick references a few interesting cases are shown here in a nut shell.

Dr. P. Sankaran mentioned a case in his book 'The Pathology in Homoeopathy'. A three year-old boy had an ulcer on his lips. The diagnosis was 'cancrum oris'. Sulphonamide ointment was applied on the affected parts. Ulcer disappeared in no time, but left a black patch on the lips. After a couple of months the black spot also vanished. Some days after this incident, mental abnormality was perceived in the behavior of the boy. After four years the boy was taken to Dr. Sankaran . Doctor prescribed a selected homoeopathic medicine and the boy recovered. Mental problem was gone but the old ulcer of the lips reappeared. Then the ulcer was treated by homoeopathic method. The result was that the boy remained well in mind as well as in the skin [43].

Carrol Dunham, in the book, 'Science of Therapeutics', recorded a case of deafness caused by suppressed Psora. Dunham treated a seventeen year old young man for his hearing trouble which started when he was four years of age. Past history revealed that at the age of three he suffered from eczema of thick, whitish scabs, hard, almost horny, covering the whole scalp. The eruption was suppressed by external application. From that time the child faced the problem of hearing. Dunham prescribed not for direct deafness. He selected homoeopathic medicine Mezerium on the basis of skin eruption which remained in the past. The deafness was completely cured [44].

Nash noted an interesting case in his book 'Leaders in Homoeopathic Therapeutics'. Dr. Nash treated a lady suffering from Gastritis. She became skeleton-like. Nash found after much questioning that about fifteen years ago' she had eczema on the nape and occiput. The eczema was suppressed by the application ointment. Dr.Nash prescribed Sulphur 200th. Her stomach trouble completely removed but the eruption reappeared [45].

Dr. Nash mentioned another case. He treated a case of very severe gastralgia caused by suppression of eczema on the hands. Dr. Nash prescribed Arsenicum because the pain came on at midnight, lasting until 3 A.M. during which time the patient had to walk the floor in agony, and there was great burning in stomach. She had but one slight attack after taking Arsenicum but old suppressed eczema came back [45].

Dr. S. P. Dey of Calcutta noted a case in his book, 'Clinical Case Reports on Constitutional Prescribing'. He treated a student aged 19 years, suffering from Rheumatoid Arthritis. He had skin disease in childhood. The eruption was suppressed by local application of ointments. Considering the totality of the symptoms of the case, Dr. Dey prescribed Medorrhinum 1 M. The patient's condition was remarkably improved. But three months later there was severe aggravation of the old skin condition. Through constitutional treatment for one year, the patient was cured. He had no pain anywhere no skin symptom [46].

To my own interest, when I had been house surgeon of D. N. De Homoeopathic Medical College Kolkata I had gone through the old case record books of indoor departments thereof. It was interestingly observed that a fair number of patients suffering from chronic diseases gave the history of suppression of skin disease in the past.

Total number of cases recorded in one year was 266. Out of them, history of suppression of skin disease of 110 patients was found. Among 266 total cases 72 patients were of Asthma of which 56 patients had a history of suppressed skin disease (mainly eczema); 58 patients were of Gastritis of which 22 patients gave history of suppression of skin disease (mainly scabies); 25 cases were of Kidney dysfunction of which 8 persons had suppressed skin ailments (either psoriasis or eczema); 84 cases exhibited Rheumatoid Arthritis of which 12 patients revealed as past suppression of psoriasis; 28 cases were of Cardio Vascular Disease of which only 2 were found of suppression of skin disease (Tables 1 and 2).

Name of Hospital	Total number of cases in one year	History of suppression of skin disease in the past	Percentage (%)
D. N. De Homoeopathic Medical college and Hospital Calcutta.	266	110	41.4

Table 1: Percentage of cases, revealed history of suppressed skin disease in the past in respect to total number of cases treated in one year.

Type of diseases	Total number of cases	History of suppression of skin disease in the past	Percentage (%)
Asthma	72	56(eczema,48 and others,8)	76.66
Gastritis	58	22(scabies, 18 and others,4)	38
Kidney disorder	24	8 (psoriasis,5 and eczema,3)	33.33
Rheumatoid Arthritis	84	12 (psoriasis, 9 and other 3)	14.25
Cardio Vascular Diseases	28	2 (eruption, allergic)	7.14

Table 2: Percentage of different type of diseases, influenced by suppression of skin disease in the past.

Conclusion

Hahnemann considered Psora as a disease or disposition to disease transmitted from generation to generation for thousands of years. Health is the result of the dynamic equilibrium among the disease agent, human host and the environment. The latest conception about the causation of disease reveals clearly that disease is due to the effect of 'multiple factors' those are directly or indirectly related to the agent, host and environment, viz., biological, nutrient, chemical, physical, mechanical, psycho-social, cultural, hereditary factors etc. According to recent opinion, the hereditary factors among these are the most predominant or fundamental cause as Hahnemann had indicated [47]. Refuting the former belief of hereditary factors in playing a role in the causation of only of a few chronic diseases, it is established that they have an immense role in the production of large number of diseases. Evidently in case of epidemic or endemic diseases, we find a variable susceptibility in the human population remaining the same risk factors to viral, bacterial or parasitic infections. Studies on twins [both identical and non-identical] indicate that heredity is partly responsible for various forms of insanity, for cancer and for other human disorders. Most tumour biologists believe that there are multiple mechanisms that influence the growth and spread of cells transformed to the neoplastic state and that most of them are, in a broad sense, genetically influenced. Diabetes mellitus, obesity, gout, essential hypertension, peptic ulcer, cancer, neuroses, psychoses, mental retardation, many infectious diseases such as acute rheumatic fever and tuberculosis are few examples where hereditary predisposition plays an important part. Therefore to bring cure to any disease especially chronic disease, one should focus one's attention towards the patient [host] to find out the fundamental cause without ignoring the disease agents and the environmental factors acting as exciting or maintaining causes.

Hahnemann's theory of Psora was very simple as it was based on practical observations. Hahnemann standing on the basement of his power of his perfect observation and foresight, perceived the close connection lying between skin and rest of the body. What Hahnemann emphasized in his Psora theory that the serious complication might develop from suppression of skin disease is no longer denied by modern science. It's not the only efficacy of Psora theory, but it serves as a pioneer to the key of ideal cure of innumerable non venereal chronic diseases. In treatment of chronic diseases, to achieve success by means of homoeopathic method, there is need of proper 'Anti Miasmatic' treatment. Hahnemann opines that the fundamental cause of all natural diseases is the Miasm. Until and unless, Miasm is done away with by dint of Anti Miasmatic treatment, the permanent cure of chronic disease is a far cry. According to Hahnemann's 'Psora Theory', Psora is the mother of almost all chronic diseases. Consequently in some of the stages of treatment of any type of chronic disease, it is necessary to bring Psora under control. Anti Psoric remedies are selected according to the general principles of homoeopathy. It is administered one dose at a time, the effect of which as a rule allowed passing away completely before being repeated. Over hasty repetition of anti-psoric remedies is to be avoided as much as the employment of too large doses. Dr. J. H. Allen, the author of 'The Chronic Miasms Psora and Pseudo-Psora', concluded, "we cannot select the most similar remedy possible unless we understand the phenomenon of the acting and basic miasms; for the true similar is always based upon the basic miasm, whether we be conscious or unconscious of the fact."

Therefore Hahnemann's 'Theory of Chronic Disease' should be perceived and it must be implemented in practical field so that a physician may achieve his mission i.e. "to restore the sick to health to cure."

References

1. Samuel H (1981) The Chronic Diseases: Their Peculiar Nature and Their Homoeopathic Cure New Delhi: Jain publishing Co. Vol: 1.
2. Roberts HA (1976) The Principles and Art of Cure by Homoeopathy. New Delhi: B. Jain publishers, p. 184.
3. Richard H (1993) Samuel Hahnemann His Life & Work. New Delhi: B. Jain publishers, p. 149
4. Richard H (1992) Samuel Hahnemann His Life & Work. New Delhi: B. Jain publishers, Vol. II., Reprinted in India, p. 167.
5. Sankaran P (1961) Pathology in homoeopathy: A New Look at Chronic Diseases. Santa Cruz Bombey-54: The Homoeopathic Medical Publishers, p. 39.
6. Richard H (1992) Samuel Hahnemann His Life & Work. p. 177.
7. Clarke JH. The Prescriber The Homoeopathic Publishing Co. p. 29.
8. Stuart C (1979) The Genius of Homoeopathy: 'The Identity of Psora and Tuberculosis' New Delhi: B. Jain publishers p. 102.
9. Roberts HA (1976) The Principles and Art of Cure by Homoeopathy. New Delhi: B. Jain publishers p. 182.
10. Kent JT (1977) Lectures on Homoeopathic Philosophy. New Delhi: B. Jain publishers, p. 137.
11. Lesser O Text Book of Homoeopathic Materia Medica.
12. Richard H (1992) Samuel Hahnemann His Life & Work. New Delhi: B. Jain publisher, p. 168.
13. Mackenzie (1933) Journal of the American Institute of Homoeopathy, p. 716.
14. Bach Edward Chronic Disease-A Working Hypothesis.
15. Patersion J (1950) The Bowel Nosodes. Brit. Hom. J.
16. Chandran KC (2013) Miasms: Understanding Its Biological Mechanism, Homoeopathy Articles.
17. Bodman FH (1939) Constitutions and Chronnic Disease, Brit Hom J, p. 224.
18. Clignett PO (1965) Natural Defenses against viruses, Brit Hom J, p. 239.
19. Eardley AWR (1962) Heredity and Homoeopathy, Brit Hom J, p. 68.
20. Gordon Ross AC (1962) Chronic Disease, Brit Hom J, p. 84.
21. Ross TD (1962) Miasmatic thoughts: Brit Hom J, p. 71.
22. Twentyman LR (1952) Miasms and Archetypes, Brit. Hom. J. 42: 130.
23. Zissu Roland (1961) The evolution of Ideas on Constitution and Temperament from the Homoeopathic Standpoint, Brit. Hom. J. pp: 50-55.
24. Watson Ian. The Homoeopathic Miasm-A Modern View. eBook Amazon.co.uk
25. Vithoulkas George (2002) The Science of Homoeopathy New Delhi: B. Jain publishers.
26. Obermayer M (1955): Psychocutaneous Medicine. Spring field, III.
27. Thomas B. Fitzapatrick, Arthur Z.Eisen, Irwin M, Fredberg K (1979) Dermatology in General Medicine New York: McGraw-Hill Co. p. 1358
28. Griesemer RD (1978) The incidence of emotionally triggered disease in dermatologic practice, Psychiartr Ann 8: 49-56.
29. Alexander F, French TM, Pollock GH (1968) Psychosomatic specificity. Chicago: Univ. of Chicago Press p. 4-11.
30. Hahnemann Samuel (1981) The Chronic Diseases, Their Peculiar Nature and Their Homoeopathic Cure New Delhi: Jain India publishing Co. p. 18-31.
31. William Wood and Co. (1909) Moris Sir Malcolm: Diseases of the skin. New York.
32. William Wood and Co. (1908) Moris Sir Malcolm: Diseases of the skin. New York.
33. Gaucher, Earnest (1910) Diseases of the skin, including radiotherapy and radium therapy. London: John Murray Publishing House. p. 11.
34. Gordon C (1982) Sauer: Manual of skin diseases, Lippincott Williams, (4thedn) p. 223-225.
35. Wyngarden James B (1982) Cecil Text Book of Medicine Elsevier. Health Science Division 2: 2271.
36. Arthur Rook, Wikinson DS, Ebling FJG (1982) Text Book of Dermatology London: Black Well Science Ltd. (3rdedn) p. 306.
37. Arthur Rook, Wikinson DS, Ebling FJG (1982) Text Book of Dermatology London: Black Well Science Ltd. (3rdedn) p. 144.
38. BBC NEWS (2009)Eczema's link to asthma uncovered.
39. Eczema and asthma: the link (2010) kidspot.
40. Atkinson F (2009) Middleton's allergy: Principle and Practice (7thedn).
41. Holgate S, Lamnske R, Simson (2009) FER Publisher Mosby , an affiliate of Elsevier, Inc.
42. Leslie C (2009) Grammar and Greenberger Paul A. Patterson's Allergic Diseases, Philadelphia: Lippincott Williams & Wikins, (7thedn).
43. Sankaran P (1961) Pathology in homoeopathy. Santa Cruz, Bombey-54, The Homoeopathic Medical Publishers pp: 18.
44. John Henry C (1983) A Dictionary of Practical Materia Medica, New Delhi: Jain publishing Co. p. 482.
45. Nash EB (1959) 'Leaders in Homoeopathic Therapeutics' Set Dey & Co. p. 89.
46. Dey SP (1979) Clinical Case Reports on Constitutional Prescribing C. Ringer & Co.
47. Skamene Emil (1980) Genetic Control of Natural Resistance to Infection & Malignancy. Elsevier Inc.

3

Salutary Effects of Germinated *Glycine max* Seeds on Post Prandial Hyperglycemia and Dyslipidemia - Evidence from *In-vivo* and *In-vitro* Studies

Richa Gupta[1], **Suman Bala Sharma**[1*] **and Usha Rani Singh**[2]

[1]*Department of Biochemistry, University College of Medical Sciences, University of Delhi, India*

[2]*Department of Pathology, University College of Medical Sciences, University of Delhi, India*

[*]**Corresponding author**: Suman Bala Sharma, Director-Professor Department of Biochemistry, University College of Medical Sciences, University of Delhi, India, E-mail: drsbs08@hotmail.com

Abstract

Background: Germinated *Glycine max* seeds have been known to have anti-hyperglycemic effects; however, a comprehensive study pertaining to this has never been experimentally determined.

Methods: The aqueous extract of 12 h germinated *Glycine max* seeds (gGmax) were orally administered to Streptozotocin induced diabetic rats for 28 days and the effects were observed on glycemic index, lipid profile, antioxidant parameters alpha amylase and alpha glucosidase activity. Further the histomorphological changes were seen in the rat's pancreas. Finally, the metabolite profiling was done.

Results: There was a significant improvement in FBG and OGTT in diabetic rats treated with gGmax after a period of 28 days. The extract also led to a substantial increase in the levels of insulin and c-peptide as compared to diabetic control rats with marked improvement in insulin resistance. Lipid profile and atherogenic factors were significantly improved. Histomorphological examination of pancreatic tissue revealed increased number of islets and β-cells in treated rats as compared to diabetic controls. Subsequently, marked suppression in the activity of alpha-amylase and alpha- glucosidase was observed.

Conclusion: The antidiabetic property of the extract is attributed through the improvement in insulin secretion, suppression of post- prandial hyperglycemia and β-cell regeneration. Besides its antidiabetic properties, *Glycine max* seeds also demonstrated salutary effects on the management of dyslipidemia which may be mediated through scavenging of free radicals as well as suppression of atherogenic lipid variants and apolipoproteins. Overall this study represents *Glycine max* seeds as a promising therapeutic agent for diabetes and dyslipidemia.

Keywords: Diabetes; *Glycine max*; Post-prandial hyperglycemia; β-cell regeneration; Dyslipidemia

Abbreviation:

gGmax: 12 h Germinated *Glycine max* seeds; FBG: Fasting Blood Glucose; OGTT: Oral Glucose Tolerance Test; CVD: Cardio Vascular Disease; STZ: Streptozotocin; AYUSH: Ayurveda, Yoga and Naturopathy, Unani, Siddha and Homoeopathy; IAEC: Institutional Animal Ethical Committee; Hb1Ac: Glycosylated Hemoglobin; HOMA-IR: Homeostatic Model Assessment-Insulin Resistance; TG: Triglycerides; HDL: High Density Lipoprotein; LDL: Low Density Lipoprotein; VLDL: Very Low Density Lipoprotein; Ox LDL: Oxidized Low Density Lipoprotein; IC_{50}: Half maximal Inhibitory Concentration; FRAP: Ferric Reducing Ability of Plasma; TPTZ: 2,4,6-Tris(2-pyridyl)-s-triazine; GC-MS: Gas Chromatography-Mass Spectrometry; ANOVA: Analysis of Variance

Introduction

Diabetes is a metabolic disorder characterized by chronic hyperglycemia resulting from defects in insulin secretion, insulin action, or both [1]. It has caused significant morbidity and mortality due to microvascular and macrovascular complications [2]. It is one of the largest global health emergencies of the 21st century. Although the prevalence of diabetes is increasing at an alarming rate throughout the world, the occurrence and consequences associated with it is found to be high in countries like China (109.6 million), India (69.2 million), and United States (29.3 million). Several pathogenic processes are involved in the development of diabetes. These range from autoimmune destruction of the β-cells of the pancreas with consequent insulin deficiency to abnormalities that result in resistance to insulin action [3].

Recently, considerable research has been focused on postprandial hyperglycemia because it doubles the risk of death from cardiovascular disease [4]. In diabetes, the postprandial phase is characterized by a rapid increase in blood glucose levels after meals [5]. The present day studies highlights on the possibility that postprandial "hyperglycemic spikes" may be relevant to the pathophysiology of late diabetes complications. In-fact Asian population displays marked increase in post-prandial hyperglycemia [6]. It has also been shown that, apart from oral glucose tolerance test (OGTT), activity of pancreatic α-amylase and α- glucosidasecorrelates to an increase in post-prandial glucose levels, the control of which is therefore an important aspect in treatment of type 2 diabetes [7].

Another important consequence of diabetes is exacerbated atherosclerosis and its recognized complications, which ultimately leads to the development of cardio vascular diseases (CVD). Several mechanisms have been suggested to play a role in mediating the additive effects of hyperglycemiaon atherogenesis. These include increased oxidative stress and derangement in lipid and lipoprotein metabolism [8].

Currently there are several classes of synthetic drugs available to achieve better glycemic control but most of them are still not used for prevention of atherosclerosis, because of their potential toxicity and intolerance, thus the management of diabetes and its threatening complications are still a challenge. In this scenario, herbal drugs are offering great potential, as they exhibit multifarious approach. Moreover, they are considered to be safeand cost effective when compared to synthetic anti-hyperglycemic agents.

Compounds with both antidiabetic and anti-atherosclerotic properties are considered to be stupendous. Therefore, the present study demonstrates theantihyperglycemicand anti-atherosclerotic potential of aqueous extract of 12 h germinated *Glycine max* (gGmax) seeds in Streptozotocin (STZ)-induced diabetic rats models. The study elucidates its mechanism of action by observing its effect on glycemic index, insulin resistance, lipid profile, oxidized LDL, apolipoprotein and free radical suppression. Moreover, histomorphological studies of pancreas were also performed to assess the effect on islets of langerhans. Further, the role ofα amylase and α-glucosidase inhibition was also studied in order to assess its potential on post-prandial blood sugar control. Subsequent metabolite profiling was also performed.

Material and Methods

Plant material

The seeds of *Glycine max* were procured, and identified by department of Ayurveda, Yoga and Neuropathy, Unani, Siddha and Homoeopathy (AYUSH), Government of India. The voucher of the specimen was deposited in Botanic Garden of Indian Republic (BGIR), Noida and number was provided (Voucher specimen no-264).

Preparation of plant extracts

The seeds were germinated for 12 h at 37°C after which they were grinded to a fine paste. The seed paste was suspended in 500 ml of distilled water overnight, filtered and then lyophilized. The yield of aqueous extract was approximately 10% of the dried seeds. The stock solutions for inhibition assays were prepared by dissolving up to 1 mg of extract in 1 ml of DMSO and appropriately diluting it before use.

Preliminary screening of germinating *Glycine max* seed extracts: *In-vivo* studies

Induction of diabetes in rats

Diabetes was induced by injection of STZ [Sigma Aldrich, USA] (45 mg/kg body weight in 0.1 M citrate buffer, pH 4.5, intra peritoneally) to overnight fasting rats [9]. After 48 h of STZ administration, fasting blood glucose (FBG) levels were monitored and repeated twice at intervals of three days. The animals with blood glucose level above 200 mg/dL were considered to be diabetic. Institutional approval (IAEC) was taken for the study as per as the CPCSEA guidelines (Reg. No 508/2001/ CPCSEA, IAEC Approval no: UCMS/IAEC/27, dated 30th December 2009).

Experimental studies

The rats were divided into four groups, where group I was labeled as normal control. Group II was labeled as diabetic control and group III and IV comprised of diabetic rats. Group III rats were treated with glibenclamide (600 mg/kg b.wt.) and group IV rats were treated with gGmax seed extracts (200 mg/kg b.wt.).

The control rats received vehicle, i.e. distilled water, and the treated rats received gGmax seed extracts or glibenclamide in 1 ml of distilled water. The treatment was given daily for a period of 28 days using standard orogastric cannula. The blood was drawn from retro orbital plexus of overnight fasted rats by using micro capillary technique [10]. The blood collected in plain vial, was allowed to clot for separation of serum.

Glycemic control

The FBG level was measured by glucose oxidase peroxidase enzymatic method [11]. The estimation of Glycosylated hemoglobin (Hb1Ac) was done by method described by Goldstein et al. [12]. For OGTT, glucose (2 g/kg) was administered to non-diabetic control rats and was treated with glibenclamide (600 µg/kg) as well as gGmax (200 mg/kg) and improvement in glucose tolerance was estimated at an interval of 0, 60 and 120 minutes respectively. Serum insulin and C-peptide levels were measured by ELISA kits from Mercodia.

Calculation of insulin resistance indices [13,14]

- HOMA-IR=[fasting blood glucose (FBG; mg/dl)] × [fasting insulin; µU/ml)]/405.
- 20/(fasting C-peptide × fasting blood glucose)

Management of dyslipidemia

All the lipid profile parameters were performed in serum. Triglycerides (TG) were measured as per the method described [15]. Total cholesterol (TC) was assayed as per the method of Allain et al. [16]. High-density lipoprotein (HDL) was determined bythe method of Burstein [17]. Low-density lipoprotein (LDL) and very low-density lipoprotein (VLDL) were calculated by using the formula from Friedwald et al. [18]. ApoB was estimated by immunoturbidity method. LDL/ApoB ratio was used to measure small-dense LDL. oxLDL was estimated by the baseline levels of diene conjugates in lipid fraction of LDL as described [19].

Histomorphological studies

Pancreas was dissected from rats and fixed in 10% neutral formaldehyde for histopathological evaluation. Tissue samples were processed, embedded in paraffin, sectioned (5 µ thick), and stained with haematoxylin and eosin.

In-vitro studies

Screening of gGmax for α-amylase inhibitory activity: Starch-Iodine colour assay

Screening of gGmax for α-amylase inhibitors was carried out in a microtitre plate according to Xiao et al. [20] based on the starch-iodine test. The total assay mixture composed of 40 µl 0.02 M sodium phosphate buffer (pH 6.9 containing 6 mM sodium chloride), 0.02 units of PPA solution and gGmax at concentration from 10-100 µg/ml (w/v) were incubated at 37°C for 10 min. Then soluble starch (1%, w/v) was added to each reaction well and incubated at 37°C for 15 min. 1 M HCl (20 µl) was added to stop the enzymatic reaction, followed by the addition of 100 µl of iodine reagent (5 mM I2 and 5 mM KI). The color change was noted and the absorbance was read at 620 nm on a microplate reader. The control reaction representing 100% enzyme activity did not contain any plant extract.

To eliminate the absorbance produced by plant extract, appropriate extract controls without the enzyme were also included. The known PPA inhibitor, acarbose [Sigma Aldrich, USA; purity ≥ 95%], was used a positive control at a concentration range of 10-100 µg/ml. A dark-blue color indicates the presence of starch; a yellow color indicates the absence of starch while a brownish color indicates partially degraded starch in the reaction mixture. In the presence of inhibitors from the extracts the starch added to the enzyme assay mixture is not degraded and gives a dark-blue color complex whereas no color complex is developed in the absence of the inhibitor, indicating that starch is completely hydrolysed by α-amylase.

In-vitro α-amylase inhibitory assay

The assay was carried out following the standard protocol by Hansawasdi [21] with slight modifications. Starch azure (2 mg) was suspended in a tube containing 0.2 ml of 0.5 M Tris-HCl buffer (pH 6.9) containing 0.01 M calcium chloride (substrate). The tube was boiled for 5 min and then pre-incubated at 37°C for 5 min. gGmax (1mg) was dissolved in 1ml of 0.1% of dimethyl sulfoxide in order to obtain concentrations of 10, 20, 40, 60, 80 and 100 µg/ml. Then 0.2 ml of extract of a particular concentration was put in the tube containing the substrate solution. 0.1 ml of porcine pancreatic amylase in Tris-HCl buffer (2 units/ml) was added to the tube containing the extract and substrate solution. The process was carried out at 37°C for 10 min.

The reaction was stopped by adding 0.5 ml of 50% acetic acid in each tube. The reaction mixture was then centrifuged at 3000 rpm for 5 min at 4°C. The absorbance of resulting supernatant was measured at 595 nm using spectrophotometer. The concentration of the extract required to inhibit 50% of alpha amylase activity under the conditions was defined as the IC_{50} value. The experiments were repeated thrice with the same protocol. The α-amylase inhibitory activity was calculated as follows:

The α-amylase inhibitory activity = (Ac+) – (Ac-) – (As-Ab) / (Ac+) – (Ac-) × 100

Where, Ac+, Ac-, As, Ab are defined as the absorbance of 100% enzyme activity (only solvent with enzyme), 0% enzyme activity (only solvent without enzyme), a test sample (with enzyme) and a blank (a test sample without enzyme) respectively.

In-vitro α-glucosidase inhibitory assay

The assay was performed with the standard protocol by Brueggeman [22]. α-glucosidase (2U/ml) was premixed with 20 µl of gGmax at various concentrations (10, 20, 40, 60, 80 and 100 µg/ml) and incubated for 5 min at 37°C. 1 mM para-nitrophenylglucopyanoside (20 µl) in 50 mM of phosphate buffer (pH 6.8) was added to initiate the reaction. The mixture was further incubated at 37°C for 20 min.

The reaction was terminated by addition of 50 µl of 1 M sodium carbonate and the final volume was made up to 150 µl. α-glucosidase activity was determined spectrophotometrically at 405 nm by measuring the quantity of para-nitrophenol released from pNPG. The concentration of extract required to inhibit 50% of alpha glucosidase activity under the conditions was defined as the IC_{50} value. The assay was performed in triplicate.

Antioxidant activity

Ferric reducing ability of plasma (FRAP) was determined as described previously [23]. Briefly, the working FRAP reagent was prepared by adding 300 mmol/l acetate buffer (pH 3.6), 10 mmol/l TPTZ in 40 mmol/l HCl and 20 mmol/l FeCl3.6H2O in the ratio of 10:1:1 respectively. Sample was added, thoroughly mixed and the absorbance was monitored at 593 nm for 4 min. The values are expressed as µmol/ml.

Preliminary Phytochemical Analysis

The gGmax extract was subjected to phytochemical analysis using Gas Chromatography-Mass Spectrometry.

GC-MS Analysis

Analysis of the gGmax extract was performed on a GC-MS-Triple quad (Agilent 7890 A) gas chromatograph equipped with DB 5 ms capillary column (30 m × 0.25 mm ID). Helium was the carrier gas with flow rate of 1 ml/min, the injector mode-split (1:11), the injection volume 2 µl, the temperature program used is as follows: 80°C (3 min), then increased to 280°C at 10°C/min, held at 280°C (10 min) and temperature scan, m/z 35-300 amu. Appropriate solvent controls were also run. The identification of the components was based on the comparison of their mass spectra with those of NIST-Wiley 2008 library.

Statistical analysis

Statistical analysis was done by PRISM-6 and MS-EXCEL. Values are expressed as the mean ± SEM for five animals in each group. The data was analysed by using repeated measure analysis of variance (ANOVA) followed by Dunnett's multiple comparison test and one-way ANOVA followed by Tukey's multiple comparison test. The results were considered significant at $P<0.05$. The experiments for α-amylase and α- glucosidase were done in triplicate. IC_{50} values were calculated by plotting Lineweaverburk plot.

Results and Discussion

Oral administration of gGmax extract at dose of 200 mg/kg body weight for the period of 28 days exhibits remarkable glycemic control in the diabetic rats. The results summarized in the Table 1 shows statistically significant decrease in FBG ($p<0.0001$) and Hb1Ac ($p<0.001$) levels in diabetic rats treated with gGmax extract after a period of 28 days. Glucose tolerance was also found to be significantly improved after the treatment duration.

The effect of gGmax extract on serum insulin and C-peptide levels is recapitulated in Figure 1A. A significant decrease ($p<0.0001$) in the levels of insulin was observed in diabetic control rats as compared to normal rats. Administration of gGmax extract significantly increased ($p<0.001$) the levels of insulin. The drug glibenclamide also produced significant elevation in the insulin levels ($p<0.001$) in diabetic rats. However, in gGmax extract treated rats the increase in insulin level was found to be significantly higher when compared to ($p<0.001$) glibenclamide ($p<0.01$) treated rats. A significant depletion ($p<0.001$)

in the C-peptide levels was also observed in diabetic control (Figure 1B). The gGmax extract treated diabetic rats showed significant increase in ($p<0.01$) the C-peptide levels. The elevation in the level of insulin in gGmax extract treated rats suggests that it is able to potentiate the release of insulin from pancreatic β-cells. The antihyperglycemic activity of gGmax extract could be due to its insulinogenic action as increased levels of insulin and C-peptide were found in gGmax extract treated diabetic rats.

Insulin resistance indices are paraphrased in Figure1C and 1D. Both the indices indicate the improvement in insulin resistance after administration of the extract for 28 days. The improvement was significant when compared to the diabetic control ($p<0.001$).

The effect of gGmax extract on serum lipidprofile is summarized in (Table 2). A significant increase in the serum lipids, except HDL-c, was observed in diabetic rats when compared with the healthy rats ($p<0.001$). Treatment with gGmax extract for 28 days shows a marked reduction ($p<0.001$) in levels of TC, TG, LDL and VLDL. This lipid lowering effect produced by gGmax was found to be better than that of glibenclamide. The increased TG and TC levels and decreased HDL levels were known factors associated with coronary heart disease. Recent studies suggest that TG itself is independently related to CVD and most of the anti-hypercholesterolemic drugs do not decrease TG levels [24]. As the gGmax produced favourable effect on these factors, this suggests that the extract may help to prevent the progression of cardiovascular diseases.

Experimental groups	F86 (mg/dl)	GHb (%)	Body Weight (grams)		OGTT (mg/dl)
			Initial	Final	
Normal Control	107.6 ± 7.12	3.42	252 ± 2.00	301 ± 7.80	146 ± 332
Diabetic Control	265.8 ± 9.65$^{\#}$	5.94	175 ± 11.61	170 ± 6.89	390.6 ± 5.75$^{\#}$
Glib. treated	115.6 ± 9.34***	4.80	192 ± 6.63	243 ± 8.60	298.4 ± 13.96***
gGmax treated	114.4 ± 11.10***	4.12*	188 ± 4.63	246 ± 10.41	255 ± 8.83***

Values are given as means ± SEM. #$p<0.0001$ as compared with normal control group, $^{*}p<0.01$, $^{***}p<0.001$ as compared with diabetic control group.

Table 1: Effect of gGmax on glycemic response and body weight in STZ induced diabetic rats.

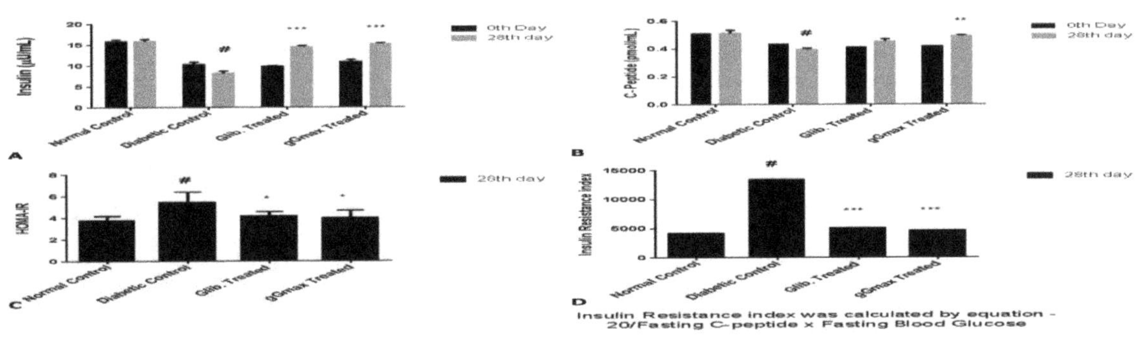

Figure 1: Effect of gGmax on (A) serum insulin, (B) serum c-peptide levels (C) HOMA- IR and (D) 20/Fasting C peptide X Fasting blood glucose in STZ induced diabetic rats. Values are given as means ± SEM. #$p<0.0001$ as compared with normal control group, *$p<0.01$, **$p<0.001$, ***$p<0.0001$ as compared with diabetic control group.

Groups	Serum Lipid profile (mg/dl)				
	TG	TC	HDL	LDL	VLDL
Normal control (veluele)	72.08 ± 6.91	77.8 ± 7.2	36.4 ± 3.3	26.84 ± 3.5	14.56 ± 1.23
Diabetic control (vehicle)	211.6 ± 9.3*	176.8 ± 8.7	21.4 ± 3.1*	113.08 ± 5.6*	42.32 ± 4.5*
Diabetic+Glib. (600 µg/kg)	100.8 ± 4.6****	97.6 ± 5.5	34 ± 3.6****	43.44 ± 6.03****	20.16 ± 1.9****
Diabetic+12 gGmax (200 mg/kg)	90 ± 2.7****	89.4 ± 3.7	32 ± 3.3****	39.4 ± 2.1****	18 ± 0.97****

Values are given as means ± SEM. # $p<0.0001$ as compared with normal control group, ****$p<0.0001$as compared with diabetic control group.

Table 2: Effect of gGmax on serum lipid profile in STZ induced diabetic rats.

A significant reduction in Ox-LDL, sd-LDL and apoB levels was observed ingGmax extract treated rats (Figure 2). Moreover the antioxidant power of gGmax extract was found to be 136.35 μmol/ml (Figure 3).

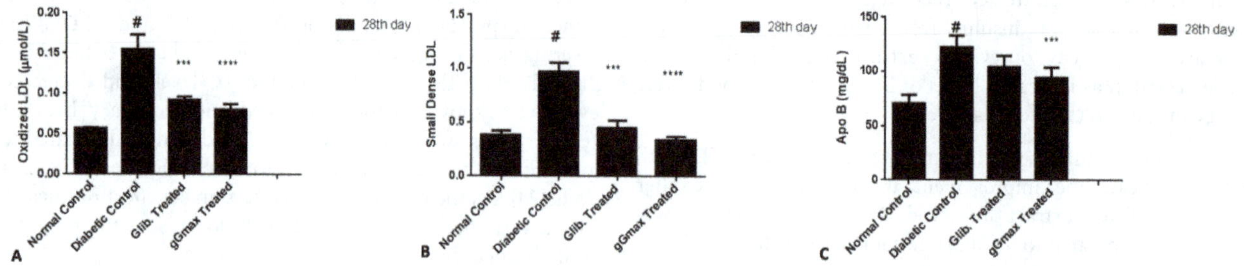

Figure 2: Effect of gGmax on (A) Ox LDL, (B) sd LDL, (C) Apo B in STZ induced diabetic rats. Values are given as means ± SEM. #p<0.0001 as compared with normal control group, ****p<0.0001, ***p<0.001 as compared with diabetic control group.

Histomorphological examination of pancreatic tissue from STZ-induced diabetic control rats (Figure 4A) showed reduction in the number of islets and β-cells, however pancreatic tissues of gGmax extract treated rats (Figure 4B) revealed an increase in the number of islets and β-cells as compared to the diabetic control rats. The reports suggest that STZ, a beta cytotoxin, acts through rapid depletion of pancreatic β-cells which leads to reduction in insulin secretion [25]. However, treatment with gGmax extract leads to the increased number of islets and β-cells. This interprets that gGmax extract produces insulinogenic effect through the regeneration of β-cells.

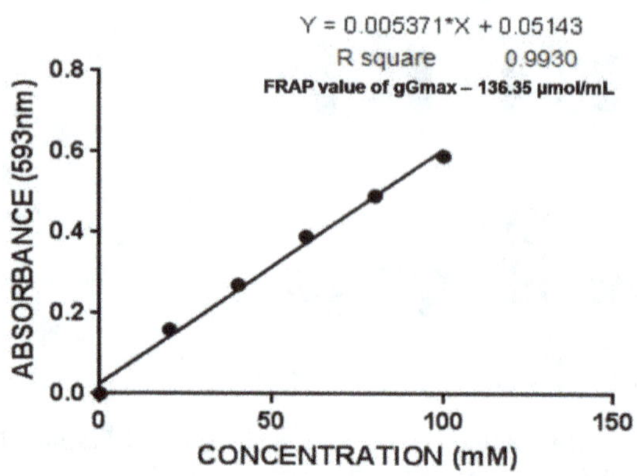

Figure 3: Linear nature of FRAP standards and antioxidant power of gGmax in STZ induced diabetic rats.

Screening for α-amylase inhibition was performed based on starch-iodine color complex formation. The rats treated with gGmax extract tested positive for inhibition of α-amylase and was further quantified with respect to PPA inhibition as per modified method given by Hansawasdi et al. [21]. It was noted that it exhibited significant α-amylase inhibitory activity. The percentage inhibition at varied concentrations (10, 20, 40, 60, 80, 100 μg/ml) of gGmax extract showed concentration dependant reduction in percentage inhibition (Figure 5A). The highest concentration of 100 μg/ml of gGmax extract showed maximum inhibition of 79.2%. Acarbose was taken as a positive control with a maximum inhibition of 81.1%. The IC_{50} values for the acarbose and gGmax extract were also calculated by plotting lineweaverburk plot. The IC_{50} of acarbose is found to be 67.77 μg/ml whereas gGmax extract exhibited an IC_{50} value of 28.01 μg/ml which is less than acarbose (Figure 5B and 5C).

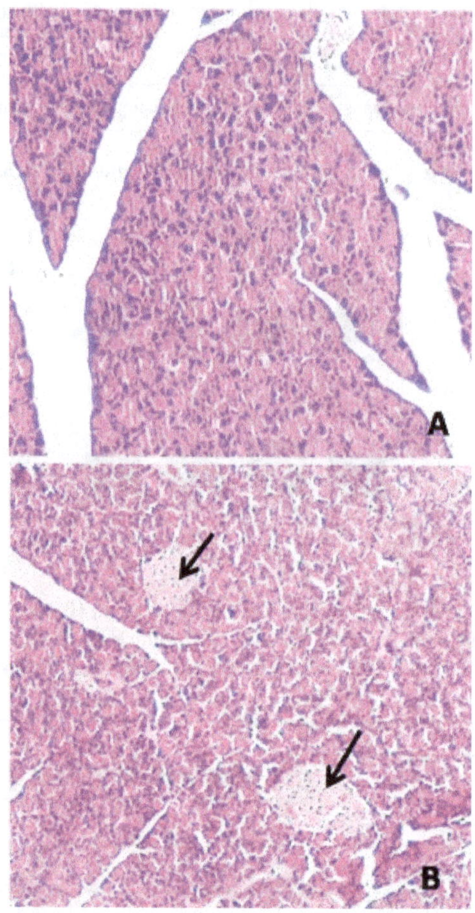

Figure 4: Histopathological findings of pancreas (haematoxylin and eosin stained figures). (A) Diabetic control rats showing reduced islets, (B) Diabetic rats treated with gGmax showing regeneration of islets.

Subsequently, the effect of gGmax was studied on inhibition of α-glucosidase activity. The *in-vitro* assay confirmed the powerful alpha glucosidase inhibitory activity of gGmax when compared with that of acarbose. The IC_{50} values were found to be 14.01 µg/ml and 18.51 µg/ml of acarbose and gGmax respectively (Figure 6A-6C). The results confirmed that gGmax extracts hold a promising therapeutic value in controlling post-prandial hyperglycemia.

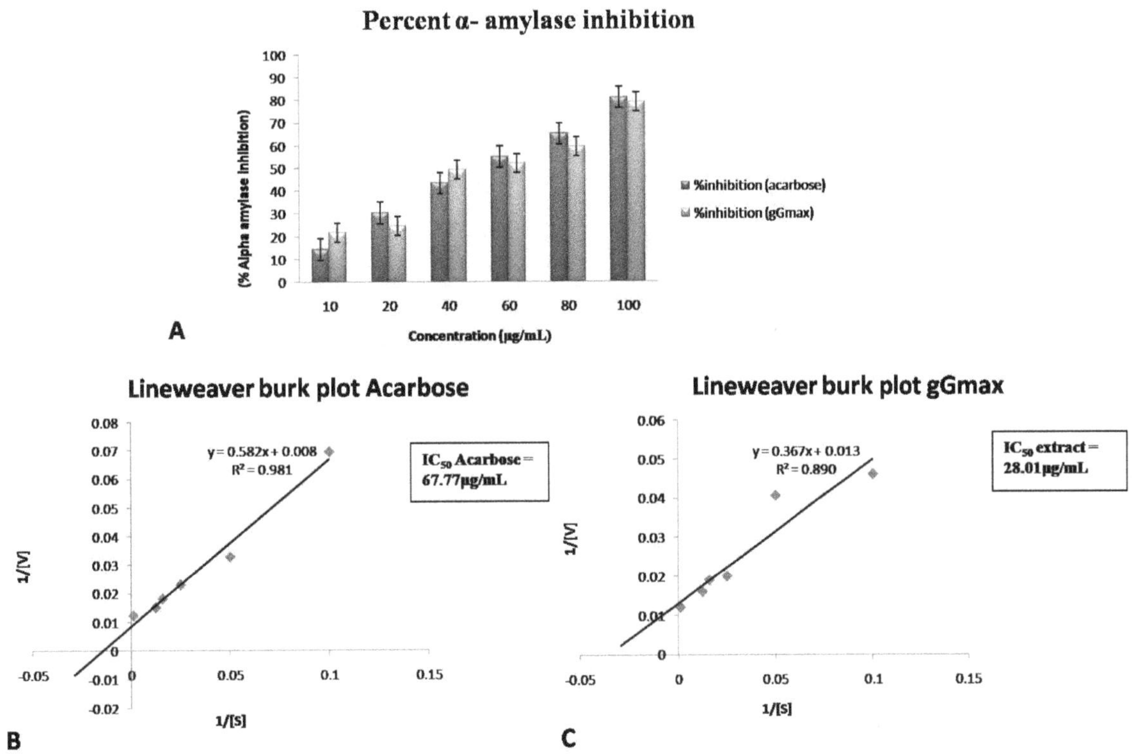

Figure 5: (A) The percentage inhibition of α-amylase at varied concentrations (10, 20, 40, 60, 80, 100 µg/ml) of plant gGmax and acarbose, (B) Lineweaverburk plot of Acarbose (standard drug) with calculation of IC_{50} which is 67.77 µg/ml for acarbose, (C) Lineweaverburk plot of gGmax with calculation of IC_{50} which is 28.01 µg/ml for gGmax.

Compounds	Molecular weight	Retention time	Area %
Undecanoic acid	186	20.35	96.02
Hexadecanoic acid or	256	27.82	5.33
Palmitic acid	270	28.32	7.13
Genistein Daidzein	254	28.51	5.12
Cinnamic acid ester	652	28.71	5.69
Isoquinoline alkaloid	403	29.1	48.74
4- ethoxy Benzoic acid, ethyl ester	194	29.23	16.28
Myristic acid	228	28.45	7.5
3-eicosene	280	29.67	6.15
Phthalic acid ester	278	31.46	50.01

Table 3: GC- MS analysis: Major identified phytochemicals present in gGmax.

The phytochemical analysis of gGmax extract was done toelucidate the major chemical constituents present in it. The extract prominently comprises of several fatty acids, alkaloids, saponins and flavonoids. The major identified constituents of gGmax extract are summarized in Table 3.

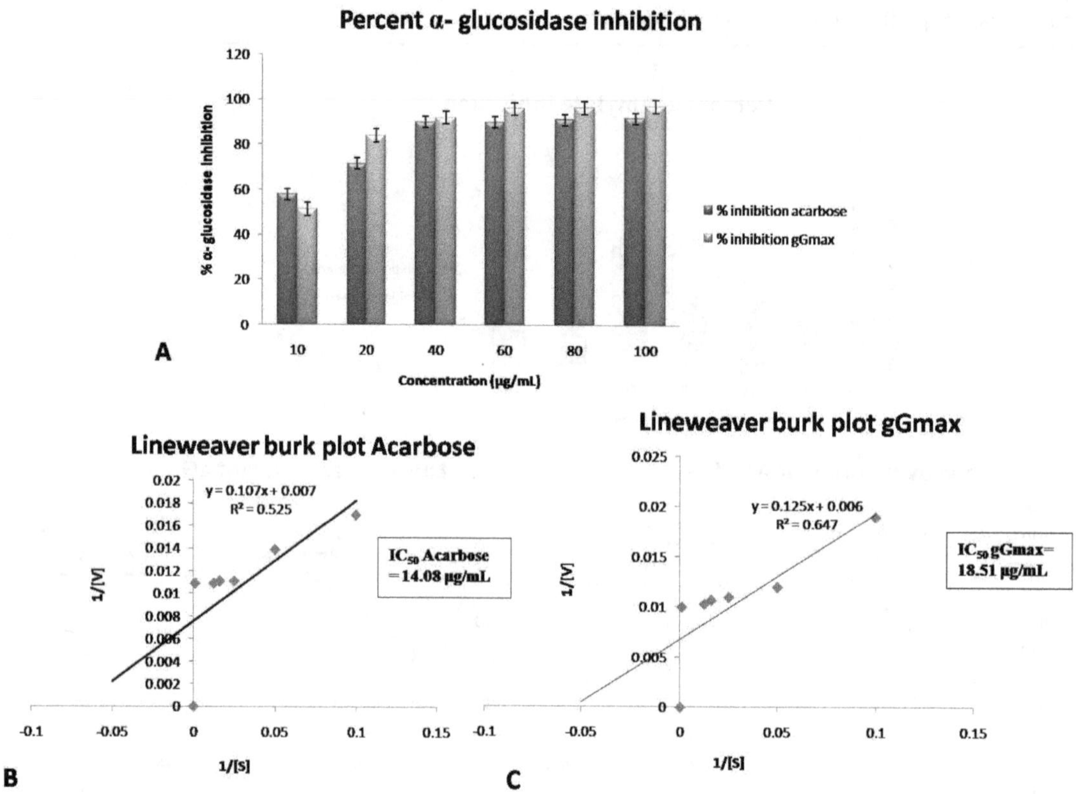

Figure 6: (A) The percentage inhibition of α-glucosidase at varied concentrations (10, 20, 40, 60, 80, 100 µg/ml) of plant gGmax and acarbose, (B) Lineweaverburk plot of Acarbose (standard drug) with calculation of IC_{50} which is 14.08 µg/ml for acarbose, (C) Lineweaverburk plot of gGmax with calculation of IC_{50} which is 18.51 µg/ml for gGmax.

Therefore, it is concluded that, gGmax extract exhibits a strong antihyperglycemic activity. It suppresses postprandial glycemic response by controlling OGTT as well as inhibiting α- amylase and α-glucosidase activity. It improves the glycemic response by regeneration of β- cells. It is evident from the results that gGmax possesses anti-hyperlipidemic and antioxidant potential also. These activities indicate the role of gGmax as a potent anti-atheroscleroctic agent and thus may prevent the progression of cardiovascular diseases. Plant based therapeutics are prospective medications of future and gGmax presents a strong candidate in this pipeline.

Acknowledgements

The authors acknowledge UGC for financial support and Indian Pharmacopoeia Commission (IPC) for their assistance in preliminary screening of samples.

References

1. American Diabetes Association (2011) Diagnosis and classification of diabetes mellitus. Diabetes Care 34: 62-69.
2. Cade WT (2008) Diabetes-related microvascular and macrovascular diseases in the physical therapy setting. Phys Ther 88: 1322–1335.
3. International Diabetes Federation (2015) IDF Diabetes Atlas,7th edition.
4. Bonora E, Muggeo M (2001) Postprandial blood glucose as a risk factor for cardiovascular disease in Type II diabetes: The epidemiological evidence. Diabetologia 44: 2107-2114.
5. Chiu CJ, Taylor A (2011) Dietary hyperglycemia, glycemic index and metabolic retinal diseases. Prog Retin Eye Res 30: 18-53.
6. Dickinson S, Colagiuri S, Faramus E, Petocz P, Brand-Miller JC (2002) Postprandial hyperglycemia and insulin sensitivity differ among lean young adults of different ethnicities. J Nutr 132: 2574-2579.
7. Eichler HG, Korn A, Gasic S, Pirson W, Businger J (1984) The effect of a new specific alpha-amylase inhibitor on post-prandial glucose and insulin excursions in normal subjects and Type 2 (non-insulin-dependent) diabetic patients. Diabetologia, 26: 278-281.
8. Rask-Madsen C, King GL (2005) Proatherosclerotic mechanisms involving protein kinase C in diabetes and insulin resistance. Arterioscler Thromb Vasc Biol 25: 487-496.
9. Siddiqui O, Sun Y, Liu JC (1987) Facilitated transdermal transport of insulin. J Pharm Sci 76: 341-345.
10. Sorg DA, Buckner B (1964) A simple method of obtaining venous blood from small laboratory animals. Exp Biol Med 115: 1131-1132.
11. Barham D, Trinder P (1972) An improved colour reagent for the determination of blood glucose by the oxidase system. Analyst 97: 142-145.
12. Goldstein DE, Little RR, Wiedmeyer HM, England JD, McKenzie EM (1986) Glycated hemoglobin: methodologies and clinical applications. Clin Chem 32: 64-70.
13. Matthews DR, Hosker JP, Rudenski AS, Naylor BA, Treacher DF, et al. (1985) Homeostasis model assessment: Insulin resistance and beta-cell

function from fasting plasma glucose and insulin concentrations in man. Diabetologia 28: 412-419.

14. Ohkura T, Shiochi H, Fujioka Y, Sumi K, Yamamoto N, et al. (2013) 20/(fasting C-peptide × fasting plasma glucose) is a simple and effective index of insulin resistance in patients with type 2 diabetes mellitus: A preliminary report. Cardiovasc Diabetol 12: 21.
15. Fossati P, Prencipe L (1982) Serum triglycerides determined colorimetrically with an enzyme that produces hydrogen peroxide. Clin Chem 28: 2077-2080.
16. Allain CC, Poon LS, Chan CSG, Richmond W, Fu PC (1974) Enzymatic determination of total serum cholesterol. Clin Chem 20: 470-475.
17. Burstein M, Scholnick HR, Morfin R (1970) Rapid method for the isolation of lipoproteins from human serum by precipitation with polyanions. J Lipid Res 11: 583-595.
18. Friedewald WT, Levy RI, Fredrickson DS (1972) Estimation of the concentration of low-density lipoprotein cholesterol in plasma, without use of the preparative ultracentrifuge. Clin Chem 18: 499-502.
19. Ahotupa M, Ruutu M, Mantyla E (1996) Simple methods of quantifying oxidation products and antioxidant potential of low density lipoproteins. Clin Biochem 29: 139-144.
20. Xiao Z, Storms R, Tsang, A (2006) A quantitative starch-iodine method for measuring alpha-amylase and glucoamylase activities. Anal Biochem 351: 146-148.
21. Hansawasdi C, Kawabata J, Kasai T (2000) Alpha-amylase inhibitors from roselle (Hibiscus sabdariffa Linn.) tea. Biosci Biotechnol Biochem 64: 1041-1043.
22. Pistia-Brueggeman G, Hollingsworth RI (2001) A preparation and screening strategy for glycosidase inhibitors. Tetrahedron 57: 8773-8778.
23. Benzie IF, Strain JJ (1996) The ferric reducing ability of plasma (FRAP) as a measure of "antioxidant power": the FRAP assay. Anal Biochem 239: 70-76.
24. Bainton D, Miller NE, Bolton CH, Yarnell JW, Sweetnam PM, et al. (1992) Plasma triglyceride and high density lipoprotein cholesterol as predictors of ischaemic heart disease in British men. The caerphilly and speedwell collaborative heart disease studies. Br Heart J 68: 60-66.
25. El-Hazmi MAF, Warsy AS (2001) Evaluation of serum cholesterol and triglyceride levels in 1-6-year-old Saudi children. J Trop Pediatr 47: 181-185.

4

Molecular Modeling Studies of Some Substituted 2-Phenyl-benzimidazole Derivatives as Inhibitors of IgE Response

Mukesh C. Sharma*

Drug Research Laboratory, School of Pharmacy, Devi Ahilya University, Takshila Campus, Khandwa Road, Indore, M.P, India

***Corresponding author**: Sharma MC, Drug Research Laboratory, School of Pharmacy, Devi Ahilya University, Takshila Campus, Khandwa Road, Indore, M.P, India, E-mail: mukeshcsharma@yahoo.com

Abstract

We perform the two-dimensional (2D) QSAR studies of a series of substituted 2-phenyl-benzimidazole analogues to elucidate the structural properties required inhibitors of IgE response. The 2D-QSAR studies were performed using three statistical methods: the multiple linear regressions, giving square of correlation coefficient r^2=0.8386, cross validated squared correlation coefficient q^2=0.7218 and predictable ability pred_r^2=0.7525; Multiple linear regression (MLR). The results show that the proposed 2D-QSAR models are valid and that they can be applied to predict the activities of substituted 2-phenyl-benzimidazole inhibitors of IgE response.

Keywords: 2D QSAR; Multiple linear regression; Benzimidazole analogues; IgE responses; Asthma

Introduction

Asthma is a chronic respiratory disease that affects 300 million adults and children worldwide, including 15.7 million adults and 6.5 million children in the United States [1]. The prevalence has increased by 50% in the past few decades, particularly in Westernized countries. Although corticosteroids and β2-agonists are effective in managing asthma symptoms, there is no curative therapy. There are also concerns regarding the side effects from chronic use of current drugs, particularly by children. The chronic nature of asthma and the lack of preventive and curative therapy are leading patients with asthma in Western societies to seek complementary and alternative medicine (CAM) treatment [2,3]. Human allergic disorders (type I hypersensitivity responses) ranging from hay fever, excema, and food allergies to potentially life threatening asthma and anaphylactic shock are increasing worldwide [4]. Central to the cascade of events that lead to these clinical allergic manifestations are protein-protein binding events between human immunoglobulin E (hIgE) and its class specific Fc receptors on effector cells [5-7]. Allergic asthma is a multifactorial disease, influenced by genetic and environmental factors, and is characterized by bronchial hyperresponsiveness, the presence of IgE antibodies to inhalant allergens and often also by enhanced total serum IgE levels. A switch recombination of antibodies to IgE requires two signals from activated T cells: the expression of the ligand for CD40 and the secretion of IL-4 or IL-13. Both IL-4 and IL-13, independently of each other, are able to induce IgE antibody [8-10]. The allergen-IgE interactions on the mast cell surface initiate a complex series of downstream signaling cascades, including phosphorylation of the immunoreceptor tyrosine-based activation motifs (ITAMs) in the β- and γ-chains of FcεRI, resulting in mast cell degranulation [11,12]. While there are a number of pharmacological agents available for the treatment of asthma and allergic rhinitis, a major shortcoming of many of these therapeutic alternatives is that they impact the disease state by targeting a single mediator that modifies a response at the target organ. By acting on effecter molecules, these drugs provide some symptomatic relief but do not modulate the course of the disease. Anti-histamines, for example, continue to be the drugs of choice for allergic rhinitis because they are somewhat effective and are linked to few side effects [13].

QSAR refers to a discipline in computational chemistry that addresses the modeling of biological activities or chemical reactivity based on the quantitative description for the chemical structure of molecules. QSAR relies on the basic assumption that molecules with similar physicochemical properties or structures will have similar activities [14].

Quantitative structure activity relationship (QSAR) is one of the most important areas in chemometrics, and is a valuable tool that is used extensively in drug design and medicinal chemistry. Once a reliable QSAR model is established, we can predict the activities of molecules, and know which structural features play an important role in biological processes [15]. Since the QSAR model and properties of molecules can be obtained based on descriptors, choosing the most relevant descriptors is necessary. Therefore, using a technique as variable selection for extent number of descriptors is the most essential step in QSAR study [16]. The present paper deals with the novel development of drugs for the category, substituted 2-phenyl-benzimidazole derivatives inhibitors of IgE response.

The main purpose of quantitative structure–activity relationship (QSAR) analyses is to make activity predictions for unknown compounds to guide the structure-based design of new analogues. Multiple linear regression (MLR) models have been developed as a mathematical equation which can relate chemical structure to the activity. The results obtained will be helpful to pharmacologists, chemists and medicinal chemists to come up with improved IgE responses drugs.

Materials and Method

A dataset of ninety four 2-phenyl-benzimidazole derivatives [17] (Richards et al.) for their IgE response have been taken for present QSAR work given in Table 1. Total of ninety four molecules were considered for this study out of which twenty four molecules were used as test set.

The test set was chosen so as to accommodate compounds with activities in a different range. QSAR models were developed for both the training and the test set molecules, and the test set was used to validate the developed models.

In logIC_{50} values were converted to -logIC_{50} in order to bring out better linear correlations and reduce clustering of compounds while generating QSAR regression lines. The experimental information associated with biological activity, which is used as dependent variables in building a QSAR model. In this study, computational work (2D-QSAR) was performed using Vlife MDS QSAR plus software [18] on a HP computer with Core2 Duo processor and a window XP operating system.

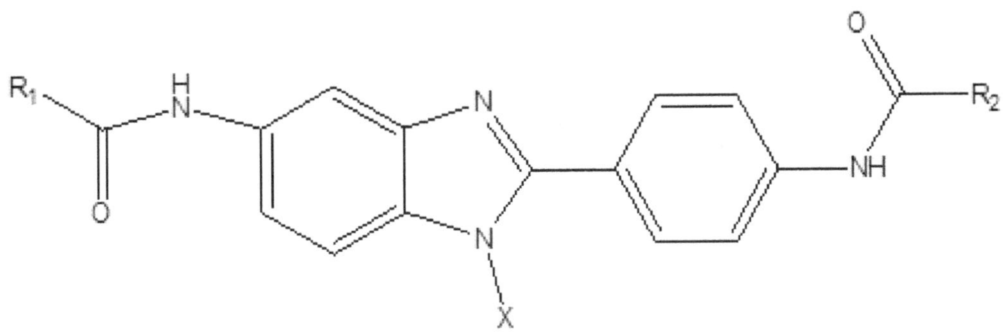

S.No	R1	R2	X	Y	IC_{50}	pIC_{50}
1	Phenyl	Phenyl	H	H	20	7.698
2	4-Bromopheny	4-Bromophenyl	H	H	200	6.698
3	3-Chlorophenyl	3-Chloropheny	H	H	25	7.602
4	2-Chlorophenyl	2-Chloropheny	H	H	45	7.346
5	3,4-Dichlorophenyl	3,4-Dichlorophenyl	H	H	40	7.397
6*	2,3-Dichlorophenyl	2,3-Dichlorophenyl	H	H	10	8.000
7	3,5-Dichlorophenyl	3,5-Dichlorophenyl	H	H	70	7.154
8	2,4-Dichlorophenyl	2,4-Dichlorophenyl	H	H	30	7.522
9	2,6-Dichlorophenyl	2,6-Dichlorophenyl	H	H	400	6.397
10*	Penta-fluoro-phenyl	Penta-fluoro-phenyl	H	H	4	8.397
11	Phenyl	4-Chlorophenyl	H	H	90	7.045
12	4-Nitrophenyl	4-Nitrophenyl	H	H	150	6.823
13*	4-Cyanophenyl	4-Cyanophenyl	H	H	100	7
14	4-Methoxyphenyl	4-Methoxyphenyl	H	H	30	7.522
15	3,4-Dimethoxyphenyl	3,4-Dimethoxyphenyl	H	H	700	6.154
16	4-S-methyl-phenyl	4-S-methyl-phenyl	H	H	150	6.823
17*	4-Methylphenyl	4-Methylphenyl	H	H	20	7.698
18	1-Naphthalene	1-Naphthalene	H	H	80	7.096
19	CH2-2-thiophene	CH2-2-thiophene	H	H	500	6.301
20	Cyclohex-3-ene	Cyclohex-3-ene	H	H	400	6.397

21*	Phenyl-	Cyclohexyl	H	H	10	8
22	CH3	Cyclohexyl	H	H	100	7
23	3,4-Dichlorophenyl	Cyclohexyl	H	H	0.8	9.096
24	4-Chlorophenyl	Cyclohexyl	H	H	6	8.221
25*	Cyclohexyl	3,4-Dichlorophenyl	H	H	0.4	9.397
26	Cyclohexyl	4-Chlorophenyl	H	H	8.0	8.096
27	1-Adamanty	2-Fluorophenyl	H	H	10	8
28	1-Adamanty	4-Fluorophenyl	H	H	10	8
29	2-Pyridyl	1-Adamanty	H	H	6	8.221
30*	3-Pyridyl	1-Adamanty	H	H	20	7.698
31	Cyclohexyl	Cyclohexyl	H	H	4	8.397
32	1-Adamantyl	1-Adamantyl	H	H	4	8.397
33	Cycloheptyl	Cycloheptyl	H	H	1.5	8.823
34*	Cyclobutyl	Cyclobutyl	H	H	400	6.397
35	Cyclopropyl	Cyclopropyl	H	H	1000	6
36	4-Methyl-cyclohexyl	4-Methyl-cyclohexyl	H	H	4	8.397
37	Cinnamyl	Cinnamyl	H	H	70	7.154
38*	Phenyl	Phenyl	CH_3	H	800	6.096
39	Cyclohexyl	Cyclohexyl	$COOCH_2CH_3$	H	7	8.154
40	Cyclohexyl	Cyclohexyl	$COCH_3$	H	1.5	8.823
41	Cyclohexyl	Cyclohexyl	H	H	2	8.698
42*	4-Methyl-phenyl	4-Methyl-phenyl	H	H	40	7.397
43	4-Fluorophenyl	4-Fluorophenyl	H	H	150	6.823
44	4-Methoxyphenyl	4-Methoxyphenyl	H	H	100	7
45	Phenyl	3,4-Dichlorophenyl	H	H	100	7
46*	Phenyl	5-Methyl-2-pyridyl	H	H	300	6.522
47	Cyclohexyl	Phenyl	H	H	9	8.045
48	1-Adamantyl	Phenyl	H	H	25	7.602
49	Phenyl	1-Adamantyl	H	H	8	8.096
50*	1-Adamantyl	4-Chlorophenyl	H	H	9	8.045
51	1-Adamantyl	3,4-Dichlorophenyl	H	H	1.5	8.823
52	2-Adamantyl	3,4-Dichlorophenyl	H	H	16	7.795
53	Cyclohexyl	4-Fluorophenyl	H	H	5	8.301
54	Cyclohexyl	4-Chlorophenyl	H	H	3	8.522
55*	2-Adamantyl	4-Methoxyphenyl	H	H	7	8.154
56	4-Methoxyphenyl	1-Adamantyl	H	H	40	7.397

57	4-Fluorophenyl	2-Adamantyl	H	H	40	7.397
58*	1-Adamantyl	2-Pyridyl	H	H	10	8
59	2-Adamantyl	2-Pyridyl	H	H	10	8
60	2-Adamantyl	3-Pyridyl	H	H	20	7.698
61*	2-Adamantyl	4-Pyridyl	H	H	40	7.397
62	2-Pyridyl	2-Adamantyl	H	H	40	7.397
63	2-Pyridyl	1-Adamantyl	H	H	40	7.397
64	2-Adamantyl	5-Methyl-2-pyridyl	H	H	20	7.698
65*	Cyclohexyl	Cyclohexyl	H	H	80	7.096
66	1-Adamantyl	1-Adamantyl	H	H	16	7.795
67	4-Methyl-cyclohexyl	4-Methyl-cyclohexyl	H	H	35	7.455
68	1-Adamantyl	Cyclohexyl	H	H	8	8.096
69*	2-Adamantyl	2-Methyl-cyclohexyl	H	H	4	8.397
70	2-Methyl-cyclohexyl	1-Adamantyl	H	H	4	8.397
72	Phenyl	Phenyl	H	H	400	6.397
72	3,4-Dichlorophenyl	Phenyl	H	H	50	7.301
73*	Phenyl	Cyclohexyl	H	H	70	7.154
74	Cyclohexyl	Phenyl	H	H	130	6.886
75	1-Adamantyl	Phenyl	H	H	150	6.823
76*	Phenyl	1-Adamantyl	H	H	4	8.397
77	3,4-Dichlorophenyl	1-Adamantyl	H	H	0.7	9.154
78	3,4-Dichlorophenyl	Bicycloheptyl	H	H	40	7.397
79*	3,4-Dichlorophenyl	Cyclohexyl	H	H	15	7.823
80	Cyclohexyl	Cyclohexyl	H	H	50	7.301
81	1-Adamantyl	1-Adamantyl	H	H	6	8.221
82	Cycloheptyl	Cycloheptyl	H	H	3	8.522
83	Cycloheptyl	Cycloheptyl	H	H	500	6.301
84*	Bicycloheptyl	Bicycloheptyl	H	H	30	7.522
85	2-Methyl-cyclohexyl	2-Methyl-cyclohexyl	H	H	60	7.221
86	4-Methyl-cyclohexyl	4-Methyl-cyclohexyl	H	H	3	8.522
87	1-Adamantyl	Cyclohexyl	H	H	60	7.221
88*	Cyclohexyl	1-Adamantyl	H	H	4	8.397
89	4-Methyl-cyclohexyl	1-Adamantyl	H	H	3	8.5228
90	Cyclohexyl	Bicycloheptyl	H	H	30	7.522
91*	1-Adamantyl	Bicycloheptyl	H	H	20	7.698
92	1-Adamantyl	Cycloheptyl	H	H	3	8.522

93	1-Adamantyl	Cycloheptyl	H	H	70	7.154
94	2-Pyridyl	1-Adamantyl	H	H	40	7.397
*Test compound						

Table 1: Structures and activities of benzimidazole derivatives as inhibitors of IgE response.

All the 2D descriptors were calculated for QSAR analysis using Vlife MDS 3.5 software. Energy minimization and geometry optimization were conducted using Merck molecular force field as force field and charge, maximum number of cycles were 1,000, convergence criterion (RMS gradient) was 0.01 and medium's dielectric constant of 1 by batch energy minimization method. The dataset of 94 molecules was divided into training set (71 compounds) and test set (23 compounds) by Sphere Exclusion (SE) method [19] for multiple linear regression (MLR) model with dissimilarity value of 11.2 using pEC50 activity field as dependent variable and various 2D descriptors as independent variables.

Energy-minimized geometry was used for calculation of descriptors, a total of 208 2D descriptors were calculated which encoded different aspects of molecular structure and consists of electronic, thermodynamic, spatial, and structural descriptors, e.g., retention index (chi), atomic valence connectivity index (chiV), path count, chain path count, cluster, path cluster, element count, estate number, semi-empirical, molecular weight, molecular refractivity, logP, and topological index.

Multiple linear regression (MLR)

MLR is a method used for modeling linear relationship between a dependent variable Y (pIC_{50}) and independent variable X (2D descriptors). MLR is based on least squares: the model is fit such that sum-of-squares of differences of observed and a predicted value is minimized. MLR estimates values of regression coefficients (r^2) by applying least squares curve fitting method. The model creates a relationship in the form of a straight line (linear) that best approximates all the individual data points. In regression analysis, conditional mean of dependant variable (pEC50) Y depends on (descriptors) X. MLR analysis extends this idea to include more than one independent variable. Regression equation takes the form

$$Y=b1 * x1+b2 * x2+b3 * x3+c$$

Where Y is dependent variable, 'b's are regression coefficients for corresponding 'x's (independent variable), 'c' is a regression constant or intercept [20,21].

Results and Discussion

For QSAR analysis regression was performed using pIC_{50} values as dependent variables and calculated parameters as independent variables. In any thorough investigation of the effects of molecular properties, it is essential to prove that the results are both statistically valid. 2D-QSAR equations were selected by optimizing the statistical results generated along with variation of the descriptors in this model.

pIC_{50}=0.3821(±0.0259) SsOHE-index+0.1694(±0.0117) ChiV3Cluster +0.4181(±0.0356) SssCH2E-index -0.2025(±0.0011) T_C_F_2+ 0.3689(±0.0770) SsClE-index

Ntraining=71, Ntest=23, r^2=0.8386, q^2=0.7218, F test=43.3584, r^2_se=0.1236, q^2_ se=0.1733, pred_r^2=0.7525, pred_r^2se=0.4268.

In above QSAR models, r^2 is a correlation coefficient that has been multiplied by 100 gives explained variance in biological activity. Predictive ability of generated QSAR models was evaluated by q^2 employing LOO method. F value reflects ratio of variance explained by models and variance due to error in regression. High F value indicates that model is statistically significant. Eq. (1) shows 84 % variance in the observed activity values. The low standard error of r^2_se=0.1236 demonstrates accuracy of the model.

Cross validated q^2 of this model 0.7218, indicates good internal prediction power of the model. Another parameter for predictivity of test set compounds is high pred_r^2=0.7525, which shows good external predictive power of the model. The electro-topological parameter SsClcount define the total number of chlorine atoms connected with one single bond. The positive coefficient of the descriptor suggests that IgE responses of Substituted 2-phenyl-benzimidazole may be increased by increasing the number of chlorine atoms present in the nucleus.

The positive coefficient of the molecular connectivity index descriptor in the model suggests that the decrease in branching in the molecule and the presence of heteroatoms increases the IgE responses. An estate contribution electro-topological state descriptor SssCH2E-index, which represents the indices for number of -CH_2 group connected with two single bonds, is inversely proportional to the activity. The positive coefficient of T_C_F_2 in the QSAR model reveal that the presence of [fluoro-phenyl at the end terminal of benzimidazole increases activity. The contribution charts of selected descriptors are represented in Figure 1a. The Observed activity and Predicted activity pIC_{50} along with residual values are shown in Table 2 and plots of observed vs. predicted values of pIC_{50} are shown in Figure 1b.

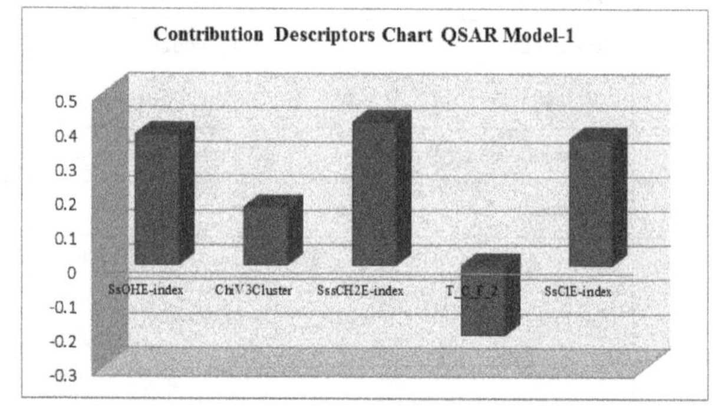

Figure 1a: Plot of contribution chart of 2D QSAR Model.

Com	pIC_{50}	2D-QSAR Model-1	
		Pred.	Res.
1	7.698	7.5014	0.1966
2	6.698	6.1844	0.5136
3	7.602	7.1742	0.4278
4	7.346	7.1565	0.1895
5	7.397	7.2394	0.1576
6*	8	8.1913	-0.1913
7	7.154	7.1385	0.0155
8	7.522	7.3699	0.1521
9	6.397	6.317	0.08
10*	8.397	8.3898	0.0072
11	7.045	7.3238	-0.2788
12	6.823	6.38	0.443
13*	7	6.9905	0.0095
14	7.522	7.3895	0.1325
15	6.154	6.3705	-0.2165
16	6.823	6.3512	0.4718
17*	7.698	7.349	0.349
18	7.096	7.4522	-0.3562
19	6.301	6.308	-0.007
20	6.397	6.2796	0.1174
21*	8	8.2619	-0.2619
22	7	7.3976	-0.3976
23	9.096	9.3444	-0.2484
24	8.221	8.4161	-0.1951
25*	9.397	9.3997	-0.0027
26	8.096	8.445	-0.349
27	8	8.378	-0.378
28	8	8.3608	-0.3608
29	8.221	8.395	-0.174
30*	7.698	7.3062	0.3918
31	8.397	8.3479	0.0491
32	8.397	8.2606	0.1364
33	8.823	8.3629	0.4601
34*	6.397	6.3113	0.0857

35	6	6.2892	-0.2892
36	8.397	8.2849	0.1121
37	7.154	7.1138	0.0402
38*	6.096	6.1735	-0.0775
39	8.154	8.1753	-0.0213
40	8.823	8.1666	0.6564
41	8.698	8.2351	0.4629
42*	7.397	7.1904	0.2066
43	6.823	6.1705	0.6525
44	7	7.3229	-0.3229
45	7	7.3268	-0.3268
46*	6.522	6.3362	0.1858
47	8.045	8.2932	-0.2482
48	7.602	7.3312	0.2708
49	8.096	8.3279	-0.2319
50*	8.045	8.3315	-0.2865
51	8.823	8.3254	0.4976
52	7.795	7.2976	0.4974
53	8.301	8.3018	-0.0008
54	8.522	8.364	0.158
55*	8.154	8.2889	-0.1349
56	7.397	7.2641	0.1329
57	7.397	7.2266	0.1704
58*	8	8.3328	-0.3328
59	8	8.3162	-0.3162
60	7.698	7.3431	0.3549
61*	7.397	7.3523	0.0447
62	7.397	7.3951	0.0019
63	7.397	7.3285	0.0685
64	7.698	7.3244	0.3736
65*	7.096	7.336	-0.24
66	7.795	7.2644	0.5306
67	7.455	7.2963	0.1587
68	8.096	8.2371	-0.1411
69*	8.397	8.278	0.119
70	8.397	8.2609	0.1361

72	6.397	6.242	0.155
72	7.301	7.238	0.063
73*	7.154	7.093	0.061
74	6.886	6.9321	-0.0461
75	6.823	6.4323	0.3907
76*	8.397	8.3511	0.0459
77	9.154	9.3763	-0.2223
78	7.397	7.4799	-0.0829
79*	7.823	7.4276	0.3954
80	7.301	7.4261	-0.1251
81	8.221	8.4405	-0.2195
82	8.522	8.4509	0.0711
83	6.301	6.4649	-0.1639
84*	7.522	7.4487	0.0733
85	7.221	7.4676	-0.2466
86	8.522	8.5002	0.0218
87	7.221	7.4985	-0.2775
88*	8.397	8.4923	-0.0953
89	8.522	8.4921	0.0299
90	7.522	7.5365	-0.0145
91*	7.698	7.571	0.127
92	8.522	8.3909	0.1311
93	7.154	7.4208	-0.2668
94	7.397	7.4738	-0.0768
*Test compound			

Table 2: Predicted activities according to 2D QSAR models results of benzimidazole with bacterial strains.

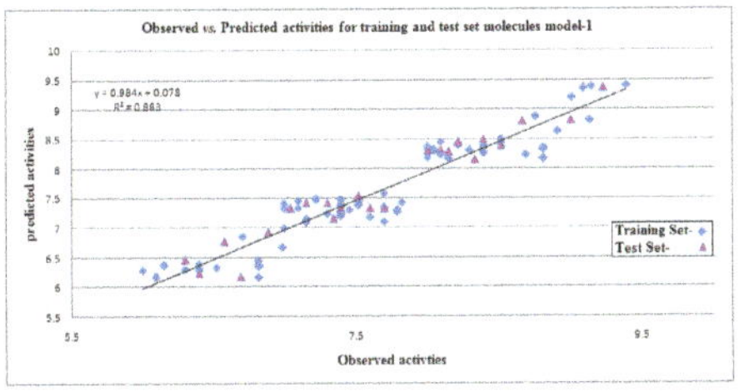

Figure 1b: Graphs of observed vs. predicted activity of 2D QSAR model-1.

Conclusion

A multiple linear regression (MLR) procedure was used to model the relationships between molecular descriptors and the inhibitors of IgE response of the benzimidazole derivatives. The quantitative structure-activity relationship (QSAR) analysis of some synthesized substituted 2-phenyl-benzimidazole derivatives inhibitors of IgE response were performed to find out the structural requirements of their IgE responses activities. Various 2D descriptors were calculated and used in the present analysis. The knowledge of Structure-Activity Relationship (SAR), together with the generation of QSAR, constitutes a large body of evidence that may assist in the development of new molecules with excellent biological activity and low toxicity. The results obtained from present investigation of IgE responses studies indicate that the presence of a chloropheny, fluoro-phenyl substituent leads to increase in the activity in comparison to the presence of a methyl group. QSAR analysis has been used to study the quantitative effects of the molecular structure of the benzimidazoles on their inhibitory activity. In this model special emphasis was given to the contribution of electrotopological in predicting biological activity of 2-phenyl-benzimidazole derivatives and they were found to improve the QSAR model and make it more precisely predictive.

Acknowledgments

The author wishes to express gratitude to V-life Science Technologies Pvt. Ltd for providing the trail version software for the study. Authors are thankful to the University Grants Commission (UGC), New Delhi for awarding a Research Award No. F. 30-1/2013(SA-II)/RA-2012-14-NEW-GE-MAD-4200.

References

1. http://www.cdc.gov/nchs/fastats/asthma.htm.
2. Hassed C (2005) An integrative approach to asthma. Australian Family Physician 34: 573-576.
3. Bielory L, Russin J, Zuckerman GB (2004) Clinical efficacy, mechanisms of action, and adverse effects of complementary and alternative medicine therapies for asthma. Allergy and Asthma Proceedings 25: 283-291.
4. Holgate ST (1999) The epidemic of allergy and asthma. Nature 402: 2-4.
5. Turner H, Kinet JP (1999) Signalling through the high-affinity IgE receptor Fc epsilon RI. Nature 402: 24-30.
6. Sutton B J, Gould H J (1993) The human IgE network. Nature 366: 421-428.
7. Sayers I, Helm BA (1999) the structural basis of human IgE-Fc receptor interactions. Clinical & Experimental Allergy 29: 585-594.
8. Punnonen J, Aversa G, Cocks BG, McKenzie AN, Menon S, et al. (1999) Interleukin 13 induces interleukin 4-independent IgG4 and IgE synthesis and CD23 expression by human B cells. Proceedings of the National Academy of Sciences USA 90: 3730-3734.
9. Cocks BG, Malefyt R, Galizzi JP, Vries JE, Aversa G (1993) IL-13 induces proliferation and differentiation of human B cells activated by the CD40 ligand. International Immunology 5: 657-663.
10. Defrance T, Carayon P, Billian G, Guillemot JC, Minty A, et al. (1994) Interleukin 13 is a B cell stimulating factor. Journal of Experimental Medicine 179: 135-143.
11. Blank U, Rivera J (2006) Assays for regulated exocytosis of mast cell granules. Current Protocols in Cell Biology 15: 11.
12. Andrews NL, Pfeiffer JR, Martinez AM, Haaland DM, Davis RW, et al. (2009) Mobile Fc Epsilon R1 receptor aggregates are signaling competent. Immunity 31: 469-479.
13. Drazen J (1998) Clinical pharmacology of leukotriene receptor antagonists and 5-lipoxygenase inhibitors. American Journal of Respiratory and Critical Care Medicine 157: S233-S237.
14. Huang C, Embrechts MJ, Sukumar N, Breneman CM (2007) Data Fusion and Auto-fusion for Quantitative Structure-Activity Relationship (QSAR). Artificial Neural Networks 4668: 628-637.
15. Mungalpara J, Pandey A, Jain V, Mohan CG (2010) Molecular modelling and QSAR analysis of some structurally diverse N-type calcium channel blockers. Journal of Molecular Modeling 16: 629-644.
16. Habibi-Yangjeh A, Pourbasheer E, Danandeh-Jenagharad M (2009) Application of principal component-genetic algorithm artificialneural network for prediction acidity constant of various nitrogen-containing compounds in water. Monatshefte für Chemie 140: 15-27.
17. Richards ML, Lio SC, Sinha A, Banie H, Thomas RJ, et al. (2006) Substituted 2-phenyl-benzimidazole derivatives: novel compounds that suppress key markers of allergy. European Journal of Medicinal Chemistry 41: 950-969.
18. Vlife MDS software package (2008), version 3.5, supplied by Vlife science technologies Pvt. Ltd, Pune.
19. Golbraikh A, Tropsha A (2002) Predictive QSAR modeling based on diversity sampling of experimental datasets for the training and test set selection. Journal of Computer-Aided Molecular Design 16: 357-369.
20. Croux C, Joossens K (2005) Influence of observations on the misclassification probability in quadratic discriminant analysis. Journal of Multivariate Analysis 96: 348-403.
21. Devillers J (1996) Neuronal network in QSAR and drug design. Academic Press, London.

Estimated Effects of Whole-system Naturopathic Medicine in Select Chronic Disease Conditions

Erica B. Oberg*, **Ryan Bradley, Kieran Cooley, Heidi Fritz, Joshua Z. Goldenberg, Dugald Seely, Jane D. Saxton and Carlo Calabrese**

Pacific Pearl La Jolla, San Diego, CA 92037, USA

***Corresponding author:** Erica B. Oberg, Professor, Pacific Pearl La Jolla, San Diego, CA 92037, USA, E-mail: erica.oberg@icloud.com

Abstract

Background: Naturopathic medicine (NM) is a holistic approach to primary care that almost always employs multi-modal interventions, i.e. nutrition and lifestyle change recommendations plus dietary supplements. While evidence supports individual elements of NM, the whole practice is often critiqued for its lack of evidence.

Methods: We systematically searched PubMed/MEDLINE, EMBASE, CINAHL, Cochrane Library and AMED from inception to April, 2012 as well as conducted hand searches of existing grey literature. For inclusion, studies had to report results from multi-modal treatment delivered by North American naturopathic doctors. The effect size for each study was calculated; no pooled analysis was undertaken. Risk of bias was assessed using the Cochrane risk of bias as well as Downs and Black tools.

Results: Fifteen studies met inclusion criteria, investigating a range of chronic diseases of public health significance. Studies were of good quality and had low to medium risk of bias including acknowledged limitations of pragmatic trials. Effect sizes (Cohen's d) for the primary medical outcomes varied and were statistically significant ($p<0.05$) in 10 out of 13 studies. A quality of life metric was included in all of the randomized controlled trials with medium effect size and statistical significance in some subscales.

Conclusions: Previous reports about the lack of evidence or benefit of NM are inaccurate; a small but compelling body of research exists. Further investigation is warranted into the effectiveness of whole practice NM across a range of health conditions. [PROSPERO 2012:CRD42012002176]

Keywords: Cardiovascular disease; Chronic disease; Complementary and alternative medicine (CAM); Diabetes; Mental health; Naturopathic medicine; Pain; Pragmatic trial; Quality of life; Randomized controlled trial; Systematic review; Whole-systems research

Introduction

The burden of chronic disease on the healthcare system is well established. Estimates are that 44% of Americans (133 million people) suffer from at least one chronic disease, while 13% (63 million) suffer from three or more [1,2]. These numbers are rising, and it is estimated that by 2020, 157 million Americans will have at least one chronic disease, while a staggering 81 million are expected to have multiple chronic conditions, with the most common being hypertension, hyperlipidemia, diabetes, heart failure, arthritis, and cancer [1,3]. To take the example of type 2 diabetes, coined as the "the epidemic of the 21st century" [4], approximately 24 million Americans are currently affected, and this number is expected to double in the next 25 years [1]. According to the American Diabetes Association, "people diagnosed with diabetes incur average medical expenditures of about $13,700 per year, of which $7,900 is attributable to diabetes" [5].

A second disease of epidemic proportions, cardiovascular disease (CVD) currently affects 83.6 million Americans (greater than one in three people): 77.9 million have hypertension, and 15.4 million have coronary heart disease [6]. By 2030, over 40% of the American population is expected to have some form of CVD [6]. In 2009, 1/6th of all hospital stays in the US (six million) were attributable to CVD; the direct cost associated with this was $71.2 billion dollars [6]. Direct and indirect costs of CVD were $312 billion, and this is expected to rise to $1.48 trillion dollars by 2030 [6]. When considering the sum of healthcare expenditure, 75% of all healthcare costs in the US (equivalent to $1.7 trillion dollars annually) are attributable to chronic disease [1,3]. It is clear that new solutions are needed, including a greater emphasis on multidisciplinary, prevention oriented care [2].

Between 2002 and 2005, the Naturopathic Medical Research Agenda (NMRA) formalized the focus of a research mission for naturopathic medicine (NM), as practiced in North America. The NMRA envisioned a pathway for the development of research focused on evaluating outcomes from naturopathic practice assessed by applying appropriate "whole practice" methodologies within pragmatic clinical settings [7]. Parallel to establishing the NMRA, in 2005, the Institute of Medicine (IOM) report "Complementary and Alternative Medicine in the United States" identified important gaps in the knowledge of CAM effectiveness and utilization [8].One of the IOM's recommendations to address these gaps was to conduct outcomes research on routine care delivery.

By linking the care people get to the outcomes they experience, clinical outcomes research has become a key to developing better ways to monitor and improve the quality of care, naturopathic and otherwise. The limitations of classical medical research designs, such as the single agent placebo-controlled randomized clinical trial, have become well-appreciated, especially as they relate to CAM research [9-12]. Alternative methods, such as patient-centered outcomes research and the inclusion of metrics that assess quality of life (QOL) have become increasingly prioritized in research, as exemplified by program announcements from the Patient-Centered Outcomes Research Institute, created under Section 6301 of the Affordable Care Act of 2010 [13]. Thus, "whole practice" research has emerged as a strong, valid and relevant methodology to investigate naturopathic medicine, as well as other multi-modal practices [9].

Standard research methodology designed to test the null hypothesis often does not specifically examine the magnitude of the effect, nor the precision around the magnitude of the effect. For clinical questions, this is critical information since clinicians must be able to evaluate the relative importance or impact a given therapeutic approach may have on their patient population, not simply the statistical significance. In whole systems research, the magnitude of the effect, or the effect size, of the multi-component intervention may be most appropriate. Meta-analysis of effect sizes allows for an examination of the clinical significance of both specific and non-specific effects of a treatment in comparison to control. Here we report effect size, calculated as a standard mean difference (Cohen's d), for all studies in which data were available (two were missing data required to calculate an effect size). The standardized mean difference provides a less heterogeneous metric of the magnitude of the effect of whole-practice naturopathic medicine and the precision around the range of probable effect size of the multi-modal naturopathic approach in a given condition or disease.

The research base describing practice outcomes from NM in health and disease is typically assumed to be limited [14]. However, in the domain of patient-centered research, the field of NM has been in the vanguard, defining its priorities in patient-reported outcomes research before well-established nomenclature (and avenues for funding) came into fashion. The purpose of this review was to compile and consolidate research that has investigated the whole practice of naturopathic medicine as it is practiced in community settings in order to better assess the quantity and quality of the research, and clinical effect, if any.

Methods

Definition of naturopathic medicine

Naturopathic medicine is a distinct primary health care profession, emphasizing prevention, treatment and optimal health through the use of therapeutic methods prescribed according to a therapeutic order which encourage the inherent self-healing process of the body [15]. Clinical practice focuses on the patient as a whole person, and addresses physical, mental, emotional, spiritual, and environmental dimensions of health concurrently to promote healing. Naturopathic doctors (NDs) in Canada and the United States receive training to a common standard as defined by the Council on Naturopathic Medical Education (CNME) [15]. Graduates from accredited schools are eligible for licensing in 17 states, two US territories, the District of Columbia, and five provinces in Canada. Scope of practice and training standards differ from practitioners called naturopaths in Australia, New Zealand, and European and other countries; thus, for purposes of this review, we limited research to investigations of North American naturopathic practice.

Identification of eligible studies

In April 2012, a comprehensive search was conducted in the PubMed/MEDLINE database (1946-2012) to locate studies pertaining to North American licensed naturopathic medicine with patient-reported, clinical, and/or cost outcomes. The search included both controlled vocabulary (MeSH) terms, e.g. Naturopathy and Treatment Outcome, and natural language words and phrases, e.g. naturopathic medicine and whole practice. The PubMed/MEDLINE search query was then "translated" and the following electronic databases were searched according to their specific conventions: EMBASE (1966-2012), CINAHL with Full Text (1982-2011), the Cochrane Library (1966-2012), and AMED (1985-2012). A language filter was applied limiting citations to English, French and Spanish to reflect the emphasis on naturopathic medicine as practiced in North America. No other filters were used, in order to increase search sensitivity. Additionally, conference proceedings of the American Association of Naturopathic Physicians (AANP) and Canadian Association of Naturopathic Doctors (CAND) were scanned for relevant abstracts. Hand searches of the following journals were conducted: Journal of Naturopathic Medicine (1990-2000); International Journal of Naturopathic Medicine (2004-2012; online archive searched); Journal of Orthomolecular Medicine (1990-2012); Townsend Letter (1990-2012) as well as grey literature in the form of reference sections and citations to those studies that met inclusion criteria. The systematic review, including inclusion criteria, preliminary and final search strings, were preregistered with PROSPERO [PROSPERO 2012:CRD42012002176] [16].

Study selection

In accordance with PRISMA guidelines [17], two reviewers independently reviewed the search results to select studies that met inclusion criteria. To be included, studies had to be longitudinal clinical studies reporting longitudinal outcomes, in which North American licensed naturopathic doctors managed clinical conditions employing their full scope of practice. Observational and randomized clinical trials (RCTs) were included if they were consistent with whole practice (i.e. the naturopathic intervention consisted of at least two different treatment modalities).

Data abstraction

Data abstraction was conducted in duplicate (CC, DS), using piloted data extraction sheets. The following data items were extracted: study setting; study population, participant demographics and baseline characteristics; details of the intervention and control conditions; study methodology: recruitment and study completion rates; outcomes and times of measurement; indicators of acceptability to users; suggested mechanisms of intervention action; information of assessment of the risk of bias; information on or to calculate effect size. In the event that data was missing or unclear, a request for information was sent to the original investigators. Author assessment took place independently with disagreements being resolved by consensus.

Methodological assessment and quality rating

Two authors (KC, JG) independently assessed each randomized controlled trial for risk of bias using the Cochrane risk of bias tool [18]. The use of the risk of bias tool is explained in detail elsewhere [19] and includes assessment of the following domains: sequence generation, allocation concealment, blinding of participants and personnel, blinding of outcome assessors, incomplete outcome data, selective outcome reporting, and other sources of bias (e.g. distribution of baseline characteristics, industry initiation and funding). The same two authors also used the Downs & Black checklist as a second critical appraisal tool for methodological quality of the studies included in the review [20]. This 28-item checklist is appropriate for both randomized and non-randomized studies, quantifying an overall score (out of 28; higher scores indicate greater methodological rigor) as well as domain-specific scores for reporting (11), external validity (3), internal validity (bias) (7), internal validity (confounding) (6) and power (1). Author assessment took place independently with disagreements being resolved by consensus.

Assessment of clinical outcomes and effect size

Primary outcome measures, as defined by the investigators of the original research, as well as quality of life metrics, such as the SF-36, were abstracted from reported results with the intention to compare and pool effect sizes using forest plots and standard methods for meta-analyses. When necessary, communication with authors provided missing data such as standard deviations. The heterogeneity of the studies we reviewed warranted use of a statistic that could be applied to summarize results of various study designs. Standardized mean differences were calculated for each study for the between group differences in the author-specified primary outcome [19,21]. For measures of quality of life, standardized mean differences were calculated for summary scores in physical, mental, and general health when available.

Using pooled variances for the standard deviations in point estimates of active and control group outcomes, Cohen's d effect sizes were computed. When interpreting Cohen's d values, an effect size of 0.2 to 0.3 is considered a "small" effect, whereas around 0.5 is considered a "medium" effect and 0.8 or greater is considered a "large" effect [22].

Though other measures such as Glass's Δ or Hedge's g can be used to calculate effect size, Cohen's d was selected based on popular use and that the calculation accounts for variance in non-specific effects seen in both the intervention and control group. This calculation results in a conservative effect size, weighted to maximize the impact of the control group and minimize the impact of the intervention group. Study heterogeneity (I2) was calculated and due to significantly different treatment populations and a large initial I2, the studies were not pooled for analysis.

Results

The PubMed/MEDLINE search string provided 1,257 total citations before removing duplicates. After 329 duplicates were removed, 931 citations were reviewed for inclusion. The final selection yielded 12 qualifying clinical studies, one of which had a cost-effectiveness analysis associated with the primary trial results. Results from hand searching added two additional studies: a more recently published randomized controlled trial (RCT) & companion cost-effectiveness analysis (CEA). In total, 15 studies of whole practice naturopathic medicine were included [23-37]. Figure 1 shows the literature flowchart.

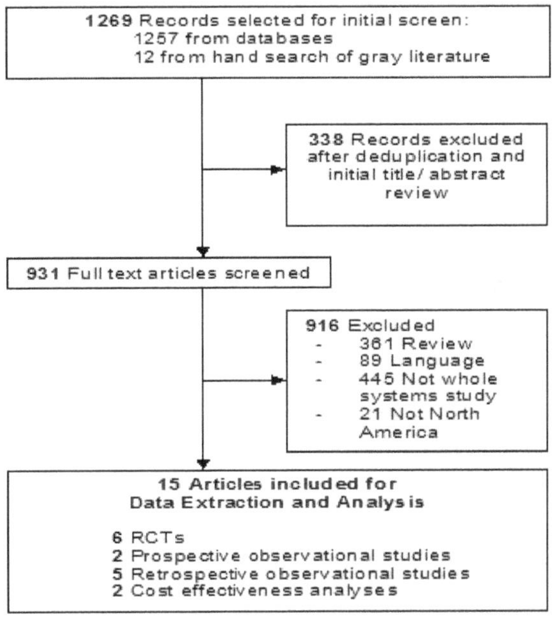

Figure 1: Literature flowchart.

Of the five retrospective studies, one included a control group [35]. Two studies were prospective observational cohort studies, of which one was comparative to an electronically created usual care control group [24], and one made comparisons to other forms of CAM [34]. Six of the studies were randomized controlled trials (RCTs) with usual care comparators [23,27-30,32], although one made comparisons to other forms of CAM as well [30].

Two cost-effectiveness analyses were identified which used data from two of the included RCTs [31,37]. All studies were in chronic disease conditions; six evaluated outcomes in diabetes or cardiovascular disease [23-25,28,33,37], five in musculoskeletal or pain conditions [26,30-32,34], and four studies were in other conditions [27,29,35,36]. Summaries of the included studies are in Table 1 [23-37].

Authors	Condition	N	Design (and comparator)	Primary Outcome	Patient-Reported outcome
Seely [23]	Cardiovascular disease	246	RCT (enhanced UC)	Framingham risk score, prevalent metabolic syndrome	SF-36
Bradley [24]	Diabetes	40	Prospective observational with controls	HbA1c, SDSCA	PHQ-8

			(UC, electronically matched from EHR)		
Bradley [25]	Hypertension	85	Retrospective cohort	Blood pressure (mm Hg systolic)	N/A
Szczurko [26]	Rotator Cuff Tendinitis	85	RCT (physical exercise active control)	SPADI	SF-36
Bradley [28]	Diabetes	37	Retrospective cohort	HbA1c, lipids, blood pressure	N/A
Cooley [27]	Anxiety	75	RCT (psychotherapy, matched breathing exercise, and placebo)	Beck Anxiety Inventory	SF-36
Shinto [29]	Multiple Sclerosis	45	3 arm RCT (UC and UC+education)	Modified Fatigue Impact Scale	SF-36
Ritenbaugh [30]	TMJ	160	3 arm RCT (UC and TCM)	Worst/average score of facial pain	Effect of pain on ADLs, social activities
Szczurko [32]	Chronic Low Back Pain	75	RCT (physiotherapy instruction, breathing exercise, and home exercise booklet)	Oswestry questionnaire	SF-36
Bradley [33]	Diabetes	16	Retrospective cohort	% HbA1c, % making glycemic improvement	N/A
Secor [34]	Pain	94	3 arm prospective observational (acupuncture, chiropractic)	Pain VAS	SF-12
Cramer [35]	Menopausal symptoms	239	Retrospective cohort with controls (UC, electronically matched in EHR)	% with improvement in 7 symptoms	N/A
Milliman [36]	Hepatitis C	41	Consecutive case series	ALT	N/A
Herman [31]	Low back pain (Szczurko)	75	Cost-effectiveness analysis	QALYs, societal health costs	N/A
Herman [37]	Cardiovascular disease (Seely)	246	Cost-effectiveness analysis	QALYs, societal health costs	N/A

NOTE:

ADLs: Activities of Daily Living; ALT: Alanine Transaminase; HbA1c: Hemoglobin A1C; PHQ-8: Patient Health Questionnaire; QALYs: Quality Adjusted Life Years; RCT: Randomized Controlled Trial; SDSCA: Summary of Diabetes Self Care Activities Assessment Scale; SF-36: Short Form-36 and 12; SPADI: Shoulder Pain and Disability Index; TMJ: Temporomandibular Joint disorders; TCM: Traditional Chinese Medicine; UC: Usual Care (biomedical care by MD/DO/NP); VAS Visual Analog Scale

Table 1: Characteristics of studies assessing whole system naturopathic medicine.

Study quality and risk of bias

In general, the RCTs included in this review were assessed as having a low risk of bias on most domains and were clearly reported. However, none of the included trials were blinded, a recognized impracticality in whole systems research [10].

Because of this limitation, as well as missing outcome data in some trials, the assessment of the overall risk of a biased effect estimate was high in all but one trial. Methodological rigor, as quantified by the Downs and Black checklist, varied among the studies, with higher rigor demonstrated by randomized controlled trials and in the more recent studies; see Figures 2 and 3 and further detail.

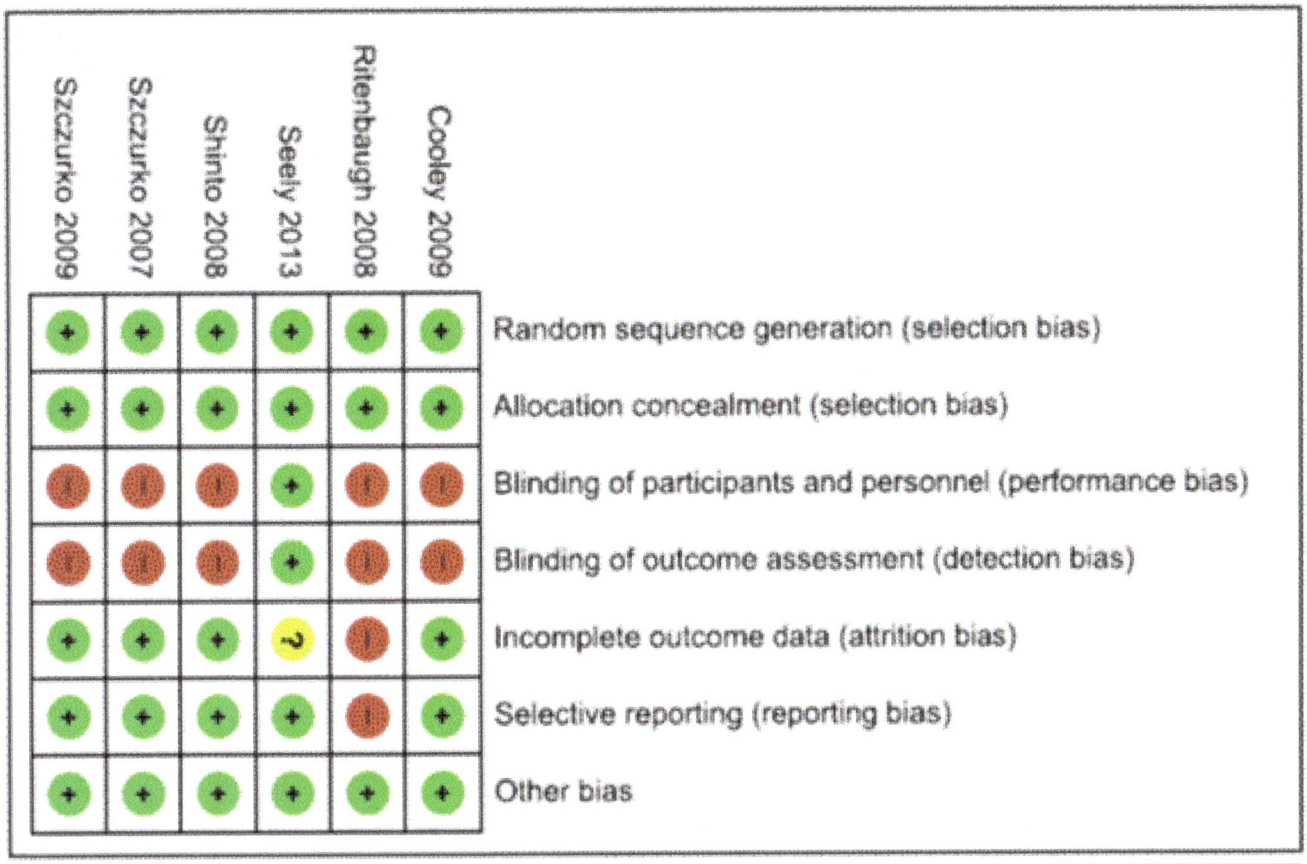

* Categories of low, unclear and high risk of bias are identified by the Cochrane Risk of Bias Tool [19]

Figure 2: Risk of bias of included studies, individually.

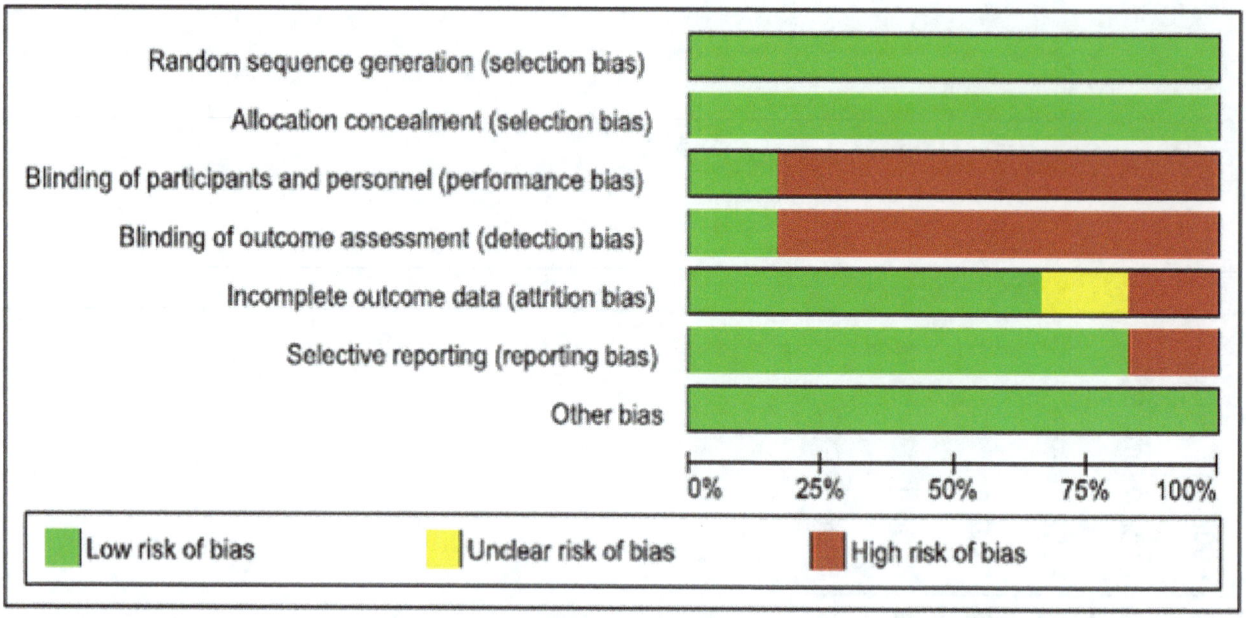

* Categories of low, unclear and high risk of bias are identified by the Cochrane Risk of Bias Tool [19]

Figure 3: Risk of bias of included studies, collectively.

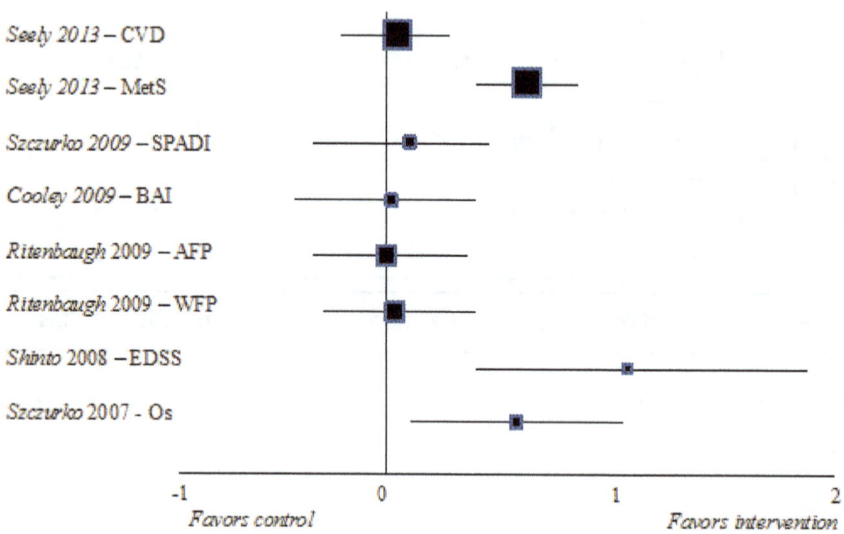

Legend: Definitions: AFP = average facial pain, WFP = worst facial pain, SBP = systolic blood pressure, DBP = diastolic blood pressure, CVD = cardiovascular disease, MetS = metabolic syndrome

Figure 4: Effect size estimates for primary outcomes.

Cardiometabolic disease (Cardiovascular disease, diabetes, hypertension, metabolic syndrome): Cardiometabolic disease represents one of the leading public health concerns in the United States, and the majority of studies of whole practice naturopathic medicine focused on these conditions. Bradley et al. conducted three observational studies in diabetes and one in hypertension [24,25,28,33] and Seely et al. conducted a pragmatic RCT and economic evaluation [23,37]. In the first retrospective evaluation of diabetes care, glycemic control and other risk factors improved during receipt of naturopathic care [33].

Primary clinical outcomes

Studies reported results in comparison to usual care controls or other CAM modalities, or reported differences between treatment groups, typically reporting mean changes and p values. To address the heterogeneity amongst the studies and the need to assess the magnitude of the observed effects systematically, we calculated effect sizes for each study, which are presented in Figure 4 for primary outcomes. No adverse events were reported.

Rates of health promotion delivery were substantially higher than national primary care averages. Evidence-based therapeutic lifestyle change recommendations (dietary) were made for 100% of patients, and 94% of patients were prescribed exercise. 69% of patients received counseling regarding stress reduction techniques. In the second retrospective evaluation of diabetes care, observations of clinical outcomes following a mean 27 month duration of care demonstrated the following significant mean changes in clinical risk factors: -0.65% for HbA1c (p=0.046), -45 mg/dL for triglyceride (TAG) (p=0.037), -7 mm Hg in Systolic Blood Pressure (SBP) (p=0.02), and -5 mm Hg in Diastolic Blood Pressure (DBP) (p=0.003) [28]. Mean changes in total cholesterol did not reach statistical significance. Three unique dichotomous outcomes were reported for this study: the percentage of patients who achieved new control (i.e. had not achieved control or within normal limits after diagnosis but prior to the study), had clinically significant risk factor improvements, or had any improvement. For HbA1c, the percent reaching new control was 26%, 42% had clinically significant improvements in risk factors, and 68% had any improvement. Respectively, percent of patients achieving these outcomes were LDL,7%, 28%, and 62% for LDL; 0%, 25%, and 39% for HDL; 14%, 38%, and 52% for TAG; 16%, 51%, and 86% for SBP; and 27%, 54%, and 70% for DBP. In the most recent study, a prospective observational cohort study conducted within a large health maintenance organization, a mean HbA1c decrease of -0.90% (P=0.02) was observed [24]. This was a -0.51% mean difference compared to usual care (P=0.07), following six-months of care. Significant improvements were found in most patient-reported measures, including glucose testing (P=0.001), healthy dietary behaviors (P=0.001), increased physical activity (P=0.02), improved mood (P=0.001), increased self-efficacy (P=0.0001) and increased motivation to change lifestyle (P=0.003).

In the 2011 retrospective evaluation of hypertension (HTN) outcomes, Bradley et al. found that patients with both stage 1 and stage 2 HTN had blood pressure reductions during receipt of naturopathic care, with stage 2 patients achieving mean reductions of 26 mmHg (P<0.0001) and 11 mmHg (P<0.0001) in systolic BP (SBP) and diastolic BP (DBP), respectively. The proportion of patients with resolution of hypertension, defined as BP less than <140/90 mmHg, was 33% (P<0.033) [25].

In 2013, Seely et al. reported results of an RCT comparing the addition of naturopathic treatment to community based usual care by a general practice medical doctor (GP) alone [23]. Composite reduction in cardiovascular disease risk as measured by Framingham risk scores demonstrated that the group receiving naturopathic care in addition to usual care experienced a 3.6% favorable difference in risk compared to usual care alone (NNT=30 for 10 year event risk). This absolute risk reduction was the equivalent to seeing a risk reduction of becoming 5.5 years "younger in CV years." A 27% absolute reduction in the prevalence of metabolic syndrome was also observed in the naturopathic care arm. A cost effectiveness analysis also accompanied this trial [37]. Of the 246 employees who consented to the trial, two-thirds gave consent to make available their claims and sick leave data. There were no statistically-significant differences between those who did and did not give this consent across baseline characteristics, outcomes, or tendency to miss study visits. The measured risk reductions came with an average net savings of $1138 in societal costs and $1187 in employer costs. There was no change in quality-adjusted life-years across the study year.

Pain

The studies summarizing naturopathic treatment of pain syndromes cover a wide range of conditions. Pain is among the top five reasons patients seek medical attention [38]. In the study by Secor et al., data obtained from an electronic outcome measures data management system at an integrative pain clinic found significant improvements in pain scores and quality of life measures [34]. Patients who received naturopathic care experienced the greatest pain reductions (60%, p ≤ 0.0001); however, the chiropractic and acupuncture treatment groups also experienced statistically significant pain reductions of 34% and 52% respectively.

A three-armed randomized controlled trial of naturopathy (NM), traditional Chinese medicine (TCM), or standard care (SC) for temporal mandibular jaw pain was undertaken in a large health maintenance organization in Portland [30]. TCM and NM both demonstrated significantly greater in-treatment reductions for worst facial pain compared to SC; reductions for NM versus SC were greatest (p=0.019).

In the RCT by Szczurko et al. investigating rotator cuff tendinitis, pain scores decreased by 54.5% (P<0.0001) in the NM group and by 18% (P=0.0241) in the comparison group which received physical therapy exercise recommendations [26]. The same team's 2007 RCT of naturopathic vs. standard physiotherapy for chronic low back pain also found significant benefits in the naturopathic treatment group (-6.89, 95% CI. -9.23 to -3.54, p=<0.0001) as measured by the Oswestry questionnaire. An additional finding of this trial included a 0.5 kg/m2 reduction in Body Mass Index (BMI) (p=0.01).

Other chronic conditions

The remaining studies investigated other chronic conditions: multiple sclerosis, hepatitis C, anxiety, and menopausal symptoms. The 2008 RCT by Shinto et al. investigated outcomes in multiple sclerosis [29]. Three intervention arms were defined: usual care, naturopathic medicine plus usual care, and MS education plus usual care. While there were no significant differences between groups on any outcome measure, there was a trend favoring the naturopathic group in the General Health subscale of the SF-36 (p=0.11), Timed Walk (p=0.11), and neurologic impairment (EDSS) (p=0.07). In 2009, Cooley et al. randomized people with anxiety to receive naturopathic care or psychotherapy over a six week period [27]. Beck Anxiety Inventory scores decreased significantly in the naturopathic group compared to the psychotherapy group (p=0.003). Significant differences between groups were also observed in mental health, concentration, fatigue, social functioning, and vitality. In a retrospective study of menopausal symptoms, management by both naturopathic and conventional primary care physicians in a community health clinic was compared [35]. Multivariate analyses found that patients treated with NM were approximately seven times more likely than conventionally treated patients to report improvements for insomnia (odds ratio [OR], 6.77; 95% confidence interval [CI], 1.71, 26.63) and decreased energy (OR, 6.55; 95% CI, 0.96, 44.74). NM patients also reported improvements for anxiety (OR, 1.27; 95% CI, 0.63, 2.56), hot flashes (OR, 1.40; 95% CI, 0.68, 2.88), menstrual changes (OR, 0.98; 95% CI, 0.43, 2.24), and vaginal dryness (OR, 0.91; 95% CI, 0.21, 3.96) about as frequently as patients who were treated conventionally. Finally, in 2003, Milliman et al. reported retrospective outcomes of naturopathic treatment of Hepatitis C [36]. A statistically significant reduction in alanine transaminase (ALT), the primary liver enzyme, was reported.

Quality of life outcomes

Amongst the RCTs and prospective observational studies evaluated, all but one included a quality of life outcome measure as well as a disease-centered metric [23-29,32-36]. The outlier did assess the impact of the disease state (TMJ) on social function and activities of daily living [30]. Effect size estimates for quality life outcomes are summarized in Figure 5.

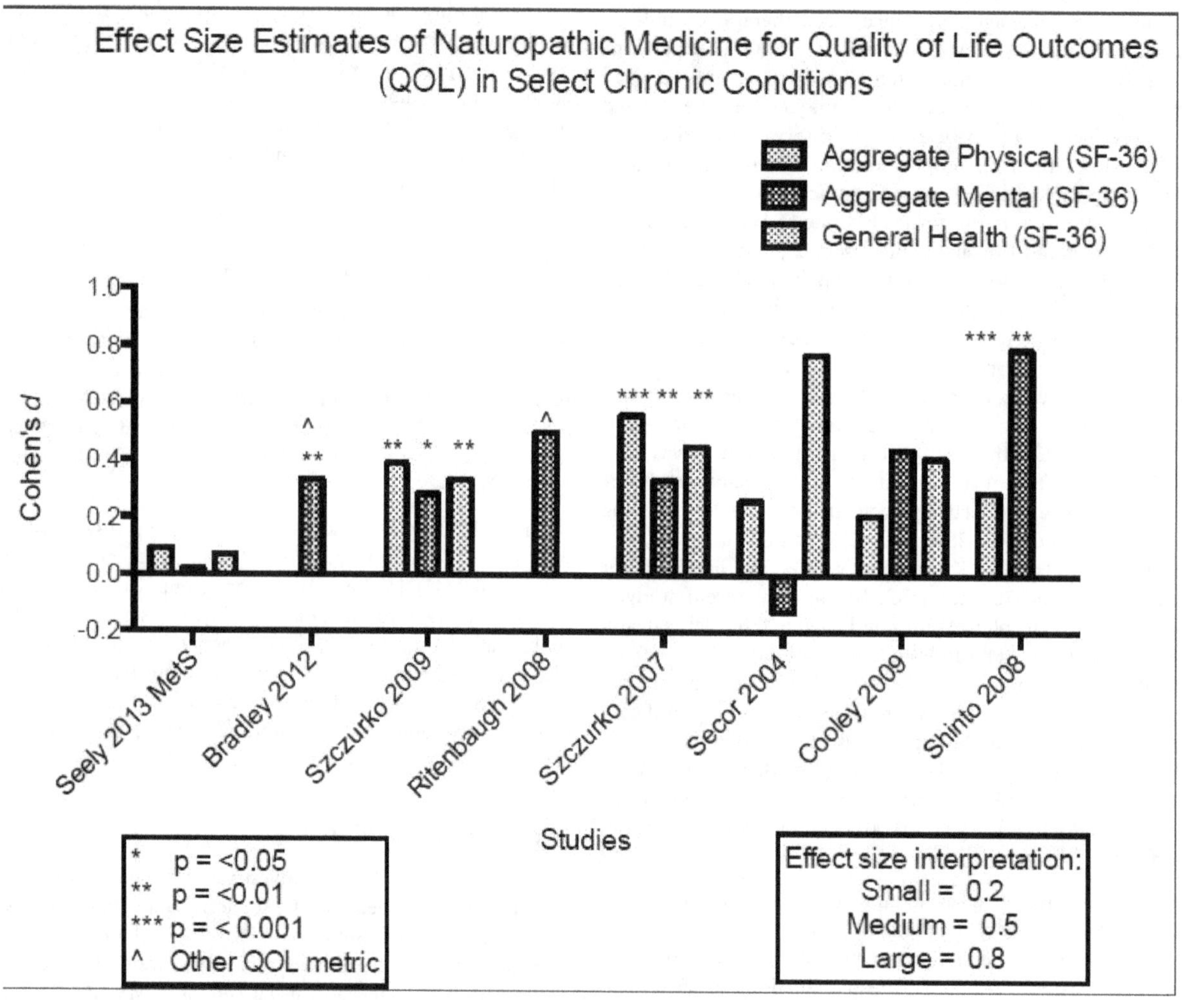

Figure 5: Effect size estimates for quality of life.

The SF-36 was the most common quality of life measure used (five RCTs), however the SF-12, PHQ-8 (a depression score), and a rating of the impact of facial pain on social functioning were also used. All eight studies using these instruments showed improvements with NM, with a majority demonstrating a medium effect size and statistical significance in some scales. In the evaluation of cardiometabolic risk reduction by Seely et al., improvements between groups were seen in all domains of the SF-36, but these did not reach statistical significance and the effect size was relatively small (<0.2) [23]. Bradley et al. found improved mood (as measured by PHQ-8) in the NM group at 6 and 12 months as compared to usual care (p=0.001, and 0.005, respectively) [24]. In their study of rotator cuff tendonitis, Szczurko et al. found statistically significant between-group differences in all SF-36 subscales; the aggregate mental and physical components demonstrated a 5.73 and 5.71 point difference respectively, favoring the NM group (p=0.01, p=0.0004 respectively) [26]. Effect size estimates were medium to small (0.39 to 0.28). In the same team's low back pain trial, QOL improved 7.0 (mental) and 8.47 (physical) points between groups (p-0.004 and <0.0001, respectively) [32]. Effect sizes were medium (0.33 for the aggregate mental component, 0.56 for the aggregate physical component). In the study by Ritenbaugh et al. measuring TMD-related psychosocial interference, NM provided significantly greater decreases than standard care or TCM ($p \leq 0.02$) with medium effect (0.5) [30]. In the comparison of NM to other CAM modalities by Secor et al., the effect size of the general health score of the SF-36 had a large effect (0.77), with the actual differences also reaching statistical significance ($p<0.001$). Cooley et al. found significant differences between groups for mental health, concentration, fatigue, social functioning, vitality, and overall quality of life, with the NC group exhibiting greater clinical benefit [27]. Effect sizes were 0.21 for aggregate physical functioning, 0.44 for aggregate mental functioning and 0.41 for general health QOL. Finally, in the study of patients with multiple sclerosis by Shinto et al., while thresholds for statistical significance were not reached, effect sizes were large (0.79 for mental health) possibly due to the generally poor QOL in this patient population [29].

Cost outcomes

Two cost-effectiveness analyses (CEAs) were performed in conjunction with two of the clinical trials [31,37]. Both trials recruited from a population of Canadian postal workers and had access to the same employment data. Both CEAs revealed societal and employer savings associated with use of NM. In one study, naturopathic treatment of LBP showed participant savings and significant benefit in quality-adjusted life years [31]. The cost-effectiveness analysis found that patients randomized to the naturopathic group improved their health status by the equivalent to 9.4 "perfect health" days over the three-month study period. In addition, naturopathic care significantly reduced societal costs by $1212 per participant. From the perspective of the employer, the intervention cost $154 per absentee day avoided. This compares favorably to employer cost of lost productivity of $172 per day, translating into a return on investment of 7.9% under the healthcare coverage limits set by this employer, assuming the employer paid the full cost of naturopathic care. Participants experienced savings related to lower expenditures on additional care of $1096 per participant [31].

Discussion

While the sample sizes of many of the studies are small, the results of this meta-analysis indicate that receiving whole-system naturopathic medicine as practiced in North America is associated with improved health outcomes, as well as improved quality of life, in patients with or at risk for chronic conditions, including cardiovascular disease, diabetes, chronic pain, anxiety, multiple sclerosis, hepatitis C, as well as menopausal symptoms. Although cost-effectiveness data are limited on naturopathic medicine in the context of chronic disease, the data thus far suggest the use of NM results in cost savings to employers as well as reductions in societal costs. This is especially relevant in the current era when healthcare resources are increasingly consumed by the management of chronic diseases and associated complications. Additional demonstrations and evaluations of licensed North American naturopathic doctors are warranted to enhance current strategies and improve health outcomes and should focus on diverse healthcare environments in generalizable populations.

Primary outcomes, patient-centered outcomes

The primary outcomes that were assessed and that showed improvement with the short-term use of NM were: reduced prevalence of metabolic syndrome by 16.9% compared to usual care [23]; improvements in glycemic control (reduced HbA1c), reductions in blood pressure (systolic and diastolic blood pressure reductions up to 26 and 11 mmHg respectively) [24,25,28]; improvement in anxiety (>50% reduction compared to active psychotherapy controls) [27]; reduced pain severity (>50% reductions in chronic low back pain and rotator cuff tendonitis compared to active physiotherapy controls) [26,32], and improvement in the pain of temporomandibular syndrome (TMJ) and other body pain compared to controls receiving other complementary modalities [30,34]. Although not statistically significant, point estimates of effect also suggest improvement in fatigue, neurologic, and cognitive impairment associated with multiple sclerosis compared to enhanced usual care [29], menopausal symptoms when compared to usual care [35], as well as ALT levels in hepatitis C patients [36]. For quality of life, patients treated with multi-modal interventions by naturopathic doctors showed small to moderate improvements in overall QOL scores as well as for physical function and mental function [26,32], and specific symptoms such as psychosocial interference [30], mental health, concentration, fatigue, social functioning, and vitality [27]. No adverse effects were reported in any of the studies. When considered collectively, the results of our study suggest that the care delivered by naturopathic doctors improves the health outcomes of patients affected by chronic disease, as measured by both clinical and patient-reported outcomes, as well as reduces direct and indirect costs.

Characterizing the NM intervention

Naturopathic doctors employ a diverse toolkit of treatment modalities which are selected based on the therapeutic order and emphasize healthy lifestyle choices and minimally invasive treatments. Details of the specific modalities used in each intervention can be found in the original studies and summarized in Table 1. In summary, the naturopathic interventions included diet counseling and nutritional recommendations, specific home exercises and physical activity recommendations, deep breathing techniques or other stress reduction strategies, dietary supplements including vitamins, hydrotherapy, soft-tissue manual techniques, electrical muscle stimulation, and botanical medicines. None of the studies included pharmaceutical agents even though these are sometimes part of naturopathic practice.

As a multi-modal system emphasizing diet and lifestyle interventions, outcomes of naturopathic medicine can be compared to other behavioral change research. For instance, a Scandinavian study with a very similar inclusion criteria had outcomes of similar effect on cardiovascular disease risk factors such as adiposity and blood pressure [39-41]. In studies based on the Diabetes Prevention Program protocol, intensive lifestyle modification reduced waist circumference -1.9 cm (-2.80 to -0.90), and diastolic blood pressure -2.3 mmHg (-4.04 to -0.51) compared to the control group [39,40]. In Seely 2013, the NM intervention reduced systolic (mean -6.55 mmHg, 95% CI -9.70 to -3.42) and diastolic (-3.33 mmHg, -5.92 to -0.75) blood pressure [23], improved lipids; LDL (-0.01 mmol/L, -0.28 to 0.25) and the ratio of total cholesterol to HDL (-0.79 points, 95% CI -1.24 to -0.35) [23].

For diabetes management, the Look AHEAD trial provides a relevant lifestyle change comparator. In the Look AHEAD trial, the intensive lifestyle intervention achieved improvements in HbA1c level (-0.36%), systolic (-5.33 mmHg) and diastolic (-2.92 mm Hg) blood pressure, HDL (3.67) and triglycerides (-25.56) compared to baseline values [42]. Similarly naturopathic care (Bradley 2009) improved

HbA1c by -0.65%, triglycerides by -45 mg/dL, as well as systolic (-7 mmHg), and diastolic (-5 mmHg) blood pressure compared to baseline [28]. And in Bradley 2012, mean HbA1c was reduced by -0.90% (p=0.02) with naturopathic care, a -0.51% HbA1c difference compared to usual care [24].

Impact of comparators

As a multi-modal system, naturopathic medicine is inherently difficult to evaluate using the single-agent placebo-controlled model. In the real world of clinical practice (independent of discipline), interventions are typically utilized in combination and patients are not blinded, are unlikely to be representative of a narrowly defined disease group, often present with co-morbidities, and typically receive other forms of care. No randomized, placebo-controlled trial is able to recruit these heterogeneous participant samples, nor mimic real world clinical settings. Therefore, objective evaluations of "whole practice" outcomes and the conduct of pragmatic trials provides the best true estimates of "real world" expectations for the effects of any new clinical service, including assessments of naturopathic medicine. However, even in pragmatic research, appropriate comparators remain necessary to assess the incremental value of an experimental health service. For evaluations of naturopathic medicine, rather than comparison to placebo or overly contrived time-attention control groups mimicking services that do not exist, the appropriate comparator is the usual care practices within the same clinical setting, i.e., the status quo.

Three of the included RCTs employed usual care/enhanced usual care comparators [23,29,30]. but one included an active control arm as well [30]. The other RCTs used active comparators [26,27,32]. Of the five retrospective studies, one included an electronically created usual care control group matched from medical records [35]. Two studies were prospective observational cohort studies, of which one was compared to an electronically created usual care control group [24]. The other made comparisons to other forms of CAM [34]. Use of enhanced usual care and active controls (acupuncture, chiropractic, education, psychotherapy) provides a useful picture of real-world effect. When most patients seek care from a naturopathic doctor, they are motivated to engage in something more and might be looking for other additions to their usual care. While heterogenous, the different comparators provide a real-world perspective about what can be expected at the population level, especially in our era of increasing valuation of patient-preferences and autonomy.

Similarly, for evaluations of non-pharmacological therapies, appropriate comparators were chosen based on customary usual care practices, such as standardized physical exercises for rotator cuff tendonitis and standardized psychotherapy for anxiety [26,27,32]. The studies analyzed here are all examples of evaluations of actual practice outcomes, i.e., pragmatic research, which most accurately estimates the effectiveness in a real world setting, and thus the results have greater external validity than could be achieved from any placebo-controlled clinical trial [43-45].

Impact of study design

Evidence now shows that unblinded studies are not inherently inferior to double blinded, placebo controlled trials with respect to internal validity, bias, and methodological rigor. In fact, contrary to common perception, evidence favors non-blinded studies utilizing objective measures [46]. Wood et al., have shown that unlike trials with subjective outcomes (which may exaggerate treatment effects when there is inadequate allocation concealment or lack of blinding) unblended trials with objective outcomes do not exaggerate treatment effects [46]. Savovic et al. conducted an analysis of 234 meta-analyses containing 1973 trials and reported similar findings, with little evidence of bias in non-randomized or non-blinded trials utilizing objective and mortality outcomes [47]. Therefore despite the lack of comparator for several of the observational studies, the emphasis on objective outcome measures of clinical risk and health status strengthens the results, and limits the bias inherent in observational studies.

The observational studies of whole practice naturopathic medicine themselves are of methodologic interest. Observational studies have been recognized as an important method for the evaluation of healthcare delivery, in part due to their generally larger size and longer duration, as well as including a more representative patient population than RCTs [48]. Research has also confirmed that well- designed observational studies can capture outcomes data that is comparable in accuracy to that reported by RCTs, without systematic overestimation of the magnitude of treatment effects [49,50]. Large analyses published in the New England Journal of Medicine have found that observational and randomized studies conducted in the same conditions and using similar outcome measures report similar estimations of treatment effects [49,50]. Yet, observational studies remain limited in their ability to control for confounders that may influence outcomes, e.g., other concurrent care services, and thus interpretation should remain conservative regarding attribution of cause and effect. Despite these limitations, the outcomes reported demonstrate no evidence of harm or worsening clinical status secondary to exposure to naturopathic medicine, and in fact suggest clinical benefit in all occasions.

Limitations

Despite finding beneficial effects on recognized predictors of cardiovascular events, the studies included in our review were not able to assess the effect of naturopathic medicine on the incidence of cardiovascular events or mortality from cardiometabolic disease. Second, due to heterogeneity among studies, we were not able to pool primary outcomes or quality of life data. It is hoped that with the growth of evidence in this area, a more rigorous synthesis of data may be possible in future. It should be noted that although the studies included here were pragmatic in nature, the delivery of care within the context of a research study may not always reflect that in the clinical field. The studies included here examined the practice of North American naturopathic medicine only, so these findings are not necessarily generalizable to the European or Australian practice of NM and also may not reflect the entirety of evidence relating to whole practice naturopathic medicine, or therapies used by naturopathic doctors in the treatment of chronic conditions. Finally, a considerable amount of time has elapsed from the date of the earliest published studies, during which naturopathic medicine has evolved to its current form.

Future Directions

Despite the results presented here in select conditions, research on the practice and outcomes of naturopathic medicine is in its infancy, and more research is required to further assess its contributions to health care. Because of the difficulties inherent in evaluating the multi-modal, non-pharmaceutical-dependent, interventions used by emerging disciplines, we recommend all future evaluations of whole practice naturopathic medicine include objective outcomes, provided they are clinically relevant and important to the patient. Additionally, extreme care should be taken to avoid (or quantify and carefully describe) participant withdrawals, losses to follow-up, and other causes of missing outcome data. Trials with large amounts of missing outcome data may benefit from sensitivity analyses especially extreme plausible analyses [51,52]. In addition to design considerations, future research on naturopathic medicine should assess its potential on additional high morbidity, high mortality chronic diseases for which usual practices results in disappointing clinical outcomes (e.g., depression, chronic kidney disease, advanced cardiovascular disease, asthma, irritable bowel syndrome, inflammatory bowel disease, fibromyalgia, chronic fatigue syndrome) as well as include larger replication studies for diabetes, CVD prevention, pain conditions and mental health.

Conclusion

When examined as a body of literature, the universally positive trends in favor of naturopathic medicine warrant increased funding to continue and expand research efforts. The quality of research assessing clinically relevant disease-oriented and patient-centered outcomes of whole practice naturopathic medicine is generally good. Naturopathic medicine appears to be a system of medicine with potentially positive public health implications for a wide variety of chronic health conditions.

Acknowledgements

With appreciation to the Naturopathic Physicians Research Institute (501(c)3) for supporting this work. The authors have no conflicts of interest to declare.

References

1. (2009) Tackling the burden of chronic diseases in the USA. Lancet 373: 185.
2. O'Connell B (2003) Controlling blood pressure with a healthy lifestyle. Diabetes Self Manag 20: 14-17, 21-23.
3. Ornish D, Scherwitz LW, Billings JH, Brown SE, Gould KL, et al. (1998) Intensive lifestyle changes for reversal of coronary heart disease. JAMA 280: 2001-2007.
4. Ginter E, Simko V (2012) Type 2 diabetes mellitus, pandemic in 21st century. Adv Exp Med Biol 771: 42-50.
5. American Diabetes Association (2013) Economic costs of diabetes in the U.S. in 2012. Diabetes Care 36: 1033-1046.
6. Go AS, Mozaffarian D, Roger VL, Benjamin EJ, Berry JD, et al. (2013) Heart disease and stroke statistics--2013 update: a report from the American Heart Association. Circulation 127: 6-245.
7. Standish LJ, Calabrese C, Snider P (2006) The naturopathic medical research agenda: the future and foundation of naturopathic medical science. J Altern Complement Med 12: 341-345.
8. (2005) Complementary and Alternative Medicine in the United States. Washington D.C: Institute of Medicine. National Academies Press. 335 p.
9. Wardle J, Oberg EB (2011) The intersecting paradigms of naturopathic medicine and public health: opportunities for naturopathic medicine. J Altern Complement Med 17: 1079-1084.
10. Ritenbaugh C, Aickin M, Bradley R, Caspi O, Grimsgaard S, et al. (2010) Whole systems research becomes real: new results and next steps. J Altern Complement Med 16: 131-137.
11. Verhoef MJ, Lewith G, Ritenbaugh C, Boon H, Fleishman S, et al. (2005) Complementary and alternative medicine whole systems research: beyond identification of inadequacies of the RCT. Complement Ther Med 13: 206-212.
12. Herman PM, Sherman KJ, Erro JH, Cherkin DC, Milliman B, et al. (2006) A method for describing and evaluating naturopathic whole practice. Altern Ther Health Med 12: 20-28.
13. (2010) Patient-Centered Outcomes Research Institute (PCORI). Patient Protection and Affordable Care Act ,U.S. Government Accountability Office.
14. Khorsan R, Coulter ID, Crawford C, Hsiao AF (2011) Systematic review of integrative health care research: randomized control trials, clinical controlled trials, and meta-analysis. Evid Based Complement Alternat Med 636134.
15. Fleming SA, Gutknecht NC (2010) Naturopathy and the primary care practice. Prim Care 37: 119-136.
16. (2012) PROSPERO:CRD42012002176. Systematic review of clinical studies of whole practice natruopathic medicine. Registered 21 Mar 2012 ed: PROSPERO.)
17. Liberati A, Altman DG, Tetzlaff J, Mulrow C, Gotzsche PC, et al. (2009) The PRISMA statement for reporting systematic reviews and meta-analyses of studies that evaluate health care interventions: explanation and elaboration. J Clin Epidemiol 62: 1-34.
18. Hartling L, Ospina M, Liang Y, Dryden DM, Hooton N, et al. (2009) Risk of bias versus quality assessment of randomised controlled trials: cross sectional study. BMJ 339: b4012.
19. Higgins G (2011) Cochrane Handbook for Systematic Reviews of Interventions Version 5.1.0 ed: The Cochrane Collaboration.
20. Downs SH, Black N (1998) The feasibility of creating a checklist for the assessment of the methodological quality both of randomised and non-randomised studies of health care interventions. J Epidemiol Community Health 52: 377-384.
21. Breaugh J (2003) Effect Size Estimation: factors to consider and mistakes to avoid. Journal of Management 29: 79-97.
22. Parker RI, Hagan-Burke S (2007) Useful effect size interpretations for single case research. Behav Ther 38: 95-105.
23. Seely D, Szczurko O, Cooley K, Fritz H, Aberdour S, et al. (2013) Naturopathic medicine for the prevention of cardiovascular disease: a randomized clinical trial. CMAJ 185: E409-416.
24. Bradley R, Sherman KJ, Catz S, Calabrese C, Oberg EB, et al. (2012) Adjunctive naturopathic care for type 2 diabetes: patient-reported and clinical outcomes after one year. BMC Complement Altern Med 12: 44.
25. Bradley R, Kozura E, Kaltunas J, Oberg EB, Probstfield J, et al. (2011) Observed Changes in Risk during Naturopathic Treatment of Hypertension. Evid Based Complement Alternat Med 2011: 826751.
26. Szczurko O, Cooley K, Mills EJ, Zhou Q, Perri D, et al. (2009) Naturopathic treatment of rotator cuff tendinitis among Canadian postal workers: a randomized controlled trial. Arthritis Rheum 61: 1037-1045.
27. Cooley K, Szczurko O, Perri D, Mills EJ, Bernhardt B, et al. (2009) Naturopathic care for anxiety: a randomized controlled trial ISRCTN78958974. PLoS One 4: e6628.
28. Bradley R, Kozura E, Buckle H, Kaltunas J, Tais S, et al. (2009) Description of clinical risk factor changes during naturopathic care for type 2 diabetes. J Altern Complement Med 15: 633-638.
29. Shinto L, Calabrese C, Morris C, Yadav V, Griffith D, et al. (2008) A randomized pilot study of naturopathic medicine in multiple sclerosis. J Altern Complement Med 14: 489-496.
30. Ritenbaugh C, Hammerschlag R, Calabrese C, Mist S, Aickin M, et al. (2008) A pilot whole systems clinical trial of traditional Chinese medicine and naturopathic medicine for the treatment of temporomandibular disorders. J Altern Complement Med 14: 475-487.
31. Herman PM, Szczurko O, Cooley K, Mills EJ (2008) Cost-effectiveness of naturopathic care for chronic low back pain. Altern Ther Health Med 14: 32-39.
32. Szczurko O, Cooley K, Busse JW, Seely D, Bernhardt B, et al. (2007) Naturopathic care for chronic low back pain: a randomized trial. PLoS One 2: e919.

33. Bradley R, Oberg EB (2006) Naturopathic medicine and type 2 diabetes: a retrospective analysis from an academic clinic. Altern Med Rev 11: 30-39.
34. Secor ER, Markow MJ, Mackenzie J, Thrall RS (2004) Implementation of outcome measures in a complementary and alternative medicine clinic: evidence of decreased pain and improved quality of life. J Altern Complement Med 10: 506-513.
35. Cramer EH, Jones P, Keenan NL, Thompson BL (2003) Is naturopathy as effective as conventional therapy for treatment of menopausal symptoms? J Altern Complement Med 9: 529-538.
36. Milliman WB, Lamson DW, Brignall MS (2000) Hepatitis C; a retrospective study, literature review, and naturopathic protocol. Altern Med Rev 5: 355-371.
37. Herman PM, Szczurko O, Cooley K, Seely D (2014) A naturopathic approach to the prevention of cardiovascular disease: cost-effectiveness analysis of a pragmatic multi-worksite randomized clinical trial. J Occup Environ Med 56: 171-176.
38. Manchikanti L, Singh V, Datta S, Cohen SP, Hirsch JA; American Society of Interventional Pain Physicians (2009) Comprehensive review of epidemiology, scope, and impact of spinal pain. Pain Physician 12: E35-70.
39. Knowler WC, Barrett-Connor E, Fowler SE, Hamman RF, Lachin JM, et al. (2002) Reduction in the incidence of type 2 diabetes with lifestyle intervention or metformin. N Engl J Med 346: 393-403.
40. Tuomilehto J, Lindström J, Eriksson JG, Valle TT, Hämäläinen H, et al. (2001) Prevention of type 2 diabetes mellitus by changes in lifestyle among subjects with impaired glucose tolerance. N Engl J Med 344: 1343-1350.
41. Eriksson KM, Westborg CJ, Eliasson MC (2006) A randomized trial of lifestyle intervention in primary healthcare for the modification of cardiovascular risk factors. Scand J Public Health 34: 453-461.
42. Look AHEAD Research Group, Wing RR (2010) Long-term effects of a lifestyle intervention on weight and cardiovascular risk factors in individuals with type 2 diabetes mellitus: four-year results of the Look AHEAD trial. Arch Intern Med 170: 1566-1575.
43. Glasgow RE, Emmons KM (2007) How can we increase translation of research into practice? Types of evidence needed. Annu Rev Public Health 28: 413-433.
44. Godwin M, Ruhland L, Casson I, MacDonald S, Delva D, et al. (2003) Pragmatic controlled clinical trials in primary care: the struggle between external and internal validity. BMC Med Res Methodol 3: 28.
45. Treweek S, Zwarenstein M (2009) Making trials matter: pragmatic and explanatory trials and the problem of applicability. Trials 10: 37.
46. Wood L, Egger M, Gluud LL, Schulz KF, Jüni P, et al. (2008) Empirical evidence of bias in treatment effect estimates in controlled trials with different interventions and outcomes: meta-epidemiological study. BMJ 336: 601-605.
47. Savovic J, Jones HE, Altman DG, Harris RJ, Juni P, et al. (2012) Influence of reported study design characteristics on intervention effect estimates from randomized, controlled trials. Ann Intern Med 157: 429-438.
48. Authors Thadhani R Formal trials versus observational studies. Formal trials versus observational studies .
49. Concato J (2013) Study design and "evidence" in patient-oriented research. Am J Respir Crit Care Med 187: 1167-1172.
50. Benson K, Hartz AJ (2000) A comparison of observational studies and randomized, controlled trials. N Engl J Med 342: 1878-1886.
51. Akl EA, Briel M, You JJ, Sun X, Johnston BC, et al. (2012) Potential impact on estimated treatment effects of information lost to follow-up in randomised controlled trials (LOST-IT): systematic review. BMJ 344: e2809.
52. A Hierarchy of Healing: The Therapeutic Order (2012) A Unifying Theory of Naturopathic Medicine. Textbook of Natural Medicine J.E. Pizzorno & M. Murray.

6

Biofield Treatment: An Alternative Approach to Combat Multidrug-Resistant Susceptibility Pattern of *Raoultella ornithinolytica*

Mahendra Kumar Trivedi[1], Shrikant Patil[1], Harish Shettigar[1], Mayank Gangwar[2] and Snehasis Jana[2*]

[1]*Trivedi Global Inc., 10624 S Eastern Avenue Suite A-969, Henderson, NV 89052, USA*

[2]*Trivedi Science Research Laboratory Pvt. Ltd, Madhya Pradesh, India*

***Corresponding author:** Jana S, Trivedi Science Research Laboratory Pvt. Ltd, Fortune City, Hoshangabad Rd., Bhopal, Madhya Pradesh, India, E-mail: publication@trivedisrl.com

Abstract

Raoultella ornithinolytica is belongs to the family of *Enterobacteriaceae,* a Gram-negative encapsulated aerobic bacillus associated with bacteremia and urinary tract infections. As biofield therapy is increasingly popular in biomedical heath care, so present study aimed to evaluate the impact of Mr. Trivedi's biofield treatment on antimicrobial sensitivity, minimum inhibitory concentration (MIC), biochemical study, and biotype number of multidrug resistant strain of *R. ornithinolytica.* Clinical sample of *R. ornithinolytica* was divided into two groups i.e. control and biofield treated which were analyzed for the above parameters using MicroScan Walk-Away® system on day 10 after treatment. Antimicrobial sensitivity assay results showed a significant increase (60.71%) in sensitivity pattern of antimicrobials i.e. changed from resistant to susceptible while 10.71% of tested antimicrobials changed from intermediate to susceptible as compared to control. MIC results showed a significant decrease in MIC values of 71.88% tested antimicrobials as compared to control.

Biochemical reaction study showed 15.15% alteration in different biochemical such as cetrimide, cephalothin, kanamycin, and ornithine after biofield treatment as compared to control. A significant change in biotype number (7775 4370) was also observed with organism identified as *Klebsiella oxytoca* after biofield treatment as compared to control (7775 5372). Overall results conclude that biofield treatment could be used as complementary and alternative treatment strategy against multidrug resistant strain of *R. ornithinolytica* with respect to improve the sensitivity and reduce the MIC values of antimicrobials. Hence, it is assumed that biofield treatment might be a suitable cost effective treatment strategy in near future, which could have therapeutic value in patients suffering from multidrug resistant pathogens.

Keywords: *Raoultella ornithinolytica*; Biofield treatment; Antimicrobial susceptibility; Biochemical reaction; Biotype; Multidrug resistant

Introduction

Genus *Raoultella* belongs to the family *Enterobacteriaceae,* mainly contains Gram-negative, aerobic, non-motile, capsulated, and facultative anaerobic bacilli [1]. Initially, genus *Raoultella* was classified in *Klebsiella,* further on the basis of 16S rRNA and rpoB genes study includes it in new genus *Raoultella.* It includes *Raoultella ornithinolytica, R. electrica, R. planticola, and R. terrigena. R. ornithinolytica* is widely distributed in aquatic flora, fishes and insects, but it was associated with histamine poisoning in fish [2]. Human infections are often less reported earlier, but different cases of bacteremia are reported due to *R. terrigena* [3], *R. planticola* [4] and *R. ornithinolytica* [5,6].

Although most of the infectious cases are often associated with underlying existing infection especially malignancies. However, other pathogenic cases such as urinary tract infection, soft issue infections in adults and neonatal infections are also reported [7]. Thus, this is very clear from the above reports that *Raoultella* genus acts as human pathogen and multidrug resistant (MDR) strain will cause a serious threat to human health causing pneumonia and other infections [8]. Broad spectrum antimicrobials and combinations therapies are the only treatment strategy to cure the infection of MDR. Antimicrobials are always associated with serious side effects [9]. Currently, no such alternative therapies apart from medicines are available against MDR microorganism infections, biofield treatment may be a new approach to improve the susceptibility pattern of *R. ornithinolytica.*

The National Center for Complementary and Alternative Medicine (NCCAM) places biofield therapy under subcategory of energy therapies as one of the five complementary medicine domain. It is scientifically preferred term for the biologically produced electromagnetic and subtle energy field that provides regulatory and communication functions within the organism. The cumulative effect of bio-magnetic and electric field that surrounds the human body is defined as biofield energy. However, the energy can exists in several forms such as kinetic, potential, electrical, magnetic, and nuclear. But human body has the power to produce measurable electric and magnetic signals [10,11].

Similarly, the human nervous system consists of the energy and chemical information in the form of electrical signals. Thus, human has the ability to harness the energy from environment or universe and can transmit into any living or nonliving object(s) around the globe. The objects always receive the energy and responding into useful way via biofield energy and the process is known as biofield treatment. Even every cell of human body will produce minute amount of magnetic and electric field, as it always covers with positive and negative charge in outer and inner cell wall respectively [12]. The biofield energy can be monitored by using electromyography (EMG), electrocardiography (ECG) and electroencephalogram (EEG) [13]. Mr. Trivedi's biofield treatment is well known and significantly studied in different fields such as altering the sensitivity pattern of different human pathogens [14-16]. It has been significantly studied in field of agriculture [17-19], biotechnology [20,21], and in material science [22-24].

Materials and Methods

Experimental design and biofield treatment

MDR strain of *R. ornithinolytica* was obtained from stored stock cultures of clinical sample in Microbiology Lab, Hinduja Hospital, Mumbai. MDR strain was divided in two groups i.e. control and treatment. In case of treatment group, sealed pack of MDR strain of *R. ornithinolytica* was handed over to Mr. Trivedi for biofield treatment under laboratory conditions. Mr. Trivedi provided the treatment through his energy transmission process to the treated group without touching the sample. The biofield treated sample was returned in the similar sealed condition and further analyzed on day 10 using the standard protocols. After biofield treatment, following parameters like antimicrobial susceptibility, MIC values, biochemical reactions, and biotype number were measured using MicroScan Walk-Away® system (Dade Behring Inc., USA) with respect to control. All antimicrobials and biochemicals were procured from Sigma Aldrich.

Evaluation of antimicrobial susceptibility assay

Antimicrobial susceptibility pattern of *R. ornithinolytica* was studied using MicroScan Walk-Away® system along with Negative Break Point Combo (NBPC 30) panel as per manufacturer's instructions. The antimicrobial susceptibility pattern (S: Susceptible, I: Intermediate, and R: Resistant) and minimum inhibitory concentration (MIC) values were determined by observing the lowest antimicrobial concentration showing growth inhibition. The antimicrobials used in the susceptibility assay viz. amikacin, amoxicillin/k-clavulanate, ampicillin/sulbactam, ampicillin, aztreonam, cafazolin, cefepime, cefotaxime, cefotetan, cefoxitin, ceftazidime, ceftriaxone, cefuroxime, cephalothin, chloramphenicol, ciprofloxacin, ESBL-a Scrn, ESBL-b Scrn, gatifloxacin, gentamicin, imipenem, levofloxacin, meropenem, moxifloxacin, nitrofurantoin, norfloxacin, piperacillin, piperacillin/tazobactam, tetracycline, ticarcillin/k-clavulanate, and tobramycin, trimethoprim/ sulfamethoxazole [25].

Biochemical study

Biochemical study of *R. ornithinolytica* was determined using MicroScan Walk-Away® system in both control and treated groups. Biochemicals used in the study are acetamide, adonitol, arabinose, arginine, cetrimide, cephalothin, citrate, colistin, esculin hydrolysis, nitrofurantoin, glucose, hydrogen sulfide, indole, inositol, kanamycin, lysine, malonate, melibiose, nitrate, oxidation-fermentation, galactosidase, ornithine, oxidase, penicillin, raffinose, rhaminose, sorbitol, sucrose, tartarate, tryptophan deaminase, tobramycin, urea, and Voges-Proskauer [25].

Identification by biotype number

The biotype number of *R. ornithinolytica* in control and treated samples were determined followed by identification of microorganism by MicroScan Walk-Away® processed panel report with the help of biochemical reaction data [25].

Results

Antimicrobial susceptibility

Results of antimicrobial sensitivity pattern and MIC values of control and biofield treated MDR strain of *R. ornithinolytica* are summarized in Tables 1 and 2, respectively. All these changes were observed on day 10 after the biofield treatment as compared to control group. Antimicrobial sensitivity assay showed that 60.71% of tested 28 antimicrobials were reported with significant increase in sensitivity pattern from R → S *viz.* amoxicillin/k-clavulanate, ampicillin/ sulbactam, aztreonam, cefazolin, cefotaxime, ceftriaxone, cefuroxime, cephalothin, ciprofloxacin, gatifloxacin, gentamicin, levofloxacin, moxifloxacin, piperacillin, tetracycline, trimethoprim/ sulfamethoxazole, and tobramycin after biofield treatment. Apart from this, 10.71% tested antimicrobials showed altered sensitivity pattern from I → S in ceftazidime, piperacillin/tazobactam, and ticarcillin/k-clavulanate as compared to control. Rest of the antimicrobials (28.7%) did not show any alteration in sensitivity pattern (Table 1).

S. No.	Antimicrobial	Control	Treated
1	Amikacin	S	S
2	Amoxicillin/k-clavulanate	R	S
3	Ampicillin/sulbactam	R	S
4	Ampicillin	R	R
5	Aztreonam	R	S
6	Cefazolin	R	S
7	Cefepime	S	S
8	Cefotaxime	R	S
9	Cefotetan	S	S
10	Cefoxitin	S	S
11	Ceftazidime	I	S
12	Ceftriaxone	R	S
13	Cefuroxime	R	S
14	Cephalothin	R	S
15	Chloramphenicol	S	S
16	Ciprofloxacin	R	S
17	Gatifloxacin	R	S
18	Gentamicin	R	S
19	Imipenem	S	S
20	Levofloxacin	R	S

21	Meropenem	S	S
22	Moxifloxacin	R	S
23	Piperacillin	R	S
24	Piperacillin/tazobactam	I	S
25	Tetracycline	R	S
26.	Ticarcillin/k-clavulanate	I	S
27.	Tobramycin	R	S
28.	Trimethoprim/sulfamethoxazole	R	S
R: Resistant; I: Intermediate; S: Susceptible			

Table 1: Effect of biofield treatment on *Raoultella ornithinolytica* to antimicrobial susceptibility.

Besides antimicrobial sensitivity assay, an overall significant decrease in MIC values were reported in 71.88% of antimicrobials (twenty three out of thirty two) against *R. ornithinolytica* as compared to control. Four folds decreased in MIC value were observed in case of cefotaxime, ceftriaxone, piperacillin, piperacillin/tazobactam, ticarcillin/k-clavulanate, and cefuroxime while two folds decreased in MIC value in case of amoxicillin/clavulanic acid, ampicillin/sulbactam, aztreonam, cefazolin, cephalothin, ceftazidime, gentamicin, norfloxacin, tetracycline, tobramycin, gatifloxacin, levofloxacin, moxifloxacin, and ciprofloxacin. Trimethoprim/sulfamethoxazole was reported with decreased MIC value (less than 2/38 μg/mL) as compared to control (Figure 1 and Table 2).

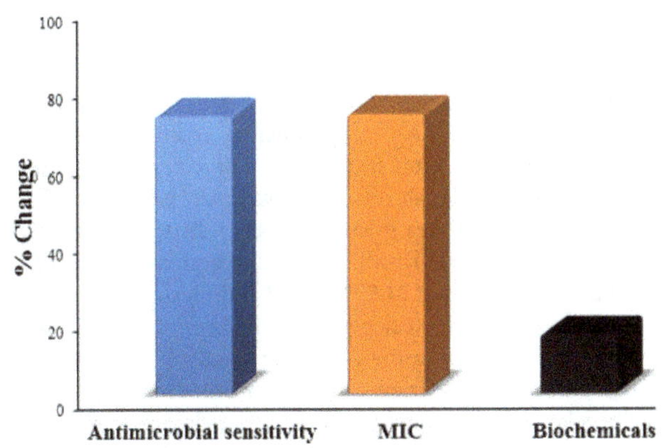

Figure 1: Percentage change in antimicrobial sensitivity pattern, minimum inhibitory concentration (MIC) values and biochemical reactions after biofield treatment of multidrug resistant strain of *Raoultella ornithinolytica.*

S. No.	Antimicrobial	Control (μg/mL)	Treated (μg/mL)
1	Amikacin	≤16	≤16
2	Amoxicillin/k-clavulanate	>16/8	≤8/4
3	Ampicillin/sulbactam	>16/8	≤8/4
4	Ampicillin	>16	>16
5	Aztreonam	>16	≤8
6	Cefazolin	>16	≤8
7	Cefepime	≤8	≤8
8	Cefotaxime	>32	≤8
9	Cefotetan	≤16	≤16
10	Cefoxitin	≤8	≤8
11	Ceftazidime	16	≤8
12	Ceftriaxone	>32	≤8
13	Cefuroxime	>16	≤4
14	Cephalothin	>16	≤8
15	Chloramphenicol	≤8	≤8
16	Ciprofloxacin	>2	≤1
17	ESBL-a Scrn	>4	≤4
18	ESBL-b Scrn	>1	≤1
19	Gatifloxacin	>4	≤2
20	Gentamicin	>8	≤4
21	Imipenem	≤4	≤4
22	Levofloxacin	>4	≤2
23	Meropenem	≤4	≤4
24	Moxifloxacin	>4	≤2
25	Nitrofurantoin	≤32	≤32
26	Norfloxacin	>8	≤4
27	Piperacillin	>64	≤16
28	Piperacillin/tazobactam	64	≤16
29	Tetracycline	>8	≤4
30	Ticarcillin/k-clavulanate	64	≤16
31	Tobramycin	>8	≤4
32	Trimethoprim/sulfamethoxazole	>2/38	≤2/38
ESBL-a, b Scrn: Extended-Spectrum β-Lactamase screen.			

Table 2: Minimum inhibitory concentration (MIC) of tested antimicrobials on *Raoultella ornithinolytica.*

Biochemical reaction

Table 3 summarizes the data related to biochemical reactions in control and biofield treated group. Results showed that, 15.15% tested biochemical reactions out of 33 were changed from positive (+) to negative (-) such as cetrimide, cephalothin, kanamycin, ornithine, and tobramycin after biofield treatment as compared with control (Figure 1).

S. No.	Code	Biochemical	Control	Treated
1	ACE	Acetamide	-	-
2	ADO	Adonitol	+	+
3	ARA	Arabinose	+	+
4	ARG	Arginine	-	-
5	CET	Cetrimide	+	-
6	CF8	Cephalothin	+	-
7	CIT	Citrate	+	+
8	CL4	Colistin	-	-
9	ESC	Esculin hydrolysis	+	+
10	FD64	Nitrofurantoin	-	-
11	GLU	Glucose	+	+
12	H2S	Hydrogen sulfide	-	-
13	IND	Indole	+	+
14	INO	Inositol	+	+
15	K4	Kanamycin	+	-
16	LYS	Lysine	+	+
17	MAL	Malonate	+	+
18	MEL	Melibiose	+	+
19	NIT	Nitrate	+	+
20	OF/G	Oxidation-Fermentation	+	+
21	ONPG	Galactosidase	+	+
22	ORN	Ornithine	+	-
23	OXI	Oxidase	-	-
24	P4	Penicillin	+	+
25	RAF	Raffinose	+	+
26	RHA	Rhaminose	+	+
27	SOR	Sorbitol	+	+
28	SUC	Sucrose	+	+
29	TAR	Tartrate	-	-
30	TDA	Tryptophan Deaminase	-	-
31	TO4	Tobramycin	+	-
32	URE	Urea	+	+
33	VP	Voges-Proskauer	+	+
- (negative); + (positive)				

Table 3: Effect of biofield treatment on *Raoultella ornithinolytica* to the vital process of microorganism.

Organism identification by biotype number

Based on the biochemical results, change in biotype number was observed in biofield treated group (7775 4370) at day 10 of *R. ornithinolytica* with respect to control (7775 5372). After alteration in biotype number the new organism was identified as *Klebsiella oxytoca* (Table 4).

Feature	Control	Treated
Biotype	77755372	77754370
Organism Identification	*Raoultella ornithinolytica*	*Klebsiella oxytoca*

Table 4: Effect of biofield treatment on *Raoultella ornithinolytica* to distinguishing feature of the genotype.

Discussion

MDR emergence of *R. ornithinolytica* is a global health problem commonly associated with bacteremia, urinary tract infection, neonatal infections, and exist in underlying existing infection [6,26,27]. Increasing resistance in microorganism for antimicrobials becomes a major threat to health and economic problem which ultimately leads to allowing survival of the resistant bacteria and death of the susceptible ones. Major mechanistic pathways associated with resistant in microorganism are cell membrane alterations, which lead to decreased uptake of drug [28]; mutation occurs, that lead to over expression of drug target enzymes and the other common mechanism being the drug efflux pump [29]. Now-a-days, *R. ornithinolytica* acquired resistance against broad range of antimicrobials. Research study suggests that most of the clinical isolates of *R. ornithinolytica* were found resistant to all class of antimicrobials such as ampicillin, amoxicillin, cephalothin, cephotaxime, chloramphenicol, penicillin, gentamicin, rifampin, and streptomycin. Nitrofurantoin and meropenam showed highest sensitivity for *R. ornithinolytica* in all the clinical samples [30]. Our experimental control sample (*R. ornithinolytica*) showed similar sensitivity and resistant pattern of tested antimicrobials. Overall results showed increase in antimicrobial sensitivity after biofield treatment in 71.4% tested antimicrobials as compared to control. Mr. Trivedi's biofield treatment has significantly decreased the MIC values of 71.87% tested antimicrobials as compared to control. As an enteric pathogen, *R. ornithinolytica* causes enteric fever associated with syndrome like fever, headache, and abdominal pain. Best treatment therapy during the infection starts with amoxicillin/clavulanic acid for 10-14 days, but therapy depends upon the sensitivity pattern of clinical strain [31]. Different class of antimicrobials showed significant effect after biofield treatment viz. β-Lactam penicillins (amoxicillin/clavulanic acid, ampicillin/sulbactam, and piperacillin), cephalosporins (cefazolin, ceftriaxone, and cefuroxime), monobactum (azetronan), fluoroquinolones (ciprofloxacin and levofloxacin), aminoglycosides (amikacin and tobramycin) and tetracycline. Lucchetti et al. studied the effect of energy therapy as an alternate medicine on growth of bacterial culture, and found a significant effect [32]. Similarly, experimental results showed improved antimicrobial sensitivity and reduced MIC values suggest that biofield treatment could be a new alternative treatment approach to inhibit the growth of pathogenic bacteria.

Several phenotypic biochemical identification tests were available to differentiate the *Raoultella* species. Identification test of *R. ornithinolytica* was performed using a series of biochemical reactions and the basic positive reactions were observed in case of urea, ornithine and lysine decarboxylase, citrate, glucose, and sucrose. It generally grown at 10°C with utilization of L-sorbose as a carbon source [33]. Experimental control group showed positive reaction in above general characteristic of *R. ornithinolytica*, but biofield treatment group showed a significant alteration i.e. negative reactions in biochemical such as cetrimide, cephalothin, kanamycin, ornithine and tobramycin. Further, these biochemical changes were studied by biotype number analysis which was performed using an automated system. A significant changed in biotype number was found in treated group on day 10, and new organism was identified as *Klebsiella oxytoca* after biofield treatment as compared to control *R. ornithinolytica* (Table 4). Biofield treatment on pathogenic microorganism had been reported, which alter the biochemical reactions, followed by change biotype number and identification of new microorganism after treatment. Current results are well supported with recent reported study [34].

Overall results of antimicrobial assay suggest that Mr. Trivedi's biofield treatment has significantly improved the sensitivity and MIC value of most of the tested antimicrobials (Figure 1). Therefore, it may be possible that lower dose of antimicrobials might require with similar response after biofield treatment, which may minimize the side effects associated with higher doses of antimicrobials. Mr. Trivedi has the ability to harness energy from environment and altered the significant changes in microorganisms [15,16]. Biofield treatment might be responsible to do alteration in microorganism at genetic level and/or enzymatic level, which may act on receptor protein. While altering receptor protein, ligand-receptor/protein interactions may alter that could lead to show different phenotypic characteristics. Biofield treatment might induce significant changes in MDR strain of *R. ornithinolytica*, so that tested antimicrobials were showed better susceptibility pattern, decreased MIC values, and altered biochemical reactions, against this microorganism.

Conclusion

Present study concludes that biofield treatment has the ability to inhibit the microbial growth, by significantly increasing the susceptibility pattern and decreasing the MIC values of 71% tested antimicrobials. Biofield treatment has significantly altered the biochemical reactions and biotype number of MDR strain of *R. ornithinolytica*. On the basis of changed biotype number after biofield treatment, new organism was identified as *Klebsiella oxytoca*. It is assumed that biofield treatment could be applied in biomedical health care system in future to improve the antimicrobial potency that enhance human well-being.

Acknowledgement

Authors gratefully acknowledged the whole team of PD Hinduja National Hospital and MRC, Mumbai, Microbiology Lab for their support.The generous support of Trivedi Science™, Trivedi Master Wellness™ and Trivedi Testimonials is gratefully acknowledged.

References

1. Drancourt M, Bollet C, Carta A, Rousselier P (2001) Phylogenetic analyses of Klebsiella species delineate Klebsiella and Raoultellagen. nov., with description of Raoultella ornithinolytica comb. nov., Raoultella terrigena comb. nov. and Raoultella planticola comb. nov. Int J Syst Evol Microbiol 51: 925-932.
2. Kanki M, Yoda T, Tsukamoto T, Shibata T (2002) Klebsiella pneumoniae produces no histamine: Raoultella planticola and Raoultella ornithinolytica strains are histamine producers. Appl Environ Microbiol 68: 3462-3466.
3. Shaikh MM, Morgan M (2011) Sepsis caused by Raoultella terrigena. JRSM Short Rep 2: 49.
4. Chun S, Yun JW, Huh HJ, Lee NY (2014) Low virulence? Clinical characteristics of Raoultella planticola bacteremia. Infection 42: 899-904.
5. Hadano Y, Tsukahara M, Ito K, Suzuki J, Kawamura I, et al. (2012) Raoultella ornithinolytica bacteremia in cancer patients: Report of three cases. Intern Med 51: 3193-3195.
6. Haruki Y, Hagiya H, Sakuma A, Murase T, Sugiyama T, et al. (2014) Clinical characteristics of Raoultella ornithinolytica bacteremia: A case series and literature review. J Infect Chemother 20: 589-591.
7. Chun S, Yun JW, Huh HJ, Lee NY (2015) Clinical characteristics of Raoultella ornithinolytica bacteremia. Infection 43: 59-64.
8. Tseng SP, Wang JT, Liang CY, Lee PS, Chen YC, et al. (2014) First report of bla(IMP-8) in Raoultella planticola. Antimicrob Agents Chemother 58: 593-595.
9. Cunha BA (2001) Antibiotic side effects. Med Clin North Am 85: 149-185.
10. Rubik B (1994) Manual healing methods. Alternative medicine: expanding medical horizons, Washington, DC, US Government Printing Office, NIH Publication No. 094-066.
11. Thomas AH (2012) Hidden in plain sight: The simple link between relativity and quantum mechanics. Swansea, UK: CreateSpace Independent Publishing Platform.
12. Dale C (2009) The subtle body: An encyclopedia of your energetic anatomy. Boulder, CO: Sounds True, Inc.
13. Movaffaghi Z, Farsi M (2009) Biofield therapies: Biophysical basis and biological regulations. Complement Ther Clin Pract 15: 35-37.
14. Trivedi MK, Bhardwaj Y, Patil S, Shettigar H, Bulbule, A (2009) Impact of an external energy on Enterococcus faecalis [ATCC-51299] in relation to antibiotic susceptibility and biochemical reactions-an experimental study. J Accord Integr Med 5: 119-130.
15. Trivedi MK, Patil S (2008) Impact of an external energy on Staphylococcus epidermis [ATCC-13518] in relation to antibiotic susceptibility and biochemical reactions-an experimental study. J Accord Integr Med 4: 230-235.
16. Trivedi MK, Patil S (2008) Impact of an external energy on Yersinia enterocolitica [ATCC-23715] in relation to antibiotic susceptibility and biochemical reactions: An experimental study. Internet J Alternat Med 6.
17. Shinde V, Sances F, Patil S, Spence A (2012) Impact of biofield treatment on growth and yield of lettuce and tomato. Aust J Basis Appl Sci 6: 100-105.
18. Sances F, Flora E, Patil S, Spence A, Shinde V (2013) Impact of biofield treatment on ginseng and organic blueberry yield. Agrivita J Agric Sci 35: 22-29.
19. Lenssen AW (2013) Biofield and fungicide seed treatment influences on soybean productivity, seed quality and weed community. Agricultural Journal 8: 138-143.
20. Altekar N, Nayak G (2015) Effect of biofield treatment on plant growth and adaptation. J Environ Health Sci 1: 1-9.
21. Patil SA, Nayak GB, Barve SS, Tembe RP, Khan RR (2012) Impact of biofield treatment on growth and anatomical characteristics of Pogostemon cablin (Benth.). Biotechnology 11: 154-162.
22. Trivedi MK, Tallapragada RR (2008) A transcendental to changing metal powder characteristics. Met Powder Rep 63: 22-28.
23. Dabhade VV, Tallapragada RR, Trivedi MK (2009) Effect of external energy on atomic, crystalline and powder characteristics of antimony and bismuth powders. Bull Mater Sci 32: 471-479.
24. Trivedi MK, Tallapragada RR (2009) Effect of superconsciousness external energy on atomic, crystalline and powder characteristics of carbon allotrope powders. Mater Res Innovations 13: 473-480.

25. Fader RC, Weaver E, Fossett R, Toyras M, Vanderlaan J, et al. (2013) Multilaboratory study of the biomic automated well-reading instrument versus MicroScan WalkAway for reading MicroScan antimicrobial Susceptibility and identification panels. J Clin Microbiol 51: 1548-1554.
26. Mau N, Ross LA (2010) Raoultella ornithinolytica bacteremia in an infant with visceral heterotaxy. Pediatr Infect Dis J 29: 477-478.
27. Garcia-Lozano T, Pascual Pla FJ, Aznar Oroval E (2013) Raoultella ornithinolytica in urinary tract infections. Clinical and microbiological study of a series of 4 oncologic patients. Med Clin (Barc) 141: 138-139.
28. Tenover FC (2006) Mechanisms of antimicrobial resistance in bacteria. Am J Infect Control 119: S3-S10.
29. Alekshun MN, Levy SB (2007) Molecular mechanisms of antibacterial multidrug resistance. Cell 128: 1037-1050.
30. Al-Hulu SM, Al-Charrakh AH, Al-Saadi MAK (2009) Isolation and characterization of Raoultella ornithinolytica from clinical specimens in hilla city. Iraq Med J Babylon 7: 42-47.
31. Morais VP, Daporta MT, Bao AF, Campello MG (2009) Enteric fever-like syndrome caused by Raoultella ornithinolytica (Klebsiella ornithinolytica). J Clin Microbiol 47: 868-869.
32. Lucchetti G, de Oliveira RF, Goncalves JP, Ueda SM, Mimica LM, et al. (2013) Effect of Spiritist "passe" (Spiritual healing) on growth of bacterial cultures. Complement Ther Med 21: 627-632.
33. Hansen DS, Aucken HM, Abiola T, Podschun R (2004) Recommended test panel for differentiation of Klebsiella species on the basis of a trilateral interlaboratory evaluation of 18 biochemical tests. J Clin Microbiol 42: 3665-3669.
34. Trivedi MK, Patil S, Shettigar H, Gangwar M, Jana S (2015) Antimicrobial sensitivity pattern of Pseudomonas fluorescens after biofield treatment. J Infect Dis Ther 3: 222.

7

The Effects of Acupuncture on Insomnia, Anxiety, and Depression in Women with Chronic Liver Disease

Seung-Mo Kim[1], **Min-Ah Kwak**[1], **Ae Ryun Choi**[2], **Im Hee Shin**[3], **Byung Seok Kim**[4] **and Chang Hyeong Lee**[4*]

[1]*Department of Internal Medicine, College of Korean Medicine, Daegu Haany University, Daegu, Korea*

[2]*Department of Sasang Constitutional Medicine, College of Korean Medicine, Daegu Haany University, Daegu, Korea*

[3]*Department of Medical Statistics, School of Medicine, Catholic University of Daegu, Daegu, Korea*

[4]*Department of Internal Medicine, School of Medicine, Catholic University of Daegu, Daegu, Korea*

[*]**Corresponding author:** Chang Hyeong Lee, Department of Internal Medicine, School of Medicine, Catholic University of Daegu, 3056-6 Daemyeong 4-dong, Nam-gu, Daegu 705-718, Korea, E-mail: chlee1@cu.ac.kr.

Abstract

Objective: To evaluate the feasibility and effects of acupuncture on insomnia, anxiety, and depression in women with Chronic Liver Disease.

Patients and Methods: Twenty-four women patients over the age of 18 years who had liver disease complicated by psychiatric disorders such as insomnia, anxiety, and depression were randomly assigned to either the treatment group (n=12) or the control group (n=12). In the treatment group, acupuncture was performed 3 times per week for 4 weeks (12 sessions in total). In control group, there was no acupuncture but the same assessment with treatment group. Insomnia, anxiety, and depression were measured using the National Cancer Center (NCC) scoring system. We assessed deterioration of liver disease using the Child score and blood tests.

Results: In the treatment group, the mean NCC insomnia, anxiety, and depression scores decreased significantly over the treatment period; control group scores did not decrease significantly. After 12 acupuncture treatments, the total NCC score for insomnia, anxiety, and depression was significantly lower in the treatment group compared with that of the control group. After the trial, liver function of neither group got worse.

Conclusions: These results suggest that acupuncture treatment may be beneficial in improving insomnia, anxiety, and depression among patients with chronic liver disease without worsening of liver function. Further study with a larger sample size including male participants is needed to confirm our findings.

Keywords: Acupuncture; Insomnia; Anxiety; Depression; Chronic liver disease

Introduction

Liver cirrhosis associated with chronic hepatitis [1-4]. and hepatocellular carcinoma (HCC) [5] has been reported to cause psychiatric problems. Chronic liver disease is associated with impaired health-related quality of life (HRQOL), depression, anxiety, and other psychological impairments [6,7]. In cases where these chronic conditions stigmatize the patient, psychological impairment becomes more pronounced. Moreover, complications of advanced liver disease may be associated with poorer HRQOL irrespective of the cause of the liver involvement. These psychiatric disorders have been attributed to the production of toxic metabolites that damage the brain, resulting in neurological and psychological problems [8].

In general, doctors should avoid prescribing long-term use of drugs for the treatment of psychiatric disorders, as it could further deteriorate liver function in patients with liver disease [8]. For instance, antidepressant drugs have been reported to be associated with several adverse drug reactions including hepatotoxicity [9]. Nevertheless, long-term use of anti-anxiety and anti-depressant drugs may be necessary, which paradoxically may exacerbate the condition [10].

Some studies suggested that acupuncture had the potential to treat psychological disorders including anxiety, insomnia, and depression [11-14]. Despite the large number of studies on this subject, few addressed the use of acupuncture to treat psychiatric problems associated with chronic liver disease. A few articles reported that acupuncture alleviated depression related to chronic hepatitis or otherwise impaired liver function. One observational study showed the improvement of depression after acupuncture in 28 patients with chronic hepatitis [7,15,16]. There were acupuncture studies with negative turnover of hepatitis B virus versus control group via examination of physiological parameters [14,15].

In our previous pilot study, acupuncture resulted in significant improvements in insomnia, anxiety, and depression in HCC patients with liver cirrhosis. Moreover, there was no worsening signs of liver function after treatment and adverse events did not occur during the trial [17].

This randomized controlled trial was parallel design and allocation ratio was 50%. This study aimed to reconfirm previous findings and establish the clinical effects of acupuncture for the alleviation of insomnia, anxiety, and depression in patients with chronic liver disease such as HCC, liver cirrhosis, and chronic hepatitis. For the evaluation of acupuncture safety, we also examined the changes of blood composition of patients.

Materials and Methods

Ethics statement

This trial was approved by the Institutional Review Board of Daegu Catholic University Hospital, and was conducted in accordance with the provisions of Declaration of Helsinki (1989) and Good Clinical Practice (GCP). It was registered on Clinical Research Information Service (KCT0001411) retrospectively. The reason for non-registration before participants recruitment was that this regulation for registration had not been strongly recommended in 2012.

Participant recruitment

Twenty-four participants were enrolled in the clinical trial between September 7, 2012 and March 16, 2013. Participants were informed of the purpose, method, anticipated adverse dangers and discomforts, disclosure of personal information, compensation, and right to discontinue the clinical trial. All patients signed an agreement to participate at one's own will. This study was approved by the Institutional Review Board of Daegu Catholic University Hospital. Participants were recruited via a recruitment notice on the web site or a poster. The required sample size was estimated to be a total 24 participants, considering a drop-out rate of 20%.

Inclusion and exclusion criteria

The subjects were female patients, over 18 years of age, diagnosed with chronic liver disease such as HCC, liver cirrhosis, and chronic hepatitis. In addition, inclusion criteria were complaints of distress with a National Cancer Center (NCC) psychological symptoms score higher than 4 points in both severity and inconvenience in one at least one of the following: anxiety, depression, or insomnia.

Other inclusion criteria included, a Child-Pugh score, a scoring system used to assess the severity and prognosis of chronic liver disease and cirrhosis, lower than 9 in classification either A or B, serum bilirubin level of 5 mg/dL or lower, aspartate aminotransferase (AST) and alanine aminotransferase (ALT) values of 100 IU/L or lower, serum creatinine value of 1.5 mg/dL or lower, and an INR) of 2.0 or lower.

The subjects underwent a washout period 3 days before the trial, in which the administration of tranquilizers and antidepressants was limited. The subjects were required to be monitored during the trial and to follow the restriction standards of the trial.

The exclusion criteria included severe neutropenia (absolute neutrophil level of 500/uL or lower), platelet count less than 50,000/uL, fever, aggravation of liver function, abdominal aneurysm, sepsis, and thrombosis. Pregnant women (positive human chorionic gonadotropin) and subjects judged by investigators to have difficulty continuing the trial were also excluded.

Intervention

In treatment group, a total of 12 sessions of acupuncture was performed, 3 sessions per week for 4 weeks. Acupuncture points, Neiguan (PC6), Gongsun (SP4), Shenmen (HT7), Yintang (EX-HN3), Hegu (LI4), Taichong (LR3) and Baihui (GV20) were applied in the treatment group to a total of 9 acupuncture points including bilateral LI4 and LR3. Stainless steel needles (0.20 × 30 mm; Dongbang acupuncture, Korea) were used and retained for 25 minutes after insertion. Acupuncture was performed by a traditional Korean medicine (TKM) physician who was registered and had at least 3 years of clinical experience. Acupuncture was manually performed with a sensation of de qi. In Control group, no acupuncture or placebo was conducted, but the same assessment with treatment group was performed.

Outcome measurements

The effects of acupuncture were assessed using the NCC scoring system for psychological symptoms. The NCC scoring system questionnaire consists of 2 questions each for the 3 symptoms of insomnia, anxiety, and depression. Question 1 inquired about the severity of the symptom, and Question 2 inquired about the inconvenience caused by one of the symptoms. Each question included a scale of 0 [none] to 10 [extremely severe], a higher score meaning greater severity and inconvenience [18].

Measurement taken at 3 points over 4 weeks included baseline, midtreatment (2weeks after initiation), and end of treatment (4 weeks after initiation). Patients were assessed through physical examination (body temperature, blood pressure, pulse, body weight), Child-Pugh score and laboratory examination, and NCC psychological symptoms scores.

Safety evaluation

To evaluate the safety of acupuncture, the body temperature, blood pressure, pulse, and body weight of the participant were assessed at each visit. Child-Pugh scores and biochemistry tests (AST, ALT, BUN, Creatinine, T-bilirubin, Albumin, prothrombin time (PT)) were performed at 0, 2, and 4 weeks for patients in the treatment and control groups. Adverse events were examined by the investigator at each visit.

To check for aggravation of liver cirrhosis, patients were evaluated for hepatic coma, hepatorenal syndrome, hemorrhage from rupture of esophageal and gastric varices, infection/sepsis, spontaneous peritonitis, and liver function failure. For patients with aggravated liver cirrhosis, the investigator decided whether to discontinue the trial and hospitalization.

Compliance was calculated from the attendance rate of more than 80%, and any participant absent for 5 consecutive appointments was regarded as a drop-out. Participants were told to immediately report any adverse events between visits. Any abnormal condition following acupuncture was to be investigated in relation to the clinical trial and followed up.

Sample size determination

Sample size was determined based on a preliminary study [17] where the difference value of NCC total score average of patients between acupuncture group and control group with mean was 9.630 and standard deviation was 7.518 is considered to be of clinical relevance. To detect this difference, we need a sample size of 10 in each group (α=0.05, β=0.20). To allow 20% for drop to follow up, our proposed trial requires 24 patients (12 for each group).

Statistical analysis

The data was analyzed using intention-to-treat approaches. Statistical analyses were carried out using the program PASW (new version of SPSS Win Ver.) 19.0. Two sample t-test and chi-square test were used to compare between treatment and control group for baseline characteristics. Repeated measure 2-factor analysis was used to analyze change of total NCC scores according to time and group and contrast was used to analyze the multiple comparison result. At last, the result was regarded as statistically significance when p-value less than 0.05.

Results

Baseline characteristics

Of the 24 women outpatients were screened and randomly assigned to the acupuncture (n=12) and control groups (n=12). There was no difference in baseline characteristics between treatment and control group except for number of cirrhotic patients (Table 1). Twenty-one patients completed the trial with drop-outs of 3 patients (Figure 1).

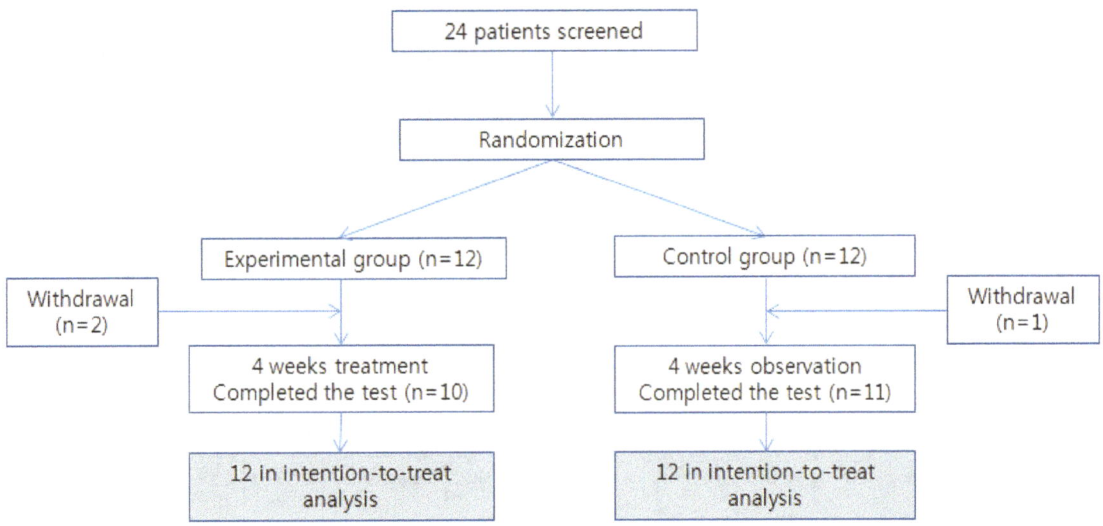

Figure 1: Study flow chart.

	Treatment group (n=12)	Control group (n=12)	P-value
Age (years)[a]	57.7 ± 10.1	61.6 ± 8.2	0.310[b]
Body weight (kg)[a]	58.3 ± 8.9	58.4 ± 8.2	0.962[b]
Height (cm)[a]	156.7 ± 4.7	154.9 ± 4.9	0.386[b]
Liver cirrhosis/chronic hepatitis, n (%)	12/0	6/6	0.014[c]
HCC, n (%)	1 (8.3)	1 (8.3)	1.000[c]
Ascites, n (%)	1 (8.3)	2 (16.7)	1.000[c]
NCC score			
Insomnia severity NCC 1-1[a]	6.8 ± 1.3	7.0 ± 1.4	0.655[b]
Insomnia inconvenience NCC 1-2[a]	6.8 ± 1.6	5.7 ± 2.1	0.139[b]
Anxiety severity NCC 2-1[a]	6.1 ± 2.6	5.1 ± 2.2	0.317[b]
Anxiety inconvenience NCC 2-2[a]	5.6 ± 2.6	4.5 ± 3.0	0.347[b]
Depression severity NCC 3-1[a]	6.6 ± 2.7	4.9 ± 2.6	0.144[b]

Depression inconvenience NCC 3-3[a]	6.0 ± 2.8	4.2 ± 3.0	0.138[b]
There was no difference in baseline characteristics between treatment and control group except for number of cirrhotic patients.			
[a]mean ± standard deviation ;[b]P-values are calculated by two sample t-test.			
[c]P-values are calculated by Chi-square test.			

Table 1: Comparison of baseline characteristics between treatment and control group.

Effects

NCC scores were evaluated at 3 time points (baseline, middle, and end of treatment; 0, 2 and 4 weeks, respectively). In treatment group, intragroup analysis revealed that the NCC scores for insomnia, anxiety, and depression all decreased significantly after 4 weeks of treatment (Figure 2).

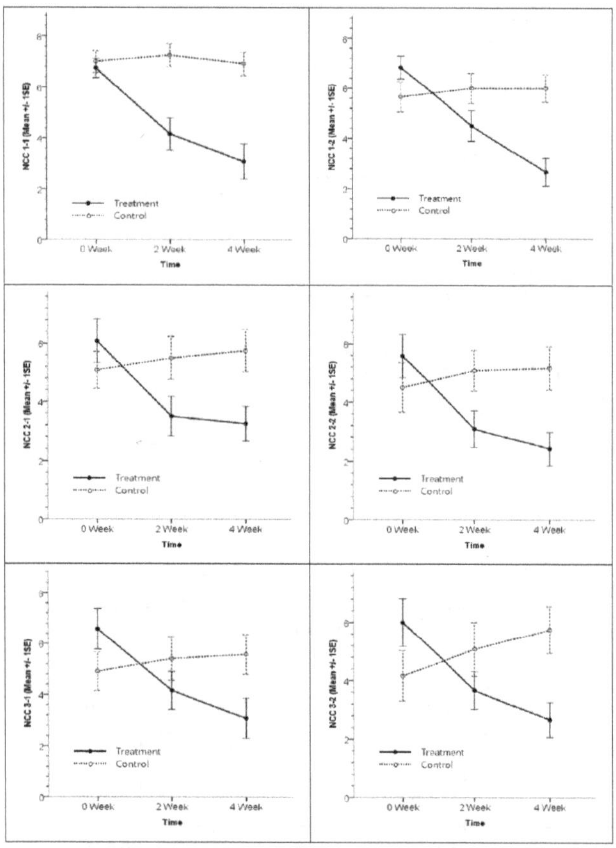

Figure 2: Change of NCC score mean value between treatment group and control group.

In treatment group, NCC scores for insomnia severity (NCC 1-1: 6.8 ± 1.3, 4.2 ± 2.2, 3.1 ± 2.4) and insomnia inconvenience (NCC 1-2: 6.8 ± 1.6, 4.5 ± 2.1, 2.7 ± 1.9) at 0, 2, and 4 weeks, respectively, decreased significantly (both, $p<0.001$). Anxiety severity scores (NCC 2-1: 6.1 ± 2.6, 3.5 ± 2.4, 3.3 ± 2.0) and anxiety inconvenience scores (NCC 2-2: 5.6 ± 2.6, 3.0 ± 2.2, 2.4 ± 1.9) at 0, 2, and 4 weeks, respectively, also decreased; these differences were significant (both, $p<0.05$). Similarly, Severity for depression (NCC 3-1) also showed a significant decrease, with 6.6 ± 2.8, 4.2 ± 2.6, 3.1 ± 2.7 ($p=0.01$). On the other hand, there were no significant changes in inconvenience of depression (NCC 3-3).

The total NCC score was calculated to evaluate the effect of acupuncture on overall psychological distress. The mean NCC score in the treatment group significantly decreased, with changes of 37.9 ± 11.9, 23.1 ± 12.4, and 17.2 ± 11.9 at 0, 2, and 4 weeks, respectively ($p<0.01$). After the last acupuncture treatment, the total NCC scores decreased 45.4%, while that of the control group tended to increase. The total NCC score of the treatment group decreased significantly compared that of the control group ($p<0.01$) (Table 2).

		Week 0	Week 2	Week 4	P-value	
Total NCC Score (Median ± SD)	Treatment	37.9 ± 11.9	23.1 ± 12.4	17.2 ± 11.9	17.070 (0.000)* 1>2>3†	20.687 (0.000)* 1>2>3†
	Control	31.3 ± 12.4	34.3 ± 13.6	35.2 ± 12.6	3.678 (0.042)* 1<2,3†	
NCC Score, National Cancer Center score						
*Statistically significant with p<0.05; †Multiple comparison result by contrast						

Table 2: Change of total NCC score mean value.

Safety

To evaluate the safety of acupuncture, we performed liver function tests. There were no significant differences in AST, ALT, BUN, Creatinine, T-bilirubin, Albumin, or PT (Table 3) between the treatment and control groups. Furthermore, aggravation of liver cirrhosis and primary complications (hepatic encephalopathy, hepato-renal syndrome) were not observed in either group. All patients showed good compliance. Adverse events were assessed every visit during the course of the trial, and no adverse event was observed in the course of study in any of the 21 patients.

Variables	Group	Week 0	Week 2	Week 4
AST	Treatment	47.5 ± 18.8	52.4 ± 30.4	45.4 ± 21.1
	Control	38.3 ± 16.4	36.8 ± 20.6	40.1 ± 23.0

ALT	Treatment	17.9 ± 4.3	19.7 ± 5.9	19.3 ± 7.0
	Control	30.1 ± 9.8	24.2 ± 5.1	27.8 ± 4.5
BUN	Treatment	13.0 ± 4.8	12.9 ± 3.3	12.9 ± 3.9
	Control	14.7 ± 3.9	13.4 ± 2.9	13.9 ± 3.9
Creatinine	Treatment	0.68 ± 0.1	0.67 ± 0.07	0.67 ± 0.08
	Control	0.68 ± 0.1	0.68 ± 0.12	0.7 ± 0.12
T-bilirubin	Treatment	1.32 ± 1.26	1.38 ± 1.44	1.34 ± 1.26
	Control	0.81 ± 0.46	0.81 ± 0.42	0.75 ± 0.39
Albumin	Treatment	3.95 ± 0.42	3.93 ± 0.39	3.98 ± 0.37
	Control	4.2 ± 0.32	4.05 ± 0.27	4.15 ± 0.29
PT	Treatment	14.6 ± 1.2	14.3 ± 1.2	14.3 ± 1.3
	Control	13.5 ± 0.8	12.6 ± 3.8	13.5 ± 1.0

AST, aspartate aminotransferase; ALT, alanine aminotransferase; BUN, blood urea nitrogen; PT, prothrombin time.
mean ± standard deviation

Table 3: Mean change of blood composition.

Discussion

This randomized, controlled trial investigated the effect of acupuncture on psychiatric problems related with chronic liver disease. Twenty-four patients had undergone chronic liver disease including HCC, liver cirrhosis and chronic hepatitis. Two patients in treatment group and one in control group were drop-out because of private reasons without any adverse events. Twenty-one patients completed the trial. Considering significant change of NCC score of insomnia, anxiety and depression, acupuncture might give positive effect on psychiatric symptoms associated with chronic liver disease. These findings concur with our previous pilot study.

The acupuncture points used in this study were selected based on previous studies. Liver disease can lead to the stagnation of liver qi, inducing emotional imbalance. Based on this pathogenesis, we chose LI4 and LR3 named 'four gates' points those were determined to regulate flow of the liver qi. In addition, we selected PC6, SP4, HT7 for regulating the overall flow of qi in the body based on those used in several studies [19-23] and GV20, EX-HN1 were added from the extra-meridian points for calming and relaxing effects [17]. The acupuncture treatment was administered 3 times a week for 4 weeks 12 sessions. Single-sided PC6, SP4, HT7, GV20, EX-HN1 and both sided LI4, LR3 total nine acupuncture points were used.

The BDI and Hamilton depression scales have been used as indices for depression, anxiety, and insomnia in clinical trials [24,25]. We used the NCC index to evaluate anxiety, depression, and insomnia. This index was developed by psycho-oncology experts in Korea using standard diagnostic principles of psychological distress and information from literature reviews. NCC includes self-reporting questionnaires to document the severity of insomnia, depression, anxiety, or limitations of daily life. Although this tool was developed to assess distress in cancer patients, it met our assessment needs, focusing on the alleviation of symptoms rather than the eradication of liver disease. At baseline, all patients recorded NCC scores greater than 4 points, which indicates the need for the aid of mental health professionals. After 2 weeks, NCC scores in the treatment group were less than 4 points, while the control group showed no improvement in psychiatric symptoms.

Except the inconvenience of depression (NCC 3-2), each NCC scores for mental stress decreased significantly compared with those of control group. There were no evident adverse events, such as subcutaneous bleeding, following acupuncture. Four weeks of acupuncture treatment improved the symptoms of insomnia, anxiety, and depression compared with that of control group, furthermore, there was no side effect such as aggravation of liver function and complications associated with liver disease.

Several studies have shown benefits of acupuncture including improvements of emotional and physical well-being in depressive disorders [26-28]. However, patients with chronic liver disease also suffer from accompanied psychiatric disorders such as anxiety, insomnia, depression et al. Unlike other disease, use of medication to treat symptoms of anxiety, depression and insomnia in patients with chronic liver disease is restricted for fear that it should progress liver dysfunction. Therefore a treatment to improve anxiety, depression and insomnia without aggravating liver disease is in much need. Acupuncture may be a safe and effective treatment for psychiatric distress of liver disease.

One study showed more improvement of irritable bowel syndrome when permitted to have a relationship with the practitioner [25]. We attempted to minimize interaction with patients, since acupuncture treatment could foster a relationship between patients and practitioners, consequently result in a placebo effect [29-31]. Therefore, we restricted talks with patients except for advice agreed upon before treatment.

The present study had several limitations. First, the study consists of small sample size and was conducted only for female patients. Second, the design of the study is not optimal. In control group, there was only observation without any sham treatment. Third, the measurement tool of psychiatric disorders was not widely known worldwide.

In spite of these limitations, this is the first study to show the feasibility and safety of acupuncture for the treatment of psychiatric disorders accompanied with chronic liver disease. The results of this study showed a mean reduction of 45.4% in total NCC scores in treatment group, whereas no reduction in control group. This study's result can provide preliminary data indicating that acupuncture can be a good alternative treatment for insomnia, anxiety, and depression accompanied with chronic liver disease patients.

Further retrospective clinical trials using a larger patient cohort will be needed to verify the effects and safety of acupuncture for insomnia, anxiety, and depression associated with liver disease. Also, research using sham control group may be warranted to investigate the effects of acupuncture.

Conclusion

In this study, we administered acupuncture to patients with liver cirrhosis, chronic hepatitis, and HCC, conditions that contraindicate the use of medications for anxiety, depression, and insomnia. We observed that acupuncture improved symptoms of insomnia, anxiety, and depression in patients with liver disease. Furthermore, we encountered no complications of acupuncture treatment or aggravation of liver cirrhosis, HCC, or impaired liver function.

Footnotes

Acknowledgements: This study was supported by a grant from the Ministry of Health and Welfare, Republic of Korea, 2012. (Project No: 090-091-3000-3033-320)

Author Disclosure Statement: No competing financial interests exist.

Provenance and peer review: Not commissioned; externally peer reviewed.

References

1. Modabbernia A, Ashrafi M, Malekzadeh R, Poustchi H (2013) A review of psychosocial issues in patients with chronic hepatitis B. Arch Iran Med 16: 114-122.
2. Orrù MG, Pariante CM (2005) Depression and liver diseases. Dig Liver Dis 37: 564-565.
3. Bianchi G, Marchesini G, Nicolino F, Graziani R, Sgarbi D, et al. (2005) Psychological status and depression in patients with liver cirrhosis. Dig Liver Dis 37: 593-600.
4. Forton DM, Thomas HC, Murphy CA, Allsop JM, Foster GR, et al. (2002) Hepatitis C and cognitive impairment in a cohort of patients with mild liver disease. Hepatology 35: 433-439.
5. Palmieri VO, Santovito D, Margari F, Lozupone M, Minerva F, et al. (2015) Psychopathological profile and health-related quality of life (HRQOL) in patients with hepatocellular carcinoma (HCC) and cirrhosis. Clin Exp Med 15: 65-72.
6. Lee K, Otgonsuren M, Younoszai Z, Mir HM, Younossi ZM (2013) Association of chronic liver disease with depression: a population-based study. Psychosomatics 54: 52-59.
7. Tufan ZK, Arslan H, Yildiz F, Bulut C, Irmak H, et al. (2010) Acupuncture for depression and myalgia in patients with hepatitis: an observational study. Acupunct Med 28: 136-139.
8. Grant BF, Stinson FS, Dawson DA, Chou SP, Dufour MC, et al. (2004) Prevalence and co-occurrence of substance use disorders and independent mood and anxiety disorders: results from the National Epidemiologic Survey on Alcohol and Related Conditions. Arch Gen Psychiatry 61: 807-816.
9. Lucena MI, Carvajal A, Andrade RJ, Velasco A (2003) Antidepressant-induced hepatotoxicity. Expert Opin Drug Saf 2: 249-262.
10. Ananth J, Swartz R, Burgoyne K, Gadasally R (1994) Hepatic disease and psychiatric illness: relationships and treatment. Psychother Psychosom 62: 146-159.
11. Wu J, Yeung AS, Schnyer R, Wang Y, Mischoulon D (2012) Acupuncture for depression: a review of clinical applications. Can J Psychiatry 57: 397-405.
12. van der Watt G, Laugharne J, Janca A (2008) Complementary and alternative medicine in the treatment of anxiety and depression. Curr Opin Psychiatry 21: 37-42.
13. Kalavapalli R, Singareddy R (2007) Role of acupuncture in the treatment of insomnia: a comprehensive review. Complement Ther Clin Pract 13: 184-193.
14. Spence DW, Kayumov L, Chen A, Lowe A, Jain U, et al. (2004) Acupuncture increases nocturnal melatonin secretion and reduces insomnia and anxiety: a preliminary report. J Neuropsychiatry Clin Neurosci 16: 19-28.
15. Chen J, Chen M, Zhao B, Wang Y (1999) Effects of acupuncture on the immunological functions in hepatitis B virus carriers. J Tradit Chin Med 19: 268-272.
16. Qiu W, Chang J, Shen SE, Shi B, Pan X (2007) Clinical observation on electroacupuncture treatment of 30 cases of chronic hepatitis B. J Tradit Chin Med 27: 108-110.
17. CH Lee, BS Kim, JS Kim (2012) The Effects of Acupuncture on the Insomnia, Anxiety and Depression of Liver Cancer patients: Pilot study. J Kor Orient Med 33:34-46.
18. National Cancer Center (2009) Development of recommendations for distress management toward improvement of quality of life in cancer patients. Seoul: The Ministry of Health-Welfare 5-13, 44-105.
19. Duan DM, Tu Y, Chen LP, Wu ZJ (2009) Efficacy evaluation for depression with somatic symptoms treated by electroacupuncture combined with Fluoxetine. J Tradit Chin Med 29: 167-173.
20. Fu WB, Fan L, Zhu XP, He Q, Wang L, et al. (2009) Depressive neurosis treated by acupuncture for regulating the liver--a report of 176 cases. J Tradit Chin Med 29: 83-86.
21. Liu LY, Lu Q, Wang LL (2009) Influence of electro-acupuncture on the side effects of fluoxetine on depression patients. J Tradit Chin Med 29: 271-274.
22. Song Y, Zhou D, Fan J, Luo H, Halbreich U (2007) Effects of electroacupuncture and fluoxetine on the density of GTP-binding-proteins in platelet membrane in patients with major depressive disorder. J Affect Disord 98: 253-257.
23. Zhang ZJ, Chen HY, Yip KC, Ng R, Wong VT (2010) The effectiveness and safety of acupuncture therapy in depressive disorders: systematic review and meta-analysis. J Affect Disord 124: 9-21.
24. Jay CL, Butt Z, Ladner DP, Skaro AI, Abecassis MM (2009) A review of quality of life instruments used in liver transplantation. J Hepatol 51: 949-959.
25. Younossi Z, Kallman J, Kincaid J (2007) The effects of HCV infection and management on health-related quality of life. Hepatology 45: 806-816.

26. Luo WZ, Zhang QZ, Lai XS (2010) [Effect of acupuncture treatment of relieving depression and regulating mind on insomnia accompanied with depressive disorders]. Zhongguo Zhen Jiu 30: 899-903.

27. Wang XY, Li XY, Deng AJ, Bo ZY (2010) [Comparative study on abdominal acupuncture and western medicine for treatment of menopause depressive disorder]. Zhongguo Zhen Jiu 30: 913-917.

28. He Q, Zhang J, Tang Y (2007) A controlled study on treatment of mental depression by acupuncture plus TCM medication. J Tradit Chin Med 27: 166-169.

29. Kaptchuk TJ, Kelley JM, Conboy LA, Davis RB, Kerr CE, et al. (2008) Components of placebo effect: randomised controlled trial in patients with irritable bowel syndrome. BMJ 336: 999-1003.

30. Garcia MK, McQuade J, Haddad R, Patel S, Lee R, et al. (2013) Systematic review of acupuncture in cancer care: a synthesis of the evidence. J Clin Oncol 31: 952-960.

31. Streitberger K, Kleinhenz J (1998) Introducing a placebo needle into acupuncture research. Lancet 352: 364-365.

8

Herbal Medicine: Yesterday, Today and Tomorrow

Paul C. Chikezie[1*] **and Okey A. Ojiako**[2]

[1]*Department of Biochemistry, Imo State University, Owerri, Nigeria*

[2]*Department of Biochemistry, Federal University of Technology, Owerri, Nigeria*

[*]**Corresponding author:** Chikezie PC, Department of Biochemistry, Imo State University, Owerri, Nigeria, E-mail: p_chikezie@yahoo.com

Abstract

Herbal medicines involve the integration of several therapeutic experiences and practices of indigenous systems of medicine that may span many previous generations, which often provides valuable guidelines to the selection, preparation and application of herbal formulation for the treatment, control and management of variety of ailments. According to World Health Organization, 60% of the world's population depends on traditional medicine and 80% of the population in developing countries depends almost entirely on traditional medicine practices and herbal medicines for their primary health care needs. As a result of increasing demand for herbal medicines, there are increasing concerns about the safety, standardization, efficacy, quality, availability and preservation of herbal products by policy-makers, health professionals as well as the general public. Improvement in the quality of herbal medicines could be achieved by deliberate implementation of good agricultural practices (GAPs) at the point of cultivation of medicinal plants and good manufacturing practices (GMPs) during the process of manufacture and packaging of finished herbal products, as well as post-marketing quality assurance surveillance. Additionally, following the current sustained improvements in quality control and regulatory measures in many countries of the world, it is envisaged that in the near future, herbal medicinal practices will be integrated into the conventional medicines.

Keywords: Herbal medicines; Herbal products; Phytochemicals; Standardization

Introduction

Herbal medicine, also called botanical medicine or phytomedicine, refers to the use of plant parts such as seeds, berries, roots, leaves, bark or flower for medicinal and therapeutic purposes [1,2]. Herbal medicines are associated with several therapeutic experiences and practices of indigenous systems of medicine, which serve as guidelines for the selection, preparation and application of herbal formulation to achieve therapeutic benefits. Alleviation of diseases and maintenance of good health using herbal medicines is as old as mankind and is the most popular form of healthcare practice known to humanity that has been practiced by all cultures in all ages throughout the history of civilization. Herbal medicine has evolved throughout the timeline of human civilization. The present commentary briefly described the existence of herbal medicine in pre-historic/ancient times and influence of government policies as well as impact of modern day science and technology in the advancement of herbal medicine, in efforts to achieve the goals of catering for the needs of human health and wellness.

Scientific search engines such as PubMed, Medline, EMBASE, Mendeley, Google Scholar, ScienceDirect and SpringerLink were used to retrieve online publications from 1983 to 2012. Keywords such as 'herbal medicines', 'pre-historic herbal medicines', 'traditional medicine practices', 'herb toxicity', and 'phytomedicine' were used to collate relevant articles. The results were then cross-referenced to generate a total number of 53 references cited in this review.

History of herbal medicine

People worldwide have been using herbal medicine for the treatment, control and management of variety of ailments since pre-historic times [3-6]. There is ample archaeological evidence to support the fact that primitive man used plant and herbs for medicinal purposes. For instance, pollen analyses of numerous plants found in the grave of Neanderthal man buried 60,000 years ago in Iraq indicated that the plants buried with the corpse were all of medicinal value [3,5]. In another instance, medicinal herbs found in the personal belongings of the 'Ice Man' whose body was frozen in the Swiss Alps for more than 5,300 years are thought to have been used to treat the parasites found in his intestine [3,5].

Other sources also provide ample historical evidence of man's use of plants for medicinal purposes over in antiquity. For example, the Sumerian clay tablet, dated about 5,000 years ago, recorded and described the medicinal uses of plants such as laurel, caraway and thyme by the ancient Sumerian of Mesopotamia [2,5,6]. These plants are still used all over the world for medicinal purposes. The *Ebers papyrus*, written about 3,500 years ago points to the fact that ancient Egyptians used plants such as mandrake for pain relief and garlic for the treatment of heart and circulatory disorders [5]. The Old Testament of the Bible (Ezekiel 47:12) also mentioned the use of plants for medicinal purposes [7,8]. Ancient China is also a source of information about the early use of medicinal plants. 'The Pen Tsao' (Canon of Herbs) a Chinese pharmacopoeia published about 1600 BC contains list of several medicinal plants and their uses- including *Ma-Huang*, the shrub that introduced the drug ephedrine to modern medicine [4]. In India herbal medicine, the Rig-Veda, a collection of Hindu sacred verses, contains most aspects of Vedic science such as yoga, meditation, mantra and Ayurveda, which are still widely practiced today [9].

Ancient western world traditional medicine systems

In the ancient western world, the development of western medicine is believed to have been influenced by the writing of Greek philosophers, in particular, Hippocrates (460-377 BC) and Aristotle (384-322 BC), and the works of Dioscorides, who compiled information on more than 600 plant species with medicinal value in his famous book *'De Materia Medica'*. This book, which was written in the first century AD, remained the standard reference in most of Europe for more than 1,500 years [5,10]. During the Renaissance (476-1500 AD) and the Middle Ages herbal medicine played an important role in health care management [11]. Additionally, the monasteries preserved information about herbal remedies in countries such as England, Ireland and Germany [4]. At the same time, the Arabs preserved much of the Greco-Roman expertise, and expanded it to include the use of their own resources, together with those of the Chinese and Indian, which was unknown to the Greco-Roman world [6]. In the United States, herbal traditions brought by the European settlers were merged with those acquired from native Americans, until the early 1900s when expansion of the pharmaceutical industries, coupled with the advancement in analytical techniques as well as increased knowledge of synthetic chemistry, led to a decline of herbal medicine practices in the in the developed world [4].

Evaluation of some African medicinal plants

Little is known about African traditional medicine in particular and the use of herbal medicine by ancient African people. Although it is difficult to state the exact period the use of medicinal plants originated in Africa, the likely earliest time was circa 1770 BC in the code of Hammurabi (Babylon) and 1550 BC in Egypt [2]. This is because African traditional systems of medicine are poorly recorded and, to a large extent, remain so to date [12-14]. African traditional systems of medicine were once believed to be primitive and wrongly derided by foreign religions especially during the colonial rule in Africa and subsequently by conventional or orthodox medicine practitioners [14]. Despite the suppression by the colonial rulers and the negative attitudes of the orthodox practitioners, traditional healers and herbalists in Africa continued to dispense herbal remedies [12,13]. Collaborative ethnobotanical studies, and subsequent experimental evaluation have confirmed the therapeutic potential of some African medicinal plants such as *Acacia senegal* (Gum Arabic), *Agathosma betulna* (Buchu), *Aloe ferax* (Cape Aloes), *Aloe vera* (North African Origin), *Artemisia afra* (African Wormwood), *Aspalanthus linearis* (Rooibos tea), *Catha edulis* (Khat), *Commiphora myrrha* (Myrrh), *Harpagophytum procumbens* (Devils Claws), *Hypaxis hamerocallidea* (African potato) and *Catharanthus roseus* (Rosy Periwinkle) [13,15]. Several authors have also reviewed the ethnomedical uses of several plants which were highly valued by ancient Egyptians and are still in use today [16-19].

Herbal medicine during the 19th and 20th centuries

Prior to the 19th century, plant medicines were administered in their crude form as infusions (herbal teas), tinctures (alcoholic extracts), decoctions (boiled extracts of roots or stem bark), and syrup or applied externally as ointments (poultices, balms and essential oils) and herbal baths [3,20]. However, from the late 19th century onwards, scientists began the isolation, purification and identification of bioactive principles from medicinal plants. This endeavour led to the discovery of some of the most important drugs that are still widely used in modern medicine [5,10,21,22]. For instance, morphine isolated from opium poppy (*Papaver somniferum*) is a powerful pain reliever and narcotic; quinine isolated from *Cinchona* plant species is an effective antimalarial drug; taxol (isolated from *Taxus brevifolius*) and vincristine (isolated from *Catharanthus rosesus*) are highly effective against certain cancers. Also, serpentine (isolated from the root of the Indian plant *Rauwolfia serpentia*) is used for the treatment of hypertension [20-23].

In addition to the biologically-active plant-derived natural products, many other plant bioactive principles had served as lead compounds for the design, synthesis and development of novel drugs [4,21,23,24]. In this contest, some plant derived natural products have been slightly modified to render them more effective or less toxic [4,5]. For instance, aspirin was developed in 1953 through structural modification of salicylic acid, which was identified as the active principle in a number of plants known for their pain relieving properties [5,23]. In the same way, due to the poor bioavailability of the anti-malarial agent artemisinin, which limits its effectiveness, various derivatives have been developed. These include artesunate, artemether, arteether and artemether. The earliest and famous discovery of an effective antimalarial agent-quinine was obtained from *Cinchona officinalis* bark dates back to 1638. In another example, the development of the current and popular oral hypoglycemic agent-metformin was based on the use of goat's rue (*Galega officinalis*) to treat diabetes [4]. The blood glucose lowering property of *G. officinalis* has been attributed to the presence of a guanidine-type of alkaloid-galegine. However, galegine was found to be toxic for human use, and therefore, several structural analogs were synthesized and clinic trials confirmed its efficacy. These efforts culminated to the development and marketing of metformin as an effective anti-diabetic drug [4,22].

Contemporary issues on herbal medicine

Although the direct use of plant extracts in developed countries continued to decline in the late 19th and early 20th centuries, medicinal plants still play a key role in health care system of many parts of the world [5,25]. However, the use of herbal supplements has increased dramatically over the past 30 years and most commonly used medicinal plants in the United States have been reviewed [1,26]. According to World Health Organization (WHO) [27] 60% of the world's population depends on traditional medicine and 80% of the population in developing countries depends almost entirely on traditional medicine practices and herbal medicines for their primary health care needs [19,28]. Furthermore, at the beginning of the 21st century, the worldwide annual market for herbal medicinal products approached US$ 60 billion [29] and the long tradition of herbal medicine continues to the present day in China, Indian and many countries in Africa and South America [5,19,25,28,30]. In many village marketplaces of these countries, medicinal herbs are sold alongside vegetables and other wares. Practitioners of herb medicines in developing countries often undergo a rigorous and extended training to learn the names, uses, and preparation of native plants [14].

Traditional medicine agenda for developing countries

In order to achieve "health for all", an effective health agenda must ensure that Western medicine is complemented with traditional medicine [19,31]. Accordingly, African Head of States declared the first ten years of the millennium (2001-2010) as the 'Decade of Traditional Medicine in Africa' that is commemorated on 31st August of every year [13,27]. This was renewed for the period 2011-2020 and the recent adoption of the Traditional Health Practitioner's Bill by the

South African legislature and commemoration of African Traditional Medicine day in Cameroon are testimonies to the fact that African governments are committed to ensuring the integration of traditional medicine into African health care systems [30,32]. For instance, the WHO in collaboration with the Cameroonian government has put in place a strategic platform for the practice and development of traditional medicine in Cameroon, with a view to harmonizing the traditional medicine practice through the creation of synergy between traditional and modern medicine practices and institutionalization of more harmonized integrated traditional medicine practices by the year 2012 [30]. In attempt to create a sustainable synergy between traditional and modern medicine practices, the WHO is now engaged in the establishment of definitive guidelines for scientific methodology of clinical research and the re-appraisal of effectiveness of herbal medicine. Couple of years ago, the Nigerian Government established a national committee on traditional medicine with the expressed desire to boost Nigeria's market share of traditional medicine [33]. These efforts are further complimented by huge investments in medicinal plant research in China, India, Nigeria, and the United States by the WHO [29] as well as renewed interest in prospecting for medicinal plants by multinational pharmaceutical companies.

In the developed countries, it has been reported that sufferers of chronic diseases are turning to herbal remedies as alternative to modern synthetic drugs [34]. This renewed interest in the use of herbal medicine is believed to be motivated by several factors including:

Unsubstantiated concerns to side effects of modern drugs: Although synthetic drugs exhibit quicker efficacy, there are at present, unsubstantiated opinion of higher incidents of adverse reactions following the use modern drugs when compared with herbal remedies [35-39].

Accessibility and availability of herbal remedies: Herbal remedies are readily available and accessible for both practitioners and especially patients in remote rural areas [19,30,31,34].

High cost of synthetic drugs: Medicinal plants used for remedies are comparatively less expensive when compared with orthodox/synthetic drugs [19].

Cultural factors: From a cultural perspective, traditional medicine has always been considered as an efficient and acceptable option even when modern health facilities are available. As a result of recent advances in biochemistry, immunology, medical botany and pharmacognosy, research findings have established the descriptive capacity, effectiveness and rationality of herbal medicines.

Research efforts on herbal medicine

The uses of drugs and dietary supplements derived from plants have accelerated in recent years. Pharmacologist, microbiologist, biochemist, botanist and natural product chemists are currently investigating medicinal plants for phytochemicals and lead compounds that could be developed for the treatment of several ailments [30,40,41], as exemplified by the plethora of publications of scientific research papers in many reputable journals. Most of these research exercises cover the areas of bio-analytical methodology, isolation, purification and characterization of the bioactive principles of medicinal plants. Furthermore, research efforts in herbal medicine are now focused on the identification of phytochemicals and elucidation of their molecular structures, and more recently, establishing their mechanism of action and potential toxicological properties. For instance, Tanaka *et al.,* [42] employed spectroscopic data to identify five phytosterols, namely, lophenol, 24-methyl-lophenol, 24-ethyllophenol, cycloartanol, and 24-methylene cycloartanol as the major anti-hyperglycemic phytochemicals in *A. vera* gel using Type II diabetic BKS.Cg-m(+/+)Lepr(db/J) (db/db) mice.

Based on the outcomes of herbal medicine research over the years, the 21st century has seen a paradigm shift towards therapeutic standardization of herbal drugs, of which their efficacies have been supported and confirmed through clinical trials [43]. A potentially far-reaching observation in terms of the safety concerns of consuming certain herbal medicine has been also evaluated and documented using in vitro and in vivo methods [37,44].

Herbal medicine: safety concerns, prospects and handicaps

The worldwide phytomedicine markets, in addition to the control and regulatory measures on the manufacture, distribution and sale of herbal medicine as well as safety concerns have been reviewed [1,37]. As a result of increasing demand for herbal healthcare products and application of traditional medicine, also referred to as complementary and alternative medicine systems, in both developing and developed countries, there are increasing concerns about the safety, standardization, efficacy, quality, availability and preservation of herbal products by policy-makers, health professionals and the general public. The problems associated with regulation, standardization and quality assurance in the manufacture of herbal medicines are prevalent both in developed and developing countries of the world [2,45,46].

Standardization and regulatory measures of herbal medicinal products

Standardization of herbal medicines is often a very difficult task because of the complexity of their diverse secondary metabolites, with therapeutic actions that may depend largely on age, genetic factors and geographical location of the plant species [47]. The variability in phytochemical contents amongst varieties of herbal products from the same plant species engenders profound differences in pharmacological activity. Also, the harvesting process and period, coupled with incidents of adulterations due to the presence of microorganisms and pesticides have profound impact on achieving uniform standards of herbal medicines worldwide [48]. Improvement in the quality of herbal medicines could be achieved by deliberate implementation of good agricultural practices (GAPs) at the point of cultivation of medicinal plants and good manufacturing practices (GMPs) during the process of manufacture and packaging of finished herbal products, as well as post-marketing quality assurance surveillance [48].

Additionally, for greater healthcare value and for commercial benefits, these concerns have to be allayed by carrying out cutting edge research to investigate these perceived drawbacks of the use of herbal remedies and the findings made available to the public. In this regard, records show that robust phytochemical and pharmacological research activities on medicinal plants and herbal medicines are actively going on in reputable Research Institutes and Universities, and efforts are being made to isolate and identify bioactive chemical constituents and to substantiate the claims of their efficacy and safety. Therefore, the presence of a vast array of phytochemicals in herbal medicines has opened up intense research activities involving the characterization of new chemical constituents, the identification and structure elucidation, biosynthesis and chemical reactivity of bioactive principles. Interestingly, life scientists are now been engaged in

Research Institutes and Universities in view of current trends in herbal medications, in order to ensure the dissemination of expertise in the analysis, uses, and recent issues on potential toxicity of herbal remedies for informed decisions and guides to herbal medicinal practice. Accordingly, most scientific evidence from randomized clinical trials has shown favourable outcomes in respect of the use of many herbal remedies [49]. Furthermore, the so-called Omic techniques have unravel the complicity associated with the understanding of mechanism of action of herbal bioactive principles, which has introduced vistas of scientific methods for the modernization and standardization of several Chinese herbal medicines [50]. It is worthwhile to note that new approaches and insights into Chinese herbal medicine through Research and Development (R&D) have led to the development of numerous traditional remedies and innovative drug discovery systems [51], which will make great impact on the mainstream biomedical science [52,53].

Aside the use of scientific methods to ensuring the quality and safety of herbal remedies, the integration of control measures during the course of production, storage and sale, which conforms to extant rules and regulations should be officially and legally applied using established Government institutions and legislative instruments. Unfortunately, in the absence of stricter regulatory controls the production and sale of herbal medicines in developing countries is a major drawback of traditional medicine.

Conclusion

In spite of the increasing demand for herbal medicines for the alleviation/management of diseases, as well as improvement of general well-being, there still remain several challenges that are hindering the efforts being made to integrate it into national health systems. Among the key challenges are poor quality control and lack of standardization, lack of pharmacological and clinical data on majority of herbal products to ascertain efficacy and address concerns about toxicity.

Nevertheless, following recent renewed interest in medicinal plant research and the use of cutting-edge analytical techniques and well thought-out research methodologies, the prospects of advancing the frontiers of knowledge in herbal medicine is now at an all-time high. Additionally, following the current sustained improvements in quality control and regulatory measures in many countries of the world, it is envisaged that in the near future, herbal medicine will be integrated into conventional medical systems.

References

1. Bent S1 (2008) Herbal medicine in the United States: review of efficacy, safety, and regulation: grand rounds at University of California, San Francisco Medical Center. J Gen Intern Med 23: 854-859.
2. Falodun A (2010) Herbal medicine in Africa-distribution, standardization and prospects. Res J Phytochem 4: 154-161.
3. Griggs B (1981) Green pharmacy: A history of herbal medicine. J Morman & Hobhouse Ltd. London.
4. Kinghorn AD, Balandrin MF (1993) Human Medicinal Agents from Plants. America Chemical Society. San Francisco. USA.
5. Kong JM, Goh NK, Chia LS, Chia TF (2003) Recent advances in traditional plant drugs and orchids. Acta Pharmacol Sin 24: 7-21.
6. Philipeon JD (2003) Phytochemistry and medicinal plants. Phytother 56: 237-243.
7. Duke JA (1983) Medicinal plants of the Bible. Trado-Medic Book. Conch Magazine Ltd. New York.
8. Zand J, Rountre R, Walton R (1994) Smart medicine for a healthier child. Avery Publishing Group. Garden City Park. New York.
9. Grover JK, Yadav S, Vats V (2002) Medicinal plants of India with anti-diabetic potential. J Ethnopharmacol 81: 81-100.
10. Goldman P1 (2001) Herbal medicines today and the roots of modern pharmacology. Ann Intern Med 135: 594-600.
11. Brater DC, Daly WJ (2000) Clinical pharmacology in the Middle Ages: principles that presage the 21st century. Clin Pharmacol Ther 67: 447-450.
12. Sowofora A (1993) Medicinal plants and traditional medicine in Africa. 2nd Edition. Spectrum Books. Ibadan. Nigeria. pp 26-100.
13. Elujoba AA, Odeleye OM, Ogunyemi CM (2005) Traditional medicine development for medicinal and dental primary care delivery system in Africa. Afr J Tradit Compl Altern Med 2: 46-61.
14. Okigbo RN, Mmeka EC (2006) An appraisal of phytomedicine in Africa. KMITL Sci Tech J 6: 83-93.
15. van Wyk B-E, van Oudtshoorn B, Gericke N (1997) Medicinal plants of South Africa. 2nd Edition. Briza Publication. Pretoria. South Africa.
16. Hammouda FM, Ismail SI, Abdel-Azim NS, Shams KA, Batanounny KH (2005) Guide to medicinal plants in North Africa. IUCN Center for Mediterranean Cooperation, Malaga, Spain.
17. Hamed AR, Abdel-Shafeek KA, Abdel-Azim NS, Ismail SI, Hammouda FM (2007) Chemical Investigation of Some Capparis Species Growing in Egypt and their Antioxidant Activity. Evid Based Complement Alternat Med 4: 25-28.
18. Mahmoud SM, Abdel-Azim NS, Shahat AA, Ismail SI, Hammouda FM (2007) Phytochemical and biological studies on Verboscum sinaiticum Benth growing in Egypt. Nat Prod Sci 12:186-189.
19. Abdel-Azim NS, Shams KA, Shahat AAA, El-Missiry MM, Ismail SI et al. (2011) Egyptian herbal drug industry: challenges and future prospects. Res J Med Plant 5: 136-144.
20. Gurib-Fakim A (2006) Medicinal plants: traditions of yesterday and drugs of tomorrow. Mol Aspects Med 27: 1-93.
21. Newman DJ, Cragg GM, Snader KM (2003) Natural products as sources of new drugs over the period 1981-2002. J Nat Prod 66: 1022-1037.
22. Gupta R, Gabrielsen B, Ferguson SM (2005) Nature's medicines: traditional knowledge and intellectual property management. Case studies from the National Institutes of Health (NIH), USA. Curr Drug Discov Technol 2: 203-219.
23. Lesney MS (2004) Nature's pharmaceuticals: Natural products from plants remain at the core of modern medicinal chemistry. TCAW 13: 26-31.
24. UNESCO FIT/504-RAF-48 (1998) Terminal reports: Promotion of ethnobotany and the sustainable use of plant resources in Africa. Paris. pp.60.
25. Tapsell LC, Hemphill I, Cobiac L, Patch CS, Sullivan DR, et al. (2006) Health benefits of herbs and spices: the past, the present, the future. Med J Aust 185: S4-24.
26. http://umm.edu/health/medical/altmed/treatment/herbal-medicine [accessed on 25 February 2015].
27. WHO (2001) Legal status of traditional medicines and complimentary/alternative medicine: worldwide review. WHO Publications pp.10-14.
28. Zhang BB, Moller DE (2000) New approaches in the treatment of type 2 diabetes. Curr Opin Chem Biol 4: 461-467.
29. Tilburt JC, Kaptchuk TJ (2008) Herbal medicine research and global health: an ethical analysis. Bull World Health Organ 86: 594-599.
30. Fokunang CN, Ndikum V, Tabi OY, Jiofack RB, Ngameni B, et al. (2011) Traditional medicine: past, present and future research and development prospects and integration in the National Health System of Cameroon. Afr J Tradit Complement Altern Med 8: 284-295.
31. WHO (2002) Traditional medicinal strategy 2002-2005. WHO Publication pp. 1-6.
32. Department of Health (2004) Traditional health practitioners' bill. Available from: http://www.doh.gov.za/docs/index.html [accessed on 25 February 2015].

33. Adelaja A (2006) Nigeria boosts research into traditional medicine. Available from: http://www.scidev.net/en/news/nigeria-boosts-research-into-traditional-medicine.html [accessed on 25 February 2015].
34. Calixto JB (2000) Efficacy, safety, quality control, marketing and regulatory guidelines for herbal medicines (phytotherapeutic agents). Braz J Med Biol Res 33: 179-189.
35. Piédrola G, Novo E, Escobar F, García-Robles R (2001) White blood cell count and insulin resistance in patients with coronary artery disease. Ann Endocrinol (Paris) 62: 7-10.
36. Yaryura-Tobias JA, Pinto A, Neziroglu F (2001) Anorexia nervosa, diabetes mellitus, brain atrophy, and fatty liver. Int J Eat Disord 30: 350-353.
37. Haq J (2004) Safety of medicinal plants. Pak J Med Res 43: 8 pages.
38. Gardhipuram PSK, Durairaji SK, Sorimuthu PS (2006) Anti-diabetic activity of fruits of Terminalia chebula on streptozotocin-induced diabetic rats. J Health Sci 54: 283-291.
39. Aronson JK (2009) Side effects of herbal medicines. Elsevier B.V. Amsterdam, Boston, Heidelberg.
40. Jiofack T, Ayissi I (2006) Floristic evaluation of the Upper Nyong valley in Cameroon, Technical report. Cameroon Wildlife Conserv Soc 3: 50.
41. Acharya D, Shrivastava A (2008) Indigenous Herbal Medicines: Tribal Formulations and Traditional Herbal Practices. 1stedn., Aavishkar Publishers, Jaipur-India. pp. 440.
42. Tanaka M, Misawa E, Ito Y, Habara N, Nomaguchi K, et al. (2006) Identification of five phytosterols from Aloe vera gel as anti-diabetic compounds. Biol Pharm Bull 29: 1418-1422.
43. Alvari A, Mehrnaz SO, Ahmad FJ, Abdin MZ (2012) Contemporary overview on clinical trials and future prospects of hepato-protective herbal medicines. Rev Recent Clin Trials 7: 214-223.
44. van de Venter M, Roux S, Bungu LC, Louw J, Crouch NR, et al. (2008) Antidiabetic screening and scoring of 11 plants traditionally used in South Africa. J Ethnopharmacol 119: 81-86.
45. Rotblatt MD1 (1999) Herbal medicine: a practical guide to safety and quality assurance. West J Med 171: 172-175.
46. Sane RT (2002) Standardization, quality control and GMP for herbal drugs. Indian Drug 39: 184-190.
47. Firenzuoli F, Gori L (2007) Herbal medicine today: clinical and research issues. Evid Based Complement Alternat Med 4: 37-40.
48. Fong HH1 (2002) Integration of herbal medicine into modern medical practices: issues and prospects. Integr Cancer Ther 1: 287-293.
49. Bubela T, Boon H, Caulfield T (2008) Herbal remedy clinical trials in the media: a comparison with the coverage of conventional pharmaceuticals. BMC Med 6: 35.
50. Buriani A, Garcia-Bermejo ML, Bosisio E, Xu Q, Li H, et al. (2012) Omic techniques in systems biology approaches to traditional Chinese medicine research: present and future. J Ethnopharmacol 140: 535-544.
51. Pan SY, Chen SB, Dong HG, Yu ZL, Dong JC, et al. (2011) New perspectives on chinese herbal medicine (zhong-yao) research and development. Evid Based Complement Alternat Med 2011: 403709.
52. Trusheim MR, Berndt ER, Douglas FL (2007) Stratified medicine: strategic and economic implications of combining drugs and clinical biomarkers. Nat Rev Drug Discov 6: 287-293.
53. Parekh HS, Liu G, Wei MQ (2009) A new dawn for the use of traditional Chinese medicine in cancer therapy. Mol Cancer 8: 21.

9

Effects of Zuogui Wan and Yougui Wan on the Expression of Learning- and Memory-related Signal Transduction Molecules

Xiangping Kang[1], Chao Liang[2], Guoqin Jin[1*], Xueli Zhang[1], Zhangbin Gong[1], Yanwu Xu[1] and Zhifen Han[3]

[1]*Department of Biochemistry, Institute of Basic Medicine, Shanghai University of Traditional Chinese Medicine (TCM), Shanghai 201203, China*

[2]*Experiment in TCM, Department, Institute of Basic Medicine, Shanghai University of Traditional Chinese Medicine (TCM), Shanghai 201203, China*

[3]*Experiment Center for Teaching & Learning, Shanghai University of Traditional Chinese Medicine (TCM), Shanghai 201203, China*

[*]**Corresponding author:** Guoqin Jin, Department of Biochemistry, Institute of Basic Medicine, Shanghai University of Traditional Chinese Medicine (TCM), Shanghai 201203, China, E-mail: jinguoqin8405@126.com

Abstract

Objective: This study aimed to determine the effect of kidney-tonifying recipe Zuogui Wan (ZGW) and Yougui Wan (YGW) on learning and memory ability, serum corticosterone (CORT), and expression of learning- and memory-related signal transduction molecules in aging rats.

Methods: Naturally aged rats (23 months) were used as animal model and were randomly divided into four groups: senile control group, senile+antagonist RU486 (antagonist of GR group, senile+ZGW group, and senile +YGW group). A fifth group was designated as the young group, composed of five-month old rats. Starting from the 21st month, rats of senile+ZGW and senile+YGW group were administered with ZGW and YGW respectively for three months.

For subcutaneous injection, RU486 (5 mg/kg body weight) was administered 2 h prior to the Morris maze test (senile+antagonist RU486 group). Spatial learning and memory abilities were observed using Morris water maze test. Contents of serum CORT were examined using enzyme-linked immunosorbent assay.

Expression of related signal transduction molecules (CaM, pCaMK II, pERK1/2, pCREB, Arc, and pSynapsin I) were tested using Western blot. Regulating effects of kidney-tonifying recipe and RU486 on above-mentioned indicators were also studied.

Results: Contents of corticosterone in serum of senile rats were significantly higher compared with the young group. Morris water maze test showed that spatial learning and memory abilities of aging rats were clearly reduced. Expression of learning- and memory-related signal transduction molecules was also visibly lowered. However, kidney-tonifying recipe and RU486 exhibited potential to improve abnormal changes of the above-mentioned indicators in senile rats to varying extent.

Conclusion: Experimental findings indicate that kidney-tonifying recipe and RU486 may improve spatial learning and memory abilities and retard the effects of aging on senile rats by down-regulating abnormally high corticosterone levels and up-regulating expression of related signal transduction proteins.

Keywords: Aging; Corticosterone; Zuogui Wan; Yougui Wan; Learning and memory

Research Highlights

(1) This study was based on a theory of TCM: "Kidney Deficiency and Aging". Naturally aged rats were used as experimental animal models. Effects of kidney-tonifying recipes (Zuogui Wan and Yougui Wan) on degradation of learning and memory were determined. This research provides scientific experimental basis for clinical application of the two recipes. Furthermore, the present study may reveal scientific connotation of the theory: "Kidney Deficiency and Aging".

(2) Several studies have investigated the disorder in the hypothalamus-pituitary-adrenal (HPA) axis in aging rats. The mechanism by which high levels of corticosterone, which is the final hormone of HPA axis, eventually leads to degeneration of learning and memory remains unclear. In the present study, the molecular mechanism of age-related learning and memory impairment was observed, and the effect of kidney-tonifying recipes was also studied. These investigations were based on the learning- and memory-related signal transduction pathway, mediated by the glucocorticoid receptor (GR).

Introduction

Aging is a natural and complex biological process during which many physiological functions may become disordered, including impairment of learning and memory ability. Increasing amount of evidence have demonstrated that the hypothalamus pituitary-adrenal (HPA) axis is one of the most important neuroendocrine systems closely related to aging [1,2]. Disorder of HPA axis may cause damage to the hippocampus and degeneration of learning and memory ability, which can consequently destroy the steady state of the body and lead to aging [3].

The present research work revealed that the HPA axis in aging rats was hyperactive, leading to high levels of corticosterone which exhibit toxic effect on the hippocampus through the glucocorticoid receptor (GR) [4,5]. Hippocampus is part of the limbic system and is highly involved in learning and memory. The hippocampus is a GR-rich region and thus it is a key to the toxic effects of high levels of corticosterone (CORT) [6,7].

Therefore, the toxic effect of hippocampus may be fundamental to learning and memory degradation.

ZGW and YGW are two classic kidney-tonifying recipes prescribed by Jingyue Zhang of the Ming Dynasty. Both recipes exhibit effects such as anti-aging and enhancement of learning and memory ability [8]. In the present study, ZGW and YGW were administered to naturally aged rats.

Effects of ZGW and YGW on learning and memory ability, corticosterone level, and expression of learning- and memory-related signal transduction molecules (such as CaM, pCaMK II, pERK1/2, pCREB, Arc, and pSynapsin I) were observed.

Furthermore, the effects of the glucocorticoid receptor (GR) antagonist RU486 on the abovementioned indicators were also investigated. Results of the present study may provide scientific experimental basis for the application of ZGW and YGW on tonifying kidney and improving intelligence in clinical treatments.

Material and Methods

Animals

Male, pathogen-free grade Sprague-Dawley rats were provided by the Animal Laboratories in Shanghai University of Traditional Chinese Medicine, China. Experimental use of animals complied with the Guidance Suggestions for the Care and Use of Laboratory Animals, issued by the Ministry of Science and Technology of China [9].

Drugs

RU486, 17-hydroxy-11-(4-dimethlaminophenyl)-17-(1-propynyl)-estra-4,9-diene-3-one (purity >98%) was provided by Sigma-Aldrich Co., St. Louis, MO, USA. Structural formula of RU486 is shown in Figure 1.

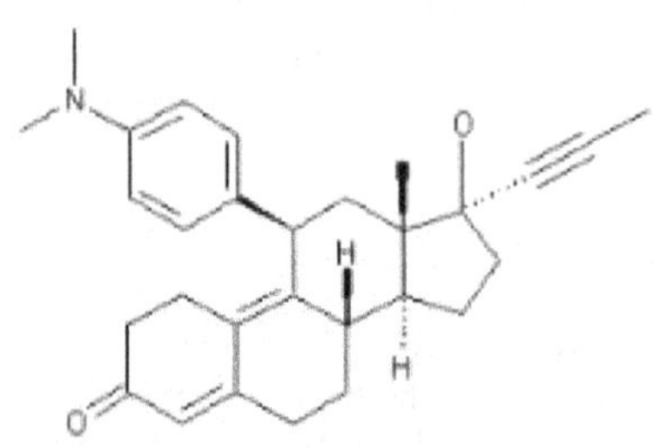

Figure 1: Structural formula of RU486.

Chinese medicine compounds

ZGW prescription: The decoction comprised *Radix rehmanniae praeparata, Rhizoma dioscoreae, Semen cuscutae, Lycium barbarum L., Cornus officinalis, Radix achyranthis bidentatae,* tortoise-plastron glue, and antler glue according to the ratio 4:2:2:2:2:1.5:2:2, immersed in eight times the volume of distilled water for 1 h. The herbs were then decocted twice in simmer water for 30 minutes each time. The decoction was condensed to 1.53 g crude drug/ml condensed decoction and was stored at −20°C and rewarmed to 25°C to 30°C before administration.

YGW prescription: The decoction comprised *Radix rehmanniae praeparata, Rhizoma dioscoreae, L. barbarum, C. officinalis, Semen cuscutae,* antler glue, *Eucommia ulmoides, Angelica sinensis, Cinnamomum cassia,* and radix aconite according to the ratio 4:2:2:1.5:2:2:2:1.5:1:1, immersed in eight times the volume of distilled water for 1 h. The herbs were then decocted twice in simmer water for 30 minutes each time.

The decoction was condensed to 1.83 g crude drug/ml condensed decoction and was stored at -20°C and rewarmed to 25°C to 30°C before administration. Drug doses: Doses of ZGW and YGW prepared were about 7 times the dose of adult body weight (mg/kg) [10,11]. Rats were administered with ZGW and YGW respectively for 90 consecutive days starting from the 21st month [12].

Establishment of aging rats and grouping

One hundred and six 23-month old, specific pathogen-free grade, male Sprague-Dawley rats weighing 900 g to 1000 g were used in this study as aging rats. Twenty five-month-old, specific pathogen-free grade, male Sprague-Dawley rats weighing 300 g to 350 g were used as control rats (young rats).

Aging rats were randomly divided into the following four groups: senile control group (aged 23 months), senile+antagonist RU486 (aged 23 months), senile+ZGW group (aged 23 months), and senile+YGW group (aged 23 months). The fifth group was the young group (aged 5 months). Starting from age 21 months [12], the senile+ZGW group and senile+YGW group were administered with ZGW and YGW, respectively for 3 months.

Systemic administration of RU486

Steroid solutions were freshly prepared before injection by dissolving the crystalline steroid in absolute ethanol and dilution in polyethylene glycol (PEG) to a final ethanol concentration of 0.2%. For subcutaneous injection, RU486 (5 mg/kg body weight) was administered 2 h prior to the Morris maze test (senile+antagonist RU486 group) [13]. Rats of other groups received equal volumes of normal saline.

Serum and brain tissue samples of rats

Rats were euthanized under 10% chloral hydrate (3.5 ml/kg weight) anesthesia, and 10-ml blood samples were collected from the abdominal aorta using a syringe. Blood samples were then centrifuged at 3000 rounds per minute for 10 minutes at room temperature to obtain the serum. The brain was divided into two parts, namely, the cortex and the hippocampus. Serum and brain tissues were preserved in liquid nitrogen for 30 minutes and stored at -70°C.

Morris water maze test [14]

Five-day spatial navigation test was performed to detect average escape latency and to assess spatial learning and memory ability. Morris water maze equipment was provided by the Shanghai Geriatric Institute of Chinese Medicine. All rats were allowed to swim freely for 2 minutes a day prior to the test to adapt to the environment.

A certain amount of ink was poured into the swimming pool to hide the platform located at the first quadrant, 1.5 cm under the water. During the whole test, the platform was maintained in the same quadrant. Rats entered the water pool from the 4th quadrant.

A computer recorded the time the rats spent to find the platform (escape latency) and the swimming route of the rats. The time limit for each test was set at 70 seconds. Rats that failed to find the platform within the designated time limit were given 70-second time records.

After test completion, rats were allowed to stay on the platform for 20 seconds. Each rat was subjected to the test twice a day, and average time of escape latency was calculated for further analysis.

ELISA

An enzyme-labeled immunosorbent assay (ELISA) kit was used to measure serum corticosterone levels in strict accordance with the manufacturer's instructions. Levels were calculated using a standard curve method.

Western blot assay for CaM, pCaMK II, pERK1/2, pCREB, Arc and pSynapsin I expression in the hippocampus

Total protein was extracted using RIPA lysis buffer (Beyotime, Shanghai, China), and total protein content was determined using a bicinchoninic acid quantitative protein detection kit (Beyotime, Shanghai, China).

Forty micrograms of hippocampus protein was mixed with sampling buffer solution and boiled in a water bath for 5 minutes. Four percent stacking gel and 10% separation gel were prepared, and electrophoresis was performed under 60 V for 60 minutes and 100 V for about 100 minutes.

Extracted proteins were transferred to polyvinylidene fluoride membrane (Millipore Corporation) using a water-bath electric transfer device at 4°C, 350-mA constant current for 80 minutes.

The membrane was blocked with 5% skimmed milk powder and shaken gently for 1 h at room temperature. After rinsing with TBST, membranes were incubated with rabbit anti-CaM, phosphor-CaMK II, phosphor-ERK1/2, phosphor-CREB, phosphor-Synapsin I, GAPDH polyclonal antibodies (1:500; Cell Signaling Technology), and mouse anti-Arc monoclonal antibody (1:200; Santa Cruz) overnight at 4°C.

The membrane was rinsed with TBST four times for 10 minutes each time, and was then incubated with peroxidase conjugated goat anti-rabbit/mouse IgG (1:2000; Santa Cruz) at 37°C for 45 minutes and rinsed with TBST four times for 10 minutes each time.

Following polyvinylidene fluoride membrane coloration, Pierce chemiluminescent substrate solutions A and B were mixed for 5 minutes at room temperature and the scanned image was analyzed with a digital gel image analysis system (Protein Simple Company, USA).

Statistical analysis

Measurement data were expressed as mean ± SD using SPSS16.0 software (SPSS, Chicago, IL, USA). Differences between groups were compared using one-way analysis of variance. Data of the water maze test were analyzed using analysis of variance of repeated data measurement [15].

For all statistical comparisons, a value of $P<0.05$ was considered statistically significant.

Results

Learning and memory abilities of experimental animals

Morris test showed that latency shortened from the 1st day to the 5th day of observation. Compared with the young rats, latency of the senile rats clearly increased from the 2nd day ($P<0.05$).

Compared with the senile rats, latency of the senile+ZGW group shortened from the 2nd day ($P<0.05$), and latency of the senile+YGW group and senile+antagonist RU486 group shortened from the 3rd day ($P<0.05$) (Table 1 and Figure 2).

Group	Latency (second)				
	1st day	2nd day	3rd day	4th day	5th day
Young group	64.5 ± 7.34	55.7 ± 9.37	42.3 ± 8.49	33.6 ± 7.52	24.7 ± 4.97
Senile control group	70.0 ± 0.00	68.8 ± 2.57*	65.0 ± 6.11*	63.0 ± 6.06*	60.4 ± 7.04*
Senile+antagonist RU486 group	68.1 ± 4.33	61.2 ± 7.51	53.4 ± 5.95∆	46.6 ± 3.86∆	42.2 ± 3.55∆
Senile+ZGW group	67.1 ± 4.50	58.8 ± 8.38∆	51.6 ± 6.38∆	45.3 ± 4.83∆	39.8 ± 3.29∆
Senile+YGW group	68.9 ± 2.33	60.2 ± 8.39	49.5 ± 3.37∆	42.7 ± 3.23∆	39.7 ± 2.50∆

*$P<0.05$, vs. young group, ∆$P<0.05$, vs. senile control group. Data are expressed as mean ± SD, n=10 for each group. Variance analysis of repeated data measurement was used for comparison of several groups [15].

Table 1: Comparison of spatial learning and memory ability in different groups.

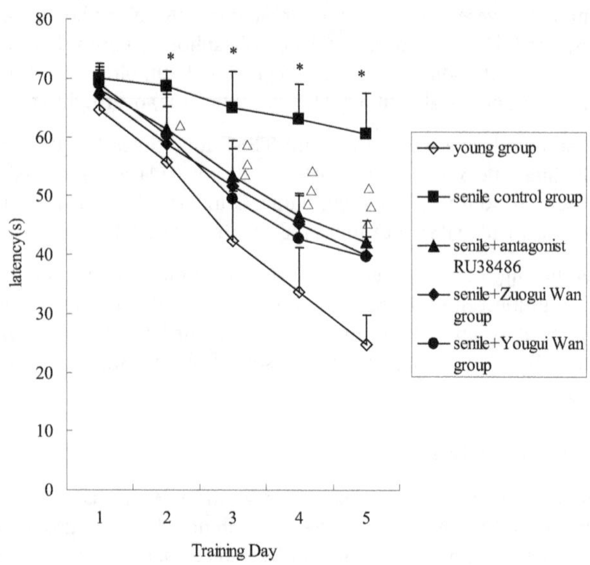

Figure 2: Escape latency (s) of experimental rats in Morris water maze test. *P<0.05, vs. young group, ΔP<0.05, vs. senile control group. Data are expressed as mean ± SD, n=10 for each group. Variance analysis of repeated data measurement was used for comparison of several groups [15].

Group	CORT level (ng/L)
young group	71.89 ± 7.63
Senile control group	195.13 ± 10.80*
Senile+antagonist RU486 group	82.55 ± 7.71Δ
Senile+ZGW group	141.61 ± 8.86Δ
Senile+YGW group	141.59 ± 15.29

Table 2: Changes of CORT level in serum of different groups. *P<0.05, vs. young group, ΔP<0.05, vs. senile control group.

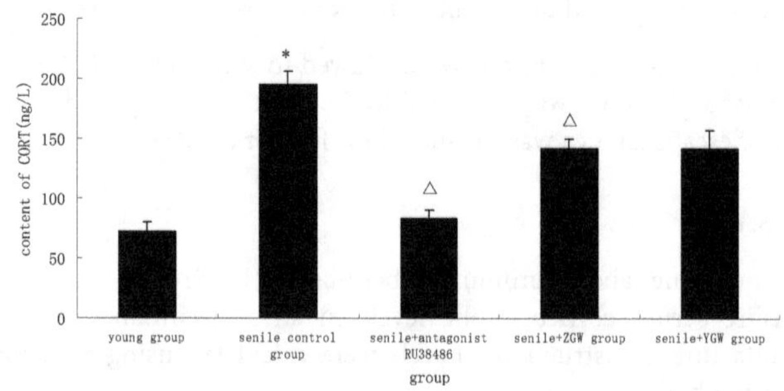

Figure 3: Changes of CORT level in serum of different groups. *P<0.05, vs. young group, ΔP<0.05, vs. senile control group. Data are expressed as mean ± SD, n=8 for each group, using one-way analysis of variance and the Student-Newman-Keuls test. CORT: corticosterone.

Serum levels of corticosterone

Results of the ELISA test demonstrated that corticosterone level in senile rats was significantly higher compared with the young rats group (P<0.05).

Compared with senile control group, content of corticosterone in senile+antagonist RU486 and senile+Zuogui Wan group clearly decreased (P<0.05).

The same trend was observed in senile+Yougui Wan group but the difference was not statistically significant (Table 2 and Figure 3).

CaM, pCaMK II, pERK1/2, pCREB, Arc and pSynapsin I expression in rat hippocampus

Semi-quantitative analysis using Western blot assay showed that CaM, pCaMK II, pERK1/2, pCREB, Arc, and pSynapsin I expression in the senile control group was significantly lower compared with the young group (P<0.05). Expression was increased to varying degrees by the kidney-tonifying recipe and RU486 (Table 3, Figures 4A and4B).

Group	CaM	pCaMK II	pERK1/2	pCREB	Arc	pSynapsin I
young group	0.578 ± 0.075	0.660 ± 0.062	0.613 ± 0.061	0.588 ± 0.072	0.568 ± 0.067	0.602 ± 0.029
Senile control group	0.221 ± 0.022*	0.250 ± 0.029*	0.287 ± 0.041*	0.185 ± 0.032*	0.226 ± 0.052*	0.206 ± 0.022*
Senile+antagonist RU486 group	0.409 ± 0.055	0.429 ± 0.038	0.432 ± 0.045Δ	0.371 ± 0.040	0.323 ± 0.047	0.391 ± 0.041
Senile+ZGW group	0.444 ± 0.073	0.536 ± 0.044Δ	0.404 ± 0.046	0.426 ± 0.049Δ	0.328 ± 0.045	0.378 ± 0.048
Senile+YGW group	0.398 ± 0.03Δ	0.515 ± 0.047Δ	0.440 ± 0.036Δ	0.421 ± 0.049Δ	0.327 ± 0.062	0.307 ± 0.043
Absorbance ratios of CaM, pCaMK II, pERK1/2, pCREB, Arc, and pSynapsin I to GAPDH are expressed as mean ± SD, n=6 for each group, using one-way analysis of variance and the Student-Newman-Keuls test. CaM: calmodulin; CaMK II: calmodulin-dependent protein kinase II; ERK: extracellular signal-regulated kinase; CREB: cAMP response-element binding protein; GAPDH: glyceraldehyde-3-phosphate dehydrogenase; *P<0.05, vs. young group, ΔP<0.05, vs. senile control group.						

Table 3: CaM, pCaMK II, pERK1/2, pCREB, Arc and pSynapsin I protein expression in hippocampus.

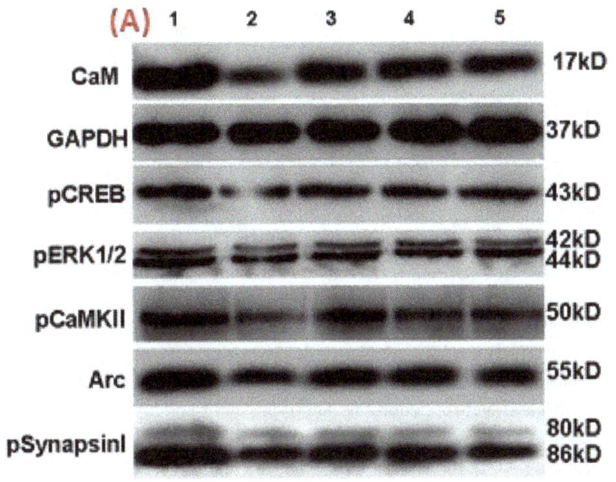

Figure 4A: CaM, pCaMK II, pERK1/2, pCREB, Arc and pSynapsin I expression in the hippocampus. Representative protein bands from Western blot for CaM, pCaMK II, pERK1/2, pCREB, Arc and pSynapsin I in hippocampus. 1-young group, 2-senile control group, 3-senile+antagonist RU486 group, 4-senile+ZGW group, 5-senile+YGW group.

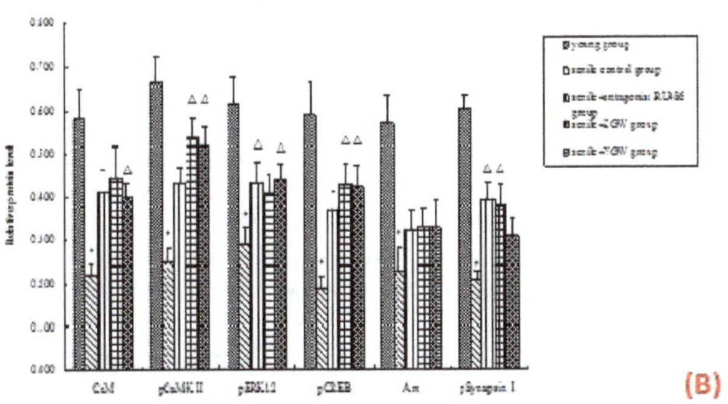

Figure 4B: CaM, pCaMK II, pERK1/2, pCREB, Arc and pSynapsin I expression in the hippocampus. Density values ratio of CaM, pCaMK II, pERK1/2, pCREB, Arc and pSynapsin I to GAPDH. Data are expressed as mean ± SD, n=6 for each group, using one-way analysis of variance and the Student-Newman-Keuls test. *P<0.05, vs. young group, ΔP<0.05, vs. senile control group.

Discussion

Aging and age-associated cognitive impairments are complex and multifactorial processes. The process of normal aging often results in cognitive decline both in human and animal models. Growing evidence have shown that memory loss with aging may be associated with high levels of glucocorticoid [16,17]. Disorder in the HPA axis can be observed in humans and rodents during the normal process of aging, such as hypersecretion of glucocorticoid. High level of glucocorticoid is related to the action of the glucocorticoid receptor (GR) [18]. The GR is a nuclear receptor abundant in the hippocampus. High levels of glucocorticoid can cause atrophy of the hippocampus and decay of memory, which is mediated by GR [19]. Results of the present study showed that corticosterone levels in aging rats were significantly higher compared with the young rats, and the high level of corticosterone led to a decrease in the expression of GR in CA1 and CA2-3 subregion of hippocampus [20]. The abnormal changes caused hyperactivity in the HPA axis, resulting to the dysfunction of learning and memory. This response may be a form of self-defense of the neurons of hippocampus to the toxic effect of corticosterone.

Calmodulin-dependent protein kinase II (CaMK II) is a kind of serine/threonine protein kinase and is regulated by Ca^{2+}/calmodulin (CaM). Many studies have shown that CaMK II is related to synaptic plasticity and memory formation [21,22]. Furthermore, the function of CaMK II in reducing long term potentiation (LTP) of the hippocampus might be relevant to extracellular signal-regulated kinase (ERK), another key molecule in memory formation [23,24]. Regulation of the mitogen-activated protein kinase (MAPK)/ERK signaling pathway activated many transcription factors, such as cAMP response-element binding protein (CREB) [25,26]. These transcription factors exhibit important functions in synaptic plasticity by regulating the expression of specific molecules, such as activity-regulated cytoskeleton-associated protein (Arc) and synapsin (Syn). Increasing evidence has indicated that Arc and Syn have important functions in refactoring cytoskeleton of neurons, which include establishing synaptic morphology, strengthening connections between neurons, and consolidating LTP [27,28]. Thus, Arc and Syn are key molecules that maintiain long-term memory.

In the present study, expression of learning- and memory-related signal transduction molecules (such as CaM, pCaMK II, pERK1/2, pCREB, Arc, and pSynapsin I) of senile rats was observed. Furthermore, effect of classic kidney-tonifying recipe (ZGW and YGW) and RU486 were also tested. Results showed that senile rats exhibited poor learning ability and high level of corticosterone. Expression of learning- and memory-related signal transduction molecules also decreased. The results suggested that high levels of corticosterone injured the hippocampus by reacting with GR. Thus, subsequent signaling pathway mediated by GR was impaired. As a result, expression of many key molecules associated with learning and memory were decreased. In addition, synaptic plasticity and establishment of LTP were also affected, which could partly explain the degradation of learning and memory ability of aging rats.

ZGW and YGW are two classic kidney-tonifying recipes that were prescribed according to "interdependence between yin and yang". Sun et al. (YEAR) suggested that ZGW inhibited apoptosis and maintained stability of the cell membrane through improving the activity of adenosine triphosphatase (ATPase) [29]. Ma et al. (YEAR) proved that YGW regulated expression of apoptosis-related genes, such as bax and bcl-2 in the CA1 subregion of hippocampus in aging rats [30]. Results of the present study also showed that Zuogui Wan and Yougui Wan could improve abnormal changes, such as high levels of corticosterone, poor learning and memory ability, and low expression of learning and memory-related molecules in senile rats to varying extent. Furthermore, GR antagonist RU486 also worked on these indicators. The abovementioned observations revealed that the kidney-tonifying recipes (ZGW and YGW) and RU486 might improve spatial learning and memory ability and retard aging of senile rats by regulating the function of HPA axis, down-regulating abnormally high level of corticosterone, and up-regulating expression of related signal transduction molecules.

Acknowledgement

This study was financially supported by the National Natural Science Foundation of China (No.30873317, 81473583), Shanghai Natural Science Foundation of China (No.15ZR1441400), the leading Academic Discipline Project of Shanghai Municipal Education Commission (No.J50301), and Scientific Program of Shanghai Education Commission (No.2012JW03).

References

1. Pulopulos MM, Hidalgo V, Almela M, Puig-Perez S, Villada C, et al. (2015) Acute stress and working memory in older people. Stress 18: 178-187.
2. Khemissi W, Farooq RK, Le Guisquet AM (2014) Dysregulation of the hypothalamus-pituitary-adrenal axis predicts some aspects of the behavioral response to chronic fluoxetine: association with hippocampal cell proliferation. Front Behav Neurosci 8: 340
3. Aguilera G (2011) HPA axis responsiveness to stress: implications for healthy aging. Exp Gerontol 46: 90-95.
4. Zhao XY, Jin GQ, Gu CY (2010) Effects of Zuogui Wan and Yougui Wan on learning and memory related signal transduction molecular mRNA expressions in the corticosterone induced rat's hippocampus neuron pathological model. China Journal of TCM and Pharmacy 25: 1983-1987
5. Dai WW, Jin GQ, Zhang XL (2004) Effects of kidney-tonifying herbs on the glucocorticoid receptor mRNA expression in hippocampal subfields of aging rats. Acta Biochimica et Biophyscia Sinica 36: 163
6. Hu P, Oomen C, van Dam AM, Wester J, Zhou JN, et al. (2012) A single-day treatment with mifepristone is sufficient to normalize chronic glucocorticoid induced suppression of hippocampal cell proliferation. PLoS One 7: e46224.
7. Chen KC, Blalock EM, Curran-Rauhut MA, Kadish I, Blalock SJ, et al. (2013) Glucocorticoid-dependent hippocampal transcriptome in male rats: pathway-specific alterations with aging. Endocrinology 154: 2807-2820.
8. Kang XP, Jin GQ, Liang C (2013) Effects of kidney-tonifying recipe on the expressions of learning and memory related signal molecules. Chinese Journal of Gerontology 33: 2064-2067
9. The Ministry of Science and Technology of the People's Republic of China. Guidance Suggestions for the Care and Use of Laboratory Animals 2006-09-30
10. Lu Y, Zhang DF (2012) Pharmacology of Chinese Materia Medica. Beijing: People's Medical Publication House.
11. Wei W, Wu XM, Li YJ (2010) Experimental Methodology of Pharmacology. Beijing: People's Medical Publication House.
12. Kang XP, Jin GQ, Gong ZB (2007) Effects of Zuogui Pill and Yougui Pill on the expression of amine acids neurotransmitter receptor in the aging rat's hypothalamus. Pharmacology and Clinics of Chinese Materia Medica 23: 6-8
13. Xu L, Holscher C, Anwyl R, Rowan MJ (1998) Glucocorticoid receptor and protein/RNA synthesis-dependent mechanisms underlie the control of synaptic plasticity by stress. Proc Natl Acad Sci U S A 95: 3204-3208.
14. Morris RJ (1984) Development of a water-maze procedure for studying spatial learning in the rats. Neurosci Methods 11: 47-60
15. Qiu H, Jin GQ, Jin RF, Zhao WK (2007) [Analysis of variance of repeated data measured by water maze with SPSS]. Zhong Xi Yi Jie He Xue Bao 5: 101-105.
16. Hasan KM, Rahman MS, Arif KM, Sobhani ME (2012) Psychological stress and aging: role of glucocorticoids (GCs). Age (Dordr) 34: 1421-1433.
17. Liston C, Gan WB (2011) Glucocorticoids are critical regulators of dendritic spine development and plasticity in vivo. Proc Natl Acad Sci U S A 108: 16074-16079.
18. Pardon MC, Sarmad S, Rattray I (2009) Repeated novel cage exposure induced improvement of early Alzheimer's like cognitive and amyloid changes in TASTPM mice is unrelated to changes in brain endocannabinoids levels. Neurobiology Aging 30: 1099-1113
19. Jeanneteau F, Chao MV (2013) Are BDNF and glucocorticoid activities calibrated? Neuroscience 239: 173-195.
20. Kang XP, Jin GQ (2012) Degradation mechanisms of learning and memory in aging rats and the effects of kidney-tonifying recipe. China Journal of TCM and Pharmacy 27: 981-986
21. Uddin RK, Singh SM (2013) Hippocampal gene expression meta-analysis identifies aging and age-associated spatial learning impairment (ASLI) genes and pathways. PLoS One 8: e69768.
22. Karthik Bodhinathan, B.Tech, Ashok Kumar (2010) Intracellular redox state alters N-Methyl D-Aspartate receptor response during aging through Ca2+/calmodulin -dependent protein kinase II. J Neurosci 30: 1914-1924
23. Steelman LS, Chappell WH, Abrams SL, Kempf RC, Long J, et al. (2011) Roles of the Raf/MEK/ERK and PI3K/PTEN/Akt/mTOR pathways in controlling growth and sensitivity to therapy-implications for cancer and aging. Aging (Albany NY) 3: 192-222.
24. Martinez-Lopez N, Athonvarangkul D, Mishall P, Sahu S, Singh R (2013) Autophagy proteins regulate ERK phosphorylation. Nat Commun 4: 2799.
25. Morris KA, Gold PE (2012) Age-related impairments in memory and in CREB and pCREB expression in hippocampus and amygdala following inhibitory avoidance training. Mech Ageing Dev 133: 291-299.
26. Hansen RT 3rd, Zhang HT (2013) Senescent-induced dysregulation of cAMP/CREB signaling and correlations with cognitive decline. Brain Res 1516: 93-109.
27. Sama DM, Norris CM (2013) Calcium dysregulation and neuroinflammation: discrete and integrated mechanisms for age-related synaptic dysfunction. Ageing Res Rev 12: 982-995.
28. Miyashita T, Kubik S, Lewandowski G, Guzowski JF (2008) Networks of neurons, networks of genes: an integrated view of memory consolidation. Neurobiol Learn Mem 89: 269-284.
29. Sun LL, Kang GS, Ma YC (2010) The effect of Zuogui pill on ATPase bcl-2 bax and caspase-3 of subacute aging rats induced by D-galactose. Chinese Archives of Traditional Chinese Medicine 28: 205-207
30. Ma SJ, Cao S, Yao JP (2011) Effect of bushen prescription on expression of apoptosis related gene-bax, bcl-2 mRNA in hippocampal CA1of natural aged rats. Pharmacology and Clinics of Chinese Materia Medica 27: 6-7.

10

Anti-Inflammatory Effects of Moxibustion on Mice with Adjuvant Arthritis: Role of TRPV1

Jie-Jun Li, Jin-Feng Jiang*, Ying Jiang and Xiao-Jing Wu

Key Laboratory of Acupuncture Combined with Medication, The Second Clinical Medical College, Nanjing University of Traditional Chinese Medicine, Nanjing 210046, China

***Corresponding author:** Jin-feng Jiang. Institutional addresses:Key Laboratory of Acupuncture Combined with Medication, The Second Clinical Medical College, Nanjing University of Traditional Chinese Medicine, Nanjing 210046, China, E-mail: Dr. acujf@njutcm. edu. cn

Abstract

Aim and Objective: This research was done to observe the anti-inflammatory effect of moxibustion and explore the role of Transient Receptor Potential Vanilloid sub type 1 (TRPV1) on Mice with adjuvant arthritis.

Method: Adjuvant arthritis (AA) was established by using the amount of 20 μL of Freund's Adjuvant Complete (FCA) intradermal injected into right hindfoot plantar. 50 KM mice were randomized into 6 groups by random number table method: control group (n=10), model group (n=8), capsaicin group (n=8), capsazepine group (n=8), moxibustion group (n=8) and Moxibustion+Capsazepine (MC) group (n=8). 16 C57BL/6 wild-type mice are randomized into 2 groups by random number table method: Wild-Type (WT) model group and WT moxibustion group with 8 in each. 14 TRPV1 knockout mice are randomized into 2 groups by random number table method: knockout (KO) model group and KO moxibustion group with 7 in each.

Each mouse in the capsaicin group is subcutaneously injected with the amount of 0.1 ml/10 g into the L5, L6 spinal cords. Each mouse in the capsazepine group was intraperitoneally injected with the amount of 0.1 ml/10 g. Similarly, each mouse in the moxibustion group, WT moxibustion group and KO moxibustion group was given a suspended moxibustion with 5 mm × 200 mm specially-made moxa stick for 20 minutes on L5 and L6 spinal cords. Kept the distance between the moxa stick and the skin where L5 and L6 spinal cords located was 10 ± 2 mm that the temperature was stabilized at 46 ± 1°C. Each mouse in MC group was intraperitoneally injected with the amount of 0.1 ml/10 g first, then after 15 minutes was given a suspended moxibustion for 20 minutes on L5 and L6 spinal cords.

All the treatments above were performed at the same day when models were successfully establishedand performed once per day for 7 days in total. During the performance, mice in the control group, model group, WT model group and KO model group were of no treatment in any way. The right hindfoot paw volumes of mice in each group were measured and recorded on Day 1, Day 2, Day 4, Day 6 and Day 8 of the experiment. After all treatments, the serum IL-1β and TNF-α level was determined by ELISA.

Results: Compared with the model group, the paw volumes in the moxibustion group was significantly decreased ($P<0.01$), simultaneously moxibustion caused a significant decrease in serum IL-1β and TNF-α levels ($P<0.01$). Compared with the model group, the paw volumes, serum IL-1β and TNF-α levels in the Moxibustion+Capsazepine (MC) group was significantly decreased ($P<0.01$); but compared with moxibustion group, the paw volumes, serum IL-1β and TNF-α levels in MC group was obviously increased with significance in between ($P<0.05$). Compared with KO control group, no changes in the paw volumes, serum IL-1β and TNF-α levels in KO moxibustion group, there was no significant difference in between ($P>0.05$).

Conclusions: TRPV1 plays a central role in the anti-inflammatory effect of moxibustion, while the effect may be lost if lacked of TRPV1-mediated.

Keywords: TRPV1; Moxibustion; Inflammation

Introduction

Moxibustion, one of tranditional Chinese medicine therapies, stimulates the body mainly in a warm/heat manner by burning moxa to alter local temperature and to activate cutaneous thermoreceptors, and thus produces its curative effect. Researchers have pointed out that the thermal stimulation is an important determination of the therapeutic efficacy of moxibustion [1]. It has been demonstrated that moxibustion of 46°Cdramatically lowered cholesterol in a mice model of acute hyperlipidemia, better than that of 38°C, indicating temperature plays a critical role in the effect of moxibustion therapy [2]. Furthermore, investigators showed there was no significant difference on the effect between medicinal cake-separated and paper pad-separated moxibustion in wheat-grain size cone moxibustion groups, implying the temperature is essential to therapeutic effect of moxibustion.

Transient receptor potential vanilloid subtype 1 (TRPV1), a heat thermoreceptor discovered in recent years, is expressed on terminals of small and medium-sized primary sensory neurons in both peripheral and central nervous system [3]. The thermal activation threshold of TRPV1 is higher than 43°C [4] and equal to the temperature of the local skin stimulated by moxibustion. The peak value of skin temperature ranged from 45.2°C to 45.5°C in ginger-separated, direct and suspended moxibustion [5]. In moxibustion applying moxibustion-box, the skin temperature averaged above 44°C when the distance was 4 cm, while ranged from 44°C to 49°C when the distance was 3 cm.

Furthermore, the animal experiments [2] showed that when the distance between the skin and the moxa stick was 35 ± 5 mm, the temperature was stabilized at 38 ± 1°C; when the distance was 10 ± 2 mm, the temperature was stabilized at 46 ± 1°C. TRPV1 was recognized as one of the thermo-sensitive cation channels [6], and such characteristic determined its necessary correlation with the therapeutic effects of moxibustion.

Inflammatory responses have been implicated in most of diseases [1], it is the main pathological basis of the therapeutic effects of moxibustion. It is universial that anti-inflammatory therapeutic effect of moxibustion is aimed at reversing the dysfunction state of inflammatory response. The universial effect is the basis of extensive clinical therapeutic function of moxibustion, which is manifested in many indications of moxibustion, including disorders of nervous, digestive, cardiocerebral vascular, and the endocrinium system, as well as the infectious diseases and tumour. It has been showed that the disease spectrum of moxibustion covered such as diarrhea, colitis, dysmenorrhea, osteoarthritis, soft tissue injury, asthma, uroschesis and herpes zoster.

Furthermore, there were studies demonstrated that long snake moxibustion can effectively relieve clinical symptoms of ankylosing spondylitis [7], while significantly downsrend I-CAM1 and TNF-α, regulating and controlling the inflammatory response. Moxibustion could up-regulate TGF-α contents expression in gastric mucosa lesion rats [8]. Atherosclerosis (AS) is a chronic inflammatory disease. Animal experiments found that moxibustion significantly decreased the levels of IL-6, IL-8 and TNF-α in chronic hyperlipidemic rats, indicating that moxibustion can effectively suppress inflammation while regulating the blood lipids [9]. Another research showed that the IL-1β and TNF-α levels in the synovial fluid of RA rabbits could be inhibited by moxibustion [10].

It has been proved that TRPV1 act as an important site of anti-inflammation and analgesia. Studies found that TRPV1 knockout mice showed enhanced LPS-induced sepsis compared with wild type [11-13]; what's more, TRPV1 showed protective effects in the inflammatory disorders of cardiovascular [12]. All of these evidences certify that TRPV1 acts to protect against the damaging impact of dieases and may influence the transition from local to a systemic inflammatory state [13].

Studies suggested administration of a TRPV1 agonist resiniferatoxin decreased TNF-α levels, and significantly attenuated the development of thermal hyperalgesia in the Streptozotocin-induced diabetes model [14]. Furthermore, application of capsaicin effectively suppressed the expression of COX-2 and mPGES-1 mRNAs, so as to attenuate the inflammatory osteoporosis and inhibit bone resorption induced by lipopolysaccharide [15].

The study was designed to study the role of TRPV1 in the anti-inflammatory effects of moxibustion. The anti-inflammatory effect of moxibustion relies on the heat stimulation; TRPV1 is an important target of anti-inflammation and analgesia, and application of TRPV1 agonists has anti-inflammatory effects; noxious heat is one of TRPV1 activators; heat stimulation higher than 43°C is in the range of the skin temperature produced by moxibustion clinically, which is equal to TRPV1 activation temperature threshold. Therefore, we made a hypothesis that TRPV1 played a central role in the anti-inflammatory effect on moxibustion. Without TRPV1 mediating, moxibustion may lose its anti-inflammatory effect.

Materials and Methods

Experimental animals

50 Kunming (KM) male mice of 32-36 g (Certificate No. of SCXK (Shanghai): 2007-0005, provided by Shanghai Slac Laboratory Animal Co., Ltd.), 16 C57BL/6 wild-type male mice of 16-20 g (Certificate No. of SCXK (Jiangsu): 2010-0001, provided by Laboratory Animal Center of Nanjing University), and 14 J003770 TRPV1 knockout male mice of 17-20 g (Certificate No. SCXK (Jiangsu): 2010-0001, provided by Laboratory Animal Center of Nanjing University). All the animals were maintained in the SPF Experimental Animals Center of Nanjing University of Chinese Medicine. Use of animals was in accordance with the Guidelines to Treat the Experimental Animals published by the Ministry of Science and Technology of People's Republic of China [16].

Reagent preparation

Freund's Adjuvant, Complete (FCA) [10 ml] Capsaicin [50 mg] Capsazepine [25 mg] 500 ml absolute ethyl alcohol, Polyoxyethylene Sorbitan (Tween80) [500 ml] and Dimethyl Sulfoxide [50 ml] were purchased from Sigma (St. Louis, MO, USA). Normal Saline [250 ml] was purchased from Guangdong Litai pharmaceutical Limited by Share Ltd (Guangdong, China). Capsaicin in powder 50 mg is dissolved in 10% polyoxyethylene sorbitan (Tween 80) and 10% ethanol before being mixed with 80% normal saline to obtain a capsaicin solution of 0.01 M [11] ; Capsazepine in powder 25 mg is dissolved in 25 ml dimethyl sulphoxide and then diluted in normal saline to obtain a capsazepine solution of 0.01 M [17].

Major experimental instruments

Paw Volume Measuring Instrument (YLS-7B, Ji Nan Yi Yan TechnologyCo., Ltd., Jinan, China), Special Moxa Stick (5 mm × 200 mm, Nanyang Chinese herbal medicine Co., Ltd., Nanyang, China), 1 ml Disposable Sterile Syringe (Changzhou medical equipment General Factory Co., Ltd., Changzhou, China), Micro Syringe (25 μL, Shanghai Precision Instrument Co., Ltd., Shanghai, China).

Experimental methods

Grouping: A total of 50 KM mice (20 ± 2 g) were randomized into 6 groups by random number table method: control group (n=10), model group (n=8), capsaicin (Cap) group (n=8), capsazepine (Cpz) group (n=8), moxibustion (Mox) group (n=8) and moxibustion+capsazepine (MC) group (n=8).

A total of 16 C57BL/6 wild-type mice (18 ± 2 g) are randomized into 2 groups by random number table method: wild-type (WT) model group and WT moxibustion group with 8 in each. Similarly, a total of

14TRPV1 knockout mice (18 ± 2 g) are randomized into 2 groups by random number table method: knockout (KO) model group and KO moxibustion group with 7 in each. Basic values of the right hindfoot paw volume of each mouse was measured and recorded.

Model establishing: Except the control group, each mouse in the other groups was intradermal injected with the amount of 20 μL of Freund's Adjuvant Complete (FCA) into right hindfoot plantar, and was observed the changes of mice paw joints.

After 24 h, the right hindfoot paw volumes of all the mice were measured and recorded by paw volume measuring instrument. According to the assessment of arthritis index score table >4 points, showing the adjuvant arthritis model in mice was successed.

Group treatments: Hair located 1 cm × 2 cm around the L5, L6 spinal cords [18] of the mice in the moxibustion group, MC group, WT moxibustion group and KO moxibustion group was cut of to expose the skin which was then disinfected by alcohol tampon. Each mouse in the capsaicin group is subcutaneously injected with the amount of 0.1 ml/10 g into the L5, L6 spinal cords.

Each mouse in the capsazepine group was intraperitoneally injected with the amount of 0.1 ml/10 g. Similarly, each mouse in the moxibustion group, WT moxibustion group and KO moxibustion group was given a suspended moxibustion with specially-made moxa stick for 20 minutes on L5 and L6 spinal cords.

Kept the distance between the moxa stick and the skin where L5 and L6 spinal cords located was 10 ± 2 mm [2]. Each mouse in MC group was intraperitoneally injected with the amount of 0.1 ml/10 g first, then after 15 minutes was given a suspended moxibustion for 20 minutes on L5 and L6 spinal cords.

All the treatments above were performed at the same day when models were successfully established and performed once per day for 7 days in total. During the performance, mice in the control group, model group, WT model group and KO model group were of no treatment in any way.

Materials: On the last day of the experiment, blood samples were taken by excising the eyeballs. Serum was extracted by centrifuging at 3000 r/min for 15 min. The supernatant was collected into a 0.5 mL Eppendorf tube and then stored at -20°C for later uses.

Indexes detection: Paw Volumes Measurement: The right hind foot paw volumes of mice in each group were measured and recorded on Day 1, Day 2, Day 4, Day 6 and Day 8 of the experiment. Serum Testing: Serum samples were sent to Nanjing KeyGen Biotech. Co., Ltd where the serum IL-1β and TNF-α level was determined by ELISA.

Statistics and analysis of datas: All data's are presented as mean ± standard deviation statistics, tested by One—Way ANOVA analysis with SPSS17.0 (SPSS, Chicago, IL, USA), and 'p' values less than 0 05 were accepted as indicating significant differences for group-group comparisons.

Results

Effect of moxibustion on AA

As shown in Tables 1, 2, Figures 1 and 2, on the eighth day, compared with the model group, the paw volumes in the capsaicin group and moxibustion group were significantly decreased (P<0.01). the serum IL-1β and TNF-α levels in the capsaicin group and moxibustion group were significantly decreased (P<0.01). Compared with the moxibustion group, the paw volume, the serum IL-1β and TNF-α levels in capsaicin group were obviously increased with significance in between (P<0.01).

	Day 1	Day 2	Day 4	Day 6	Day 8
Control group	0.255 ± 0.016	0.272 ± 0.015	0.286 ± 0.025	0.282 ± 0.039	0.280 ± 0.022
Model group	0.254 ± 0.031	0.489 ± 0.022▲	0.507 ± 0.036▲▲	0.443 ± 0.031▲▲	0.429 ± 0.028▲▲
Cap group	0.285 ± 0.016	0.485 ± 0.022▲▲	0.402 ± 0.022▲▲**	0.406 ± 0.034▲▲	0.363 ± 0.019▲▲**##
Mox group	0.273 ± 0.024	0.486 ± 0.041▲▲	0.409 ± 0.065▲▲**	0.388 ± 0.031▲▲**	0.323 ± 0.043▲▲**

Notice: Control and Model: no treatment; Cpsaicin: subcutaneous injection with the amount of 0.1 ml/10 g capsaicin into the L5-L6 segment; Moxibustion: a suspended moxibustion with a specially-made moxa stick for 20 minutes on L5-L6 segment. Compared with the control group, ▲P<0.05, ▲▲P<0.01; Compared with the model group, *P<0.05, **P<0.01; compared with the moxibustion group,#P<0.05,##P<0.01.

Table 1: Comparisons of paw volumes in each group (ml).

	Control group	Model group	Cap group	Mox group
IL-1β	31.39 ± 1.86	83.45 ± 8.61▲▲	47.76 ± 2.22▲▲**##	34.65 ± 3.74▲▲**
TNF-α	24.82 ± 1.65	66.29 ± 3.44▲▲	36.01 ± 1.31▲▲**##	31.00 ± 1.22▲▲**

Notice: Control and Model: no treatment; Cpsaicin: subcutaneous injection with the amount of 0.1 ml/10 g capsaicin into the L5-L6 segment; Moxibustion: a suspended moxibustion with a specially-made moxa stick for 20 minutes on L5-L6 segment. Compared with the control group, ▲P<0.05, ▲▲P<0.01; Compared with the model group, *P<0.05, **P<0.01; compared with the moxibustion group, #P<0.05,##P<0.01.

Table 2: Comparisons of inflammatory factors in each group (pg/ml).

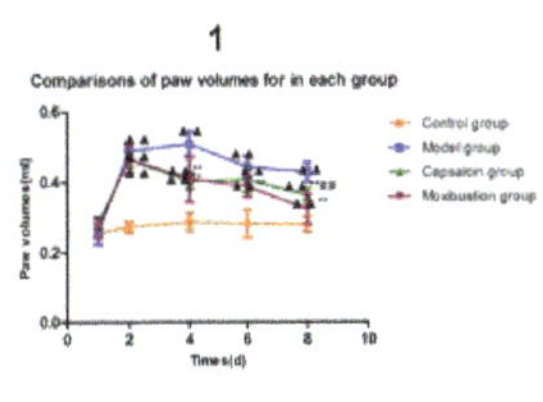

Figure 1: Data of inflammatory factors were presented as mean ± SEM (n=8) by histogram. Control and model group were of no treatment; capsaicin group was treated with subcutaneous injection of 0.1 ml/10 g capsaicin into the L5-L6 segment; moxibustion group was given a suspended moxibustion with a specially-made moxa stick for 20 minutes on L5-L6 segment. Data of paw volumes were presented as mean ± SEM (n=8) by curve graph.

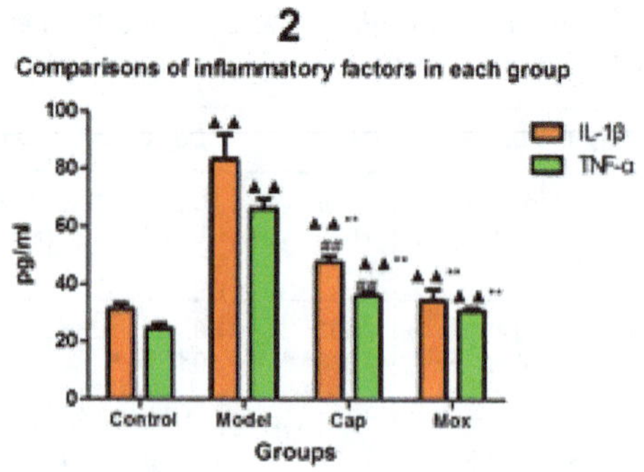

Figure 2: Significant differences compared with control group: ▲P<0.05,▲▲P<0.01; compared with model group: *P<0.05, **P<0.01, and compared with moxibustion group: #P<0.05, ##P<0.01. Control and model group were of no treatment; capsaicin group was treated with subcutaneous injection of 0.1 ml/10 g capsaicin into the L5-L6 segment; moxibustion group was given a suspended moxibustion with a specially-made moxa stick for 20 minutes on L5-L6 segment. Data of paw volumes were presented as mean ± SEM (n=8) by curve graph.

Effect of moxibustion on AA after pretreatment by capsazepine

As shown in Tables 3, 4, Figures 3 and 4, compared with the model group, the paw volumes, the serum IL-1β and TNF-α levels in the capsazepine group, moxibustion group and MC group were significantly decreased (P<0.01).

Compared with the moxibustion group, the paw volumes, the serum IL-1β and TNF-α levels in MC group was obviously increased with significance in between (P<0.01).

	Day 1	Day 2	Day 4	Day 6	Day 8
Control group	0.255 ± 0.016	0.272 ± 0.015	0.286 ± 0.025	0.282 ± 0.039	0.280 ± 0.022
Model group	0.254 ± 0.031	0.489 ± 0.022▲▲	0.507 ± 0.036▲▲	0.443 ± 0.031▲▲	0.429 ± 0.028▲▲
Cpz group	0.269 ± 0.034	0.486 ± 0.061▲▲	0.396 ± 0.043▲▲**	0.411 ± 0.036▲▲	0.343 ± 0.022▲▲**
Mox group	0.273 ± 0.024	0.486 ± 0.041▲▲	0.409 ± 0.065▲▲**	0.388 ± 0.031▲▲**	0.323 ± 0.043▲▲**
MC group	0.296 ± 0.020	0.489 ± 0.030▲▲	0.440 ± 0.015▲▲**	0.400 ± 0.031▲▲*	0.354 ± 0.023▲▲** #

Notice: Control and Model: no treatment; Capsazepine: intraperitoneal injection with the amount of 0.1 ml/10 g capsazepine; Moxibustion: a suspended moxibustion with a specially-made moxa stick for 20 minutes on L5 and L6 spinal cords; MC: intraperitoneal injection with the amount of 0.1 ml/10 g capsazepine first, and then a suspended moxibustion for 20 min on L5-L6 segment after a 15 min interval. Compared with the control group, ▲P<0.05, ▲▲P<0.01; Compared with the model group, *P<0.05, **P<0.01; compared with the moxibustion group,#P<0.05,##P<0.01.

Table 3: Comparisons of paw volumes in each group (ml).

	Control group	Model group	Cpz group	Mox group	MC group
IL-1β	31.39 ± 1.86	83.45 ± 8.61▲▲	50.55 ± 1.27▲▲** ##	34.65 ± 3.74▲▲**	71.02 ± 1.85▲▲**##
TNF-α	24.82 ± 1.65	66.29 ± 3.44▲▲	37.18 ± 1.08▲▲** ##	31.00 ± 1.22▲▲**	51.85 ± 1.61▲▲**##

Notice: Control and Model: no treatment; Capsazepine: intraperitoneal injection with the amount of 0.1 ml/10 g capsazepine; Moxibustion: a suspended moxibustion with a specially-made moxa stick for 20 minutes on L5 and L6 spinal cords; MC: intraperitoneal injection with the amount of 0.1 ml/10 g capsazepine first, and then a suspended moxibustion for 20 min on L5-L6 segment after a 15 min interval. Compared with the control group, ▲P<0.05, ▲▲P<0.01; Compared with the model group, *P<0.05, **P<0.01; compared with the moxibustion group, #P<0.05,##P<0.01

Table 4: Comparisons of inflammatory factors in each group (pg/ml).

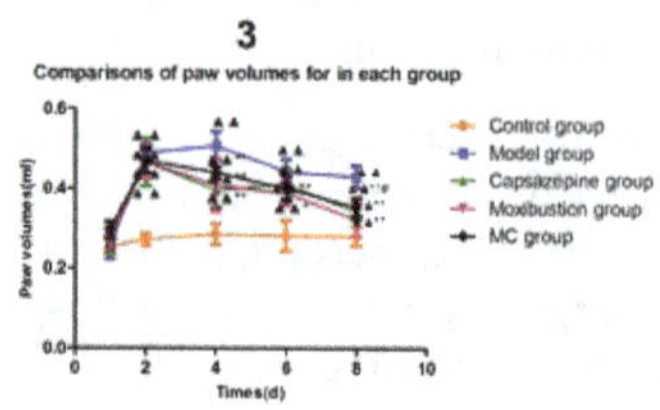

Figure 3: Data of inflammatory factors were presented as mean ± SEM (n=8) by histogram. Control and Model group: no treatment; Capsazepine: intraperitoneal injection with the amount of 0.1 ml/10 g; Moxibustion: a suspended moxibustion with specially-made moxa stick for 20 minutes on L5 and L6 spinal cords; MC: intraperitoneal injection with the amount of 0.1 ml/10 g capsazepine first, and then a suspended moxibustion for 20 min on L5-L6 segment after a 15 min interval. Data of paw volumes were presented as mean ± SEM (n=8) by curve graph.

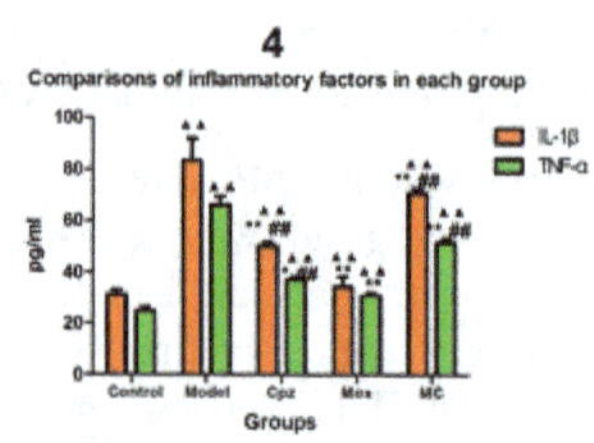

Figure 4: Significant differences compared with control group: ▲P<0.05,▲▲P<0.01; compare with model group:* P<0.05,**P<0.01, and compared with moxibustion group : #P<0.05, ##P<0.01. Control and Model group: no treatment; Capsazepine: intraperitoneal injection with the amount of 0.1 ml/10 g; Moxibustion: a suspended moxibustion with specially-made moxa stick for 20 minutes on L5 and L6 spinal cords; MC: intraperitoneal injection with the amount of 0.1 ml/10 g capsazepine first, and then a suspended moxibustion for 20 min on L5-L6 segment after a 15 min interval. Data of paw volumes were presented as mean ± SEM (n=8) by curve graph.

Effect of moxibustion on AA in wild-type groups and TRPV1 knockout groups

As shown in Tables 5, 6, Figures 5 and 6, compared with WT model group, on the eighth day, the paw volumes, the serum IL-1β and TNF-α levels in WT moxibustion group had been decreased significantly (P<0.01); compared with KO model group, no changes in the paw volumes, the serum IL-1β and TNF-α levels in KO moxibustion group, there were no significant difference in between (P>0.05).

	Day 1	Day 2	Day 4	Day 6	Day 8
WT model group	0.171 ± 0.012	0.256 ± 0.014	0.262 ± 0.018	0.311 ± 0.029	0.302 ± 0.016
WT mox group	0.177 ± 0.010	0.250 ± 0.019	0.253 ± 0.019	0.286 ± 0.014	0.259 ± 0.017**
KO model group	0.153 ± 0.011	0.283 ± 0.016	0.280 ± 0.015	0.290 ± 0.025	0.292 ± 0.003
KO mox group	0.159 ± 0.008	0.287 ± 0.033	0.288 ± 0.018	0.286 ± 0.012	0.280 ± 0.010

Notice: WT model: no treatment; WT moxibustion: a suspended moxibustion with a specially-made moxa stick for 20 min on L5-L6 segment; KO model: no treatment; KO moxibustion: a suspended moxibustion for 20 min on L5-L6 segment.

Compared with the WT model group, *P<0.05,**P<0.01; compared with the KO model group, ΔP<0.05, ΔΔP<0.01.

Table 5: Comparisons of paw volumes of mice in wild-type groups and TRPV1 knockout groups.

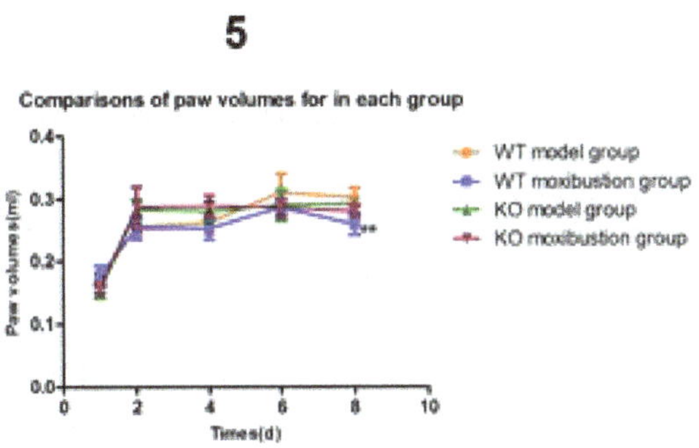

Figure 5: Data of inflammatory factors were presented as mean ± SEM (WT: n=8, KO: n=7) by histogram.
WT model group was of no treatment; WT moxibustion group was given a suspended moxibustion with a specially-made moxa stick for 20 min on L5-L6 segment; KO model group was of no treatment; KO moxibustion group was given a suspended moxibustion for 20 min on L5-L6 segment. Data of paw volumes were presented as mean ± SEM (WT: n=8, KO: n=7) by curve graph.

	WT model group	WT mox group	KO model group	KO mox group
IL-1β	82.93 ± 3.39	65.99 ± 5.45**	79.98 ± 1.67	75.44 ± 2.05
TNF-α	58.63 ± 1.96	38.06 ± 1.52**	44.98 ± 1.95	44.39 ± 2.01

Notice: WT model: no treatment; WT moxibustion: a suspended moxibustion with a specially-made moxa stick for 20 min on L5-L6 segment; KO model: no treatment; KO moxibustion: a suspended moxibustion for 20 min on L5-L6 segment. Compared with the WT model group, * P<0.05,**P<0.01; compared with the KO model group, ΔP<0.05, ΔΔP<0.01.

Table 6: Comparisons of inflammatory factors of mice in wild-type groups and TRPV1 knockout groups.

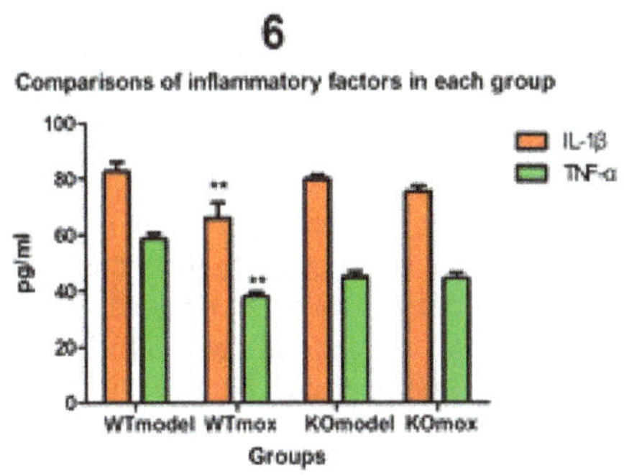

Figure 6: Significant differences compared with the WT model group: * P<0.05, **P<0.01, and with the KO model group: ΔP<0.05, ΔΔP<0.01. WT model group was of no treatment; WT moxibustion group was given a suspended moxibustion with a specially-made moxa stick for 20 min on L5-L6 segment; KO model group was of no treatment; KO moxibustion group was given a suspended moxibustion for 20 min on L5-L6 segment. Data of paw volumes were presented as mean ± SEM (WT: n=8, KO: n=7) by curve graph.

Discussion

TRPV1 has been shown to play a pivotal role in inflammatory conditions [6]. Therefore, TRPV1 is a promising target for development of inflammation [19].

AA was used as the animal model for the study. After 24 h by injection of FCA, mice appeared the acute inflammatory response, which was showed foot joint red and swollen AA and human RA have many similar clinlcal symptoms and dysimmunity, which is suitable for the study of peripheral inflammation.

TRPV1 played an important role in the progress of inflammation, which is the hub of almost all the inflammatory especially neuronal inflammatory signaling pathways. During tissue injury and inflammation, TRPV1 functions as a sensor of the detecting irritants by transmitting noxious stimuli to the central nervous system and inducing the release of a variety of pro-inflammatory neuropeptides (such as CGRP and Substance P) and regulating proinflammatory cytokines (such as IL-1β and TNF-α) at the peripheral terminal [11], at the same time, regulating the release of anti-inflammatory cytokines (such as somatostatin) [12].

Moxibustion showed anti-inflammatory effects on mice with adjuvant arthritis. TRPV1 played an important role during the progress of treatments. In the first part of our experiment, on day 8, compared with the model group, paw volumes in the capsaicin group and moxibustion group were significantly decreased (P<0.01); what's more, paw volumes of moxibustion group were much lower than that of capsaicin group. Tsuji et al. [20] found that application of TRPV1 agonist could suppress the generation of TNF-α and IL-1β as well as TNF-α and IL-1β mRNA expression, which is consisted with the results of serum TNF-α and IL-1β levels determined in our experiment.

Compared with the model group, capsaicin and moxibustion can both significantly reduce serum levels of IL-1β and TNF-α (P<0.01). In addition, compared with the capsaicin group, IL-1β and TNF-α levels of moxibustion group were much lower (P<0.01) (Table 2). Results mentioned above showed that, 1) moxibustion had an anti-inflammatory effect. Studies have found that repeated or prolonged application of TRPV1 agonists capsaicin could induce anti-inflammatory properties [21], while capsaicin and heat>43°C may have a common molecular pathway [22]. Based on what's mentioned above, we propose that repeated application of heat stimulation produced by moxibustion could generate the same anti-inflammatory effect as capsaicin did. Schumacher [23] revealed several mechanisms of anti-inflammatory and analgesic effects of TRPV1 agonists that are overlapping and complementary, including desensitization, nociceptor dysfunction, neuropeptide depletion, and nerve terminal destruction. Among these mechanisms, dysfunction of nociceptive receptors may be the most important role in the effects of analgesia therapy 2).

The anti-inflammatory effect of moxibustion may be better than that of capsaicin. In our experiment, paw volumes as well as TNF-a and IL-1β levels of moxibustion group were both much lower than that of capsaicin group. In our experiment, paw volumes as well as TNF-a and IL-1β levels of moxibustion group were both much lower than capsaicine group. The anti-inflammatory effect of capsaicin is dose-dependent [24] and the dose we administrated in the experiment may be too low to exhibit the anti-inflammatory effect of moxibustion was better than that of capsaicin.

The anti-inflammatory effects disappeared if TRPV1 antagonist was applied during moxibustion. During the second part of our experiment, we explored the effect of moxibustion on adjuvant arthritis after pretreatment by capsazepine. Some studies had demonstrated the effect of capsaicin could be completely blocked by TRPV1 antagonist capsazepine [25], so we did not set up capsaicin +capsazepine group in our experiment. Results of paw volumes showed that, on day 8, compared with model group, the paw volumes of moxibustion group, MC group and capsazepine group were significantly decreased (P<0.01), which suggested all moxibustion, capsazepine and MC group had the effect of reducing paw volumes.

MC group and moxibustion group were significantly different (P<0.05), and the paw volumes of MC group were higher than moxibustion group, prompting capsazepine might partly antagonized the effects of moxibustion (Table 3). The results of inflammatory factors IL-1β and TNF-α level showed consistent outcomes. The IL-1β and TNF-α levels of MC group was far lower than that of model group (P<0.01), but higher than moxibustion (P<0.01) and capsazepine group (P<0.01) (Table 4). The anti-inflammatory effect of moxibustion was slightly decreased by the pretreatment with capsazepine. Mcintyre Peter's [26] animal experiments and Istvan Nagy's [27] cell experiments both revealed that capsazepine was just a weak inhibitor of the heat response mediated by TRPV1 receptor, and this conclusion also supports our results. All the results indicate that TRPV1 was participated in the anti-inflammatory effect of moxibustion.

The anti-inflammatory effects disappeared too on TRPV1 knockout mice. To further confirm the anti-inflammatory effect of moxibustion was mediated by TRPV1, we used wildtype C57BL/6 mice and TRPV1 knockout mice for the third part of the experiments. Results of paw volumes showed that, on day 8, compared with WT model group, paw volumes in WT moxibustion group were significantly decreased (P<0.01), while KO moxibustion group and KO model group had no difference (P>0.05) (Table 5). Serum levels of IL-1β and TNF-α also reflected the WT moxibustion group and WT model group were significantly different (P<0.01); yet KO moxibustion group and KO model group were not (P>0.05).

TRPV1 itself is a heat sensor [22], TRPV1 knockout mice exhibited reduced thermal nociception [28], which showed that TRPV1 was necessary for reactions to noxious thermal stimuli [29]. Therefore, there was no difference between the KO model group and KO moxibustion group in our experiments, suggesting that anti-inflammatory effect of moxibustion was TRPV1-mediated, in other words, moxibustion would lose its anti-inflammatory effect if lacking TRPV1. In addition, the TRPV1-deficient mice showed impaired responses to noxious thermal stimuli only over 50°C [22], and the peak value of skin temperature was only 45.2°C ~45.5°C [5] during moxibustion, which could partly explain why there were no significant difference between KO moxibustion group and KO model group.

Sato A found that acupuncture-like stimulation can regulate various visceral functions by reflex responses, which had the segmental features via studying the neuromechanism of regulating effects of acupuncture-like stimulation on visceral functions [30]. In addition, there were studies showed that the muscles and skin of the lower limbs were controlled by nerve segments of L4~S2 spinal cord and the stimulation on the Houhui" points located on the inside of parapophysis of sixth lumbar could regulate the lower limb functions. Kelly's animal experiments [18] also revealed that ligation of L5 and L6 spinal nerve would result in partial deafferentation of the hindpaw. The researches mentioned above suggested that segmental innervations was one of the rules of how acupuncture functioned [31], according to which, we selected the area of L5 and L6 spinal cords as the point for moxibustion and capsaicin injection.

During the inflammation, the sensibilization of TRPV1 promotes the inflammatory hyperpathia [32]. A number of studies had proved that TRPV1 antagonists could increase the noxious heat pain threshold [33] and inhibit thermal hyperalgesia [34] by suppressing the expression of TRPV1 and so that it showed the anti-inflammatory effect in different inflammatory and neuropathic pain models [35]. Repeated or prolonged application of TRPV1 agonists also showed anti-inflammatory effect.

In vivo inflammatory disorders, TRPV1 agonists may play a role of anti-inflammatory and immunoregulation [20]. The inflammatory responses induced by TNF-α could be lightened via TRPV1 agonists, but aggravated by TRPV1 antagonists [36]. It had been proved that repeated capsaicin application to the skin produces a degeneration of epidermal nerve fibers [37] that may underlie the effects of TRPV1 agonists. Schumacher considered that nerve terminal destruction may be the most important role in the effects of anti-inflammatory and analgesia therapy [23].

The thermal stimulation is the most important determination of the therapeutic efficacy of moxibustion. Temperature plays a critical role in the effect of moxibustion therapy. The temperature produced by moxibustion ranges from 34°C to 57°C, consistent with the thermal activation thresholds of TRPV1-4. The peak value of skin temperature ranged from 45.2°C to 45.5°C in suspended moxibustion. In addition, synthesizing the former results of our research team, we kept the distance between the skin and the moxa stick of 10 ± 2 mm, so that the temperature was stabilized at 46 ± 1°C. A certain quantity (amount) of moxibustion is the basic guarantee of efficacy, it is common to increase moxibustion quantity to improve the curative effect in clinical.

The essence of various methods of moxibustion therapy is to achieve a certain intensity of thermal stimulation via space (area or distance) to reach the amount required in the treatment through the extension along the time axis. Accumulated times of treatment are able to increase moxibustion intensity of a single treatment, with constant temperature and area. During the experiment, we applied moxibustion 10 minutes a day for 7 days, accumulating the number of days to achieve the anti-inflammatory effect, just like the repeated application of capsaicin.

Expression of TRPV1 up-regulates in the inflammatory conditions. The therapy of anti-inflammation mediated by TRPV1 has been widely used in clinical practice. The anti-inflammation therapeutic effect of TRPV1 antagonist is mainly depending on suppressing TRPV1 expression. Application of TRPV1 agonist capsaicin in anti-inflammation currently has been presented in the circulatory system and kidney disease [38], autoimmune disease, inflammatory bowel disease [15] and so on.

However, both agonists and antagonists have inevitable side effects. Capsaicin can't be administered systemically because of its adverse effects, such as a burning sensation and Bezold-Jarisch reflex in the initial phase of bradycardia and hypopnea [35]. Likewise, the usage of TRPV1 antagonists can induce the risk of accidental burns [3], causing scald [33], meanwhile the anti-inflammatory role of TRPV1 by potent antagonists may lead to aggravation of the disease [12]. Heat stimulation of moxibustion exerts its TRPV1-mediated anti-inflammatory effect in the local place through the neuroimmunoendocrinology network, which has a great advantage of safety and no side effects.

Conclusions

TRPV1 is the target of anti-inflammatory and analgesic therapy. The TRPV1 antagonists (such as capsazepine) exert theirs anti-inflammatory effect via suppressing the TRPV1 expression, while repeated application of TRPV1 pharmacologic agonists (such as capsaicin) via producing a destruction or desensitization in the terminal of nociceptive receptors. As one of the physical agonists of TRPV1, heat stimulation of moxibustion exerts its TRPV1- mediated anti-inflammatory effect. TRPV1 plays a important role in the anti-inflammatory effect of moxibustion. Without the mediation of TRPV1, moxibustion lost its anti-inflammatory effect.

Acknowledgment

The paper was supported by National key basic research program 973 (no. 2011CB505206), 2013 Jiangsu Province Education Department of Natural Science Research of major projects (no. 13KJA360001), Academic propagate project on scientific and technical innovation team, Nanjing University of Chinese Medicine 2013 scientific and technical innovation team project. JFJ designed the study. JJL and YJcarried out the animal experiments, XJW participated in the serum IL-1β and TNF-α level decetion by ELISA. JJL performed the statistical analysis and drafted the manuscript. All authors read and approved the final manuscript.

References

1. Jiang JF, Wang LL, Bin X, Ling H, Song XG, et al. (2013) [Anti-inflammatory: effect mechanism of warming-dredging in moxibustion]. Zhongguo Zhen Jiu 33: 860-864.
2. Wang GY, Wang LL, Xu B, Zhang JB, Jiang JF (2013) Effects of Moxibustion Temperature on Blood Cholesterol Level in a Mice Model of Acute Hyperlipidemia: Role of TRPV1. Evid Based Complement Alternat Med 2013: 871704.
3. Surowy CS, Neelands TR, Bianchi BR, McGaraughty S, Kouhen REI (2008) " (R)- (5-tert-butyl-2,3-dihydro-1H-inden-1-yl)-3- (1H-indazol-4-yl)-urea (ABT-102) blocks polymodal activation of transient receptor potential vanilloid 1 receptors in vitro and heat-evoked firing of spinal dorsal horn neurons in vivo". J PHARMACOL EXP THER 326: 879-888
4. Vay L, Gu C, McNaughton PA (2012) The thermo-TRP ion channel family: properties and therapeutic implications. Br J Pharmacol 165: 787-801.
5. Dong XM, Dong QS, Xian MQ, Zheng XL, Zhang SH (1999) Observation on comparison of effects of different moxibustion to acupoint temperature. Chinese Acupuncture & Moxibustion: 22-26
6. Sooampon S, Phoolcharoen W, Pavasant P (2013) Thermal stimulation of TRPV1 up-regulates TNFα expression in human periodontal ligament cells. Arch Oral Biol 58: 887-895.
7. Li WG, Tu Q, Gu XJ (2010) [Effect on content of serum inflammatory cytokines of patients with ankylosing spondylitis in early stage treated by long snake moxibustion at Governor Vessel and functional exercise]. Zhongguo Zhen Jiu 30: 200-202.
8. Lin YP, Feng YS, Shi DM, Hou YL (2013) Effect of Moxibustion treatment on the level of cytokine in gastric tissue homogenate of the rats with Hp gastritis. Chinese Journal of Immunology 29: 900-909
9. Ji MY, Wang LL, Jiang JF, Zhou XY, Ma MY (2013) Effect of warming moxibustion on oxidative stress-inflmmatory response in rats with hyperlipemia. China Journal of Traditional Chinese Medicine and Pharmacy 28: 2301-2304
10. Yang HQ, Liu XG, Yang X, Chen T, Yu SG (2013) [Effect of different types of moxibustion intervention on expression of inflammatory cytokines IL-1 and TNF-alpha in rabbits with rheumatoid arthritis]. Zhen Ci Yan Jiu 38: 134-139.
11. Couto M, de Diego A, Perpiñi M, Delgado L, Moreira A (2013) Cough reflex testing with inhaled capsaicin and TRPV1 activation in asthma and comorbid conditions. J Investig Allergol Clin Immunol 23: 289-301.
12. Devesa I, Planells-Cases R, Fernández-Ballester G, González-Ros JM, Ferrer-Montiel A (2011) "Role of the transient receptor potential vanilloid 1 in inflammation and sepsis". Journal of Inflammation Research 4: 67-81
13. Fernandes ES, Liang L, Smillie SJ, Kaiser F, Purcell R (2012) TRPV1 Deletion Enhances Local Inflammation and Accelerates the Onset of Systemic Inflammatory Response Syndrome. The Journal of Immunology 188: 5741-5751
14. Bishnoi M, Bosgraaf CA, Abooj M, Zhong LL, Premkumar LS (2011) Streptozotocin-Induced Early Thermal Hyperalgesia is independent of Glycemic State of Rats: Role of Transient Receptor Potential Vanilloid 1 (TRPV1) and Inflammatory mediators. MOL PAIN 7: 52
15. Kobayashi M, Watanabe K, Yokoyama S, Matsumoto C, Hirata M, et al. (2012) Capsaicin, a TRPV1 Ligand, Suppresses Bone Resorption by Inhibiting the Prostaglandin E Production of Osteoblasts, and Attenuates the Inflammatory Bone Loss Induced by Lipopolysaccharide. ISRN Pharmacol 2012: 439860.

16. Wang JF, Zhou Y, Liu JH, Lu JQ, Ge LJ, et al. (2006) Guidance Suggestions for the Care and Use of Laboratory Animals. The Ministry of Science and Technology of the People's Republic of China.

17. Nguyen TL, Nam YS, Lee SY, Kim HC, Jang CG (2010) Effects of capsazepine, a transient receptor potential vanilloid type 1 antagonist, on morphine-induced antinociception, tolerance, and dependence in mice. BRIT J ANAESTH 105: 668-674

18. Kelly S, Chapman V (2002) Effects of peripheral nerve injury on functional spinal VR1 receptors. Neuroreport 13: 1147-1150.

19. Lee JY, Shin TJ, Choi JM, Seo KS, Kim HJ, et al. (2013) Antinociceptive curcuminoid, KMS4034, effects on inflammatory and neuropathic pain likely via modulating TRPV1 in mice. Br J Anaesth 111: 667-672.

20. Tsuji F, Murai M, Oki K, Seki I, Ueda K, et al. (2010) Transient receptor potential vanilloid 1 agonists as candidates for anti-inflammatory and immunomodulatory agents. Eur J Pharmacol 627: 332-339.

21. Shin YH, Namkoong E, Choi S, Bae JS, Jin M, et al. (2013) Capsaicin regulates the NF-κB pathway in salivary gland inflammation. J Dent Res 92: 547-552.

22. Tominaga M, Caterina MJ (2004) Thermosensation and pain. J Neurobiol 61: 3-12.

23. Schumacher MA (2010) Transient receptor potential channels in pain and inflammation: therapeutic opportunities. Pain Pract 10: 185-200.

24. O'Neill J, Brock C, Olesen AE, Andresen T, Nilsson M, et al. (2012) Unravelling the mystery of capsaicin: a tool to understand and treat pain. Pharmacol Rev 64: 939-971.

25. Kwak J (2012) Capsaicin Blocks the Hyperpolarization-Activated Inward Currents via TRPV1 in the Rat Dorsal Root Ganglion Neurons. Exp Neurobiol 21: 75-82.

26. McIntyre P, McLatchie LM, Chambers A, Phillips E, Clarke M, et al. (2001) Pharmacological differences between the human and rat vanilloid receptor 1 (VR1). Br J Pharmacol 132: 1084-1094.

27. Nagy I, Rang HP (1999) Similarities and differences between the responses of rat sensory neurons to noxious heat and capsaicin. J Neurosci 19: 10647-10655.

28. Cui M, Honore P, Zhong C, Gauvin D, Mikusa J, et al. (2006) TRPV1 receptors in the CNS play a key role in broad-spectrum analgesia of TRPV1 antagonists. J Neurosci 26: 9385-9393.

29. Asai H, Ozaki N, Shinoda M, Nagamine K, Tohnai I, et al. (2005) Heat and mechanical hyperalgesia in mice model of cancer pain. Pain 117: 19-29.

30. Sato A, Sato Y, Uchida S (2002) Reflex modulation of visceral functions by acupuncture—like stimulation in anesthetized rats. International Congress Series 1238: 111-123

31. Zhang Y, Yu Y, Meng Q, Li J (2011) Effects of electro-aupuncturing different neurosegmental acu-points on intragastric pressure of gastric motility abnormalities in rats. Journal of TCM Univ?of Hunan 31: 65-68

32. Vetter I, Cheng W, Peiris M, Wyse BD, Roberts-Thomson SJ (2008) Rapid, Opioid-sensitive Mechanisms Involved in Transient Receptor Potential Vanilloid 1 Sensitization. The Journal Of Biological Chemistry 283: 19540-19550

33. Brederson JD, Kym PR, Szallasi A (2013) Targeting TRP channels for pain relief. Eur J Pharmacol 716: 61-76.

34. Urano H, Ara T, Fujinami Y, Hiraoka BY (2012) Aberrant TRPV1 expression in heat hyperalgesia associated with trigeminal neuropathic pain. Int J Med Sci 9: 690-697.

35. Watabiki T, Kiso T, Kuramochi T, Yonezawa K, Tsuji N (2011) Amelioration of Neuropathic Pain by Novel Transient Receptor Potential Vanilloid 1 Antagonist AS1928370 in Rats without Hyperthermic Effect. The Journal Of Pharmacology And Experimental Therapeutics 336: 743-750

36. Zhao JF, Ching LC, Kou YR, Lin SJ, Wei J, et al. (2013) Activation of TRPV1 prevents OxLDL-induced lipid accumulation and TNF-α-induced inflammation in macrophages: role of liver X receptor α. Mediators Inflamm 2013: 925171.

37. Vyklický L, Nováková-Toušová K, Benedikt J, Samad A, Touška F (2008) Calcium-Dependent Desensitization of Vanillo id Receptor TRPV1: A Mechanism Possibly Involved in Analgesia Induced by Topical Application of Capsaicin. PHYSIOL RES 57: 59-68

38. Tsuji F, Aono H (2012) Role of transient receptor potential vanilloid 1 in inflammation and autoimmune diseases. Pharmaceuticals (Basel) 5: 837-852.

11

Tolerability and Treatment Effects of *Pelargonium sidoides* Preparation EPs 7630 in Adults Suffering from Acute *Rhinopharyngitis*

Keck T[1*], Strobl A[2] and Stracke B[3]

[1]*Department of ENT Medicine, Head and Neck Surgery, Krankenhaus, Elisabethinen GmbH Graz, Austria*
[2]*Department of ENT Medicine, Head and Neck Surgery, Krankenhaus der Barmherzigen Schwestern Linz Betriebsgesellschaft m.b.H, Linz, Austria*
[3]*Department of Clinical Research, Dr. Willmar Schwabe GmbH & Co. KG, Karlsruhe, Germany*

Abstract

Background: EPs 7630 has already been proven effective in acute rhinopharyngitis (ARP) and other acute respiratory diseases. We conducted an open-label, non-comparative, interventional multicenter study to obtain additional information on the tolerability and effectiveness of EPs 7630 in a clinical practice setting.

Methods: 120 adults with clinical ARP diagnosis and at least 2 out of a set of 10 common cold symptoms received 3 × 1 film-coated 20 mg EPs 7630 tablet daily, for 10 days. Assessment of tolerability and safety was based on adverse event (AE) elicitation and safety laboratory measures. The intensity of ARP-associated symptoms was assessed daily and treatment outcome and satisfaction were evaluated.

Results: At treatment end, 42% of patients were completely recovered, 42% showed major improvements. The majority of patients were satisfied with treatment. Over-all AE incidences were 0.017 (all AEs) and 0.010 (potentially related AEs) events/day of exposure. Most common events were gastrointestinal complaints and skin reactions. None of the events were serious.

Conclusions: The results confirm the excellent tolerability of EPs 7630. Potentially attributable AEs were limited to the drug's known spectrum of adverse effects. The majority of patients showed a favorable course of ARP which is unlikely to be explained by the natural course of the disease alone.

Keywords: *Pelargonium sidoides*; Common cold; Clinical trial; Tolerability; Bacterial and viral analysis; Treatment for the common cold

Introduction

The common cold or acute rhinopharyngitis (ARP), respectively, is characterized by nasal stuffiness and discharge, sneezing, sore throat, and cough. Symptoms peak 2-3 days after the onset of infection, with some symptoms, e.g. coughs and general discomfort, persisting for up to 3 weeks [1]. On average, adults suffer from 2-3 episodes of ARP per year, leading to time off work [2]. Consequently the economic burden resulting from lost productivity and expenditures for treatment is enormous [3,4].

It is estimated that at least 90% of ARP infections are caused by viruses [5-7] such as rhinovirus, corona virus, and respiratory syncytial virus (RSV) [8]. The pathogenesis of ARP involves a complex interplay between replicating viruses and inflammatory response of the host. Viral infection of the nasal mucosa results in vasodilatation and increased vascular permeability, which in turn cause nasal obstruction and rhinorrhea. Cholinergic stimulation leads to increased mucous gland secretion and sneezing [9]. The mechanism by which the viral infection of the common cold engenders cough is unclear [10]. However, an association among cough, throat clearing, and postnasal drip has been demonstrated [11]. Moreover, due to the inflammation of the nasal mucosa, the ostia of the paranasal sinuses and the Eustachian tubes may become obstructed, abetting the development of secondary inflammation such as sinusitis or otitis media [12].

Transmission of ARP is mostly achieved through hand-to-hand contact, with subsequent passage to the nostrils or eyes [13]. Current treatment strategies for ARP aim at relieving symptoms, shortening the illness, and reducing complications as well as the infectivity to others [2]. Due to the predominantly viral etiology of ARP, treatment with antibiotics, that is still quite common in clinical practice, is inappropriate and can be even harmful. As antibiotic treatment has the potential of causing adverse reactions and increasing antibiotic resistance [2], treatment options that are efficacious in reducing the symptom burden of the patient and accelerating remission without causing bothersome adverse effects have gained interest during recent years.

EPs® 7630[1] is a herbal drug preparation from the roots of *Pelargonium sidoides*, a medicinal plant grown in South Africa. The product is available in both tablet and liquid forms for the treatment of acute respiratory tract infections, such as ARP or acute bronchitis. It is marketed in several countries in Asia, Europe, Australia, as well as Central and South America.

Pharmacological activities of EPs 7630 and several of its isolated constituents have been demonstrated in in-vitro studies. They include

[1]EPs® 7630 is the active ingredient of the product Umckaloabo® (ISO Arzneimittel, Ettlingen, Germany)

***Corresponding author:** Tilman Keck, Krankenhaus der Elisabethinen Graz GmbH, Elisabethinergasse 14, 8020 Graz, Austria, E-mail: Tilman.Keck@elisabethinen.at

a moderate direct antibacterial and antiviral action as well as notable immune-modulatory capabilities [14]. The latter are mediated mainly by the release of tumor necrosis factor α and nitric oxides, the stimulation of interferon-β, and an increase in natural killer cell activity [15-18]. Biological activities include an improved phagocytosis, oxidative burst and intracellular killing by human peripheral blood phagocytes, as well as an inhibition of the interaction between group-A streptococci and host epithelia [19,20] and increased stress resistance [21]. A potent HIV 1 attachment inhibition by EPs 7630 has been shown by Helfer et al. [22]. Moreover, EPs 7630 was shown to interfere with the replication of seasonal influenza A virus strains (H1N1, H3N2), respiratory syncytial virus, human coronavirus, parainfluenza virus, and coxsackie virus [23]. Anti-influenza virus activity of the herbal extract was also confirmed in an animal model [24].

The efficacy of EPs 7630 in the treatment of acute respiratory tract infections has been investigated in several controlled clinical trials, the majority of which have been performed in the indication of acute bronchitis, while studies are also available for acute rhinosinusitis, acute tonsillopharyngitis, and in ARP. For these conditions, systematic reviews indicate significant advantages of EPs 7630 over placebo [25-28].The existing information regarding the tolerability and safety of EPs 7630 has been derived mainly from randomized, controlled trials whose primary objective was to investigate the efficacy of the extract, as well as from post-marketing surveillance studies [29]. Clinical trials provide a high degree of control of the experimental setting and are performed in patient populations appropriate for meeting the primary objectives of the study. Post-marketing surveillance projects, on the other hand, are non-interventional by nature and are thus subject to limitations with respect to a standardized treatment or visit schedule, etc. An interventional post-marketing trial in the registered indication may thus provide valuable safety and effectiveness information in a clinical real-life setting which we consider to be important for physicians and their patients [30]. We present the results of an open-label, non-comparative, phase IV clinical trial designed to obtain further information on the tolerability and effectiveness of EPs 7630 in a clinical practice setting, as well as to gain further insight into the bacterial and viral flora in patients suffering from the common cold. In accordance with the design, this study was not intended for demonstrating treatment efficacy, but to investigate the performance of the drug in a 'real-life' situation, yet under the well-defined conditions of an interventional trial.

Materials and Methods

Protocol and design, objectives

We present the results of an open-label, non-comparative, interventional multicenter study performed with EPs 7630 in patients suffering from symptoms of ARP.

After enrolment, eligible patients underwent 10 days of treatment with EPs 7630. Examinations were scheduled at baseline and treatment end, with an interim visit to be performed after 5 days of treatment. Moreover, the participants were asked to maintain a diary of their disease-related symptoms on a daily basis.

The protocol was reviewed and approved by an independent ethics committee. All patients provided written informed consent. The principles of Good Clinical Practice and the Declaration of Helsinki were adhered to.

Participants

The study participants were female and male out-patients with a clinical diagnosis of ARP and at least 2 out of 10 pre-defined common cold symptoms (CCS; nasal discharge, sore throat, nasal congestion, sneezing, scratchy throat, hoarseness, coughing, headache, malaise, fever). Main specific criteria for exclusion were obstructive anatomic lesions in the nasopharynx (e.g., nasal polyps), severe septal deviations, previous or planned surgery of the nose or paranasal sinuses, chronic pulmonary diseases, allergic rhinitis, conditions known to cause sore throat (e.g., tonsillo-pharyngitis, drugs, aphthous ulcers, candida), or the presence of any acute respiratory tract disease other than ARP. Concomitant intake of common cold medications that might impair the interpretation of trial results were not allowed during study participation. However, in the event of fever >38.5°C the participants were allowed to take paracetamol up to a maximum dose of 500 mg taken every 6 hours.

Intervention

EPs 7630 is a herbal preparation from the roots of *Pelargonium sidoides* (1:8-10), extraction solvent: ethanol 11% (w/w). Film-coated tablets containing 20 mg of EPs 7630 were used[§]. The study participants had to administer 3 × 1 film-coated tablets daily for 10 consecutive days (total daily dose: 60 mg EPs 7630). The investigational product was provided by the manufacturer (Dr. Willmar Schwabe GmbH & Co. KG, Karlsruhe, Germany).

Outcomes

Upon study inclusion information regarding the study participants' demographic, anthropometric and patient history data was obtained. Documented measures included sex, age, ethnic group, smoking habit and alcohol consumption, height, weight, duration of ARP symptoms, as well as previous and concomitant diseases and medication.

Tolerability was assessed by questioning patients for adverse events (AEs) of any kind during all post-baseline visits. Moreover, safety laboratory assessments, which included erythrocyte sedimentation rate (ESR), erythrocytes, thrombocytes, leucocytes, serum creatinine, alkaline phosphatase (ALP), gamma-glutamyl-transpeptidase (γ-GT), aspartate aminotransferase (AST), alanine aminotransferase (ALT), total bilirubin, albumin, prothrombin time (PT), partial thromboplastin time (PTT), and C-reactive protein (CRP), as well as general clinical and physical examinations were performed at baseline and at the end of treatment.

Outcome measures referring to treatment effectiveness and to the course of ARP during the period of observation included investigator ratings of each of a set of 10 common cold symptoms (CCS) on a 4-point verbal rating scale ranging from 0 ('not present') to 3 ('severe') which were assessed during each visit and summed up to a total score. The CCS is based on a score developed by Jackson et al. [31-33].

Observer assessments also included 8 additional ARP-associated complaints (pulmonary rales at auscultation, sputum production, chest pain during coughing, chilliness, exhaustion, loss of appetite, diarrhea, and muscle aches) which the investigators rated using the same scale and which were summed up to a separate total score. Specific guidance for the grading of each of the symptoms was given in the study protocol. Daily self-ratings for a set of 15 ARP-associated symptoms (runny nose, congested nose, sneezing, sore throat, scratchy throat, hoarseness,

§ Marketed product used in this trial: Kaloba® (Austroplant Arzneimittel, Vienna, Austria)

coughing, headache, malaise, chilliness, chest pain during coughing, loss of appetite, restless sleep, limitation of usual daily activities, muscle ache) were obtained by means of a 5-point verbal rating scale ranging from 0 ('not at all') to 4 ('severe') in the patient diary. The same scale was also used for obtaining a daily self-rating of how ill the patient felt.

The over-all recovery from ARP (rated by patients and investigators) as well as the patients' satisfaction with the treatment outcome were assessed using the Integrative Medicine Outcomes Scale (IMOS) and the Integrative Medicine Patient Satisfaction Scale (IMPSS), respectively [34]. Further effectiveness outcome measures were the number of days off work or education, the need for antibiotic treatment, and the use of paracetamol.

At baseline, a nasopharyngeal swab was taken from both nostrils for microbiological testing by means of a sterile brush. Total nucleic acid (DNA and RNA) was isolated from the samples using the QIAamp nucleic acid isolation kit (Qiagen, Hilden, Germany). The amount of isolated nucleic acid was measured by absorbance. For viral testing, an aliquot was applied to the xTAG® Respiratory Viral Panel (RVP) FAST assay (Abbott, Vienna, Austria). cDNA were generated from RNA by reverse transcription (RT) and then amplified by PCR. Subsequent to RT-PCR the amplicons were hybridized onto virus species specific DNA probes immobilized on Luminex beads. Virus species were identified using Luminex technology, with signal measurements of virus specific hybridization signals specified for the xTAG® RVP FAST assay. Viruses detectable by the assay include influenza A and B, respiratory syncytial virus (RSV), corona virus, parainfluenza virus, human metapneumovirus, entero-rhinovirus, adenovirus, and human bocavirus. Testing of bacterial DNA was done using the AIT Chip HD PathoID test (Austrian Institute of Technology).

PCR amplicons were generated from nucleic acid extracts using universal primers targeting bacterial 16S rRNA gene. The PCR products were fluorescently labelled and transferred onto a microarray. The microbial panel for oligonucleotide microarray detection, applying 20- to 30-mer probes, is capable of identifying 70 different pathogens relevant for infectious diseases with pathogen occurrence in clinical samples.

Treatment compliance was assessed by counting the number of remaining film-coated tablets at study exit.

Statistical methods, sample size

All outcome measures were analyzed descriptively using appropriate summary statistics. For change over time, descriptive p-values were determined. 95% confidence intervals (CIs) were specified for change over time as well as for AE incidence. Safety and tolerability analyses included all patients having administered the investigational treatment at least once (safety analysis set, SAF). For eligibility of the analyses of effectiveness and course of ARP, at least one post-baseline assessment of the analyzed outcome was also required (full analysis set, FAS). An additional per-protocol (PP) analysis included all patients of the FAS who completed the trial without major protocol deviations. Missing data were imputed by carrying forward the last valid observation provided that at least one post-baseline assessment had been performed.

For statistical tests two-sided p-values up to 0.05 were considered to be descriptively significant. One hundred and twenty patients were planned to be treated in this study based on practical considerations. Using confidence interval methods, the sample size assures a probability of at least 90% that an event with a true incidence rate of 2% is observed at least once.

Results

Participants

Between January 2011 and November 2012, 120 subjects were included and treated in the out-patient clinics of 8 hospitals in Austria. Three subjects (2.5%) terminated their participation in the study prematurely due to withdrawal of consent, an adverse event (allergic dermatitis), and known, pre-existing hepatitis which the subject had failed to report upon enrolment.

All patients included were analyzed for safety in the SAF and for effectiveness in the FAS, respectively. One hundred and three patients (85.8% of 120) were analyzed for effectiveness in the PP analysis data set. Major protocol deviations leading to an exclusion from the PP analysis were premature termination unrelated to (lack of) efficacy or tolerability (n=2), relevant violations of inclusion or exclusion criteria (n=2), relevant findings in the medical history (n=1), lack of treatment compliance (n=2), major deviations from the visit schedule (n=4), using an unsafe method of contraception (n=1), or use of prior or concomitant medication which was not allowed according to the protocol (n=8).

Unless otherwise noted, the results presented in the following sections apply to the SAF/FAS.

Baseline characteristics

The study participants' demographic and anthropometric characteristics are shown in Table 1. Although ethnic group was not a selection criterion, all subjects except 1 were Caucasians (99.2%). About ⅔ of the subjects reported to drink alcohol occasionally. Sixty-one patients (50.8%) had never been smokers, and 41 (34.2%) were current smokers.

At baseline, 12 patients (10.0%) reported a duration of ARP symptoms of less than 24 hours, 67 (55.8%) reported a duration of 24-48 hours, and 41 (34.2%) had been suffering for more than 48 hours. The baseline severity of CCS and other ARP-associated symptoms showed no monotonic association with symptom duration upon enrolment.

Treatment compliance

Treatment compliance was calculated as the percentage of tablets used relative to the prescribed amount. Across the entire period of observation, mean ± SD compliance was 102.7% ± 6.8%. All patients showed compliance within a pre-defined acceptable range of 75%-125%. However, 2 patients were treated for fewer than 7 days, which was considered to be a relevant protocol deviation.

Course of ARP, effectiveness

At baseline, the study participants presented with observer rated CCS total scores between 2 and 21 points (out of a maximum possible score of 30 points) and reported the presence of between 2 and all of the 10 CCS; 106 out of the 120 patients (88.3%) presented with at least 5 different symptoms at baseline. Symptom scores indicate a continuing remission of ARP-related symptoms during the course of treatment. The average total score decreased significantly from a baseline mean value of 10.8 points, over 5.1 points at the interim visit scheduled at day 5, to 2.2 points at treatment end (Table 2), corresponding to decreases by 52.8% and by 79.6% of the baseline value at day 5 and treatment end, respectively. A total of 2 patients (1.7%) were symptom free at day 5 and 28 patients (23.9%) were symptom free at day 10. Likewise, the number of patients with only one symptom remaining was 10 (8.6%) and 31

		SAF/FAS (n=120)	PPS (n=103)
Sex	Female	84 (70.0%)	72 (69.9%)
	Male	36 (30.0%)	31 (30.1%)
Age (years)		38.9 ± 13.6	39.5 ± 13.9
Height (cm)		171.3 ± 8.1	171.2 ± 8.3
Weight (kg)		73.1 ± 14.4	73.2 ± 14.8
Duration of ARP symptoms [hours]		46.2 ± 18.3	44.8 ± 18.3
SAF: Safety Analysis Set; FAS: Full Analysis Set; PPS: Per-Protocol Analysis Set			

Table 1: Baseline characteristics (number (%) of patients or mean ± SD)

	Visit	n	Total score	Change versus baseline	
			Mean SD	Mean SD	p
Common cold symptoms	Baseline	120	10.8 ± 3.6		
	Day 5	117	5.1 ± 3.4	-5.6 ± 3.8	<0.001
	Day 10 (treatment end)	117	2.2 ± 2.5	-8.6 ± 4.0	<0.001
Other ARP-associated complaints	Baseline	120	3.4 ± 2.7		
	Day 5	117	1.3 ± 1.9	-2.1 ± 2.4	<0.001
	Day 10 (treatment end)	117	0.5 ± 1.3	-2.8 ± 2.6	<0.001
Investigators' ratings; mean ± SD and Wilcoxon test for change versus baseline; FAS					

Table 2: Total scores of common cold symptoms and other ARP-associated symptoms

(26.7%) at days 5 and 10, respectively. At day 10, 55 patients out of 117 with valid data (47.0%) had a CCS total score ≤1 point and 83 (70.9%) had a score ≤2 points. A similar alleviation of symptoms was observed for the total score of other ARP-associated complaints as well (Table 2). The results in the FAS and in the PP analysis were comparable.

Figure 1 shows the time course of the 14-item summary score for the ARP symptom self-rating obtained in the patients' diary (theoretical maximum: 60 points) together with the percentage of patients who felt only mildly ill or not ill at all. The data indicate a monotonic decrease of symptom intensity. The time course resembled an exponential curve with mean values ranging from 22.1 ± 9.6 points at baseline, over 11.4 ± 9.1 points at day 5, to 3.8 ± 4.2 points at day 10. At the same time, the percentage of patients who felt only mildly ill or not ill at all increased from 15.3% at baseline to 58.6% at day 5 and to 94.6% at day 1.A total of 37 patients (30.8% of 120) were unable to attend work or school/college for at least 1 day, up to a maximum of 11 days. The average number of days off work or education was 1.7 ± 3.3 days (including patients with zero days off). According to the decision of the investigator, 2 subjects (1.7% of 120; 95% CI: 0.2%-5.9%) required antibiotic treatment, and 22 patients (18.3%) took paracetamol at least once. The average intake was 2.5 ± 2.7 tablets with a maximum intake of 12 tablets during the 10-day period of observation.

The IMOS rating scale was used for assessing the patients' and investigators' global impression of change in the intensity of ARP in comparison to baseline. Table 3 shows that according to both assessments about 84% of the patients were either fully recovered or showed major improvements of their condition at treatment end. Unchanged symptoms were reported for 3 and 5 patients according to the investigators' and patients' rating, respectively. Deteriorations were reported for none of the patients. In a subgroup analysis by onset of ARP symptoms relative to inclusion into the trial, 9 out of 12 subjects (75.0%) whose complaints had started <24 hours before inclusion were fully recovered at treatment end, compared to 29 of 66 patients (43.9%) with an onset 24-48 hours before inclusion and 11 of 39 subjects (28.2%) whose symptoms had started >48 hours before inclusion (Mantel-Haenszel $\chi 2$ statistic for the comparison of recovery rates across the three ordered categories for onset: p=0.005).

The patients' treatment satisfaction was assessed by means of the IMPSS scale (Table 3). At the final visit, about ¾ of the study participants indicated that they were satisfied or very much satisfied with the treatment received, whereas 2 patients (2.0% of 101 with valid data) expressed their dissatisfaction.

Results of Polymerase Chain Reaction (PCR) (detection of viral infection)/Microarray analysis (detection of bacterial DNA)

One hundred and nineteen swab samples were available for analysis. Virus DNA was detected in 61 of the 119 samples (51.3%). The

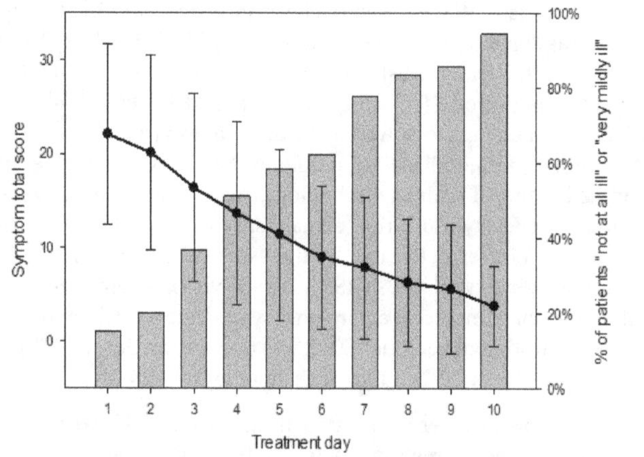

Figure 1: Patient diary ratings of ARP-associated complaints (mean ± SD) and % of patients feeling not at all ill or very mildly ill (n=119 ... 92)

most frequently detected viruses were enterovirus/rhinovirus (29% of the samples).

Bacterial DNA was identified in 118 samples (99.2%). Staphylococcus epidermidis was the organism identified most frequently.

Tolerability and safety

During treatment with EPs 7630, 15 of 120 subjects exposed (12.5%) reported 18 AEs. Ten events observed in 9 patients (7.5%) were assessed to be potentially treatment-related. Considering a cumulative exposure of 1,064 treatment days, these numbers correspond to an over-all incidence density of 0.017 AEs per day of exposure or to 1 AE in 71 days of treatment for all events, and to 0.009 events per day of exposure or 1 event in 106 treatment days for potentially related events. None of the events were serious.

Table 4 provides an overview of all adverse events according to MedDRA Preferred Terms. Among the 10 events for which a causal relationship with the investigational treatment could not be excluded, only an allergic dermatitis was assessed to be possibly related whereas all others were considered to be improbably related.

The MedDRA System Organ Class with the largest number of patients affected by an AE was gastrointestinal disorders (6, 5.0%, 95% CI: 2.3-10.5%) followed by nervous system disorders and respiratory, thoracic and mediastinal disorders (both 3, 2.5%, 95% CI: 0.9-7.1%).

		Investigators' rating	Patients' rating
IMOS	Patients with valid data	n=117	n=82
	Complete recovery	49 (41.9%)	36 (43.9%)
	Major improvement	49 (41.9%)	32 (39.0%)
	Slight to moderate improvement	16 (13.7%)	9 (11.0%)
	No change	3 (2.6%)	5 (6.1%)
	Deterioration	0 (0.0%)	0 (0.0%)
IMPSS	Patients with valid data		n=101
	Very satisfied		38 (37.6%)
	Satisfied		37 (36.6%)
	Neutral		24 (23.8%)
	Dissatisfied		1 (1.0%)
	Very dissatisfied		1 (1.0%)

Table 3: Integrative Medicine Outcome Scale (IMOS) and Integrative Medicine Patient Satisfaction Scale (IMPSS) – patients' and investigators' ratings at end of treatment/day 10 (last observation carried forward).

System Organ Class	Preferred Term	All events	Events for which a causal relationship was not entirely excluded[#]
Gastrointestinal disorders	Abdominal pain	1 (0.8%)	1 (0.8%)
	Abdominal pain upper	1 (0.8%)	1 (0.8%)
	Diarrhoea	1 (0.8%)	1 (0.8%)
	Flatulence	2 (1.7%)	2 (1.7%)
	Toothache	1 (0.8%)	–
Infections and infestations	Urinary tract infection	1 (0.8%)	–
Investigations	Activated partial thromboplastin time prolonged	1 (0.8%)	1 (0.8%)
Musculoskeletal and connective tissue disorders	Back pain	1 (0.8%)	–
Nervous system disorders	Headache	1 (0.8%)	–
	Migraine	2 (1.7%)	2 (1.7%)
Psychiatric disorders	Sleep disorder	1 (0.8%)	–
Respiratory, thoracic and mediastinal disorders	Dysphonia	1 (0.8%)	–
	Oropharyngeal pain	1 (0.8%)	–
	Sneezing	1 (0.8%)	–
Skin and subcutaneous tissue disorders	Dermatitis allergic	1 (0.8%)	1 (0.8%)
	Rash	1 (0.8%)	1 (0.8%)
Any adverse events		15 (12.5%)	9 (7.5%)

[#] Causal drug relationship: 'probable', 'possible', or 'unlikely'

Table 4: Patients with adverse events (MedDRA System Organ Classes and Preferred Terms), by causal relationship (n=120)

Except for one case of prolonged activated partial thromboplastin time (reported as an AE with unlikely causal relationship to the investigational treatment), the safety laboratory measures did not indicate any signs of intolerance, neither on a casuistic basis, nor with respect to a possible shift in the mean value.

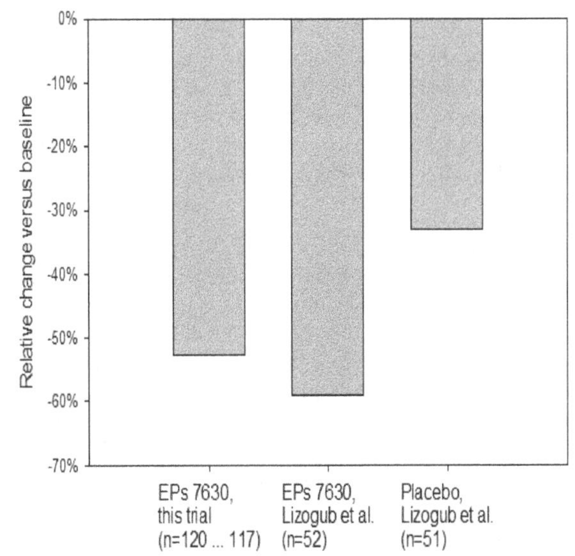

Figure 2: Relative change of ARP symptom score between baseline and treatment day 5 in this trial and in Lizogub et al. [36] (full analysis set; relative mean value difference).

Discussion

Recent reviews taking into account practically all available clinical trials and post-marketing surveillance studies with *Pelargonium sidoides* extract EPs 7630 published until early 2013 agree that a slight increase in the risk of AEs over the placebo level has to be expected, mainly due to somewhat higher rates of gastrointestinal complaints and hypersensitivity reactions, but that potentially attributable events were always non-serious, non-severe, and transient, not causing an increase in treatment-related withdrawals [28,29].

The safety and tolerability of EPs 7630 were reviewed by Matthys et al. [29] based on data from 29 clinical trials and post-marketing surveillance studies involving more than 10,000 adults and children with respiratory tract infections. Their analyses focused on adverse reactions which, according to the Summary of Product Characteristics (SmPC) of the marketed product, may occur in at least 1 patient out of 10,000 exposed. Among the 5 system groups concerned, gastrointestinal complaints showed a risk difference of +1.86% under EPs 7630 as compared to placebo and epistaxis showed a difference of +0.54%. The remaining system groups (hypersensitivity reactions, gingival bleeding, hepatic enzymes) were associated with risk differences <0.5% (data apply to events for which a causal relationship was not entirely excluded). Of note, patients exposed to EPs 7630 did not exhibit an increased risk of elevated liver enzyme or bilirubin values. In placebo-controlled clinical trials, Matthys et al. [29] reported highly variable rates of AEs (any causal relationship) ranging from 1.4% to 51.5% in patients treated with EPs 7630 compared to 0.0% to 39.6% for placebo. Higher AE rates were predominantly observed in 'smaller' trials with fewer than 100 patients in each treatment group, whereas 'larger' trials reported rates below 20% on both groups.

With an over-all AE rate of 12.5% for EPs 7630, the data from this trial are consistent with the review findings and do not indicate an under-reporting of AEs that is not uncommon in open-label trials or observational studies (e.g [35]). It is also worth mentioning that 5 of the 10 potentially attributable events in this trial were gastrointestinal complaints, and 2 were skin reactions, both of which are among the most common types of AEs noted during previous research [28,29]. On the other hand, bleeding complications (e. g., epistaxis, gingival bleeding) or elevated liver enzyme values were not observed during this study.

In a self-limiting condition like ARP, the parameter of clinical interest is not simply improvement compared to baseline, but improvement over the natural course of the disease. As an open-label trial without a control group, this trial was not designed to demonstrate treatment efficacy. It is therefore interesting to note that the extent of symptom relief in our study participants was comparable to that observed in a double-blind, randomized, trial performed by Lizogub et al. [36] in ARP, in which EPs 7630 was significantly superior to placebo. The authors' main outcome measure for efficacy was based on the change of a cold intensity score between baseline and treatment day 5. The score assessed the same 10 symptoms included in the CCS, albeit on a 5-point verbal rating scale instead of the 4-point scale used in our trial so that the absolute values cannot be compared directly.

Figure 2 shows that the ARP symptom score in Lizogub et al. [36] decreased by 59.0% and by 33.1% for EPs 7630 and placebo, respectively, after 5 days of randomized treatment, compared to a 52.8% decrease observed in the present, uncontrolled trial. We interpret this as evidence that the recovery of symptoms observed in our trial was not caused by the natural course of ARP alone, all the more since recent research indicates that placebo effects in ARP are limited and nuanced [37].

Another indicator for a beneficial effect of EPs 7630 is the observation of an association between recovery and the initiation of treatment relative to the onset of ARP. Our trial shows evidence that treatment with EPs 7630 may be most efficacious when initiated within the first 24 h after the first symptoms are noted, although the interpretation is limited by the fact that this result was observed in an exploratory post-hoc analysis.

After demonstrating the efficacy of a medicinal product in randomized placebo-controlled trials performed in rigorously standardized settings, interventional post-marketing trials in the registered indication represent a logical next step in order to gain primarily further safety information in a clinical real-life setting [30]. On the other hand, an uncontrolled trial may tend to provide an overly optimistic estimate of the efficacy of an intervention because it does not permit a separation of the pharmacological effect of a product from its placebo effect. Uncontrolled open-label studies are subject to several limitations (e.g. [35,38]), and therefore should be interpreted carefully. However, comparisons of the course of symptom recovery as well as of the rate and type of adverse events observed in this study and in controlled clinical trials with EPs 7630 in acute respiratory tract infections show that the results were in a similar range, making bias as a consequence of the uncontrolled design unlikely.

Recent studies have shown that a complex bacterial milieu exists within the human upper respiratory tract - including that of healthy individuals -, the predominant species of which are staphylococcus spp., which do usually not cause any clinical manifestations [39,40]. This is consistent with the results of the viral and bacterial analysis of the swab obtained at baseline of our trial, which showed that about half of the samples confirmed a viral infection, whereas all samples except one exhibited proof of bacterial DNA. We interpret the presence of bacterial DNA to be mainly related to the bacterial milieu found in ill and healthy individuals alike, rather than to the specific symptoms of acute rhinopharyngitis. Moreover, although ARP is considered to be almost exclusively a viral disease (e.g [41]), viral detection rates commonly range between about 43% and 63% [42,43]. The results of the viral analysis may therefore be attributable to a lack of sensitivity of the assay.

In conclusion, the study confirms the excellent tolerability of EPs 7630 during 10 days' treatment of adult patients suffering from ARP. Potentially attributable AEs were mainly limited to gastrointestinal complaints and skin reactions, which are a part of the known spectrum of adverse effects of the drug. The majority of study participants showed a favorable course of recovery from ARP which is unlikely to be explained by the natural course of the disease alone.

Acknowledgments

Medical writing services were provided by Dr. Andreas Völp, Psy Consult Scientific Services, Frankfurt, Germany. The study as well as medical writing services were funded by Dr. Willmar Schwabe GmbH & Co. KG, Karlsruhe, Germany.

Conflict of Interest

TK and AS have received honoraria from Dr. Willmar Schwabe GmbH & Co. KG, Karlsruhe, Germany; BS is an employee of Dr. Willmar Schwabe GmbH & Co. KG, Karlsruhe, Germany.

References

1. Simasek M, Blandino DA (2007) Treatment of the common cold. Am Fam Physician 75: 515-520.
2. Arroll B (2011) Common cold. Clin Evid 03: 1510.
3. Bertino JS (2002) Cost burden of viral respiratory infections: issues for formulary decision makers. Am J Med 112 Suppl 6A: 42S-49S.
4. Birnbaum HG, Morley M, Greenberg PE, Colice GL (2002) Economic burden of respiratory infections in an employed population. Chest 122: 603-611.
5. Niroumand M, Grossman RF (1998) Airway infection. Infect Dis Clin North Am 12: 671-688.
6. Dreschers S, Franz P, Dumitru CA, Wilker B, Jahnke K, et al. (2007) Infections with human rhinovirus induce the formation of distinct functional membrane domains. Cell Physiol Biochem 20: 241-254.
7. van Kempen M, Bachert C, Van Cauwenberge P (1999) An update on the pathophysiology of rhinovirus upper respiratory tract infections. Rhinology 37: 97-103.
8. Herendeen NE, Szilagy PG (2000) Infections of the upper respiratory tract. In: Behrman RE, Kliegman RM, Jenson HB (eds) Nelson Textbook of pediatrics. (16thedn) W. B. Saunders, Philadelphia 1261-1266.
9. Heikkinen T, Jarvinen A (2003) The common cold. Lancet 361: 51-59.
10. Pratter MR (2006) Cough and the common cold: ACCP evidence-based clinical practice guidelines. Chest 129: 72S-74S.
11. Curley FJ, Irwin RS, Pratter MR, Stivers DH, Doern GV, et al. (1988) Cough and the common cold. Am Rev Respir Dis 138: 305-311.
12. Pitrez PM, Pitrez JL (2003) Acute upper respiratory tract infections: outpatient diagnosis and treatment [in Portugese]. J Pediatr (Rio J) 79 Suppl 1: S77-86.
13. Lorber B (1996) The common cold. J Gen Intern Med 11: 229-236.
14. Moyo M, Van Staden J (2014) Medicinal properties and conservation of Pelargonium sidoides DC. J Ethnopharmacol 152: 243-255.

15. Kayser O, Kolodziej H, Kiderlen AF (2001) Immunomodulatory principles of Pelargonium sidoides. Phytother Res 15: 122-126.

16. Kolodziej H (2007) Fascinating metabolic pools of Pelargonium sidoides and Pelargonium reniforme, traditional and phytomedicinal sources of the herbal medicine Umckaloabo®. Phytomedicine 14 Suppl 6: 9-17.

17. Kolodziej H, Kayser O, Radtke OA, Kiderlen AF, Koch E (2003) Pharmacological profile of extracts of Pelargonium sidoides and their constituents. Phytomedicine 10 Suppl 4: 18-24.

18. Kolodziej H, Kiderlen AF (2007) In vitro evaluation of antibacterial and immunomodulatory activities of Pelargonium reniforme, Pelargonium sidoides and the related herbal drug preparation EPs® 7630. Phytomedicine 14 Suppl 6: 18-26.

19. Conrad A, Hansmann C, Engels I, Daschner FD, Frank U (2007) Extract of Pelargonium sidoides (EPs® 7630) improves phagocytosis, oxidative burst, and intracellular killing of human peripheral blood phagocytes in vitro. Phytomedicine 14 Suppl 6: 46-51.

20. Conrad A, Jung I, Tioua D, Lallemand D, Carrapatoso F, et al. (2007) Extract of Pelargonium sidoides (EPs® 7630) inhibits the interactions of group A-streptococci and host epithelia in vitro. Phytomedicine 14 Suppl 6: 52-59.

21. Rezaizadehnajafi L, Wink M (2014) EPs 7630® from Pelargonium sidoides increases stress resistance in Caenorhabditis elegans probably via the DAF-16/FOXO pathway. Phytomedicine 21: 547-550.

22. Helfer M, Koppensteiner H, Schneider M, Rebensburg S, Forcisi S, et al. (2014) The Root Extract of the Medicinal Plant Pelargonium sidoides Is a Potent HIV-1 Attachment Inhibitor. PloS one 9: e87487.

23. Michaelis M, Doerr HW, Cinatl J, Jr. (2011) Investigation of the influence of EPs® 7630, a herbal drug preparation from Pelargonium sidoides, on replication of a broad panel of respiratory viruses. Phytomedicine 18: 384-386.

24. Theisen LL, Muller CP (2012) EPs® 7630 (Umckaloabo®), an extract from Pelargonium sidoides roots, exerts anti-influenza virus activity in vitro and in vivo. Antiviral Res 94: 147-156.

25. Agbabiaka TB, Guo R, Ernst E (2008) Pelargonium sidoides for acute bronchitis: a systematic review and meta-analysis. Phytomedicine 15: 378-385.

26. Agbabiaka TB, Guo R, Ernst E (2009) Erratum to "Pelargonium sidoides for acute bronchitis: A systematic review and meta-analysis" [Phytomedicine 15 (2008) 378–385]. Phytomedicine 16: 798-799.

27. Matthys H, Malek FA, Kamin W (2014) EPs® 7630 in Acute Respiratory Tract Infections – a Systematic Review and Meta-Analysis of Randomised Clinical Trials. Forsch Komplementärmed 21: 57-58.

28. Timmer A, Gunther J, Motschall E, Rucker G, Antes G, et al. (2013) Pelargonium sidoides extract for treating acute respiratory tract infections. Cochrane Database Syst Rev 10: Cd006323.

29. Matthys H, Köhler S, Kamin W (2013) Safety and tolerability of EPs 7630 in clinical trials. Adv Pharmacoepidemiol Drug Saf 2: 142.

30. Ray WA, Stein CM (2006) Reform of drug regulation--beyond an independent drug-safety board. N Engl J Med 354: 194-201.

31. Jackson GG, Dowling HF, Spiesman IG, Boand AV (1958) Transmission of the common cold to volunteers under controlled conditions. I. The common cold as a clinical entity. AMA Arch Intern Med 101: 267-278.

32. Mossad SB, Macknin ML, Medendorp SV, Mason P (1996) Zinc gluconate lozenges for treating the common cold. A randomized, double-blind, placebo-controlled study. Ann Intern Med 125: 81-88.

33. Prasad AS, Fitzgerald JT, Bao B, Beck FW, Chandrasekar PH (2000) Duration of symptoms and plasma cytokine levels in patients with the common cold treated with zinc acetate. A randomized, double-blind, placebo-controlled trial. Ann Intern Med 133: 245-252.

34. Steinsbekk A, The Data Collection Group (1999) Data Collection in Homeopathic Practice. A Proposal for an International Standard, European Committee for Homeopathy.

35. Hakobyan L, Haaijer-Ruskamp FM, de Zeeuw D, Dobre D, Denig P (2011) A review of methods used in assessing non-serious adverse drug events in observational studies among type 2 diabetes mellitus patients. Health and quality of life outcomes 9: 83.

36. Lizogub VG, Riley DS, Heger M (2007) Efficacy of a pelargonium sidoides preparation in patients with the common cold: a randomized, double blind, placebo-controlled clinical trial. Explore (NY) 3: 573-584.

37. Barrett B, Brown R, Rakel D, Rabago D, Marchand L, et al. (2011) Placebo effects and the common cold: a randomized controlled trial. Annals of family medicine 9: 312-322.

38. Lopez-Gonzalez E, Herdeiro MT, Figueiras A (2009) Determinants of under-reporting of adverse drug reactions: a systematic review. Drug Saf 32: 19-31.

39. Ramakrishnan VR, Feazel LM, Gitomer SA, Ir D, Robertson CE, et al. (2013) The microbiome of the middle meatus in healthy adults. PloS one 8: e85507.

40. Wos-Oxley ML, Plumeier I, von Eiff C, Taudien S, Platzer M, et al. (2010) A poke into the diversity and associations within human anterior nare microbial communities. The ISME journal 4: 839-851.

41. Mäkelä MJ, Puhakka T, Ruuskanen O, Leinonen M, Saikku P, et al. (1998) Viruses and bacteria in the etiology of the common cold. J Clin Microbiol 36: 539-542.

42. Brittain-Long R, Westin J, Olofsson S, Lindh M, Andersson LM (2010) Prospective evaluation of a novel multiplex real-time PCR assay for detection of fifteen respiratory pathogens-duration of symptoms significantly affects detection rate. J Clin Virol 47: 263-267.

43. Lam WY, Yeung AC, Tang JW, Ip M, Chan EW, et al. (2007) Rapid multiplex nested PCR for detection of respiratory viruses. J Clin Microbiol 45: 3631-3640.

12

The Joint Moment Distribution of the Lower Extremity During Tai Chi Gait

Richard Pearlman[1], John E. Kovaleski[2], Jonathan Wolfe[1] and Wei Liu[3*]

[1]*School of Medicine, University of South Alabama, Mobile, Alabama, USA*

[2]*Department of Health, Physical Education, University of South Alabama, Mobile, Alabama, USA*

[3]*Edward Via College of Osteopathic Medicine Auburn, Auburn, Alabama, USA*

[*]**Corresponding author:** Wei Liu, Edward Via College of Osteopathic Medicine Auburn, Auburn, Alabama, USA, E-mail: wliu@auburn.vcom.edu

Abstract

Background: As an alternative and complementary practice, Tai Chi is becoming increasingly popular in the United States, especially among the elderly. Although several interventional and qualitative biomechanical studies have been performed, a quantitative approach, such as multi-joints kinetics synergy of ankle, knee and hip, has yet to be performed. To better understand the biomechanics of Tai Chi, the characteristics of the total support moment synergy were studied during Tai Chi gait and compared to normal gait.

Methods: Ten healthy, experienced (two years) Tai Chi Chuan practitioners performed normal walking and Tai Chi gait while data was collected using high-speed infrared motion analysis cameras. The joint distributions of the ankle, knee, and hip were calculated by ratio between individual joint moment impulse and total support moment impulse. Using a paired t-test, the joint moment distributions of the lower limb were compared between Tai Chi gait and normal walking.

Results: The total support moment of Tai Chi walking was predominated by the contribution of the knee (ankle: 32.78 ± 1.25%; knee: 58.68 ± 1.84%; hip: 8.54 ± 1.91%) whereas the ankle was the primary contributor to support in normal walking (ankle: 67.86 ± 2.76%; knee: 26.18 ± 2.69%; hip: 5.96 ± 1.83%). The contributions of all three joints studied differed significantly ($p<0.05$) between Tai Chi gait and normal gait.

Conclusion: This study demonstrates different kinetics synergy patterns between Tai Chi gait and normal gait. Importantly, Tai Chi gait places a high mechanical demand on the knee joint. Our results provide biomechanical basis of Tai Chi's benefits on increasing knee joint range of motion and muscle strength, also suggest that prescribing Tai Chi as a potential therapy for people with joint disease, it needs a careful consideration of evaluating mechanical response of people with joint disease during Tai Chi exercise due to higher mechanical demand on the knee joint.

Keywords: Tai chi; Total support moment; Gait; Support strategy

Background

Tai Chi Chuan (TCC) exercise is becoming an increasingly popular complementary and alternative approach for both healthy people and patients with a variety of medical conditions in the United States [1]. In the past two decades, promising evidence suggests that TCC provides multiple beneficial effects that include improved balance, increased postural stability, and decreased fall risk [2]. Increased muscular strength, pain reduction for patients with arthritis, reduction of stress, and enhanced cardiovascular function have been proposed as potential benefits of TCC [3-6].

Although TCC has been shown to have many benefits, the mechanism of TCC at the neuromuscular and musculoskeletal levels is less understood. As a form of physical activity, TCC is a continuous, slow and rhythmic movement, involving dynamic weight shifting strategies between two limbs during loading and unloading. These characteristics of TCC require coordinated control of the ankle, knee, and hip [7]. Quantifying the biomechanical characteristics of TCC will aid in our understanding of the movement strategies used in TCC, provide direct evidence of the neuromuscular and musculoskeletal responses of the human body during TCC, and lead to the development of more effective TCC treatment.

Previous studies on the biomechanical quantifications of TCC mainly focused on essential and basic TCC movements such as Tai Chi gait (TCG) due to the fact that TCC has varieties of forms and styles. We believe TCG to be an ideal movement to study for biomechanical analysis because TCG and walking are both a means of bipedal forward locomotion and each have distinct double support and single stance phases.

Since the same gait analysis terminology has been used to describe TCG, it has been referred to as a specific gait strategy. Past research has examined temporal and spatial measures of TCG, such as stride length; basic kinematic descriptive information, such as range of motion (ankle, knee, and hip joints); and kinetics, such as the ground reaction force (GRF), joint moment, and contact force of the lower extremities [8,9].

This biochemical information gives insight into the movements of TCC by isolating individual joints. The main motor function of walking and TCG is to support the body and prevent lower limb collapse, which is described as vertical support. Vertical support of the body during gait requires synergistic muscle moments around the hip, knee, ankle.

The total support moment (TSM) has been used to determine joint distributions of this kinetic synergy effect [10]. The total support moment is a summation of the moments of the individual segments of the limb. Despite considerable variability at individual joints, the total support moment shows decreased variability due to the nature of the limb to act as a system whose individual segments can accommodate changes within that system [10]. As a method of analysis that considers the limb as a single unit comprised of individual parts, the support moment synergy is ideal for studying multi-joint movements. Based on our knowledge, few studies have investigated the multi-joint coordination and distribution of lower extremity joint moments during TCG.

In this paper, we quantify the lower limb joint moment distributions of TSM during TCG compared to walking. We hypothesized that joint moment distributions of TSM during TCG will be different than normal walking (NW).

Methods

Subjects

Ten healthy participants (5 women, mean age 58 years) were enrolled from local Tai Chi clubs and martial art schools. A minimum of two years of TCC (24 simplified forms derived from Yang Style) experience was required.

Exclusion criteria included significant orthopedic and/or chronic pain conditions, depression, and pulmonary or renal failure. Written informed consent was obtained in compliance with the Institutional Review Board requirements at the University. Subjects were asked to stand quietly in a neutral position to capture calibration trial for five seconds. They were then instructed to perform four NW and TCG trials, respectively.

Data collection

Seven VICON MX-10 high-speed infrared motion analysis cameras (VICON Technology, CA) were used to record TCG and NW with a sampling rate at 100 Hz. Reflective cluster markers were attached to the bony landmarks at the trunk, pelvis, thigh, shank, and foot (Figure 1).

Two force platforms (Advanced Mechanical Technology Inc., Watertwon, MA, USA) embedded in a 3 m (width) × 10 m (length) walkway were used to record ground reaction forces (GRF) at 1000 Hz during the stance phase of gait.

The two force plates were synchronized with the VICON cameras so that the coordinates of each marker and GRF were simultaneously collected. Three-dimensional marker data were collected by VICON Nexus Software (VICON, CA) and filtered with a Butterworth low-pass filter (6 Hz cutoff).

Right-handed local segmental and lab coordinate systems were constructed so that the x-axis was directed laterally to the right, the y-axis was directed anteriorly, and the z-axis was directed superiorly. Figure 1 illustrates the experimental set up and the orientation of the global and local coordinate systems.

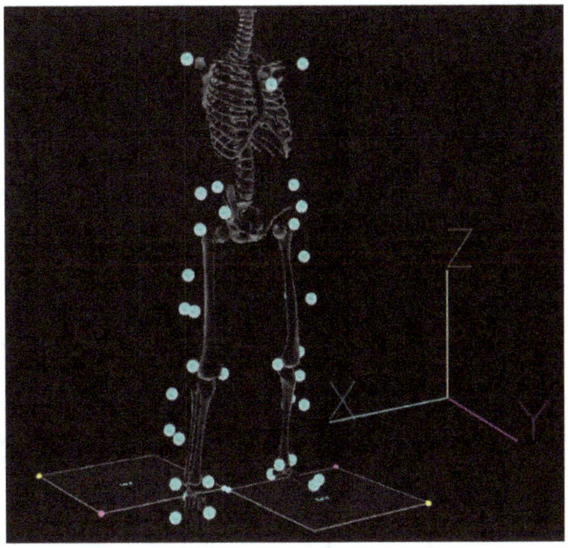

Figure 1: Experimental set-up and marker placement on lower extremity.

Data analysis

The dependent variables used were distributions of ankle, knee, and hip joint moments of the total support moment. Firstly, 3-D segmental Euler kinematics (x-y-z sequence) angles were computed based on the rotation matrix between global and local coordinate systems of each segment. Consequently, joint angular displacement, velocity, and segmental angular velocity were derived from 3-D Euler angles [10]. A traditional inverse dynamics approach was used to compute internal joint moment by using the above kinematic and ground reaction force information [10].

The total support moment (TSM) was calculated by summation of the ankle, knee, and hip moments in the sagittal plane [10]. The area under the TSM, called the TSM impulse, was derived by integration of the TSM over the gait cycle.

Finally, the ankle, knee, and hip moment impulses were derived and divided by the TSM impulse. The ratios were then normalized by 100%. A paired t-test was used to compare the ankle, knee, and hip joint distributions to the TSM impulse differences between NW and TCG. The statistical significance level for all comparisons was set at $p<0.05$.

Results

Normal gait findings

Study of ten healthy subjects showed consistent support strategies (Figure 2). The ankle (67.86 ± 2.76%) was found to be the primary contributor to the total support moment.

The knee (26.18 ± 2.69%) participated less than the ankle, and the hip (5.96 ± 1.83%) contributed the least (Figure 3).

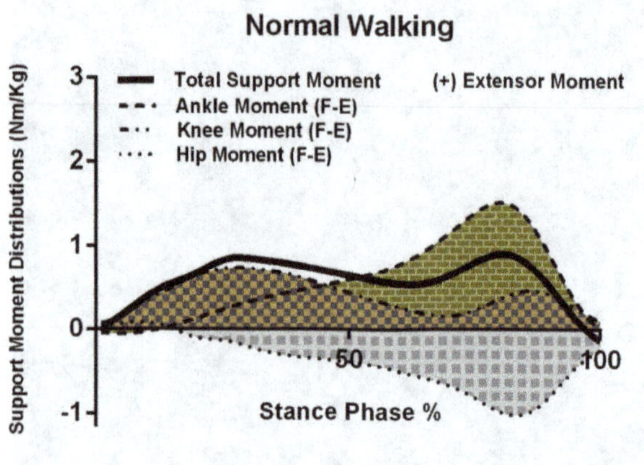

Figure 2: Illustration of time series of Individual joint distributions of total support moment during Normal Walking (NW). Extensor moment (+).

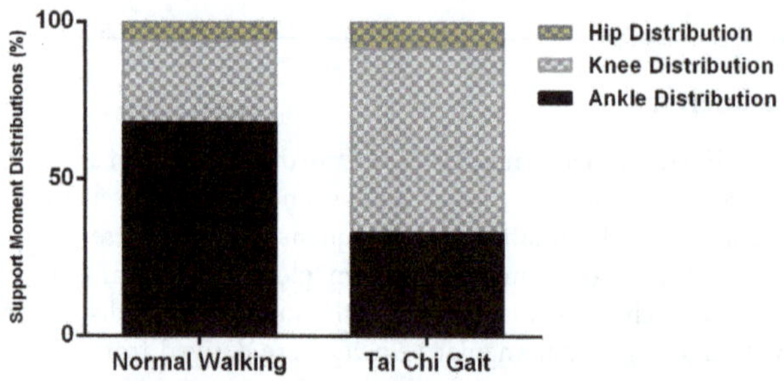

Figure 3: Bar plots of Individual joint distributions of total support moment during normal walking (NW) and Tai Chi Gait (TCG).

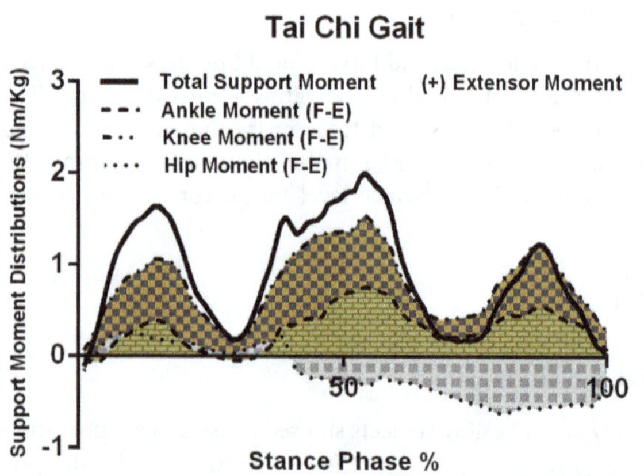

Figure 4: Illustration of time series of Individual joint distributions of total support moment during Tai Chi Gait (TCG). Extensor moment(+).

Tai Chi gait findings

While performing TCG, subjects showed little variation in support strategy as shown in Figure 4. During TCG, knee involvement was greater in TCG (58.68 ± 1.84%). Following the knee, the ankle (32.78 ± 1.25%) was the second most dominant contributor, and the hip (8.54 ± 1.91%) participated the least (Figure 3).

Normal gait vs. Tai Chi gait

Using a paired t-test, the contributions of each joint (ankle, knee, and hip) in NW and TCG were compared. In contrast to NW, TCG showed significantly different involvement of all three joints (Figure 5). The contributions of the knee (mean difference: 32.50 ± 2.87%) and hip (mean difference: 2.58 ± 1.03%) were found to be significantly greater in TCG than in NW ($p<0.05$). The ankle (mean difference: 35.08 ± 2.87%) contributed less in TCG compared to NW ($p<0.05$).

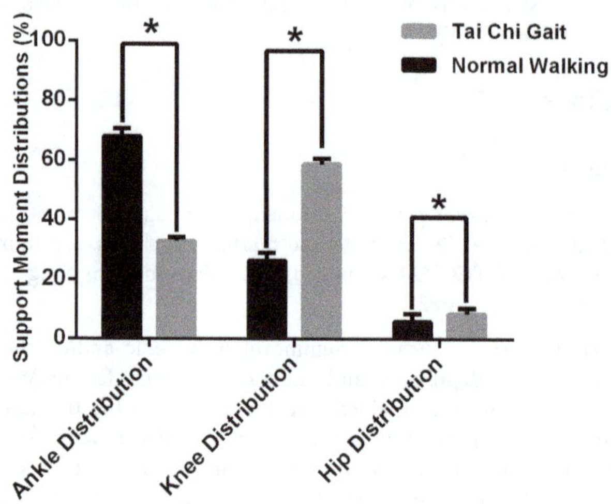

Figure 5: Comparison of the ankle, knee and hip joint moment distributions of total support moment between normal walking (NW) and Tai Chi gait (TCG). *Significant difference between NW and TCG ($P<0.05$).

Discussion

Our results for NW are consistent with those found in the literature. In our study, the ankle (67.86 ± 2.76%) was the primary contributor to the total support moment followed by the knee (26.18 ± 2.69%) and hip (5.96 ± 1.83%). Similar results were obtained by Torry et al. who determined the ankle, knee, and hip contributions(71.73 ± 14.90%, 15.59 ± 14.32%, and 12.73 ± 8.83%, respectively) to the total support moment in a control group of healthy women [11]. DeVita and Hortobagyi also reported that the ankle is the dominant contributor to the total support moment [12].

Compared to normal walking, TCG was found to utilize a significantly different support pattern: the knee showed greatly increased contribution to the total support moment. Although there are no known studies of TCG using the total support moment, other studies have compared TCG to normal walking and inferences can be made from these findings.

Several studies have noted the increased knee flexion required to perform TCG in comparison to NW. Wu reported an increase in duration and magnitude of knee and hip flexion by 139% and 66% respectively in elderly subjects performing TCG compared to NW [13]. In a similar study comparing TCG and NW, knee flexion in normal walking (7.4° - 46.0°) was observed to be less than in TCG (13.1° - 46.5°). During TCG, the knee was observed to be constantly flexed as compared to NW, which showed variable flexion over the gait cycle [14]. Taking into consideration that TCG requires constant knee flexion and is thus mechanically different in nature compared to NW, it is reasonable to see changes in the composition of the total support moment. As indicated by this study, a greater contribution of the knee is required to support the leg in the flexed stance that is necessitated by TCG. This pattern is further supported by electromyographic data of the various muscles of the leg.

Electromyographic evidence further corroborates the increased support moment contribution of the knee during TCG. The increased flexion of the knee in TCG has been shown to be correlated with increased activation of the knee extensors [14]. In one study, both the rectus femoris and tensor fasciae latae showed markedly increased activation magnitudes (403% and 252%, respectively) in comparison to normal gait [13]. Greater peak muscle activity during TCG has also been observed in other knee extensor muscles, such as the vastus lateralis and vastus medialis [14]. The results of these electromyographic studies are further supported by observations of increased knee extensor strength in experienced Tai Chi practitioners [15].

While performing TCG, increased flexion of the knee and use of the knee extensors results in greater shear forces on the knee. Between the ankle, knee, and hip joints, the knee experiences the greatest peak shear force. Increased shear force during TCG is due to the greater knee flexion and displacement of the knee from the center of gravity. Although the peak shear force is increased in the knee during TCG, compressive force is reduced [9]. These increased forces on the knee further support our results, which indicate that the knee is the primary contributor to the total support moment during TCG. Because the contribution of the knee to the total vertical support is markedly increased when performing TCG, a strikingly high mechanical demand is placed on the knee joint.

Considering the load experienced by the knee, it is not surprising that research has shown Tai Chi to be beneficial to knee health. Both greater knee strength and proprioception have been documented. In Tai Chi intervention studies using healthy, elderly subjects, increased knee extensor strength in comparison to controls has been reported [15-17]. In addition to increased knee strength, Tai Chi training has been associated with improved proprioception about the knee compared to controls [17]. Several studies have examined the biomechanics of Tai Chi in healthy adults and have provided insight into the biomechanical mechanisms underlying the changes seen in practitioners of Tai Chi [7-9,13].

Surprisingly, all biomechanical Tai Chi research to date has focused on healthy subjects. Although understanding the biomechanics of Tai Chi in people free of injury or disease is an important first step towards the evolution of Tai Chi as a therapy, if it is to be used for therapeutic purposes, the biomechanics of Tai Chi in subjects with disease must be elucidated. It is unclear how these people would handle the increased mechanical demand placed upon the knee during Tai Chi. For example, how would a person with knee osteoarthritis (OA) handle the increased knee mechanical stress associated with Tai Chi? Interestingly, there is evidence that Tai Chi is an effective therapy for people with knee OA. Interventional studies have shown that Tai Chi can reduce knee pain and stiffness as well as improve physical function [4,18]. These results are quite perplexing. Based on the current research, it would seem that the increased mechanical demand on the knee during Tai Chi would prove to be detrimental in people with knee OA. However, randomized controlled trials have provided evidence contrary to this conclusion. Future research into the biomechanics of Tai Chi in people with joint disease is required to answer these puzzling questions.

Conclusions

This study demonstrates different kinetics synergy patterns between Tai Chi gait and normal gait. Importantly, Tai Chi gait places a high mechanical demand on the knee joint. Our results provide biomechanical basis of Tai Chi's benefits on increasing knee joint range of motion and muscle strength, also suggest that prescribing Tai Chi as a potential therapy for people with joint disease, it needs a careful consideration of evaluating mechanical response of people with joint disease during Tai Chi exercise due to higher mechanical demand on the knee joint.

Competing Interests

None declared.

Acknowledgements

This study was supported by University Faculty Development Council Research Grant (W. Liu, PI). We thank Deana Rumble for her assistance on data collection.

References

1. Nahin RL, Barnes PM, Stussman BJ, Bloom B (2009) Costs of complementary and alternative medicine (CAM) and frequency of visits to CAM practitioners: United States, 2007. Natl Health Stat Report 18: 1-14.
2. Li F, Harmer P, Fitzgerald K, Eckstrom E, Stock R, et al. (2012) Tai Chi and postural stability in patients with Parkinson's disease. N Engl J Med 366: 511-519.
3. Li JX, Xu DQ, Hong Y (2009) Changes in muscle strength, endurance, and reaction of the lower extremities with Tai Chi intervention. J Biomech 42: 967-971.
4. Wang C, Schmid CH, Hibberd PL, Kalish R, Roubenoff R, et al. (2009) Tai Chi is effective in treating knee osteoarthritis: A randomized controlled trial. Arthritis Rheum 61: 1545-1553.
5. Jimenez PJ, Melendez A, Albers U (2012) Psychological effects of Tai Chi Chuan. Arch Gerontol and Geriatr 55: 460-467.
6. Jahnke R, Larkey L, Rogers C, Etnier J, Lin F (2010) A comprehensive review of health benefits of Qigong and Tai Chi. Am J Health Promot 24: e1-e25.
7. Chan SP, Luk TC, Hong Y (2003) Kinematic and electromyographic analysis of the push movement in Tai Chi. Br J Sports Med 37: 339-344.
8. Wu G, Liu W, Hitt J, Millon D (2004) Spatial, temporal and muscle action patterns of Tai Chi gait. J Electromyogr Kines 14: 343-354.
9. Wu G, Millon D (2008) Joint kinetics during Tai Chi gait and normal walking gait in young and elderly Tai Chi Chuan practitioners. Clin Biomech 23: 787-795.
10. Winter DA (2009) Biomechanics and Motor Control of Human Movement. 4th edition, John Wiley & Sons, Inc. Hoboken, New Jersey.

11. Torry MR, Decker MJ, Ellis HB, Shelburne KB, Sterett WI, et al. (2004) Mechanisms of compensating for anterior cruciate ligament deficiency during gait. Med Sci Sport Exer 36: 1403-1412.
12. DeVita P, Hortobagyi T (2000) Age causes a redistribution of joint torques and powers during gait. J Appl Physiol 88: 1804-1811.
13. Wu G (2008) Age-related differences in Tai Chi Gait kinematics and leg muscle electromyography: A pilot study. Arch Phys Med Rehabil 89: 351-357.
14. Tseng SC, Liu W, Finley M, McQuade K (2007) Muscle activation profiles about the knee during Tai-Chi stepping movement compared to the normal gait step. J Electromyogr and Kines 17: 372-380.
15. Wu G, Zhao F, Zhou XL, Wei L (2002) Improvement of isokinetic knee extensor strength and reduction of postural sway in the elderly from long-term Tai Chi exercise. Arch Phys Med Rehab 83: 1364-1369.
16. Tsang WWN, Hui-Chan CWY (2005) Comparison of muscle torque, balance, and confidence in older Tai Chi and healthy adults. Med Sci Sport Exer 37: 280-289.
17. Li JX, Xu DQ, Hong Y (2008) Effects of 16-week Tai Chi intervention on postural stability and proprioception of knee and ankle in older people. Age Ageing 37: 575-578.
18. Brismee JM, Paige RL, Chyu MC, Boatright JD, Hagar JM, et al. (2007) Group and home-based tai chi in elderly subjects with knee osteoarthritis: a randomized controlled trial. Clin Rehabil 21: 99-111.

13

Suitability for Consumption of Chyawanprakash-A Herbal Formulation in Controlled Type II Diabetics-A Open Label Clinical Study

Satyendra Kumar[1*], **Arun Gupta**[1], **Raman Ghungralekar**[2] **and Vaishali Shailesh Deshpande**[3]

[1]*Medical Affairs and Clinical Research Division, Dabur Research and Development Centre, Dabur India Limited, Uttar Pradesh, India*

[2]*Department of Kayachikitsa, R A Podar Medical (Ayurvedic) College and M A Podar hospital, Mumbai, Maharashtra, India*

[3]*Department of Kayachikitsa, Sumatibhai Shah Ayurved Mahavidyalya, Malwadi, Mumbai Pune, Maharashtra, India*

[*]**Corresponding author:** Satyendra Kumar, Medical Affairs and Clinical Research Division, Dabur Research and Development Centre, Dabur India Limited, Uttar Pradesh, India, E-mail: satyendra.kumar@mail.dabur

Abstract

Objective: Chyawanprakash, a Chyawanprash based proprietary Ayurvedic formulation in which conventional sugar and honey are replaced by permitted alternate sweeteners in diabetic population.

Design: This was a randomized open label clinical study conducted across two study sites in Maharashtra (India). 121 male and female subjects in the age range of 18-70 years who were suffering from Type II Diabetes mellitus for more than one year and were stabilized on either exercise/diet regimen or oral hypoglycemic agents were recruited in the study and advised 1 teaspoonful of Chyawanprakash twice daily orally after meals for 90 days. They were advised to continue their anti-diabetic medicines under the supervision of the Investigator. Results were assessed basis pre and post treatment changes in glycosyated hemoglobin (HbA1c) and the Physician global assessment of overall safety. Clinical symptoms, laboratory parameters like blood sugar and insulin levels, microalbuminuria, liver and renal function tests, lipid profiles etc and changes in dose of oral hypoglycemic agents were also assessed.

Results: Oral administration of Chyawanprakash in recommended dosage in controlled Type II diabetics did not show any safety concern which was evident by no statistically significant change in HbA1c levels and the clinical as well as laboratory parameters (blood sugar, microalbuminuria, liver and renal function tests, lipid profiles etc). 97% excellent safety was reported on the Physician's global assessment of overall safety. Moreover, a statistically significant improvement was also observed in energy levels of subjects.

Conclusion: Results concluded the suitability of Chyawanprakash in controlled Type II diabetics.

Keywords: Ayurveda; Diabetes; Herbal; Sugar free; Suitability; HbA1c

Introduction

The prevalence of diabetes mellitus in India is predicted to double globally from 171 million in 2000 to 366 million in 2030 posing a significant health care burden [1,2]. Patients with diabetes mellitus have infections more often than those without DM. The course of the infections is also more complicated in this patient group. One of the possible causes of this increased prevalence of infections is poor immunity [3,4].

Ayurveda has suggested rejuvenative therapies or the Rasayanas for leading a healthy and active life. Modern pharmacology interprets Rasayana as a product having antioxidant, immunomodulatory, antistress and nootropic properties and the one promoting health [5]. Chyawanprash is an Ayurvedic Rasayana formulation used in Indian traditional medicinal system for its beneficial effect on human health viz.; maintaining youth, vigour and vitality [6,7] via antioxidant and immunostimulatory actions [8,9]. However, its use in diabetic population is restricted due to sugar contents.

Chyawanprakash is Chyawanprash based proprietary product. Though, Chyawanprash is renowned as a time tested immunity booster, its use in diabetic population is restricted due to its sugar contents. Chyawanprakash is Chyawanprash based product in which sugar and honey are replaced by sorbitol and sucralose. It is intended to be used by people with diabetes irrespective of treatment regimen. Sorbitol is a nutritive sweetener providing dietary energy and often used in diet foods and cough syrups [10]. Sucralose is no-calorie sweetener, safe for consumption by diabetics as it does not affect blood glucose level [11]. Previously, safety of Chyawanprakash has been established in animal model via 28 day repeated dose oral toxicity study [12]. In another study, Chyawanprakash at doses of 1.2 g/Kg did not show significant effect on blood glucose levels in non-diabetic and streptozotocin induced diabetic animals when compared to the non-diabetic vehicle control [13]. The current study conducted between the years 2013-2014 aimed to establish the clinical safety and suitability for consumption of Chyawanprakash in controlled Type II diabetic patients.

Objective

Suitability assessment of Chyawanprakash in controlled Type 2 diabetics.

Primary outcomes

1. Assessment of pre and post treatment changes in glycosylated hemoglobin (HbA1c) values.

2. Post-treatment Physician global assessment of overall safety of Chyawanprakash

Secondary outcomes

1. Monthly assessment of changes in fasting and postprandial plasma glucose levels, adverse drug reactions, clinical symptoms of diabetes (polyuria, polydipsia, polyphagia and fatigue), changes in microalbuminuria, changes in dose of OHAs and the Quality of Life

2. Assessment of changes in pre and post treatment of serum insulin levels in fasting state

3. Assessment of post-treatment clinically significant abnormal laboratory parameters

Material and Methods

Study product

Chyawanprakash (Mfd. Dabur India Limited), Batch No. PN0201 and PN0189, Mfd.11/2012, was used in the present study. The composition details of Chyawanprakash are given in Table 1.

Contents*	Quantity (g)
Pterocarpus marsupium	3.52
Aegle marmelos, Premna integrifolia, Oroxylum indicum, Stereospermum suaveolens, Gmelina arborea, Desmodium gangeticum, Uraria picta, Vitis vinifera, *Solanum indicum, Solanum xanthocarpum, Tribulus terrestris, Phaseolus trilobus, Teramnus labialis, Pistacia integerrima, Phyllanthus niruri, Inula racemosa, Aquilaria agallocha, Terminalia chebula, Tinospora cordifolia, Curcuma zedoaria, Cyperus rotundus, Boerhavia verticillata, Nymphaea stellata, Adhatoda vasica, Glycyrrhiza glabra, Maritima annua,*	0.38
Sida cordifolia	0.684
Leptadenia reticulata	0.076
Dioscorea bulbifera	0.76
Asparagus racemosus	0.76
Withania somnifera	0.76
Pueraria tuberosa	1.14
Emblica officinalis	82.0
Sesamum indicum	0.82
Clarified butter	0.91
Bambusa bambos	1.34
Piper longum	1.84
Cinnamomum zeylanicum	0.194
Elettaria cardamomum	1.008
Cinnamomum tamala	0.205
Mesua ferrea	0.190
Syzygium aromaticum	0.212
Glycyrrhiza glabraGlabra	1.0
* Each 100 g of Chyawanprakash	

Table 1: Composition details of Chyawanprakash.

Study design

Current trial was an open labeled, prospective, and interventional, Phase III clinical study conducted across two sites in Maharashtra, India *viz.*; (1) R.A. Podar Medical (Ayurvedic) College & M.A. Podar Hospital, Worli, Mumbai and (2) Sumatibhai Shah Ayurved Mahavidyalya, Malwadi, Hadapsar, Pune; through an independent CRO. The study was conducted with prior approval from respective Institutional Ethics Committees, and in accordance with GCP guidelines, the ICMR ethical guidelines for biomedical research on human participants and Declaration of Helsinki. The clinical study was registered with the Clinical Trial Registry of India (CTRI) on 15/04/2013. The CTRI number for the study is CTRI/2013/04/003553.

Inclusion criteria

Male and female subjects in the age range of 18-70 years, suffering from Type II Diabetes mellitus for more than one year, and stabilized on diet and exercise regimen or mono/polydrug anti-diabetic therapy/ oral hypoglycemic agents (OHA). In addition, patients who had their fasting blood glucose level in a range of 90-150 mg/dl and postprandial glucose in the range of 110-180 mg/dl, HbAIC below 8%, and ECG not demonstrating any signs of uncontrolled arrhythmia/acute ischemia and X-ray chest not showing any active lesion of tuberculosis at screening visit were included.

Female subjects who entered the study were either non-pregnant or at least six weeks postpartum and non-lactating. A urine pregnancy test was done for all the female subjects of childbearing potential unless subject had had a hysterectomy, tubal ligation, or was>2 years postmenopausal. All the recruited subjects were willing to follow the study procedures and had voluntarily signed an informed consent form.

Exclusion criteria

Subjects on insulin therapy, Subjects suffering from Type I Diabetes or other than Type II Diabetes, known major complications of diabetes like ketoacidosis, nephropathy, neuropathy, retinopathy and diabetic wounds or hepatic/renal/ significant cardiovascular disease event<12 weeks prior to randomization, active metabolic or gastrointestinal diseases excluding diabetes that may interfere with nutrient absorption, metabolism or excretion, active malignancy, contagious infectious diseases such as active tuberculosis, Hepatitis B or C or HIV, subjects using any other investigational drug within 1 month prior to recruitment, known hypersensitivity to any of the ingredients used in study drug, participating in another clinical study, pregnancy, lactation or any other condition due to which patients were deemed to be unsuitable by the investigator for reason(s) not specifically stated in the exclusion criteria.

Study visits

Subjects were called to the study center for visits on every 15th day till 90 days from the baseline visit. The visit schedule was- Screening Visit (Day-5), Baseline Visit (Day 0), Visit 1(Day 15), Visit 2 (Day 30), Visit 3 (Day 45), Visit 4 (Day 60), Visit 5 (Day 75) and Visit 6 (Day 90).

Methodology

Controlled Type II diabetics attending the outpatient clinic of respective sites were screened for eligibility criteria. On screening visit, a written informed consent was obtained from subjects for their participation in the study. Subject's history was recorded and their physical examination was carried out. Clinical symptoms of diabetes viz.; polyuria, polydipsia, polyphagia and fatigue were assessed and graded on clinical symptom scoring scale.

Subjects who fulfilled all the inclusion and exclusion criteria were screened on day -5 (5 days before baseline) where subject's venous blood 8-10 ml fasting and 2 ml post prandial (one and half hour post meal) samples and fasting urine sample were collected for estimation of fasting and postprandial plasma sugar levels. If fasting blood sugar was between 90 to 150 mg/dl and postprandial blood glucose was between the ranges of 110-180 mg/dl, then HbA1c % was estimated. If the value of HbA1c% was below 8%, then CBC, ESR, Hb%, microalbuminuria, serum insulin (fasting state), Liver and Renal function Tests, Lipid profile, routine and microscopic examinations of urine, Urine pregnancy test (only if the subject was female of child bearing potential) and HIV test (I & II) were carried out. If all the lab investigations were within the prescribed limits, subject's X- ray chest (PA View) and ECG were done. If X-ray and ECG were within normal limits, then, the subject was recruited in the study (baseline visit) if he/she met all the inclusion and none of the exclusion criteria.

Intervention and treatment duration

A container containing 900 g of Chyawanprakash was given to subjects at baseline visit, on day 30 and 60. Subjects were advised 1 teaspoonful of Chyawanprakash orally twice daily after meals for 90 days continuing their anti-diabetic medicines (OHAs) under the supervision of the investigator. They were advised to continue the diabetic diet and exercise regimen (which they had been following) during the entire study period. Drug compliance was assessed at every follow-up visit.

Statistical analysis

Mean differences of continuous variables were examined by paired 't' test to evaluate if there was any statistically significant difference between the values at the initial visit and subsequent follow up visits or the final visit. All p-values were reported based on two-sided significance test and all the statistical tests were interpreted at 5% level of significance level. Safety analysis was done of all the subjects who had been administered at least one dose of Chyawanprakash.

Evaluation analysis

Subjects underwent general and systemic examinations and Subject's Quality of life was evaluated on WHO Quality of Life Questionnaire at the baseline visit. Drug compliance, general and systemic examinations and assessment of clinical symptoms of Type II DM were carried out at every visit. Assessment of dose of OHAs and Quality of life on WHO Quality of Life Questionnaire was done on monthly basis. If required, the dose of OHAs was reduced or increased by investigator after assessing subject's blood sugar levels. Subject's Fasting and PP blood sugar levels, microalbuminuria were checked every month. Overall safety of the study drug was assessed by the investigator and by the subject at the end of the study. All the subjects were closely monitored for any Adverse Events starting from baseline visit till the end of the study visit. All laboratory parameters were assessed initially and at day 90. After completion of 90 days of study treatment, all the subjects were asked to stop study medication and take advice of investigator for further treatment.

Results

A total of 151 subjects suffering from DM were screened, 121 subjects were recruited of which 101 completed the study. Twenty subjects dropped out prematurely due loss to follow up. No adverse event was reported by any of the dropped out subjects. Maximum patients (22.77%) enrolled in the study were in the age range of 61-65 years followed by 56-60 years (21.78%). The Male: Female ratio in the study was 37:64. The participant flow chart for the study is shown in Figure 1.

The Prakriti or Ayurvedic phenotype-based constitution of subjects showed majority Pitta-kaphaj phenotypes (Table 2).

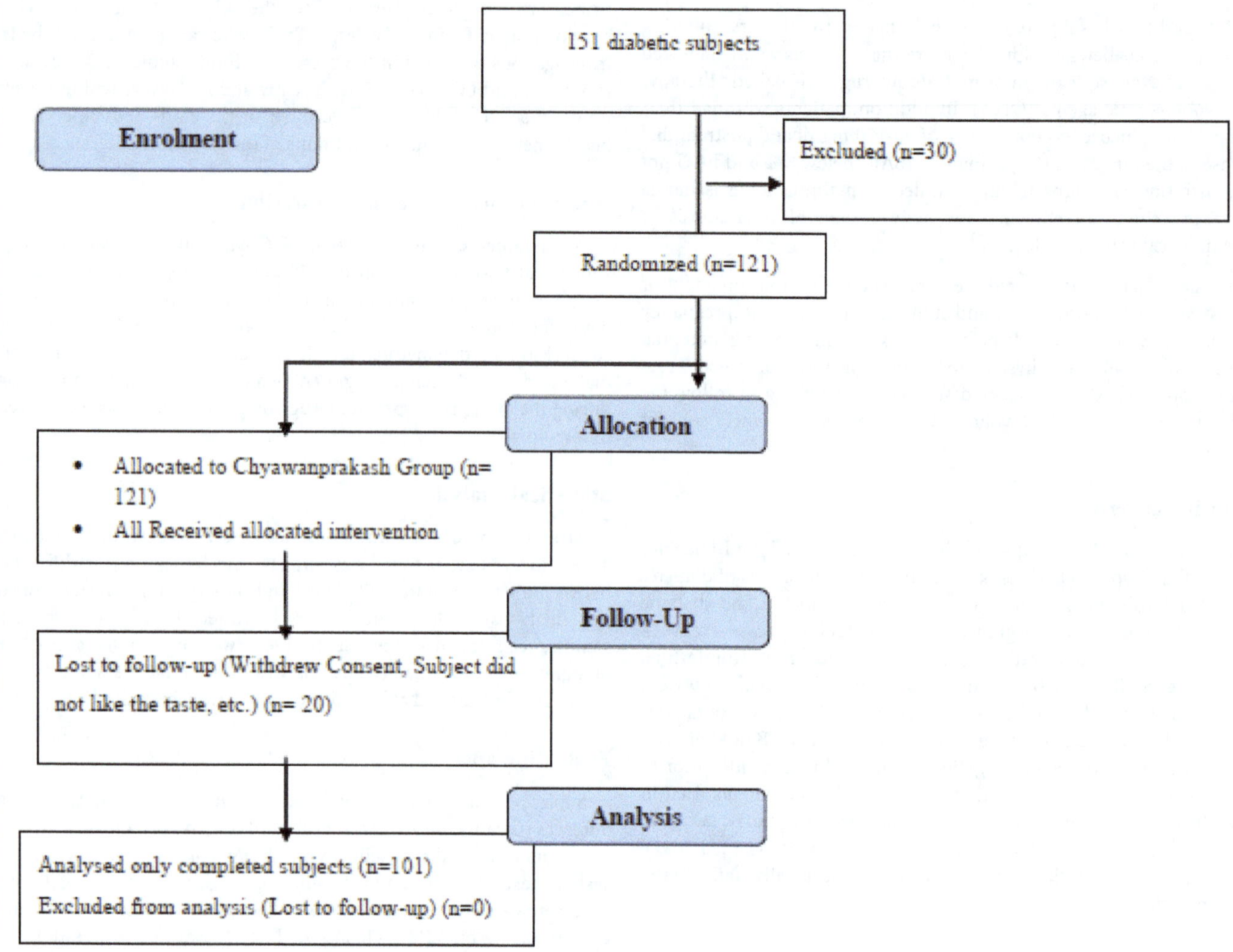

Figure 1: Patient enrolment flow chart.

S. No	Prakriti	No. of Subjects
1	Vata Pittaj	26
2	Vata Kaphaj	14
3	Pitta -Vataj	12
4	Pitta Kaphaj	35
5	Kaph a Vataj	05
6	Kapha-Pittaj	09
7	Total	101

Table 2: Prakriti wise distribution of subjects.

Parameter	Baseline Visit (0 day)	Visit VI (Day 90)
HbAlc%	6.94 ± 0.69	7.03 ± 0.94

Serum insulin	6.51 ± 4.72	9.38 ± 7.21*
*Significant p<0.05		

Table 3: Effect on glycosylated Hemoglobin (HbA1c%) values.

Efficacy Assessment

Initially the mean HbA1c% value was 6.94, while at the end of the study it was found to be 7.03, showing a statistically non-significant change ($p<0.05$, Table 3). The mean values of fasting and PP blood sugar at baseline did not show any statistical difference at the end of the study (Table 4). The mean serum insulin value was 6.51, which increased significantly ($p<0.05$) to 9.38 at the end of the study. This increase was, however, within the normal range of serum insulin. The mean increase in microalbuminuria level was non- significant from 13.69 at baseline to 17.05 at the end of the study. The mean body weight, hemoglobin and ESR values did not show any statistically significant difference at the end of the study (Table 5).

Statistically significant reduction ($p<0.05$) in the symptoms of diabetes such as polydipsia, polyphagia and fatigue were observed at the end of the study. Polyuria, however, showed a statistically significant increase ($p<0.05$) at the end of the study (Table 6). There was no change in most of the questions of WHO QOL from baseline visit to the end of the study visit. However, statistically significant improvement ($p<0.05$) was observed in energy level from baseline to end of the study visit (Table 7).

The biochemical laboratory parameters including Cholesterol, Triglycerides (TG), Low Density Lipoprotein (LDL), High density lipoprotein (HDL), Very Low Density Lipoprotein, TC/HDL, LDL/HDL, Serum Creatinine, BUN/Creatinine, Serum Uric Acid, Serum Calcium, SGOT, SGPT and bilirubin (direct and indirect), serum alkaline phosphate, total protein, serum globulin, serum albumin/globulin, were done at the initial visit and at the end of 90 days. There were significant change in serum SGOT, alkaline phosphate, albumin and LDL levels and the Albumin/ Globulin and the LDL/HDL ratio. These changes were, however, in the normal reference range at both these visits (Tables 8-11). Almost 95% subjects did not require their oral hypoglycemic medications or doses to be increased from exiting medication that they were taking. Patients who were stabilized on diet and exercise continued to do the same and there was no need to introduce OHA for diabetes management.

Blood Sugar	Baseline Visit (Day 0)	Visit II (Day 30) (Mean ± SD)	Visit IV (Day 60) (Mean ± SD)	Visit VI (Day 90) (Mean ± SD)
Fasting	104.75 ± 19.96	105.87 ± 22.45	113.09 ± 45.54	109.61 ± 35.11
Post prandial	143.19 ± 26.15	142.68 ± 35.57	158.23 ± 50.93,	153.02 ± 52.30
Micro albumin urea	13.69 ± 16.83	13.73 ± 17.12	17.31 ± 30.21	17.05 ± 29.14

Table 4: Effect on fasting and post prandial blood sugar.

S. No.	Parameters	Baseline (Day 0) (Mean ± SD)	Visit VI(Day 90) (Mean ± SD)
1	Body Weight	61.88 ± 9.37	61.87 ± 9.49
2	Hemoglobin %	12.36 ± 1.58	12.24 ±1.81
3	ESR	22.00 ±16.67	24.42 ±17.76

Table 5: Effect on body weight, Hemoglobin% and ESR.

Symptoms	Baseline	Visit I	Visit II	Visit III	Visit IV	Visit V	Visit VI
Polyuria	0.34 ± 0.59	0.37 ± 0.59	0.36 ± 0.61	0.36 ± 0.56	0.31 ± 0.50	0.29 ± 0.50	0.46 ± 0.66 *
Polydypsia	0.52 ± 0.74	0.56 ± 0.74	0.60 ± 0.73*	0.46 ± 0.62	0.46 ± 0.64	0.40 ± 0.61	0.22 ± 0.41**
Polyphasia	0.36 ± 0.59	0.40 ± 0.63	0.24 ± 0.46	0.21 ± 0.41	0.2 ± 0.40 **	0.22 ± 0.425 *	0.15 ± 0.38 **
Fatigue	0.41 ± 0.62	0.35 ± 0.61	0.28 ± 0.58 **	0.27 ± 0.54	0.19 ± 0.42 **	0.20 ± 0.42 **	0.15 ± 0.38 **
*Significant p<0.05, **Significant p<0.01							

Table 6: Mean change in symptoms of diabetes at each follow up.

Visit	How Would you rate your quality of life?	How satisfied are you with your health?	To what extent do you feel that physical pain prevents you from doing what you need to do?	Do you have enough energy for everyday life?	How satisfied are you with your sleep	How satisfied are you with your ability to perform your daily living activities?	How satisfied are you with your capacity for work?
Baseline	3.7 ± 0.46	3.67 ± 0.59	3.7+0.86	3.28+0.67	3.54 ± 0.83	3.76+0.47	3.72 ± 0.49
Final Visit	3.7 ± 0.50	3.76 ± 0.51	3.86 ± 0.80	3.42 ± 0.57**	3.56 ± 0.76	3.78 ± 0.50	3.8 ± 0.45
*Significant p<0.05, **Significant p<0.01							

Table 7: WHO QOL reading at baseline and final visits.

Visits	Baseline visit (Day 0}	Visit VI (Day 90)
Total Cholesterol	187.43 ± 45.87	193.14 ± 42.51
Triglycerides	136.30 ± 75.00	139.54 ± 77.33
HDL	47.37 ± 11.39	47.82 ± 11.37
LDL	102.57 ± 40.59	134.29 ± 39.43*
VLDL	25.99 ± 13.24	27.07 ± 14.93
TC/HDL	4.05±1.01	4.09 ± 1.06
LDL/HDL	2.20 ±0.80	2.41 ± 0.81*
*Significant p<0.05		

Table 8: Effect on lipid profile.

Visits	Baseline visit (Day 0}	Visit VI (Day 90)
Total Bilirubin	0.61 ± 0.30	0.58 ± 0.25
Direct Bilirubin	0.177 ± 0.058	0.172 ± 0.056
Indirect Bilirubin	0.44 ± 0.26	0.413 ± 0.214
SGOT	25.49 ± 7.69	23.37 ± 7.65**
SGPT	21.83 ± 9.19	22.47 ± 11.36
Alkaline Phosphate	98.64 ± 28.86	94.74 ± 30.16*
Total Protein	7.77 ± 0.48	7.71 ± 0.44
Serum Albumin	4.29 ± 0.25	4.37 ± 0.28 *
Serum Albumin/ Globulin	1.25 ± 0.21	1.33 ± 0.20
*Significant p<0.05, **Significant p<0.01		

Table 9: Effect on liver functions.

Visits	Baseline visit {Day O)	Visit VI (Day 90)
BUN	11.42 ± 4.05	10.86 ± 4.03
S. Creatinine	0.68 ± 0.18	0.67 ± 0.18

BUN/CREATININE	16.90 ± 4.36	16.22 ± 4.77
S. URIC ACID	4.99 ± 1.26	4.87 ± 1.29
S. CALCIUM	9.54 ± 0.64	9.45 ± 0.40
*Significant p<0.05, **Significant p<0.01		

Table 10: Effect of drug on renal profile.

Usage of OHAs	Baseline Visit (Day 0)	Visit II (Day 30)	Visit IV (Day 60)	Visit VI (Day 90)
Not taking any OHA	11(10.89%)	8 (7.92%)	11(10.89%)	11(10.89%)
Taking single OHA	25 (24.75%)	30 (29.70%)	22 (21.78%)	22 (21.78%)
Taking combination OHA	65 (64.36%)	63 (62.38%)	68 (67.33%)	68 (67.33%)

Table 11: Effect on oral hypoglycemic agents (oha) usage.

Safety Assessment

Of the 101 subjects who completed the study, none of the patients had any severe adverse event (SAE). Only 4 patients complained of mild adverse events like fullness of abdomen, mild pain in abdomen, skin rashes in Chyawanprakash group, however, none of the event is related to study product. These events resolved at their own and did not require stopping the intervention or administration of any medication.

The overall safety of the study drug was graded on global assessment scale by the investigator and by subject as excellent/good/fair or poor overall safety. As per physician's opinion, 97% subjects reported overall excellent safety and 3% reported overall good safety. As per patients' opinion, 94% subjects reported overall excellent safety and 6% reported overall good safety. Excellent compliance and tolerability to Chyawanprakash was observed in completed subjects. It was observed that even after consumption of Chyawanprakash for 3 months, their diabetic conditions did not worsen.

Chyawanprash is an age old formulation described in classical Ayurvedic texts due to beneficial effects on human health. It comprises multiple Ayurvedic ingredients which possess rejuvenating, strength promoting, nourishing and antioxidant properties. The beneficial effects of Chyawanprash have been mentioned in authoritative Ayurvedic literature like the Compendium of Charaka (Charaka Samhita), Bhaishajyaratnavali and The Ayurvedic Formulary of India that are mentioned in first schedule of The Drug & Cosmetic Act, 1940 of India. As per Charaka Samhita and The Ayurvedic Formulary, Chyawanprash is beneficial in various respiratory conditions, weakness and debility, in improving the quality of life and as a rejuvenator. It is also reported to exhibit immunomodulatory properties [6-9]. Chyawanprakash is a Chyawanprash based Ayurvedic Rasayana formulation intended to be used by people with diabetes in which sugar is replaced by sorbitol and sucralose. Ingredients of Chyawanprakash like Asana (*Pterocarpus marsupium* Roxb.) [14], Bilva *(Aegle marmelos (L.)* Corrêa) [15], Tvak *(Cinnamomum zeylanicum* Blume*)* [16], Kachura *(Curcuma zedoaria (Christm.)* Roscoe) [17], Amla *(Phyllanthus emblica L.)* [18] and Tejapatra *(Cinnamomun tamala* Nees.) [19] etc. are traditionally known and have been reported to possess antidiabetic properties. Herbs and replacement of sugar and honey by sorbitol and sucralose in Chyawanprakash may have contributed to its effects. Further studies to evaluate the effects of Chyawanprakash in different Ayurvedic phenotypes may be carried out in future studies

Conclusion

Oral administration of Chyawanprakash in recommended dosage in Type II controlled diabetics did not show any safety concern which was evident by no statistically significant change in clinical parameters as well as laboratory parameters like blood sugar, HbA1c, microalbuminuria, liver function tests, renal function tests, lipid profiles etc. A statistically significant improvement was observed in energy levels of subjects. Results concluded the suitability of Chyawanprakash in Type II diabetic patients controlled by Oral Hypoglycemic Agents.

References

1. Joshi SR, Parikh RM (2007) India - diabetes capital of the world: now heading towards hypertension. J Assoc Physicians India 55: 323-324.
2. Kaveeshwar SA, Cornwall J (2014) The current state of diabetes mellitus in India. Australias Med J 7: 45-48.
3. Deresinski S (1995) Infections in the diabetic patient: Strategies for the clinician. Infect Dis Rep 1: 1-12.
4. Geerlings SE, Hoepelman AI (1999) Immune dysfunction in patients with diabetes mellitus (DM). FEMS Immunol Med Microbiol 26: 259-265.
5. Govindarajan R, Vijayakumar M, Pushpangadan P (2005) Antioxidant approach to disease management and the role of Rasayana herbs of Ayurveda. J Ethnopharmacol 99: 165-178.
6. Sastri K, Chaturvedi GN (2011) Agnivesha. Charaka Samhita of Aginivesa. Rasayanadhikara. Varanasi (India): Chaukhambha Bharati Academy, pp.16-18.
7. The Ayurvedic Formulary of India, Part I Vol.1. Ministry of Health and Family Welfare, Govt. of India.
8. Madaan A, Kanjilal S, Gupta A, Sastry JLN, Verma R, et al. (2015) Evaluation of immunostimulatory activity of Chyawanprash using in vitro assays. Indian J Experimental Biol 53: 158-163.
9. Sastry JLN, Gupta A, Brindavanam NB, Kanjilal S, Kumar S, et al. (2014) Quantification of Immunity Status of Dabur Chyawanprash - A Review Part- 2 (Clinical Studies). Indian J Applied Res 4: 205-211.

10. Campbell F (2011) Biochemistry International Edition, 7th Edn, Publisher Brooks/Cole.
11. Grotz VL, Henry RR, McGill JB, Prince MJ, Shamoon H, et al. (2003) Lack of effect of sucralose on glucose homeostasis in subjects with type 2 diabetes. J Am Diet Assoc 103: 1607-1612.
12. Singh P, Wahid S, Jha KK (2010) 28-Days Repeated Dose toxicity Study of DRDC/AY/8048 (Dabur Chyawanprakash) in Wistar Rats by Oral Route. Data on files, Althea Lifesciences Limited. New Delhi, India, pp. 1-22.
13. Mani K, Sakat S, Goswami G (2011) Role on test item on blood glucose level using non diabetic and experimentally induced diabetic rats. Data on files, Althea Lifesciences Limited, New Delhi, India, pp. 1-26.
14. Devgan M, Nanda A, Ansari SH (2013) Comparative evaluation of the anti-diabetic activity of Pterocarpus marsupium Roxb. heartwood in alloxan induced diabetic rats using extracts obtained by optimized conventional and non conventional extraction methods. Pak J Pharm Sci 26: 973-976.
15. Panaskar SN, Joglekar MM, Taklikar SS, Haldavnekar VS, Arvindekar AU (2013) Aegle marmelos Correa leaf extract prevents secondary complications in streptozotocin-induced diabetic rats and demonstration of limonene as a potent antiglycating agent. J Pharm Pharmacol 65: 884-894.
16. IM K, Issac A, NM J, Ninan E, Maliakel B, et al. (2014) Effects of the polyphenol content on the anti-diabetic activity of Cinnamomum zeylanicum extracts. Food Funct 5: 2208-2220.
17. Rahmatullah M, Azam NK, Pramanik S, Jahan R (2012) Antihyperglycemic activity Evaluation of Rhizomes of Curcuma zedoaria (Christm.) Roscoe and Fruits of Sonneratia caseolaris. Internat J PharmTech Res 4: 125-129.
18. Fatima N, Hafizur RM, Hameed A, Ahmed S, Nisar M, et al. (2015) Ellagic acid in Emblica officinalis exerts anti-diabetic activity through the action on β-cells of pancreas. Eur J Nutr [Epub ahead of print].
19. Kumar S, Vasudeva N, Sharma S (2012) GC-MS analysis and screening of antidiabetic, antioxidant and hypolipidemic potential of Cinnamomum tamala oil in streptozotocin induced diabetes mellitus in rats. Cardiovasc Diabetol 11: 95.

14

Brief Review on the Causes, Diagnosis and Therapeutic Treatment of Gastritis Disease

Mohamed M Elseweidy*

Faculty of Pharmacy, Zagazig University, Zagazig, Egypt

***Corresponding author:** Mohamed M Elseweidy, Faculty of Pharmacy, Zagazig University, Zagazig, Egypt, E-mail: mmElseweidy@yahoo.com

Abstract

Gastritis represent a state of inflammation, irritation, or erosion of the stomach lining which may occur suddenly (acute) or gradually (chronic). Generally there is no universally accepted classification of gastritis and early classification was based mainly on the morphology, but recently pathogenic mechanisms have also been incorporated. The gastric mucosa is continuously exposed to many noxious factors, and Gastric protection aimed mainly to reduce or prevent the chemically induced acute hemorrhagic erosions which is exerted by compounds such as prostaglandins (PG) and SH derivatives without inhibiting acid secretion.

Common causes of gastritis are excessive alcohol consumption or prolonged use of non-steroidal anti-inflammatory drugs (NSAIDs) such as aspirin or ibuprofen. It may also develop after major surgery, traumatic injury, burns, or severe infections. Chronic causes are infection with bacteria, primarily *Helicobacter pylori* (HP), chronic bile reflux, stress additionally certain autoimmune disorders can cause gastritis as well. The most common symptom is abdominal upset or pain, indigestion, abdominal bloating, nausea, vomiting and pernicious anemia. The current study here is focusing on the causes, clinical profile, inflammatory, immune response and autoimmune atrophic gastritis in affected individuals. Additional focuses are on different diagnostic tools for *Helicobacter pylori* infection (HP) and current therapeutic treatment.

Keywords: Gastritis; Clinical profile; Inflammatory and immune response; Autoimmune atrophic gastritis; *Helicobacter pylori*; Diagnosis and current medications

Introduction

Overview and pathogenesis

The term "gastritis" refer usually to inflammation, erosive state to the stomach lining tissue which may occur either instantly (acute) or gradually as chronic state [1]. Early classification of the disease was based on tissue morphology which has been changed now with the incorporation of the pathological mechanism. Classification of gastritis was introduced by the Sydney system in 1990, updated in 1995 and included both endoscopic and histological categories [2]. Exposure of the gastric mucosa to noxious factors are continually occur and its resistance to auto digestion by gastric secretion is remarkable and mainly attributed to the presence of mucus gel layer lining the inner surface and acting as tissue protective [3]. Many compounds like prostaglandins (PG) and SH derivatives can induce acute hemorrhagic erosions which can be prevented by the gastro protective mechanism as exerted by the lining mucous. The latter is referred to as complex aqueous mixture of mucin, Electrolytes, Enzymes, bacterial products and scared cells [4]. Its physiological mechanisms are multiple; include formation of thick mucus gel which protects the epithelial surface against noxious factors, irritation or through coating the ingested food for subsequent digestion.

Causes of gastritis

Common causes of gastritis are many like continued intake of alcoholic beverages or long intake of non-steroidal anti-inflammatory drugs (NSAIDS), Aspirin for Rheumatoids and Osteoarthritis patients [5] while Stress, chronic bile reflux, autoimmune disorders and HP infection are causal for chronic gastritis. The symptoms observed her are many like nausea, vomiting, indigestion, burning sensation and abdominal bloating [6]. Blood, stool tests and gastro endoscopy are mostly requested for Diagnosis.

Morphological Patterns

Acute type

Acute gastritis is mostly induced by many agents like certain drugs, bile, Ischemia, viral, fungal, radiation acute stress (shock) and direct trauma. Alcohol consumption does not cause chronic gastritis, but it erode however the mucosal lining of the stomach. Although low doses of alcohol, not the higher one which stimulate hydrochloric acid secretion. Long intake of NSAID may induce an acute erosive gastritis, mostly due to injury and reduced prostaglandin synthesis. Duodenum-gastric bile reflux, long NSAID intake are causal factors for reactive or chemical gastritis (tortosity). Symptoms of the latter are many like cellular irritation of gastric surface associated with vasodilatation, congestion of gastric lamina propria, inflammatory cells and edema [7].

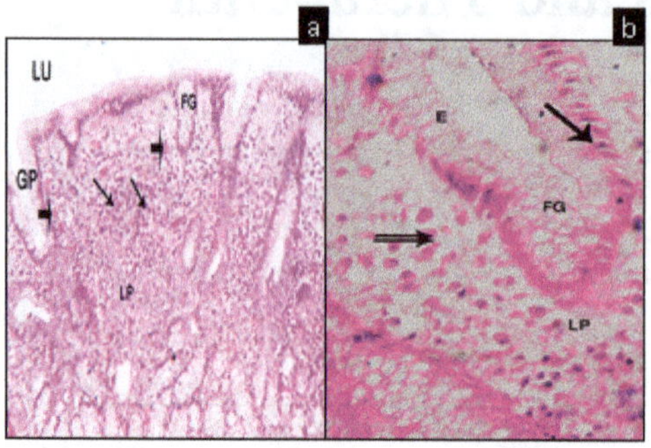

Figure 1: Histological section of human fundic gland of patient suffering from gastritis with anti *H. pylori* IgM positive group showing (a) X100 irregular short fundic gland (FG), wide gastric pit (GP), multiple inflammatory cells (arrows) and blood vessels (double arrows) filling lamina propria (LP), (b) X400 showing irregular simple columnar epithelium (E), small pyknotic nuclei (arrows) of cells lyningfundic gland (FG) and multiple inflammatory cells (double arrows) filling lamina propria (LP)[10].

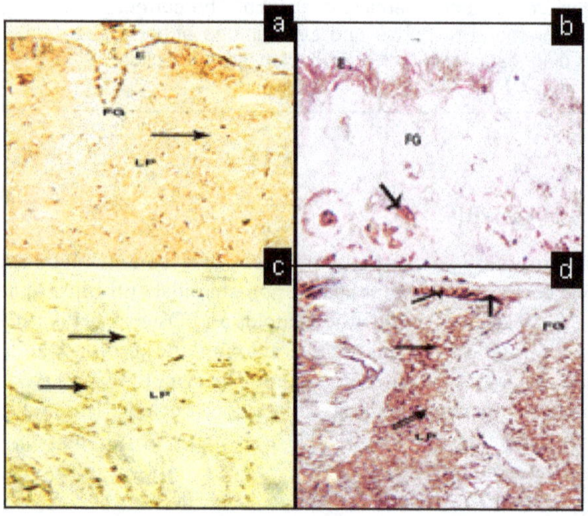

Figure 2: Immunostaining section of Gastritis patients IgM(+) category for (a) nitrotyrosine showing strong positive reaction in the epithelial (E) lining fundic gland (FG) and inflammatory cells (arrows) filling lamina propria (LP), (b) myeloperoxidase showingstrong positive reaction in the surface columnar epithelial cells (E) and other cells (arrows) lining fundic gland (FG) (c) iNOS showing strong positive reaction in the inflammatory cells (arrows) filling lamina propria (LP), (d) DNA fragmentation factor (DFF) showing strong positive reaction in the epithelial (arrows) lining fundic gland (FG) and inflammatory cells (double arrows) fill lamina propria (LP) (X200)[10].

Chronic type

Infiltration of inflammatory cells like plasma cells, lymphocytes represents an inflammatory changes (chronic type) in gastric mucosa, mainly attributed to HP infection along a disturbances in the secretion of pepsinogen enzyme, HCL additionally gastrin and somatostatin hormones. Increased apoptosis, hyper proliferation of the gastric epithelium are also observed during HP infection and is subsequently reduced upon treatment of the infection or eradication of HP [8]. Disturbances between the aggressive and cyto protective factors which maintain the integrity of the gastric mucosa represent a common mechanism of the injury. Inflammatory pattern her include massive increase of oxidative stress (high ROS), pepsinogen, gastrin and nitric acid synthesis (iNOS) with subsequent atrophy and G cells damage. Final apoptosis formation in different cell varieties may be attributed to peroxynitrite formed due to an interaction between NO and reactive oxygen species (ROS) (Figure 1 and 2) [9].

Atrophic Gastritis

Two main categories are known for chronic gastritis, namely atrophic and non-atrophic one [11]. Atrophy her represents the loss of the appropriate glands due to long exposure to HP infection and usually expressed as major risk factor for gastric cancer. Two types of which are recognized, one represented by fibrosis or proliferation of fibro muscular region in the lamina propria while the other represent intestinal metaplasia [12] due to normal mucosa replacement by the of intestinal type.

H. pylori-associated Atrophic Gastritis

Helicobacter pylori (HP) is spiral-shaped, flagellated, Gram-negative bacterium which colonizes the stomach of affected individuals [1,13]. The bacteria induces dyspepsia, peptic ulcers, acute, chronic gastritis, and mainly responsible for gastric-adenocarcinoma, pancreatic cancer [14,15] additionally several autoimmune diseases.

Routs of Transmission

Primary transmission rout is through individual exposure to vomit, (fecal-oral) way additionally contaminated water and food participated with family members [16].

Clinical profile

Infection with HP resulted in symptoms like nausea, vomiting, epigastric pain, hypochlorhydria malaise, fullness and flatulence which may extends to one week regardless any drugs intake or eradication of the bacteria from its location. Chronic gastritis however may appear during persistence of HP infection either asymptomatically or may be manifested as epigastric pain, anorexia additionally nausea and vomiting [17]. Atrophic gastritis may be developed later and characterized by gastric ulcers and adencarcinoma as complications of HP infection. Duodenal ulcer is manifested by burning sensation which may be developed few hours either after meal or at night and disappeared by intake of food.

Relation between HP infection and Oxidative Stress

Oxidative stress is mainly due to increased Free radical synthesis which is usually manifested in many diseases like chronic gastritis, peptic ulcers, gastric cancer [18,19] and HP infection is mainly responsible for such gastric disorders [20]. Specific HP bacterial strains having certain genotype like cag A+/Vac As1 may appear more virulent than the others [20,21]. Inflammatory response by the gastric epithelium her may lead to the production of interleukin-8 (IL-8) and subsequent generation of ROS additionally other cytokines like TNF-α, interferon ϒ (INF-ϒ), IL-12 and IL-6 (1). Increased level of NO synthesis was also found in certain diseases like duodenal ulcer, gastritis and gastric cancer [22,23]. This is mostly attributed to certain stimuli like bacterial lip polysaccharides, cytokines that are derived from the bacterial wall [24].

The Inflammatory and Immune Response to HP Infection

Pathologically gastric inflammation represents the main mediator her since the immune and inflammatory responses have no effect which allow bacterial persistence for long time. Immune response may be only evident with specific virulence factor which increase gastric inflammation, and stimulate the innate immunity. Local immune effectors in addition may be up regulated by an acquired T helper 1 response [25].

Host response to *H. Pylori*

The immune response towards bacterial pathogens can be divided into an innate and an adaptive response. The innate response towards bacterial infection is generally initial one as non-specific process, which reacts quickly with several bacterial molecules and directed to kill the bacteria. The adaptive immune response however is delayed and antigen-specific leading to the activation of T, B memory cells and is shaped by the innate immune response.

Innate immunity

Recognition of bacterial molecules by the innate immune system is mediated by TLRs (Toll-like receptors) expressed on APCs (antigen-presenting cells) such as monocytes and DCs (dendrite cells). Bacterial contact with monocytes and other APCs leads to the secretion of pro-inflammatory cytokines such as TNF- α (tumor necrosisfactor- α), IL (interleukin)-1β and IL-8. *H. pylori* infection has been shown to be associated with increased levels of these cytokines and acting as local chemo attractants [26,27] and inducing granulocytic infiltration [28]. Accordingly many of the studies on innate immune responses to *H. pylori* in epithelial cells have focused onTLR4, the specific 'pathogen-recognition molecule (PRM) of Gram-negative LPS (lipopolysaccharide).

However, gastric epithelial cell lines were non-responsiveto *H. pylori* LPS, even when relatively high concentrations of this endotoxin were added to the cells [29] and Consistent with this, a TLR4-neutralizing antibody did not block *H. pylori*-induced secretion of the proinflammatory cytokine IL-8 in AGS cells [30].

Humoral response

Individuals colonized with *H. pylori* elicit a strong specific systemic and local antibody response to the infection. Tosi and Czinn reported that binding of IgG to *H. pylori* promoted phagocytosis and killing *in vitro* by polymorph nuclear leucocytes. *H. pylori* strains are susceptible to complement and activate it either via the classical pathway, even in the absence of specific antibodies or by the alternative pathway [31]. Despite this vigorous immune response, *H. pylori* is not eradicated unless an infected individual is treated with a combination of antibiotics, and lifelong chronic infection usually develops. These observations suggest that gastric mucus may be a protective site in which *H. pylori* exist and are relatively inaccessible to specific antibodies or their effector functions.

H. Pylori Vaccine

Whole formalin-inactivated HP is the only vaccine tested in humans [32] and HP0231 prepared vaccine showed no function [33-35]. Collective vaccine from recombinant cag A, vacuolating cytotoxin A and neutrophil activating protein (NAP) represent a well-known trivalent vaccine [36].

Heat shock proteins (Hsp), highly conserved molecules expressed by both bacteria and mammalian species, possess a range of functions, acting as chaperones for cellular proteins and can activate innate immune receptors. Hsp complex (HspC) vaccines, containing Hsp derived from pathogenic bacteria, are immune stimulatory without addition of exogenous adjuvant and can induce immunity against their chaperoned proteins [37]. Expression of HP adhesin (HP0410) was reported in food grade bacteria Lactobacillus acidophilus and was used as oral vaccine in experimental mice. This vaccine has proved to be an effective and promising candidate (vaccine antigen) taken in consideration its low cost of preparation [38].

Autoimmune Atrophic Gastritis

Anti-gastric auto antibodies are detectable in about 30% of *H. pylori* infected patients. Two major in situ binding sites have been found: first at the luminal membrane in antrum, corpus mucosa and secondly at canalicular membranes. The presence of the latter type of autoantibodies is correlated with the histological and clinical parameters of corpus mucosa atrophy. The gastric H+/K(+)-ATPase, which is already known as an auto antigen in classic autoimmune gastritis represents also a major target in atrophic *H. pylori* gastritis [39].

Progressive inflammatory state leading to replacement of parietal cells by atrophic and metaplastic mucosa represents autoimmune gastritis. Autoantibody interaction with parietal cell proton pump and T cells resulted in breakdown of parietal cells which may resulted firstly to decreased HCL levels and lastly a chlorhydria. Its interaction however with intrinsic factor will affect vitamin B_{12} absorption leading to megaloplastic anemia which is collectively termed pernicious anemia [40]. Chronic atrophic gastritis patients additionally develop hyper gastrinemia leading to certain carcinoid tumors. Gastrin is expressed by certain studies as cancer risk biomarker and growth factor for certain malignant tumors in stomach, colon, pancreas and liver cancer. Vaccination with antigastrin for individuals having gastrointestinal cancer represents a simple, low cost tool and promising treatment [41].

Tests for *H. pylori*

Several methods are available to test for *H. pylori* infection.

Breath test (Carbon Isotope-urea Breath Test, or UBT)

Up to 2 weeks before doing the test intake of antibiotics, bismuth medicines such as Pepto-Bismol and proton pump inhibitors (PPIs) must be stopped.

During the test, a special substance like radioactive urea (harmless) is given [42]. If *H. pylori* are present, the bacteria convert the urea into carbon dioxide, which is detected and recorded in exhaled breath after 10 minutes. This test can identify almost all people who have *H. pylori* and to trace the treatment of the infection.

Blood tests

Blood tests are used her to measure antibodies to *H. pylori* and not the current infection where the test can be positive for years even if the infection is cured [43].

Stool test

A stool test can detect traces of *H. pylori* in the faeces in turn it is a diagnostic tool for the infection and confirm the treatment success [44].

Biopsy

Biopsy taken through endoscopy from the stomach lining is the most accurate way to confirm *H. pylori* infection and recommended also to diagnose dyspepsia. Testing for *H. pylori* without endoscopy is done only when the indigestion is new, the person is younger than 55, and there are no other symptoms [45,46]. However Convential PCR and multiple Genetic analysis system (MGAS) could be a potential alternative method for clinical detection and to monitor the effectiveness of HP therapy.

Treatments and Drugs

Depending on the causal factors of gastritis especially acute type due to long intake of non-steroidal anti-inflammatory drugs or alcohol, this can relieved by stopping their use while treatment of the chronic type may require different antibiotics additionally metronidazole.

Gastritis medications

Generally it is recommended to use a combination of antibiotics with metronidazole for 10-14 days [47]. Proton pump inhibitors like omeprazole are also recommended to decrease gastric acid production and facilitate quick healing [48]. Randomized clinical trial for HP gastritis patients using lansoprazole in combination with clarithromycin, amoxicillin, jinghuaweikang gelatin pearl for 10 days followed by additional 14 days using the gelatin pearl alone showed symptomatic improvement dealing with epigastric pain, bloating and belching [49].

Histamine blockers (H-2) are also recommended like ranitidine and cimetidin additionally antacid although side effects of the latter must be taken in consideration.

Natural products as medication for gastritis

Tannins and Flavonoids (Phenolic compounds), mostly found in several medicinal plants have usually certain therapeutic effects. Anti-inflammatory, antioxidant, anti ulcerogenic and wound healing are mostly attributed to these constituents [50].

Antioxidants content of Fresh vegetables and fruits have beneficial effect on GIT mucosa. Curcumin and black seed oil have significant effect on specific mucosal lesions (ulcers) due to their flavonoids content [51]. Many plants like quassin artichoke, quarcetin have inhibitory influence on cytokine mediated inflammatory mechanism, ulcer healing and suppression of NO synthesis (iNOS). The quassionoidisobrucein B (isoB), one of the main constituent of Picrolemmasprucei has proved to provide protective effect against NSAID -induced gastritis. This was attributed to reduction in 1L-1β, TNFα, prostaglandins additionally leukocyte rolling and migration [52].

Licorice extracts have significant effect on HP gastritis and gastric cancer due to its potent ant oxidative, anti-inflammatory, and anti-mutagenic actions. The expressions of COX-2, iNOS, VEGF, and IL-8 were increased after *H. pylori* infection, turned to be significantly decreased with s-lico in a dose-dependent manner [53]. Croton campestris A. St.-Hill., popularly known as "vela me do campo", is a species native from savannah area of Northeast Brazil and used by traditional communities in folk medicine for a variety of health problems, especially detoxification, inflammation and gastritis. CCRE a traditional Brazilian medicine against gastric disorders have antinuclear activity, mostly due to its stimulation of NO synthesis and activation of endogenous prostaglandin production [54].

Discussion and Conclusion

The above article represent a survey on causes, diagnostic tools additionally panel of gastritis treatment. Focus is done on agents inducing acute, chronic types and that in consequence to HP infection. Causes which affect the integrity of gastric mucosa leading to injury and in relation to inflammatory pattern, oxidative stress, hormonal, Enzymes secretion and NO synthesis were also discussed. Role of HP in association with atrophic gastritis, its routes of transmission, symptoms observed in relation to oxidative stress were also reported. Different types of immunity in concern and autoimmune atrophic gastritis were also discussed. Lastly common tests for HP, gastritis medication with special focus on natural products were also outlined.

References

1. Marshall BJ, Warren JR (1984) Unidentified curved bacilli in the stomach of patients with gastritis and peptic ulceration. Lancet 1: 1311-1315.
2. Dixon MF, Genta RM, Yardley JH, Correa P (1996) Classification and grading of gastritis. Am J Surg Pathol 20: 1161-1181.
3. Szabo S, Trier JS, Frankel PW (1981) Sulfhydryl compounds may mediate gastric cytoprotection. Science 214: 200-202.
4. Hotta K (2000) "Gastric mucus", a mysterious and interesting substance. Trends Glycosci Glycotechnol 12: 59-68.
5. Kasper DL, Braunwald E, Fauci AS, Hauser A, Longo DL, et al. (2006) Harrison. Principios de Medicina Interna.
6. Andersen LP (2007) Colonization and infection by Helicobacter pylori in humans. Helicobacter 12 Suppl 2: 12-15.
7. Voutilainen M, Juhola M, Färkkilä M, Sipponen P (2002) Foveolar hyperplasia at the gastric cardia: prevalence and associations. J Clin Pathol 55: 352-354.
8. Kozlowski W, Jochymski C, Markiewicz T (2011) Gastritis and gastric cancer - New insights in gastroprotection, diagnosis and treatments. Chronic gastritis.
9. Elseweidy MM, Taha MM, Younis NN, Ibrahim KS, Hamouda HA, et al. (2010) Gastritis induced by Helicobacter pylori infection in experimental rats. Dig Dis Sci 55: 2770-2777.
10. Elseweidy MM, Taha MM, Younis NN, Ibrahim KS, Hamouda HA, et al. (2010) Pattern of gastritis as manipulated by current state of Helicobacter pylori infection. BIBIEN 4: 1-9.
11. Rugge M, Fassan M, Pizzi M, Pennelli G, Nitti D, et al. (2011) Operative Link for Gastritis Assessment gastritis staging incorporates intestinal metaplasia subtyping. Hum Pathol 42: 1539-1544.
12. Rugge M, Meggio A, Pennelli G, Piscioli F, Giacomelli L, et al. (2007) Gastritis staging in clinical practice: the OLGA staging system. Gut 56: 631-636.
13. Bruce MG, Maaroos HI (2008) Epidemiology of Helicobacter pylori infection. Helicobacter 13 Suppl 1: 1-6.

14. Atherton JC (2006) The pathogenesis of Helicobacter pylori-induced gastro-duodenal diseases. Annu Rev Pathol 1: 63-96.
15. Trikudanathan G, Philip A, Dasanu CA, Baker WL (2011) Association between Helicobacter pylori infection and pancreatic cancer. A cumulative meta-analysis. JOP 12: 26-31.
16. Graham DY, Opekun AR, Osato MS, El-Zimaity HM, Lee CK, et al. (2004) Challenge model for Helicobacter pylori infection in human volunteers. Gut 53: 1235-1243.
17. Fischer W, Püls J, Buhrdorf R, Gebert B, Odenbreit S, et al. (2001) Systematic mutagenesis of the Helicobacter pylori cag pathogenicity island: essential genes for CagA translocation in host cells and induction of interleukin-8. Mol Microbiol 42: 1337-1348.
18. Yamaoka Y, Kwon DH, Graham DY (2000) A M(r) 34,000 proinflammatory outer membrane protein (oipA) of Helicobacter pylori. Proc Natl Acad Sci USA 97: 7533-7538.
19. Ding SZ, Goldberg JB, Hatakeyama M (2010) Helicobacter pylori infection, oncogenic pathways and epigenetic mechanisms in gastric carcinogenesis. Future Oncol 6: 851-862.
20. Chen G, Takeuchi Y, Kikuchi R, Arai D, Fukuchi K, et al. (2005) The cause of failure of eradication treatment of Helicobacter pylori. Rinsho Byori 53: 692-697.
21. Moss SF, Legon S, Bishop AE, Polak JM, Calam J (1992) Effect of Helicobacter pylori on gastric somatostatin in duodenal ulcer disease. Lancet 340: 930-932.
22. Mason JM, Delaney B, Moayyedi P, Thomas M, Walt R (2005) North of England Dyspepsia Guideline Development Group, Managing dyspepsia without alarm signs in primary care: new national guidance for England and Wales. Aliment Pharmacol Ther 21: 1135-1143.
23. Delaney B, McColl K (2005) Helicobacter pylori and gastro-oesophageal reflux disease. Aliment Pharmacol Ther 22 Suppl 1: 32-40.
24. Janssen M, Dijkmans BA, Vandenbroucke JP, van Duijn W, Peña AS, et al. (1992) Decreased level of antibodies against Helicobacter pylori in patients with rheumatoid arthritis receiving intramuscular gold. Ann Rheum Dis 51: 1036-1038.
25. Robinson K, Argent RH, Atherton JC (2007) The inflammatory and immune response to Helicobacter pylori infection. See comment in PubMed Commons below Best Pract Res Clin Gastroenterol 21: 237-259.
26. Antos D, Enders G, Rieder G, Stolte M, Bayerdörffer E, et al. (2001) Inducible nitric oxide synthase expression before and after eradication of Helicobacter pylori in different forms of gastritis. FEMS Immunol Med Microbiol 30: 127-131.
27. Kawahara T, Teshima S, Oka A, Sugiyama T, Kishi K, et al. (2001) Type I Helicobacter pylori lipopolysaccharide stimulates toll-like receptor 4 and activates mitogen oxidase 1 in gastric pit cells. Infect Immun 69: 4382-4389.
28. Crabtree J (1996) Immune and inflammatory responses to Helicobacter pylori infection. Scand J Gastroenterol Suppl 31: 3-10.
29. Bäckhed F, Rokbi B, Torstensson E, Zhao Y, Nilsson C, et al. (2003) Gastric mucosal recognition of Helicobacter pylori is independent of Toll-like receptor 4. J Infect Dis 187: 829-836.
30. Su B, Ceponis PJ, Lebel S, Huynh H, Sherman PM (2003) Helicobacter pylori activates Toll-like receptor 4 expression in gastrointestinal epithelial cells. Infect Immun 71: 3496-3502.
31. Berstad AE, Høgåsen K, Bukholm G, Moran AP, Brandtzaeg P (2001) Complement activation directly induced by Helicobacter pylori. Gastroenterology 120: 1108-1116.
32. Kotloff KL, Sztein MB, Wasserman SS, Losonsky GA, DiLorenzo SC, et al. (2001) Safety and immunogenicity of oral inactivated whole-cell Helicobacter pylori vaccine with adjuvant among volunteers with or without subclinical infection. Infect Immun 69: 3581-3590.
33. Aebischer T, Bumann D, Epple HJ, Metzger W, Schneider T, et al. (2008) Correlation of T cell response and bacterial clearance in human volunteers challenged with Helicobacter pylori revealed by randomised controlled vaccination with Ty21a-based Salmonella vaccines. Gut 57: 1065-1072.
34. Sachs G, Weeks DL, Melchers K, Scott DR (2003) The Gastric Biology of Helicobacter pylori. Annu Rev Physiol 65: 349-369.
35. Michetti P, Kreiss C, Kotloff KL, Porta N, Blanco JL, et al. (1999) Oral immunization with urease and Escherichia coli heat-labile enterotoxin is safe and immunogenic in Helicobacter pylori-infected adults. Gastroenterology 116: 804-812.
36. Malfertheiner P, Schultze V, Rosenkranz B, Kaufmann SH, Ulrichs T, et al. (2008) Safety and immunogenicity of an intramuscular Helicobacter pylori vaccine in noninfected volunteers: a phase I study. Gastroenterology 135: 787-795.
37. Chionh YT, Arulmuruganar A, Venditti E, Ng GZ, Han JX, et al. (2014) Heat shock protein complex vaccination induces protection against Helicobacter pylori without exogenous adjuvant. Vaccine 32: 2350-2358.
38. Hongying F, Xianbo W, Fang Y, Yang B, Beiguo L (2014) Oral immunization with recombinant Lactobacillus acidophilus expressing the adhesin Hp0410 of Helicobacter pylori induces mucosal and systemic immune responses. Clin Vaccine Immunol 21: 126-132.
39. Kirchner T, Faller G (1999) Helicobacter pylori infections and autoimmunity: the interplay in the pathogenesis of gastritis. Verh Dtsch Ges Pathol 83: 56-61.
40. Neumann WL, Coss E, Rugge M, Genta RM (2013) Autoimmune atrophic gastritis--pathogenesis, pathology and management. Nat Rev Gastroenterol Hepatol 10: 529-541.
41. Maddalo G, Spolverato Y, Rugge M, Farinati F (2014) Gastrin: from pathophysiology to cancer prevention and treatment. Eur J Cancer Prev 23: 258-263.
42. Broide E, Shirin H (2015) Evaluation of exalenz bioscience's breathid for helicobacter pylori detection. Expert Rev Mol Diagn 15: 299-312.
43. Feldman M, Friedman LS, Brandt LJ (2010) Sleisenger and Fordtran's gastrointestinal and liver disease: pathophysiology, diagnosis, management, expert consult premium editionenhanced online features: Elsevier Health Sciences.
44. Korkmaz H, Findik D, Ugurluoglu C, Terzi Y (2015) Reliability of stool antigen tests: investigation of the diagnostic value of a new immunochromatographic Helicobacter pylori approach in dyspeptic patients. Asian Pac J Cancer Prev 16: 657-660.
45. Siavoshi F, Saniee P, Khalili-Samani S, Hosseini F, Malakutikhah F, et al. (2015) Evaluation of methods for H. pylori detection in PPI consumption using culture, rapid urease test and smear examination. Ann Transl Med 3: 11.
46. Uotani T, Graham DY (2015) Diagnosis of Helicobacter pylori using the rapid urease test. Ann Transl Med 3: 9.
47. Scherübl H, Fischbach W, Glocker E, Malfertheiner P (2015) What is new in treating Helicobacter pylori infection? Dtsch Med Wochenschr 140: 277-280.
48. Sakamoto Y, Shimoyama T, Nakagawa S, Mikami T, Fukuda S (2014) Proton pump inhibitor treatment decreases the incidence of upper gastrointestinal disorders in elderly Japanese patients treated with NSAIDs. Intern Med 53: 1107-1111.
49. Wang TT, Zhang YM, Zhang XZ, Cheng H, Hu FL, et al. (2013) Jinghuaweikang gelatin pearls plus proton pump inhibitor-based triple regimen in the treatment of chronic atrophic gastritis with Helicobacter pylori infection: a multicenter, randomized, controlled clinical study. Zhonghua Yi Xue Za Zhi 93: 3491-3495.
50. Elseweidy MM (2011) "Gastritis and Gastric Cancer - New Insights in Gastroprotection, Diagnosis and Treatments", Role of Natural Antioxidants in Gastritis. INTECH Open Access Publisher.
51. Elseweidy MM, Younis NN, Amin RS, Abdallah FR, Fathy AM, et al. (2008) Effect of some natural products either alone or in combination on gastritis induced in experimental rats. Dig Dis Sci 53: 1774-1784.
52. Vieira SM, Silva RL, Lemos HP, Amorim RC, Silva EC, et al. (2014) Gastro-protective effects of isobrucein B, a quassinoid isolated from Picrolemma sprucei. Fitoterapia 95: 8-15.

15

Homeopathy against Malaria: It's Potential as a Third Millennium Drug

Aswathy Rajan[1*], Ramanibai Ravichandran[1] and Upma Bagai[2]

[1]*Department of Zoology, University of Madras, Chennai, India*

[2]*Department of Zoology, Panjab University, Chandigarh, India*

***Corresponding author:** Aswathy Rajan, Department of Zoology, University of Madras, Guindy Campus, Guindy, Chennai-600025, India, E-mail: zoology1808@gmail.com

Abstract

Malaria is the most devastating infectious disease in the world, and increasing numbers of multi drug resistance parasites are making it worse. The rising problem of morbidity and mortality justify the search and adoption of new tools and measures to minimize the impact of malaria. World Health Organization stated that homoeopathy is the second most used medical system internationally which is a nontoxic form of alternative medicine and can be combined with classical treatment methods for avoiding the risk of adverse effects. Innumerous scientific researches have been carried out to sustain homoeopathy as a complete scientific system to combat antagonism. Establishment of classical homeopathic drugs for malaria can prove as a next generation therapy, as homeopathy doesn't give any scope of resistance. The most important and significant aspect of homeopathic medicines is that they are developed after direct proving on human beings and not on animals. Each homeopathic medicine is therefore more akin to human nature and human system. This is a quality unshared by most medicines in other systems. This review will give scientific basis to classical homeopathic doctrine of ultra-high dilutions and their use as antimalarials. Homeopathic medicines are used against malaria since last two decades and this review provides a data of all homeopathic antimalarials and the ongoing researches. The review is supported by latest research in this field which can provide a base for designing better methodologies in the field of homeopathic antimalarial therapy.

Keywords: Homeopathy; Malaria; Potency; Antimalarial; Ultrahigh dilutions

Introduction

Mentions of malaria can be found in the ancient Roman, Chinese, Indian and Egyptian manuscripts. Morton presented the first detailed description of the clinical picture of malaria and its treatment with *Cinchona*. He also suggested that the disease is produced by some poison which enters the body [1]. The *Cinchona* (china) bark testing for malaria patient gave birth to homeopathy. Dr. Hahnemann (Father of homeopathy) theorized that because the bark produced symptoms similar to malaria, taking a small amount of bark would stimulate the body to heal itself of malaria, after which the principle of "similia simibilus currentur"-like cures like was established in homeopathy [2]. Homeopathy has been cited by the World Health Organization as one of the systems of traditional medicine that should be integrated with conventional medicine to ensure adequate global healthcare [3,4]. According to homeopathy, the body's symptoms of illness are an expression of the body trying to heal itself and should not be suppressed. Homeopathic remedies help in establishing balance in body and promote its ability to heal itself. It intervenes at the level of person's reactive, self-curative powers with a goal to bring about a change in the total functioning of the body. Homeopathy regards disease as deranged vital process, caused by dynamic influences of noxious agents of the vital principle, as manifested through perceptible sign and symptoms. According to homeopathic thought the pathogens are carriers of dynamic specific traits of respective disease force which only can affect the vital force of the susceptible living host in a suitable environment producing corresponding change in the function and structure of the physical body of the host, totality of which is named as particular disease [5].

The homeopathic approach may be useful specifically because it does not focus on the cause of the disease but on the teleonomy of the patient's reaction. It is therefore not being considered an alternative approach by many homeopaths, but complementary to effective drug use [6]. From the time of its birth, in recent years homeopathy has evolved in clinical, physical, chemical, biological and medical levels with acceptable scientific norms. Homeopathic drugs have been claimed for their efficacy, without side effects and low cost and they have been evaluated for their suitable candidature as potent antimalarials. This review gives an insight about the growth of ancient homeopathy which was based on human proving to cellular/subcellular level studies.

Materials and Methods

The data was collected from all the published research articles, reviews and newsletters available during the period of 2007-2015. Various articles were collected from E-journals like Homeopathy 4 everyone and Homeopathy Ezine. The books related to organon and philosophy, therapeutics and Materia Medica were consulted and all the data were collected from them.

The collected data were thoroughly studied and documented year wise. The list of homeopathic remedies used for malarial/malaria like fevers were taken from various homeopathic repertories by different homeopaths for the preparation of the table.

Malaria in history of homeopathy

Malaria generally presents a multifaceted expression, typically by the three phase paroxysm associated with auxiliary symptoms besides cachexia or background symptoms on becoming chronic. This is due to the different developmental stages of the parasite in the human body. Each of the stages could contribute its respective toxins, resulting in the typical paroxysmic phases and their concomitants. Consequently, selection of similimum has been problematic which continues even today. Hahnemann having himself been the first formal prover of quinine which led him to found homoeotherapeutics, was quite seized of the problem [7].

Cinchona was the first antimalarial medicine based on similia principle; later on it was established as quinine. There was a continuous but unnoticed progress in homeopathic antimalarial research since its birth. It is important to know the background and its course of development during the past to establish the identity of the ultra-high dilutions of homeopathy.

Late 18-19th century

Allen reported over 100 malarial cases cured by 50 homeopathic medicines based on a review of the literature in 1884 [8] (Table 1). Temple and Hoyne likewise dealt with results of over 50 cases treated by about 25 homeopathic drugs in 1878 [9], while Clarke listed out over 100 drugs clinically confirmed as curing intermittent fevers in 1904 [10].

Many others also provided periodical reviews of literature in homeopathic treatment for intermittent fever. Most frequently used homeopathic remedies for malaria treatment include: Arsenicum album, *Bryonia, Ipecacuanha, Eucalyptus globulus, Natrum muriaticum* and *Veratrum album* [11,12]. Fenner has listed 45 homeopathic remedies which can be used for malaria [13] and Puhlmann has added few more to the list [14]. Recent data bases lists 130 remedies which can be used for the treatments depending upon the individual's symptoms, as every patient can have different accompanying signs to his classical symptoms of malaria. The treatment is individualized according to the inter-individual differences. Kent also prescribed Ars., Calc- ar., Ferr., Psor., Sulph. and Tub. For relapsing fever whereas; Ars., Bell., Chin., Eup- per., Verat., Sulph. and Rhus- t. are recommended for remittent fever [15]. Malaria like many other ailments in chronic state becomes metastatic, expressing itself in different forms in different parts of the body and in such cases the chill may be experienced in only certain body parts.

According to Hughes, malarial toxaemia essentially involves silencing of the oxidative mechanism in one or more parts of the body and leads to sensation of chills in the parts concerned and finally their dysfunctioning due to non-availability of the energy supplies, which has potential to bring an end to the life of the host. Therefore such drugs which can review the oxidation in varied parts of the body would form the appropriate remedies. Apparently polychrests like Ars., Calc- ar., Chin- a. (remedies for malarial cachexia) which can kindle oxidation would be useful. Ars. is more deep acting and helped in successful treatment of malarial cachexia. Thus in chronic cases such drugs could be effective than not only polychrests, high oxidants but also deep acting being able to penetrate remote parts of the body like the nerves, bones and various glands [16].

In an open-double blind randomized clinical trial for malaria in Ghana following homeopathic remedies were used: Arsenicum album, china, *Eupatorium perfoliatum, Natrum muriaticum, Nux vomica, Pulsatilla, Rhus toxicodendron* and Sulphur. Chloroquine was used as standard drug in placebo control group. The percentage of 90.7% improvement in open study and 83.3% in double blind study has been attributed to the homeopathic treatment, during the four week study period. However, a definite conclusion can be drawn if study is extended for a longer follow-up period (minimum 6 months) to access the number of episodes comparing the chloroquine group with homeopathic group [17].

Patients with *P. falciparum* malaria showed rapid response in the medication with Sulphur 200 and 1M and for over 3 months no relapse was reported [18]. For irregular types of cases which are already treated with allopathic or homeopathic or any drug therapy, and in such cases more often two or more remedies are recommended. In such cases it is essential to antidote the picture of the earlier drugs. Ip. or Ars. or Nux- v. can be useful. He also reported *Chininum arsenicosum* (1X, 2X, 3X, 6X), *Chininum sulphuricum* (1X, 2X, 3X, 6X) and *Chininum purum* (Q, 1X, 2X, 3X, 6X) against malarial poisoning. *Natrum suphuricum* (3X, 6X), *Aranea diadema* (Q, 6C) and *Ceanothus americanus* (Q) which act as drainage in malaria, *Echinaecia angui* (Q), *Nyctanthes arbortristis* (Q), *Baptisia tinctoria* (Q), *Melia azardichata* (Q) and *Eupatorium perfoliatum* (Q) are prescribed for relieving concomitant peripheral and toxic symptoms of malaria are used to remove *Plasmodium* species from blood. They also act as blood purifier and drainage remedy [19].

Central council for research in homeopathy and AYUSH, India gave homeopathic medicines: *Eupatorium perfoliatum, Alstonia constricta*, Chin- a., Chin- s., Ars. as preventive medicines for malaria in Rajasthan (Jaipur, Bikaner, Jodhpur, Barmer and Jaisalmer), whereas one more drug Verat was given for the treatment. For the persons going to malarious regions, homeopathic medicines Chin- a. 3X with Nat- s. 6X and Ferr. 12X two times in day or the same at increasing intervals during the stay is recommended as preventive dose [19].

In 20th century

Robin Murphy recommended in his homeopathic medical repertory, Abies-n., Arg- n., Aran., Carb- ac., Chin., Chin- a., Chin-s., Eup-per., Ferr., Ip., Nat- m., Nat- s., Nux-v., Psor., Sulph., Ter., Verat. for the malarial fever, Eucal., for chronic and relapsing malaria. Malaria co nosode 30 is also recommended for recurring parasite which lingers in liver for months [20].

S. No.	Name of Authors	Year	Proposed Drugs
1	Nash EB	1807-1913	Ars., Chin., Eup- perf., Gels., Ip., Nat- m., Podo., Puls., Rhus- t., Sabad.
2	Temple & Hoyne	1878	Apis., Aran., Arn., Ars., Cact., Calc- ar., Camph., Caps., Chin., Cina., Gels., Helle., Ip., Lyc., Mer- c., Nat- m., Nux- v., Op., Petr., Puls., Rhus- t., Sars., Sep., Stram., Sulph., Thuj.

3	Allen HC	1879 & 1884	Apis., Ars., Bapt., Bry., Chin., Chin-.s., Eup- perf., Gels., Ign., Lach., Nat- m., Nux- v., Op., Sulph.
4	Farrington EA	1880	Apis., Ars., Arn., Camph., Carb- ac., Chin- a., Chin., Crot- h., Ipec., Lyc., Mur- ac., Nux- v., Psor., Pyr., Sulph., Sulph- ac., Verat.
5	Kent JT	1888	Ant- c., Arn., Ars., Bapt., Bry., Colch., Eup- perf., Gels., Hyos., Ip., Lyc., Mur-ac., Rhus- t.
6	Wrumb	-	Ars., Ign., Ip., Nux- v., Puls., Verat.
7	Clarke	1904	Apis., Aran., Ars., Aza., Bry., Cact., Calen., Carbo- v., Carb- ac., Cean., Ced., Chin- a., Chin.,Chin- m., Chin- s., Corn., Elat., Eup- perf., Eup- purp., Ferr., Gels., Lach., Lyc., Malar., Meny., Nat- m., Nux- v., Puls., Rhus- t., Sulph., Verat.
8	Boger CM	1905	Aran., Ars., Caps., Ced., Eup- perf., Ign., Nat- m., Nux- v., Ph- ac., Puls., Sulph., Verat.
9	Mills	1915	Ars., Alst- s., Am- pic., Aran., Caps., Chin., Chin- a., Chin- s., Corn., Helianth., Ip., Nat- m.
10	Josset	-	Ars., Caps., Ip., Nux- v.
11	Boericke W	1927	Ars., Alston., Am- pic., Aran., Caps., Chin., Chin- a., Chin- s., Corn., Helianth., Ip., Nat- m.
12	Bernoville	1936	Ars., Cean., Chin., Chin- a., Nat- m.
13	Kichlu & Boss	1988	Ars., Bry., Chin., Chin- s., Eup- perf., Ferr., Gels., Nat- m., Nux- v., Puls.

Table 1: Homeopathic drugs proposed by various authors as the most effective antimalarials.

It is also reported that a 3 week course of Neem 2X tincture can neutralize the parasite, expel it and help eliminate the chronic malaria. The follow-up monthly dose of Malaria nosode is a backup to further protect the person and help to remain free of malaria [21]. There is also in the recent literature, some works designed to explore the behavior of the body after to be stimulated by parasitic stressor and treated with homeopathic medicines. It is also recommended to take a homeopathic first aid kit for travelers to Africa containing Chin- s, Chin. with Art. and quinine [22].

Some other homeopathic formulations like *Calcarea arsenicosum, Capsicum, Carbolicum acidum, Cedron, Ferrum picricum* and *Ignatia* are also recommended for intermittent fevers [23]. The nosode Malaria Co., a compilation of malarial parasites species (*P. falciparum, P. vivax, P. ovale* and *P. malariae*) is a prescription remedy that can be used alternately with Chin., Nat- m., Phosphorus, Ars. and Eup- pru. Starting with a single dose of Nat- m. 30C, single dose of Chin. 30C in the following week, followed by a dose of Phosphorus 30C in next week with a final single dose of Arsenicum 30C in the last week of the cycle can be very effective. If one stays for an extended time in a high-risk area, these remedies can be administered in a 200C less frequently [23]. These remedies in a 30C dose can be alternated weekly prior to visiting an endemic area. A complex mixture of 'Malaria X', a preparation of 30C remedies which contains 5 ingredients (Malaria nosode and 4 other remedies- *China officinalis, Natrum muriaticum,* Arsenicum album and *Eupatorium perfoliatum*) is very effective in malarial attacks and also in preventing malaria. Other remedies useful for the prevention of malaria include *Natrum muriaticum*, Phosphorus or Arsenicum. Malaria officinalis and *Eupatorium prupurem*, have also been used as preventative remedies [23].

In Kenya, Abha Light Foundation has been working in the field of malaria for 10 years, treating the disease with homeopathy and natural medicines. They developed a protocol of homeopathic medicines for all-round prophylaxis treatment. According to them, homeopathic formulation of Neem (2X or D2) has proven its effectiveness in eliminating recurring malaria. Five drops a day for 2-3 weeks is believed to destroy any parasite that may remain in the body and breaks the cycle of recurrent malaria. Neem 2X still continues to be given successfully to thousands of Masai tribals in Tanzania [24]. It was also reported that, at many clinics in Kenya, Malaria X is a regular prescription for hundreds of patients. In a Kendu Bay Malaria prevention project in Kenya, Malaria X (3-step program) was distributed to 1500 families. Six months before starting the program, 100% of participants had attacks of malaria or malaria-like symptoms at least once in their lifetime. Of the 34 participants 71% used to get malaria or malaria like symptoms once a month or every two weeks. Since starting the 3-step program, only 12% (4 out of 34) respondents had an attack of malaria or malaria like symptoms [24].

For the treatment of malaria, depending on the specific Plasmodium species and the mainifestation of disease, Phosphorus, *China sulphuricum*, Chin., Ferrum metallicum, Arsenicum, *Lycopodium, Tuberculinum, Natrum muriaticum* and Malaria officinalis are more indicated. Phosphorus is indicated if there is marked liver involvement and yellowing of the skin; *China sulphuricum* when there is marked destruction of the red blood cells; Chin. where the periodicity of fever chills and perspiration is more marked; Ferrum metallicum when there is complete exhaustion from the anemia; *Lycopodium* when the disease has caused a weakening of the liver and kidneys and there is gas and abdominal bloating; *Tuberculinum* with intermittent fever, cachexia and weak lungs; *Natrum muriaticum* in cases of cachexia, chlorosis, emaciation and irregular intermittent fevers; Malaria officinalis to reduce the amount of live *Plasmodium* in the blood [23].

An embracing change was witnessed in the field of homeopathic research in the beginning of 20th century. Till now homeopathy was based on human provings, but use of other animal models for homeopathic research was a boon to researchers. Mice (*Mus musculus*) have been used as experimental model in homeopathic research in relation to cytotoxicity, genotoxicity and carcinogenesis studies as they share a high degree of homology with humans [25]. Salazar et al. demonstrated the effect of *Eupatorium perfoliatum* 30C and Arsenicum album 30C on *Plasmodium berghei* infected mice. Parasite multiplication was inhibited, but the most interesting observation was the increase in the number of schizonts suggesting an interruption of *Plasmodium* life cycle in this intracellular phase [26]. But this study was not able to find a mechanism of action of the treatment. In another study, a homeopathic medicine *Eucalyptus* was given in combination with allopathic medicine artesunate for clearing blood stage infection of *P. berghei* in BALB/c mice. The combination has been reported to provide a mutual protection and also protected recrudescence up to the one month follow up period [27]. Rats are also commonly used animal for homeopathic research featuring in around 67 experiments indexed in HomBRex database [28]. Both isopathic and *Similia* principle models seem useful to understand complex biological phenomena, such as host-parasite intractions and the effects of high dilutions seem to tend to restore living systems to a 'stable state', recovering normal parameters similar to control, as seen in several experimental models from both, descriptive and mathematical modeling points of view [29].

Within a decade many preliminary studies were carried out to check antimalarial activities of various homeopathic formulations. In a pre-clinical study, the combination it was confirmed that oral administration of china φ and china 30C in monotherapy for 7 days lead to complete inhibition of parasite load in *P. berghei* infected BALB/c with increased survival rate (26.8 ± 1.2 days) of mice. Both showed high efficacy when given in combination with artesunate (100 mg/kg). The therapeutic efficacy of the combination was confirmed by the stable levels of hepatic and renal markers in serum after treatment. This homeopathic regimen was reported to be better than the standard ACT (Artesunate+Sulphadoxine/Pyrimethamine) [30]. The homeopathic remedies were found to be effective on various parameters of study on mice. The viability and integrity of blood cells were also studied using Scanning electron microscopy and acridine orange staining and were found normal after the treatment [30]. Histochemical studies also revealed hepatoprotective and nephroprotective role of homeopathic formulations in P. berghei infected BALB/c mice [31].

In a similar study, mother tincture of *Chelidonium majus* and its potencies i.e., 6, 30 and 200 were found to exhibit considerable antiplasmodial activity against blood stage infection of *P. berghei* in mice and 30C was reported to enhance the maximum Mean Survival Time (MST) of mice [32]. Another homeopathic medicine, Malaria Co Nosode 30 was also reported to possess considerable antimalarial potential with 87.02% chemosuppression against *P. berghei* infection in BALB/c mice. Nosode is a homeopathic preparation of the secretion from the affected area/tissue. The drug was also found to be safe on liver and kidney functions of the host as observed by the normal levels of liver and kidney markers in serum of treated mice [33]. Contrary to homeopathic principle, recently another research proved that the combination of homeopathic formulations can be used for therapeutic purposes. The combination of 30C of china and Chelidonium was reported to possess potent antiplasmodial effect in mice [34].

In vitro techniques with homeopathic potencies are newer and more convenient method of checking efficacy of various homeopathic antimalarials. In recent times many such notable studies have been undertaken. Rajan and Bagai have also reported effective schizont maturation inhibition by some homeopathic drugs in *in vitro* system [35]. This kind of studies clearly shows that homeopathy can be coupled with latest techniques to procure more valuable scientific data.

Discussion

From the available literature and data from countable research publications on antimalarial homeopathic formulations, it is evident that classical documentation is still not practically followed everywhere. The publication of laboratory investigations of ultra-high dilutions in homeopathy has produced considerable controversy and mixed results on attempted replication [36,37]. Still, unusual effects of ultra-high dilutions in rigorous laboratory studies continue to be reported [38,39]. Multiple independent replications of this research have not yet been done because there are few investigators in the field [40]. Future research should focus on simple clinical or laboratory models that can be easily attempted by multiple investigators. In addition, better data are needed to examine the use and effects of homeopathy by the public and in actual practice [41-43]. The classically documented doctrine need to prove its potential through evidence based scientific research.

The scientific community entirely misses the boat on the treatment of infectious diseases. The approach itself is defective. One of the major defects in the conventional approach is the futile search for the so-called 'active ingredient' in any natural substance in order to isolate it, analyze it and then chemically synthesize it in order to mass produce it. Whereas, herb or natural substances (as used in homeopathy) has not one but thousands of active ingredients working together, that make whole herbs still the most effective means of treating infectious diseases, including so-called resistant malaria [24].

Homeopathy is the second largest system in the world, widely used and economical but lacks some evidence based research and data in order to prove its efficacy to the scientific community. Despite of so many latest developments in the field of homeopathic research there is certainly a missing link between the existence of active molecules in these ultra-high dilutions and its efficacy. According to hypothesis given by Khuda-Bhuksh, potentized homeopathic drugs have also been tested against many toxic chemical compounds. These potentized homeopathic medicines are capable of acting by triggering the regulatory action of master genes which initiates a series of reactions, resulting in many cellular and subcellular changes [25].

Conclusion

Despite being successfully used in many countries, homeopathy still gives a scope of doubt because of some scientific loop holes. As a result it is not accepted by whole scientific community. The modes of action of homeopathic dilutions are still a darker area in homeopathic research. Need of Randomized control trials on human subjects to prove safety and efficacy of homoeopathic drugs is the only way to get answers to many hypothesizes. In future strong scientific basis will be needed to establish homeopathy as a medicine of the 3rd millennium.

Acknowledgments

This study was supported by young scientist startup grant (YSS/2014/000290) to Aswathy Rajan from SERB (DST), New Delhi, India.

References

1. Morton R (1696) Exercitationes de morbis universalibus acutis. Ed ult Venice; Typis Hieronymi Albuzzi.
2. Hahnemann S (1960) Introduction to homeopathy. In: Organon of Medicine. (First Indian edn). Haehl R, M. Bhattacharyya and Co. (eds), Pub, Calcutta, pp. 1-300.
3. Bannerman RH, Burton J, Wen Cheih C (1983) Traditional medicine and health care coverage. World Health Organization, Geneva Switzerland.
4. World Health Organization (2000) The Priscriber. Promoting rational use of drugs and correct case management in basic health services. UNICEF's Programme Division in cooperation with the World Health Organization 18: 1-16
5. Shah H (1999) Intermittent Fever. In: Malaria and Homeopathy. Shah H and Jain M, (eds), Indian Books and Periodicals Pub, New Delhi, pp. 1-233.
6. Bellavite P, Ortolani R, Pontarollo F, Pitari G, Conforti A (2007) Immunology and Homeopathy, The Rationale of the 'Similie'. Evid Based Compl Alternat Med 4: 149-163.
7. Ramayya N (1994) Perspectives in Homeopathic Treatment of Malaria. National J Homeo 3: 1-6.
8. Allen HC (1884) Malarial fever. In: The therapeutics of intermittent fever. Claude RN, (ed), Hahnemann Pub, Calcutta pp. 1-342.
9. Temple S, Hoyne AM (1878) Therapeutics for intermittent fevers. In: Clinical therapeutics in homeopathy, Vol. 1, Richard D and Dake ES (eds), B Jain Pub, New Delhi pp. 1-583.
10. Clarke JH (1904) Malarial fever. In: Clinical Repertory to the Dictionary of Materia Medica. Clarke JH, (ed), B Jain Pub, New Delhi pp 1-325.
11. Kent JT (1974) Malaria. In: Repertory of the Homeopathic Materia Medica, Kent JT, (ed), Harjeet and Co Pub, New Delhi pp 1-115.
12. Farrington EA (1989) Fever. In: Comparative Materia Medica, Farrington EA, (ed), B Jain Pub, New Delhi pp. 30.
13. Fenner G (1925) Malaria. In: Tropenkrankheiten, Gaucher C, (ed), Schwabe Pub, Leipzig pp. 220-435.
14. Puhlmann (1920) Homeopathic remedies for malaria. In: Handbuch der homeoÖpathischen praxis, Hangstebeck T. (ed), Schwabe Pub, Leipzig, pp. 112-118.
15. Kent JT (1989) Relapsing Fever. In: Reportory of the homeopathic Materia Medica. Kent JT, (ed), B Jain Pub, New Delhi pp. 1-233.
16. Clarke JH (1986) Intermittent fevers. In: A dictionary of practical material medica, Vol. 1, Clarke JH, (ed), B Jain Pub, New Delhi pp. 1-951.
17. Van Erp VMA, Brands M (1993) Malaria and homeopathic remedies in Ghana, an open study and a double-blind randomized clinical trial. Homeopathy 5: 312-316.
18. Ramayya N (1994) Perspectives in homeopathic treatment of malaria. National J Homeo 3: 1-6.
19. Shah H (1999) Intermittent Fever. In: Malaria and Homeopathy. Shah H and Jain M, (ed), Indian Books and Periodicals Pub, New Delhi pp. 1-233.
20. Robin Murphy (2004) Fever-heat. In: Homeopathic Medical Repertory. Robin Murphy, (ed), B Jain Pub, New Delhi pp. 822-861.
21. Partington T, Ruchira DA, Hennel L, Pittendrigh A, Taylor J (2006) Silent and deadly, prophylaxis and treatment of malaria. Homeo in prac Spring 14-19.
22. Peter C (2007) Interviews with Homeopaths. Homeopathy 4 everyone 5: 11-13.
23. Birch K (2007) Malaria. In: vaccine free prevention and treatment of infectious contagious disease with homeopathy. Burch M, Über R, Robert Lee D, (eds), Trafford Pub, Bloomington pp. 351.
24. Ruchira DA (2010) The use of homeopathic prophylaxis and treatment for malaria in endemic areas of Kenya. Homeopathy 4 everyone 7: 23-26.
25. Khuda-Bukhsh AR (2009) Mice as a model for homeopathy research. Homeopathy 98: 267-279.
26. Salazar GL, Montiel EM, Monzon JT, Hernandez FH, Salasbenito JS (2006) Effects of homeopathic medications Eupatorium perfoliatum and Arsenicum album on parasitaemia of Plasmodium berghei infected mice. Homeopathy 95: 223-228.
27. Bagai U, Rajan A, Chandel S (2008) Efficacy of Eucalyptus (a homeopathic medicine) in combination with artesunate to clear Plasmodium berghei infection in BALB/c mice. In: Tandon V, Yadav AK, Roy B (eds) Current Trends in Parasitology, Proceedings, 20th National Congress of Parasitology, November 3-5-2008, NEHU, Shillong, India pp. 203-211.
28. Fisher P (2009) Biological models of homeopathy. Homeopathy 98: 183-185.
29. Bonamin LV, Endler PC (2010) Animal models for studying homeopathy and high dilutions: Conceptual critical review. Homeopathy 99: 37-50.
30. Rajan A, Bagai U (2011) SEM studies on blood cells of Plasmodium berghei infected BALB/c mice treated with artesunate and homeopathic medicine china. J Parasit Dis 35: 134-139.
31. Rajan A, Bagai U, Chandel S (2013) Effect of artesunate based combination therapy with homeopathic medicine china on liver and kidney of Plasmodium berghei infected mice. J Parasitic Dis 37: 62-67.
32. Rajan A, Bagai U (2013) Ameliorating effect of homeopathic medication Chelidonium majus 30c on Plasmodium berghei infected balb/C mice. AJHM 106: 125-131.
33. Bagai U, Rajan A, Kaur S (2012) Antimalarial potential of nosode 30 and 200 against Plasmodium berghei infection in BALB/c mice. J Vector Borne Dis 49: 72-77.
34. Rajan A, Bagai U (2013) Antimalarial potential of China 30 and Chelidonium 30 in combination therapy against lethal rodent malaria parasite: Plasmodium berghei. J Complement Integrated Med 10: 1-8.
35. Rajan A, Bagai U (2012) Antimalarial potential of homeopathic medicines against schizont maturation of Plasmodium berghei in short-term in vitro culture. Int J High Dilution Res 11: 224-236.
36. Davenas E, Beauvais F, Amara J, Oberbaum M, Robinzon B, et al. (1988) Human basophil degranulation triggered by very dilute antiserum against IgE. Nature 333: 816-818.
37. Ovelgönne JH, Bol AW, Hop WC, van Wijk R (1992) Mechanical agitation of very dilute antiserum against IgE has no effect on basophil staining properties. Experientia 48: 504-508.
38. Linde K, Jonas WB, Melchart D, Worku F, Wagner H, et al. (1994) Critical review and meta-analysis of serial agitated dilutions in experimental toxicology. Hum Exp Toxicol 13: 481-492.
39. Jonas WB, Kaptchuk TJ, Linde K (2010) Academia and clinic: A critical overview of homeopathy. Ann Intern Med 1-11.
40. Vickers AJ (1999) Independent replication of pre-clinical research in homeopathy: A systematic review. Forsch Komplementarmed 6: 311-320.
41. Linde K, Clausius N, Ramirez G, Melchart D, Eitel F, et al. (1997) Are the clinical effects of homeopathy placebo effects? A meta-analysis of placebo-controlled trials. Lancet 350: 834-843.
42. Linde K, Jonas WB (1999) Evaluating complementary and alternative medicine: the balance of rigor and relevance. In: Essentials of Complementary and Alternative Medicine. Jonas WB and Levin JS (eds), Lippincott Pub, Philadelphia pp. 57-71.
43. Jonas WB, Anderson RL, Crawford CC, Lyons JS (2001) A systematic review of the quality of homeopathic clinical trials. BMC Complement Altern Med 1: 12-17.

16

Safety of Chiropractic Spinal Manipulations

A Timucin Atayoglu[1,2*], Ayten Guner-Atayoglu[2], Gulcin Kuran-Cetinkale[2] and M Ali Cetinkale[2]

[1]*Medipol University, Department of Family Medicine, Istanbul, Turkey*
[2]*Holistic and Integrative Medicine Association, Istanbul, Turkey*

***Corresponding author:** A Timucin Atayoglu, Medipol University, Department of Family Medicine, Istanbul, Turkey. President of Holistic & Integrative Medicine Association, Turkey, E-mail: atayoglu@gmail.com

Abstract

Healthcare providers do consider the potential risk of harm that any treatment can cause. Chiropractic healthcare is a system of complementary medicine based on the manipulative treatment of misalignments of the joints, especially those of the spinal column. Recently, the use of chiropractic spinal manipulation has increased considerably while its safety has been debated and estimates vary widely for the incidence of serious complications. Some vascular and neurological incidents account for the criticism surrounding chiropractic. The aim of this review is to investigate the risk of serious complications of chirporactic spinal manipulations to enlighten further understanding on their prevention.

Keywords: Chiropractic; Complementary medicine; Complication; Safety; Spinal manipulation

Introduction

The healthcare professionals must consider the possible complications that any intervention might have. Primum non nocere or "first, do no harm" is a guiding dictum for all healthcare providers that whatever the intervention or procedure is performed, the patient's safety and well-being is the primary consideration [1].

Chiropractic is a form of complementary medicine concerned with the treatment of the neuromusculoskeletal system disorders [2]. The chiropractic practitioners often refer to their main technique as an adjustment of the spine and it involves manipulation that is the introduction of a high velocity and low amplitude thrust into a joint [3].

Chiropractic spinal manipulation (CSM) gained mainstream recognition in the 1960s, and today it is a very popular treatment option especially for neck and back pain [4]. If appropriately practiced, it is considered as relatively safe but as with all interventions, adverse incidents can happen [4].

Chiropractors commonly treat neck and back pain problems with CSM and there are a number of case studies show that to be effective [5]. However, its safety has been debated and there is controversy regarding the degree of risk of serious complications after CSM [6]. Unexpected strokes, myelopathies, radiculopathies or osteoarticular accidents have been considered as responsible for the criticism of CSM in the literature [5,7].

In this review we aim to search the literature on safety issues of CSM and the predictability of the adverse events. On the bases of relevant literature, we attempted to enlighten further understanding on the major risks associated with CSM and their prevention.

Method

Computerized literature searches were performed in the issue. The search terms used were 'adverse events', 'chiropractic', 'complications', 'risk', 'safety', 'spinal manipulation'. All reports, irrespective of language of publication, which contained data about risks associated with chiropractic spinal manipulation, were included, regardless of the profession of the therapist or the research methodology used for the report.

Result

In the literature, spinal manipulation has been associated with some serious vascular and neurological accidents after CSM, mostly of the upper spine [8]. On the other hand, to evaluate the safety of chiropractic procedures, a search on the articles that reported adverse reactions associated with chiropractic for the years 1966 to 2007 concluded that there was no strong data concerning the incidence or prevalence of adverse reactions after chiropractic intervention [9].

Eder and Tilscher [10] performed a survey of 168,000 CSM without a significant serious incident. Henderson and Cassidy [11] offered a report of more than a 500,000 CSM without a serious complication. Jaskoviak [12] reported approximately 5 million CSM of neck from 1965 to 1980 without any serious complications. Thiel et al. [13] obtained data from more than 50,000 cervical spine manipulations and there were no reports of serious adverse events, and estimates for serious cervical vascular accidents varied from 5 incidents per 100,000 CSM to 1 death per 4 million CSM. It was determined that there was inadequate data to be conclusive [13].

Among approximately 1.5 million cervical manipulations, Dvorak [14] found a rate of 1 serious complication per 400,000 neck manipulations, without any reported deaths. Patjin [15] found an overall rate of 1 serious complication in nearly 518,000 manipulations. According to Haldeman et al. [16], the risk of serious complications from cervical manipulation was about 1-2 per 1 million neck manipulations. In another study they estimated rate of Vertebral Basilar Accidents (VBAs) after manipulation of 1 in about 5 million cervical manipulations [17]. Lee et al. [18] found 55 reported serious adverse events in about 50 million CSM. According to Carey [19], estimate risk of serious complications is 1 per 3 million neck manipulations.

Klougart et al. [20] concluded an estimated risk of 1 event of vascular accidents per 1.320,000 cervical spine treatments sessions. Ernst [21] concluded that CSM can result in adverse events such as VBAs followed by stroke or death, but the incidence of such events is not known, however, he concluded that the risk-benefit spinal manipulation is not evidently favorable [22]. Estimate of the risk of death according to Terrett [23], is about 1 fatality per 4 million cervical manipulations. A review analyzed cases that were reported between 1925 and 1997 concluded that no deaths have been attributed to CSM provided by licensed physical therapists [24].

In the literature, there are some case reports of very rare adverse events. Struewer et al. [25] described a case with hematothorax due to an intercostal venous lesion following thoracic spinal manipulation. Phrenic nerve injury causing diaphragmatic palsy was reported as a very rare complication of cervical chiropractic manipulation [26].

There are also case reports of neuropraxic injury of radial nerves and a cervical epidural haematoma after CSM for neck pain. In all the cases there were criteria to consider a causality relation between the neurological adverse events and the CSM [27]. According to Biller et al. [28], there is low evidence supporting an association between CSM and internal carotid artery accident as well.

According to data that was reviewed by Patijn [15], there was a risk of one lumbar disc hernia (LDH) in more than 8 million CSM and one cauda equina syndrome (CES) in more than 4 million CSM. According to data found by Haldeman and Rubinstein [29], estimates of the risk of causing LDH or CES with CSM ranged from one in 1 million to one in over 100 million. Shekelle et al. [30] estimated the rate of occurrence of CES as an adverse event of CSM to be about one per 100 million manipulations.

Michaeli [31] surveyed 153 practitioners in South Africa who reported one minor or transient complication per 38,137 CSM. According to Stern et al. [32], the risk of complication of CSM for patients with low back pain and sciatica was less than 5%. Assendelft et al. [33] estimated the incidence of CES to be less than one per 1 million CSM. Oliphant [34] evaluated the safety of CSM and showed that an estimate of the risk of CSM causing a deteriorated LDH or CES in a patient presenting with LDH was calculated from published data to be less than 1 in 3.7 million.

Discussion

Although they are very rare, CSM can result in serious complications [7]. However, dissimilar results have been published in the literature on the incidence of serious risks associated with CSM [26] and there is insufficient data to be decisive [9].

The risk factors demonstrated in the literature associated with complications of CSM include misdiagnosis, failure to recognize the onset or progression of neurological signs or symptoms, improper technique, CSM performed in the presence of a coagulation disorder or herniated nucleus pulposus [35].

Complications associated with CSM remain rare and most of the adverse effects reported in literature are benign and remain transitory [36]. On the other hand, some life-threatening complications have been reported after CSM [26,37]. VBAs and CES are the leading causes of claims as serious complications of CSM [7,38]. However, estimates vary widely regarding the serious complications.

Some authors have encountered cases of vascular events such as VBAs after CSM of neck and it has been believed to account for 6-9% of cervical artery accidents [39] whereas according to some other researchers the causality is not strongly documented [40]. Practitioners should also be careful not to perform CSM on an already-dissected artery, since the patient with vertebral artery dissection can present with neck pain as the only symptom [41].

A variety of pre-manipulation tests are used for determining the effect of spinal motion on vertebral artery patency. In George's test, the bilateral blood pressure and pulse rates are measured first, and the subclavian and carotid arteries are auscultated. Then the patient is asked to rotate the head right and left, and then rotate, laterally bend and extend, each side for 15 seconds in the seated position (Maigne's test) and in the supine position (DeKleijn's test). A test is positive if it provokes signs or symptoms of vertebrobasilar insufficiency e.g. nystagmus or symptoms of vertigo, dizziness, tinnitus, visual blurring, slurring of speech, nausea, or faintness and may indicate vascular compromise or stenosis of the carotid or vertebral arteries. Arteriosclerosis, osteophytes or congenital atresia of the artery might be possible causes of vertebrobasilar insufficiency [42].

CES consists of neurogenic bowel and bladder disturbances, saddle anesthesia, bilateral leg weakness and sensory changes [43,44]. There have been case reports of CES observed in which an association between CSM [43]. CES represents a surgical emergency and CSM is contraindicated in the presence of CES [45]. CES has been seen as an adverse event of physical procedures performed on patients affected by LDH [43-45]. However, according to some authors some cases of CES reported in the literature might have been incorrectly attributed to CSM [11,46-48]. According to WHO guidelines the presence of an acute CES represents an absolute contraindication to CSM (Table 1) [4].

1	Anomalies such as dens hypoplasia, unstable os odontoideum, etc.
2	Acute fracture
3	Spinal cord tumor
4	Acute infection such as osteomyelitis, septic discitis, and tuberculosis of
5	Meningeal tumor
6	Haematomas, whether spinal cord or intracanalicular

7	Malignancy of the spine
8	Frank disc herniation with accompanying signs of progressive neurological deficit
9	Basilar invagination of the upper cervical spine
10	Arnold-Chiari malformation of the upper cervical spine
11	Dislocation of a vertebra
12	Aggressive types of benign tumours, such as an aneurismal bone cyst, giant cell tumour, osteoblastoma or osteoid osteoma
13	Internal fixation/stabilization devices
14	Neoplastic disease of muscle or other soft tissue
15	Positive Kernig's or Lhermitte's signs
16	Congenital, generalized hypermobility
17	Signs or patterns of instability
18	Syringomyelia
19	Hydrocephalus of unknown aetiology
20	Diastematomyelia
21	Cauda equina syndrome
NOTE: In cases of internal fixation/stabilization devices, no osseous manipulation may be performed, although soft-tissue manipulation can be safely used. Spinal manipulative therapy may also only be absolutely contraindicated in the spinal region in which the pathology, abnormality or device is located, or the immediate vicinity. [4]	

Table 1: Absolute contraindications to spinal manipulative therapy according to WHO guidelines [4].

The guidelines are usefull, because CSM should be avoided in the presence of any absolute complications accordingly and most of the complications can be prevented by excluding patients with contraindications for CSM. According to some guidelines [4] anomalies such as dens hypoplasia, unstable os odontoideum, etc., acute fracture, spinal cord tumor, acute infection such as osteomyelitis, septic discitis, and tuberculosis of the spine, meningeal tumor, haematomas, whether spinal cord or intracanalicular, malignancy of the spine, frank disc herniation with accompanying signs of progressive neurological deficit, basilar invagination of the upper cervical spine, Arnold-Chiari malformation of the upper cervical spine, dislocation of a vertebra, aggressive types of benign tumors, such as an aneurismal bone cyst, giant cell tumor, osteoblastoma or osteoid osteoma, internal fixation/stabilization devices, neoplastic disease of muscle or other soft tissue, positive Kernig's or Lhermitte's signs, congenital, generalized hypermobility, signs or patterns of instability, syringomyelia, hydrocephalus of unknown aetiology, diastematomyelia, cauda equina syndrome are considered as absolute contraindications for CSM [4]. However, in the relevant literature whether a condition is an absolute or a relative contraindication is a contraversial issue. Multiple sclerosis, which has Lhermittes sign, is commonly treated with spinal manipulation. The cause must be elicited but it is not always a contraindication for spinal manipulation. Instability may negate spinal manipulation at one segment but not the adjacent segments. In fact, as in degenerative spondylolisthesis, spinal manipulation may be given for alignment while specific stabilization exercises are given to stabilize the segment. Syringomyelia again must be diagnosed for etiology but is not always a contraindication for spinal manipulation. For example, scoliosis may be accompanied with a synrinx, not Arnold-Chiari, or other etiology found and spinal manipulation given. The great majority of neck pain patients will show degenerative disc disease. Therefore proper clinical diagnosis is required prior to performing cervical spine manipulation to identify specific levels of degenerative processes. There are also some studies on spinal cord stimulators and post-surgical spines treated with low velocity low amplitude spinal manipulation with no serious adverse reactions [49,50].

The safety of CSM in the treatment of neck or lumbar problems might be compared with other commonly accepted treatments for the similar conditions. It was reported that, significant complications may occur in 1-4% of NSAID using patients [51]. It has been shown that the risk of CES in surgically treated LDH patients is about 0.5% [52] and the complication rate with cervical spine surgery in the US is about 2% [53].

Conclusion

Safety concern of CSM is an important topic. Treatments must be safe in order to practice in a manner reflecting the principles of "primum non nocere." There should be an emphasis on evidence-based care.

CSM should be practiced only by qualified and well-experienced practitioners. They must be aware of the adverse events and should be cautious when recommending CSM for the treatment of neck pain, especially in the presence of preexisting degenerative disease of the cervical spine [26]. The described serious adverse events promptly recommend the implementation of a risk alert system [27]. All patients should be clearly informed about the potential complications, although they are rare. Information about the risks should be included in an informed consent procedure for CSM.

The evidence-based advantage of CSM should be presented. Therefore, a full medical history and correct diagnosis are important to be able to rule out contraindications to CSM. Most of the complications can be prevented by excluding patients with contraindications for CSM. Therefore, it is recommended that the procedures described in the updated guidelines be applied prior to CSM, and that CSM be avoided in the presence of any absolute complications. Chiropractic practitioners should be aware of the absolute contraindications, where any use of CSM is inappropriate because it places the patient at undue risk (Table 1). In the presence of the relative contraindication, treatment can be modified so that the patient is not at undue risk. In such a case, mobilization or low-force and soft-tissue techniques can be preferred.

Proper clinical diagnosis is required prior to performing cervical spine manipulation to identify specific levels of degenerative processes. It is important to include a neurologic examination on all CSM patients. Neurological tests such as George, DeKelyn, etc are standard tests for vertebral artery insufficiency sensitivity. A positive test is considered a contraindication to cervical manipulation even though their absence does not rule out the possibility of vertebral artery insufficiency. Such tests may help screen for patients who may be at greater risk for vertebral artery dissection following cervical spine manipulation. However, it is important to be alert that their use has potential to cause harm too [43,54].

The ability to recognize a lesion to a specific spinal region by clinical examination may help prioritize diagnostic imaging decisions. Magnetic resonance imaging (MRI) is not accepted as a must for neck and back pain patients before conservative treatments [36]. However, it is useful to be able to compare the outcomes of patients undergoing CSM interventions. If there are significantly deteriorated signs in patients further investigation should be performed and MRI is a reliable method for diagnosing most of the spinal cord pathologies. Therefore, it should be assessed especially for patients with sudden aggravated or new onset of symptoms. Today MRI is not anymore as expensive as it used to be in the past; hence the practitioners may consider requiring it easily.

Whether the adverse events related to CSM are unpredictable events with no predictive indicators or that prediction can be possible, CSM should remain under very strict control. In the literature, estimates vary widely regarding the complications of CSM.

This review has several limitations. Some relevant published articles might have been missed. We need objective data on the relationship between CSM and complications. Therefore, population-based nested case-control studies are required to determine accurately the incidence of complications following CSM.

References

1. Smith CM (2005) Origin and uses of primum non nocere--above all, do no harm! J Clin Pharmacol 45: 371-377.
2. Chapman-Smith DA, Cleveland CS (2005) International status, standards and education of the chiropractic profession. In: Haldeman S, Dagenais S, Budgell B, et al. Principles and Practice of Chiropractic McGraw-Hill. 3rd edn, 111-134.
3. Maitland GD (2005) Vertebral Manipulation. 5th edn. Butterworths, London: 1986.
4. World Health Organization (2005) WHO guidelines on basic training and safety in chiropractic.
5. Jagbandhansingh MP (1997) Most common causes of chiropractic malpractice lawsuits. J Manipulative Physiol Ther 20: 60-64.
6. Ernst E, Posadzki P (2012) Reporting of adverse effects in randomised clinical trials of chiropractic manipulations: a systematic review. N Z Med J 125: 87-140.
7. Evans DP, Burke MS, Lloyd KN, Roberts EE, Roberts GM (1978) Lumbar spinal manipulation on trial. Part I--clinical assessment. Rheumatol Rehabil 17: 46-53.
8. Ernst E (2001) Life-threatening complications of spinal manipulation. Stroke 32: 809-810.
9. Gouveia LO, Castanho P, Ferreira JJ (2009) Safety of chiropractic interventions: a systematic review. Spine (Phila Pa 1976) 32: 2375-2378.
10. Eder M, Tilscher H (1990) Chiropractic therapy: diagnosis and treatment. Rockville, Md: Aspen Publishers, p: 61.
11. Henderson DJ, Cassidy JD (1988) Vertebral Artery syndrome. In: Vernon H. Upper cervical syndrome: chiropractic diagnosis and treatment. Baltimore: Williams and Wilkins, pp: 195-222.
12. Jaskoviak P (1980) Complications arising from manipulation of the cervical spine. J Manip Physiol Ther 3: 213-219.
13. Thiel HW, Bolton JE, Docherty S, Portlock JC (2007) Safety of chiropractic manipulation of the cervical spine: a prospective national survey. Spine (Phila Pa 1976) 32: 2375-2378.
14. Dvorak J, Orelli F (1985) How dangerous is manipulation to the cervical spine? Manual Medicine 2: 1-4.
15. Patijn J (1991) Complications in Manual Medicine: A Review of the Literature. J Manual Medicine 6: 89-92.
16. Haldeman S, Chapman-Smith D, Petersen DM (1993) Guidelines for chiropractic quality assurance and practice parameters. Gaithersburg, Md: Aspen Publishers 170-172.
17. Haldeman S, Carey P, Townsend M, Papadopoulos C (2002) Clinical perceptions of the risk of vertebral artery dissection after cervical manipulation: the effect of referral bias. Spine J 2: 334-342.
18. Lee KP, Carlini WG, McCormick GF, Albers GW (1995) Neurologic complications following chiropractic manipulation: a survey of California neurologists. Neurology 45: 1213-1215.
19. Carey PF (1993) A report on the occurrence of cervical cerebral vascular accidents in chiropractic practice. J Can Chiropr Assoc 37: 104-106.
20. Klougart N, Leboeuf-Yde C, Rasmussen LR (1996) Safety in chiropractic in practice, part 1: the occurrence of cerebrovascular accidents after manipulation to the neck in Denmark from 1978-1988. J Manipulative Physiol Ther 19: 371-377.
21. Ernst E (2007) Adverse effects of spinal manipulation: a systematic review. J R Soc Med 100: 330-338.
22. Ernst E (2011) Response to critiques of deaths after chiropractic. Int J Clin Pract 65: 106.
23. Terrett AG, Kleynhans AM (1992) Cerebrovascular complications of manipulation. In: Haldeman S edn. Principals and Practice of Chiropractic. Norwalk, Ct: Appleton & Lang, pp.579-98.
24. Di Fabio RP (1999) Manipulation of the cervical spine: risks and benefits. Phys Ther 79: 50-65.
25. Struewer J, Frangen TM, Ziring E, Hinterseher U, Kiriazidis I (2013) Massive hematothorax after thoracic spinal manipulation for acute thoracolumbar pain. Orthop Rev (Pavia) 5: e27.
26. John S, Tavee J (2015) Bilateral diaphragmatic paralysis due to cervical chiropractic manipulation. Neurologist 19: 65-67.
27. Gouveia LO, Castanho P, Ferreira JJ, Guedes MM, Falcão F, et al. (2007) Chiropractic manipulation: reasons for concern? Clin Neurol Neurosurg 109: 922-925.
28. Biller J, Sacco RL, Albuquerque FC, Demaerschalk BM, Fayad P, et al. (2014) Cervical arterial dissections and association with cervical manipulative therapy: a statement for healthcare professionals from the american heart association/american stroke association. Stroke 45: 3155-3174.

29. Haldeman S, Rubinstein SM (1992) Cauda equina syndrome in patients undergoing manipulation of the lumbar spine. Spine (Phila Pa 1976) 17: 1469-1473.
30. Shekelle PG, Adams AH, Chassin MR, Hurwitz EL, Brook RH (1992) Spinal manipulation for low-back pain. Ann Intern Med 117: 590-598.
31. Michaeli A (1993) Reported occurrence and nature of complications following manipulative physiotherapy in South Africa. Aust J Physiother 39: 309-315.
32. Stern PJ, Côté P, Cassidy JD (1995) A series of consecutive cases of low back pain with radiating leg pain treated by chiropractors. J Manipulative Physiol Ther 18: 335-342.
33. Assendelft WJ, Bouter LM, Knipschild PG (1996) Complications of spinal manipulation: a comprehensive review of the literature. J Fam Pract 42: 475-480.
34. Oliphant D (2004) Safety of spinal manipulation in the treatment of lumbar disk herniations: a systematic review and risk assessment. J Manipulative Physiol Ther 27: 197-210.
35. Powell FC, Hanigan WC, Olivero WC (1993) A risk/benefit analysis of spinal manipulation therapy for relief of lumbar or cervical pain. Neurosurgery 33: 73-78.
36. Senstad O, Leboeuf-Yde C, Borchgrevink C (1997) Frequency and characteristics of side effects of spinal manipulative therapy. Spine (Phila Pa 1976) 22: 435-440.
37. Hurwitz EL, Morgenstern H, Vassilaki M, Chiang LM (2005) Frequency and clinical predictors of adverse reactions to chiropractic care in the UCLA neck pain study. Spine (Phila Pa 1976) 30: 1477-1484.
38. Kirkaldy-Willis WH, Cassidy JD (1985) Spinal manipulation in the treatment of low-back pain. Can Fam Physician 31: 535-540.
39. Haneline MT, Lewkovich GN (2005) An analysis of the etiology of cervical artery dissections: 1994 to 2003. J Manipulative Physiol Ther 28: 617-622.
40. Ernst E (2010) Vascular accidents after neck manipulation: cause or coincidence? Int J Clin Pract 64: 673-677.
41. Mas JL, Henin D, Bousser MG, Chain F, Hauw JJ (1989) Dissecting aneurysm of the vertebral artery and cervical manipulation: a case report with autopsy. Neurology 39: 512-515.
42. Greenstein GM (1997) Clinical Assessment of Neuromusculoskeletal Disorders. Saint Louis: Mosby.
43. Tamburrelli FC, Genitiempo M, Logroscino CA (2011) Cauda equina syndrome and spine manipulation: case report and review of the literature. Eur Spine J 20 Suppl 1: S128-131.
44. Kostuik JP, Harrington I, Alexander D, Rand W, Evans D (1986) Cauda equina syndrome and lumbar disc herniation. J Bone Joint Surg Am 68: 386-391.
45. Quon JA, Cassidy JD, O'Connor SM, KirkaldyWillis WH (1989) Lumbar intervertebral disc herniation: treatment by rotational manipulation. J Manipulative Physiol Ther 12: 220-226.
46. Terrett AG, Kleynhans AM (1992) Complications from manipulation of the low back. Chiropr J Aust 27: 129-140.
47. Ernst E (2001) Prospective investigations into the safety of spinal manipulation. J Pain Symptom Manage 21: 238-242.
48. Lisi AJ, Holmes EJ, Ammendolia C (2005) High-velocity low-amplitude spinal manipulation for symptomatic lumbar disk disease: a systematic review of the literature. J Manipulative Physiol Ther 28: 429-442.
49. Perrucci RM, Coulis CM (2017) Chiropractic management of post spinal cord stimulator spine pain: a case report. Chiropr Man Therap 25: 5.
50. Gudavalli MR, Olding K, Joachim G, Cox JM (2016) Chiropractic Distraction Spinal Manipulation on Postsurgical Continued Low Back and Radicular Pain Patients: A Retrospective Case Series. J Chiropr Med 15: 121-128.
51. Bjorkman DJ (1999) Current status of nonsteroidal anti-inflammatory drug (NSAID) use in the United States: risk factors and frequency of complications. Am J Med 107: 3S-8S.
52. Kardaun JW, White LR, Shaffer WO (1990) Acute complications in patients with surgical treatment of lumbar herniated disc. J Spinal Disord 3: 30-38.
53. Fineberg SJ, Oglesby M, Patel AA, Pelton MA, Singh K (2013) Outcomes of cervical spine surgery in teaching and non-teaching hospitals. Spine (Phila Pa 1976) 38: 1089-1096.
54. http://www.chirocolleges.org/georges_test.html

17

Systematic Review about the Effects of Qigong Therapeutic Exercise on Balance

Elena Mejías Gil[1*] **and María Victoria González López-Arza**[2]

[1]*University of Extremadura, Avda de Elvas S/N, 06006 Badajoz, España, Spain*

[2]*Medicine and Surgery Department, University of Extremadura, Spain*

[*]**Corresponding author:** Elena Mejías Gil, Physiotherapist, University of Extremadura, Avda de Elvas S/N, 06006 Badajoz, España, Spain, E-mail: elenamejias92@gmail.com

Abstract

Objectives: The aim of this study was to review the effects achieved by the Qigong on balance in the last 17 years publications.

Design: The performed search included quantitative researches about the effects of Qigong on balance. There was no language restriction and reviews were not included in the analysis.

Databases: PubMed, CSIC, Cochrane Library, Scopus, PEDro, Dialnet, JSTAGE, JTCM.

Results: A total of 2966 studies were founded, 11 of them were selected after having applied the established inclusion and exclusion criteria.

Conclusion: Currently, there is not enough evidence to conclusively demonstrate the benefits of Qigong in improving balance. However, based on the analyzed studies, we can say that there are signs of an improvement.

Keywords: Qigong; Qi Gong; Balance; Exercise

Introduction

Balance can be defined as the posture in which an ideal body mass distribution is achieved. Postural balance provides the body carriage stability and conditions for normal functions in stationary position or in movement, such as sitting, standing, or walking [1].

We can observe, through the literature, how balance is regulated by the vestibular, visual and proprioceptive systems, all of them working together in order to maintain body stability. The different components making up these systems collect information about our position and our posture in the environment and sent it to the centres of balance located into the brain. There, this information is processed in order to provide an integrated response according to the needs. Signals are sent through the spinal cord to regulate the interaction between facilitation and inhibition of the antigravity muscles [2-6].

Due to this complex interaction, balance can be altered in different ways and in some diseases such as Parkinson's disease (PD) and multiple sclerosis (MS) [7-19]. Apart from pathological condition and sedentary habits a bad proprioception can also modify balance capacity in a healthy person. Aging can also affect it because over time, our joints and muscles deteriorate, we lose vision and hearing ability and all this has negative effects on the sense of balance [20,21].

In any of these situations, the individual finds their functional capacity for daily life activities reduced, which, in addition to decrease their quality of life, makes them more prone to falls, increasing the risk of injury and even death [16,20,22,23]. The latest figures from National Statistics Institute quantified deaths from accidental falls during 2013 in 2,672 deceased [24].

Studies show that exercise can be a great help in maintaining and improving balance [22,25-27]. It has been shown to improve physical abilities such as strength and muscular endurance, cardiovascular rhythm, flexibility and proprioception [25,26]. However, adherence to treatment is often the main problem to achieve the objectives, because some exercises can be too demanding or difficult to include in the daily routine [27-29]. Therefore, it is still investigating therapies equally effective but less physically demanding.

Qigong is a therapeutic exercise based on the principles of traditional Chinese medicine (TCM) whose culture has practiced for over 3000 years [13,16]. His name can be interpreted as "breathing training" [16,30,31], meaning that relates to the basic techniques that are part of Qigong: postural, mental and breath control [13-19].

The scientific evidence gathered by Jahnke [31] suggests that Qigong has beneficial effects on the balance, and improve the cardiopulmonary system, bone density, coordination and proprioception, among others. However, few studies concerning balance were found.

As Blake et al. [15] outlained, Qigong practice has some advantages, e.g it does not require specific instruments and the quietness of its movements represents a low-impact exercise that can be practiced by a wide range of patients. This gives a great potential as an adjunct to conventional treatment methods.

Considering the above, the aim of this study was to review the effects achieved by the Qigong on balance in the last 17 years publications.

Material and Methods

Eligibility criteria

To be included in this systematic review, studies should be quantitative researches about the effects of Qigong on balance, published between January 01, 2000 and December 31, 2016.

Publication who had not studied the improvement of balance or not used Qigong as technique were excluded as well as those which did not follow the typology of selected studies. There was no language restriction and reviews were not included in the analysis.

Data sources

The following data bases were used to conduct literature searches: MEDLINE-PubMed, Spanish National Research Council [Consejo Superior de Investigaciones Científicas, CSIC], Cochrane Library, Scopus, Physiotherapy Evidence Database (PEDro), Dialnet, Japan Sicience and Technology Information Agregator Electronic (J-STAGE) and the website of Journal of Traditional Chinese Medicine (JTCM).

Search strategy

We use several combinations of MeSH terms "Qigong", "Qi Gong", "balance", "balance disorders", "brain injuries," "stability", "Parkinson" and "multiple sclerosis" as well as the terms "elder adults "and" older adults" using the Boolean operators AND and OR. We use the same combinations for all databases and their Spanish equivalent for Dialnet.

Study selection

Two independent authors reviewed the selected articles to be included. In case of disagreement, results were discussed in order to reach a consensus between both researchers. As a general rule, we performed a screening of those studies that followed the line of the chosen issue.

After having selected the articles, we proceeded to read their summaries, excluding those items that did not meet the above reflected inclusion and exclusion criteria. Studies that successfully passed this stage, went to the last one, which included their complete reading for analysis and inclusion in the review.

Data extracted from reading were: author, objective, number of participants, intervention, assessment tools, assessment and results.

Methodological quality

The methodological quality of the included studies was assessed using the PEDro scale [32]. It consists of 11 items with answers "yes" (Y) or "no" (N), and a total score range of 0-10 which means low or excellent methodological quality.

The 11 items assessed by PEDro scale were: 1. Specification of eligibility criteria; 2. Random assignment; 3. Hidden allocation; 4. Similar baseline; 5. Blind subjects; 6. Blind therapist; 7. Blind assessors; 8. Measurement of key outcomes (at least, from 85% of the subjects); 9. Analysis of intention to treat; 10. Statistical comparisons between groups; 11. Measures of variability and point measures.

The values obtained are considered high quality if the score is greater than 5 (6-8: good, 9-10: excellent); moderate quality, if the score is 4 or 5 (limited study); low quality, if the score is less than 4 (poor study) [33].

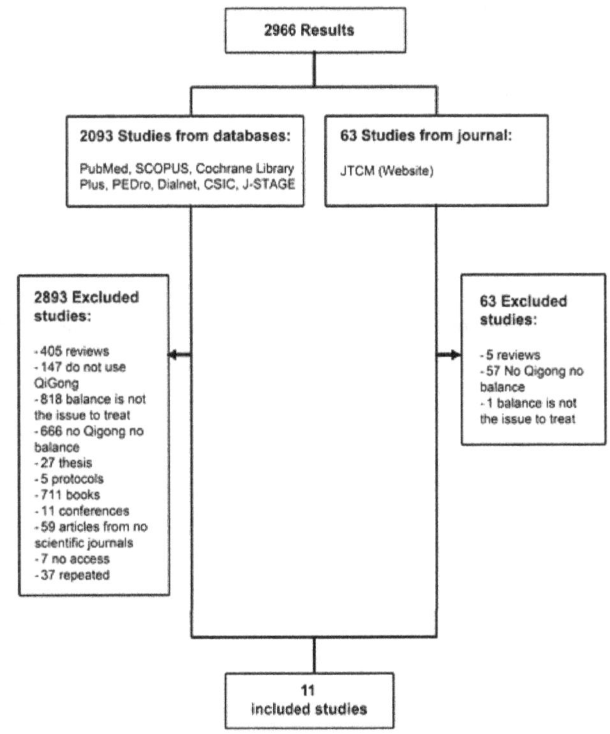

Figure 1: Selection procedure of the studies from the literature search.

Results

A total of 2966 studies were founded, 11 of them were selected after having applied the established inclusion and exclusion criteria. The process of search and selection of studies is detailed in Figure 1 Selection procedure of the studies from the literature search. The main characteristics of the selected studies are reflected in Table 1 Summary of included studies.

Studies description

Subjects

A total of 45% of these publications were pilot studies with a small sample size in some cases [9]. This means that the number of subjects in the articles ranged between 8 and 120, which focuses the average in 41 and gave us a total of 591 participants. Only three of these studies referred to have calculated the sample size needed to be representative [10,15,17]. Total 561 subjects had balance problems, due either to illness or age (80.4 ± 8.6 years). The remaining 30 were young healthy individuals without any associated pathology. Among diseases we founded: Parkinson's (PD), Fibromyalgia (FM), Muscular Dystrophy (MD), Traumatic Brain Injuries (TBI), nasopharyngeal cancer (NPC) and coronary artery disease (CAD).

Intervention period

The length of the treatment periods ranged from one to six months, without rest or follow-up stages. This clarification is necessary because one of the articles was a crossover study and it applied a rest period in between each treatment phase [11].

Measurement instruments

Just a few studies agree to use the same balance assessment scale. The most used was a single leg stance test [9,12,16,17] but other preferred to use other forms of measurement as the Berg Balance Scale [11,18,19] or a sensory organization test [14].

Effects on balance

Most studies points to a significant improvement of balance after using Qigong as training [9,12-14,16-19].

Mills and Loftus, who worked without a control group, compared the results before and after the treatment among their patients with MS and PD respectively. In the first case, they used a single leg stance test, in which they saw an improvement from 5.63 seconds in stance to 11.88. The second author used the Berg Balance Scale and he detected and improvement from 32.79 to 37.06 points (P=0.001).

The remaining authors compared their results with a control group. Among them, only Yang et al. [14] used a Sensory Organization Test, which allowed them to detect a bigger improvement at balance controlled by vestibular area (P>0.01).

Blake et al. [15] found no significant differences between the results before and after the treatment of Qigong nor any related improvement.

Regarding the remaining two authors, they are in an intermediate position between these two outcome groups. Both Wenneberg et al. [11] and Mannerkorpi et al. [10] saw in their studies, although there was no significant difference between before and after treatment results, the Qigong group did not get worse in its scores while the control group did it. This deterioration was reported as significant by both Mannerkorpi (P<0.04) and Wenneberg (P<0.025).

Wenneberg et al. [11] calculated that a sample of 54 patients would provide significant differences between the study groups. Moreover, Mannerkorpi detected an improvement of proprioception and movement harmony at the end of treatment (P=0.03).

Methodological quality

The methodological quality scores got by the articles according to the PEDro scale [32] are reflected in Table 1. The mean of these scores is around 5 point; the lowest score is 2 and the highest 8.

AUTHOR	OBJETIVE	SAMPLE	INTERVENTION	MEASURING INSTRUMENTS	MAIN BALANCE RESULTS	PEDro SCALE
Mils 2000	To provide some preliminary data on the usefulness of TJ/QG for people with MS	N=8 (MS)	Single-sample 2 months baseline 2 months intervention (TJ-QG 30 min/day)	1) Check-list of physical symptoms 2) One leg-standing test	1) Participants improvement responses: 32% 2) ↑ (P<0.05)	2/10
Mannerkorpi 2004	To evaluate the effects of body awareness therapy combined with QG for FM	N=36 (FM)	G1: QG and body awareness therapy (n=19) G2: Body awareness therapy (n=17) *Both: 1 t/w, 3 months	1) Body Awareness Rating Scale 2) Physical Function Test	1) G1↑(P=0.03) 2) NS	5/10
Wenneberg 2004	To evaluate the effects of QG for MD patients	N=36 (MD)	Phase 1: (3 months) G1: QG (n=16) G2: Control(n=15) Phase 2: (3 months) G1a:Control (n=7) G1b QG (n=9) G2: QG (n=12)	Berg's Balance Scale	Inter-group: NS Intra-group: QG remain, control worsen (p=0.025)	6/10
Stenlund 2005	To investigate whether the QG would increase physical ability for elderly patients with CAD	N=95 (CAD)	G1: QG: 1 h, 1 t/w, 3 months (n=48) G2: Control (n=47)	1) Self-estimated level of physical activity scale 2) Falls Efficacy Scale 3) Berg's Balance Scale 4) One leg-standing test 5) Coordination	Inter-group: 1) G1 improve (P<0.01) 2) and 3) NS 4) G1 improve (P=0.029) RL 5) G1 improve Intra-group:	5/10

					4) G1 improve both legs	
Schmitz–Hübsch (2006)	To evaluate the effects of QG on motor and no-motor symptoms of PD	N=56 (PD)	G1: QG: 60 min, 1 t/w for 2 months + rest for 2 months + 2 months intervention (same conditions). G2: Control	1) UPDRS-III	1) Improvement due to QiGong at 3 months (P=0.008) and at 6 months (P=0.05)	5/10
Yang 2007	To evaluate changes in balance mechanisms of healthy older adults as consequence of TJ-QG sequence	N=49	G1: TJ-QG: 1 h, 3 t/w for 6 months (n=33) G2: Control (n=16)	1) SOT 2) BoS	1) ↑vestibular score (T2:+22%, T6:+47%) for G1 2) ↑ stability at G1	5/10
Blake 2009	To examine the effects of a TJ-QG sequence on individuals with TBI	N=20 (TBI)	G1: QG: 1 h/w, 8w G2: Control	1) PSDQ a. Coordination b. Self-esteem c. Flexibility	1) NS	6/10
Gonzalez Lopez-Arza 2013	To describe the change in balance in young, healthy women after Practising QG	N=30	G1: QG: 1 h 2 t/w, 4w G2:Control	1) One leg-standing test	Intra-group G1↑ from 40.15% to 56.46% Inter-group NS	4/10
Fong 2014	To compare the one-leg-stance time and the 6MWT distance among TJ-QG-trained NPC survivors, untrained NPC survivors, and healthy individuals	N=120 (50 NPC, 68 healthy people)	G1: NPC-QG (n=25) G2: NPC-Control (n=25) G3: Healthy control (n=68) * Cross-sectional exploratory study	1) 6MWT 2) One leg-standing test in different conditions of viewing and surface	1) NS 2) G1 similar to G3 (eyes closed, stable surface) (P=0.168)	4/10
Loftus 2014	To examine the effects of QG on postural stability and PD-related falls	N=41 (PD)	One group QG: 1 h, 2 t/w, 3 months	1) Parkinson's Disease Fall Profile 2) Berg Balance Scale 3) Pull test	1) ↓ falls after QG (P=0.004) 2) ↑balance after QG (P=0.001) 3) NS	4/10
Xiao 2015	To investigate the effectiveness of QG on symptoms related to gait, functional mobility and sleep in PD patients	N=100 (PD)	G1: QG: 45 min, 4t/w + 30 min walk, 6 months G2:30 min walk, 6 months	1) Berg's balance scale 2) 6MWT 3) Time Up&Go	1) G1 improves (P=0.041) 2) G1 improves (P=0.042) 3) G1 improves (P=0.046)	8/10

TJ-QG: Taiji-Qigong sequence; G: Group; NS: Not Significant; T: Time of evaluation; min: minute; h: hours; t/w: times per week; RL: Right Leg; UPDRS: Unified Parkinson's Disease Rating Scale; SOT: Sensory organization test; BoS: Base of Support; PSDQ: Physical Self-Description Questionnaire; 6MWT: 6 Minute Walk Test; FM: Fibromyalgia; MS: Multiple Sclerosis; MD: Muscular Dystrophy; PD: Parkinson Disease; TBI: Traumatic Brain Injury; CAD: Coronary Artery Disease; NPC: Nasopharyngeal Cancer.

Table 1: Summary of included studies.

No one of the participants and therapists of these studies were blinded, although four of the researchers blinded the assessors collecting data [10,11,18,19]. Apart from two articles [9,17], all authors have mentioned that they randomized their sample and explained the procedure by which it was performed by randomization. Only Mills et al. [9], Fong et al. [17] and Loftus et al. [18] do not included a flow diagram of subjects throughout the study.

Discussion

Results of this review indicate that Qigong can induce an improvement on balance. This statement is supported by a 72.7% of the revised trials with only a 9% of them against. However, we must be cautious when interpreting these results because of the limitations founded through the analyzed studies as well as through this review.

First, the search shows a significant shortage of studies involving Qigong as a technique for improving balance. This may be due to the inclusion criteria, to the lack of knowledge about this modality of exercise or a compendium of both. Bearing in mind that this search covered seventeen years of publications, the lack of studies linking these two topics and the fact that half of the collected researches were pilot studies, it provides an idea of what unexploited field it is.

Moreover, there are very few good quality articles on the topic due to the fact that only one of them was over 6 points on the PEDro scale [19]. One of the weaknesses in the design of the articles is the lack on blinding. It is true that in this type of therapy it is impossible to blind the sample or the therapist. However, some studies could have increased the methodological quality blinding assessors as it was done, for example, in the study of Wenneberg et al. [11].

The small sample size is another important aspect of the limitations of some articles that included eight [9] or twenty participants only [15].

On the other hand, one of the strengths shared by all articles was the specification of the sequence of performance of Qigong exercise, an important fact to allow the replication of the work.

We also found a lack of homogeneity in the pathologies that makes a comparison difficult. At this point, it is noteworthy that counting with so little written on this topic, we found only two publications that aim to test the effects of Qigong in the balance of healthy subjects [14,16]. Based on only two studies we cannot say that there is clear scientific evidence that Qigong improves balance. However, other authors go on to test it directly as a treatment in patients affected by other pathologies. It is notable that in these studies the effects of Qigong could have be modified by other symptomatology, as well as by the medication these patients were taking and which was not detailed.

Finally, it would be interesting for future researches to assess the level of effectiveness of Qigong separately in different types of balance. If the study by Yang et al. [14] was correct and Qigong has greater benefits for the balance controlled by the vestibular area, when being used as a treatment, Qigong may have a different efficiency depending on the origin of the disease.

Further publication should consider these limitations to provide a more scientific and objective approach to the use of Qigong as an exercise for improving balance.

The conclusions of this work have been carried out from the studies founded by the search strategy as well as by the inclusion criteria proposed. It is necessary to consider the possibility that, due to search limits, other studies have been left out of this review.

Conclusion

Currently, we do not have enough evidence to allow us to conclusively demonstrate the benefits of Qigong in improving balance. However, based on the analyzed studies, we can say that there are signs of an improvement.

More researches are needed with a more homogeneous methodology and technique as well as with larger sample sizes and improved monitoring, in order to get a better approach to the real degree of effectiveness of Qigong therapeutic exercise for balance improvement.

References

1. MeSH Database. Nacional Center Biotechnology Information.
2. Hoffman S (2010) How does the balance system works? American Physical Therapy Association.
3. Matsuo T, Yamasaki H, Yasuhara H, Hasebe K (2013) Postural stability changes during large vertical diplopia induced by prism wear in normal subjects. Acta Med Okayama 67: 177-183.
4. Guyton A, Hall J (2006) Medical physiology. 11th edn, Elsevier, Philadelphia, Pennsylvania, pp. 692-696.
5. Quitschal RM, Fukunaga JY, Ganança MM, Caovilla HH (2014) Evaluation of postural control in unilateral vestibular hypofunction. Braz J Otorhinolaryngol 80:339-345.
6. Tomomitsu MS, Alonso AC, Morimoto E (2013) Static and dynamic postural control in low-vision and normal-vision adults. Clinics (Sao Paulo) 68: 517-521.
7. Fukunaga JY, Quitschal RM, Doná F (2014) Postural control in Parkinson's disease. Braz J Otorhinolaryngol 80: 508-514.
8. Oh B, Butow P, Mullan B (2012) A critical review of the effects of medical Qigong on quality of life, immune function and survival in cancer patients. Integr Cancer Ther 11:101-110.
9. Mills N, Allen J, Carey Morgan S (2000) Does Tai Chi/Qi Gong help patients with Multiple Sclerosis? J Bodyw Mov Ther 4: 39-48.
10. Mannerkorpi K, Arndorw M (2004) Efficacy and feasibility of a combination of body awareness therapy and qigong in patients with fibromyalgia: a pilot study. J Rehabil Med. 36: 279-281.
11. Wenneberg S, Gunnarsson LG, Ahlström G (2004) Using a novel exercise programme for patients with muscular dystrophy. Part II: a quantitative study. Disabil Rehabil 26: 595-602.
12. Stenlund T, Lindström B, Granlund M, Burell G (2005) Cardiac rehabilitation for the elderly: Qi Gong and group discussions. Eur J Cardiovasc Prev Rehabil 12: 5-11.
13. Schmitz-Hübsch T, Pyfer D, Kielwein K (2006) Qigong exercise for the symptoms of Parkinson's disease: a randomized, controlled pilot study. Mov Disord 21: 543-548.
14. Yang Y, Verkuilen JV, Rosengren KS (2007) Effect of combined Taiji and Qigong training on balance mechanisms: a randomized controlled trial of older adults. Med Sci Monit 13: 339-348.
15. Blake H, Batson M (2009) Exercise intervention in brain injury: a pilot randomized study of Tai Chi Qigong. Clin Rehabil. 23: 589-598.
16. González López-Arza MV, Varela-Donoso E, Montanero-Fernández J (2013) Qigong improves balance in young women: a pilot study. J Integr Med 11: 241-245.
17. Fong SS, Chung LM, Tsang WW (2014) Balance performance in irradiated survivors of nasopharyngeal cancer with and without tai chi qigong training. Evid Based Complement Alternat Med 2014: 1-7.
18. Loftus SL (2014) Qi Gong to improve postural stability (QTIPS) for Parkinson fall prevention. Top Geriatr Rehabil 30: 58-69.
19. Xiao CM, Zhuang YC (2015) Effect of health Baduanjin Qigong for mild to moderate Parkinson's disease. Geriatr Gerontol Int 16: 911-919.
20. Suarez H, Arocena M (2009) Balance disorders in the elderly. Rev Med Clin Counts 20: 401-407.
21. Suttanon P, Hill KD, Said CM (2012) Balance and mobility dysfunction and falls risk in older people with mild to moderate Alzheimer disease. Am J Phys Med Rehabil 91: 12-23.
22. Wong-Yu IS, Mak MK (2015) Multi-dimensional balance training programme improves balance and gait performance in people with Parkinson's disease: A pragmatic randomized controlled trial with 12-month follow-up. Parkinsonism Relat Disord 21: 615-621.
23. Fernández-Cuenca R, Llácer A, López-Cuadrado T, Gómez-Barroso D (2014) Mortality from external causes in Spain. Boletín epidemiológico seminal Vol. 22.
24. http://www.ine.es/en/prodyser/pubweb/anuarios_mnu_en.htm
25. Sharma A, Geovinson SG, Singh SJ (2012) Effects of a nine-week core strengthening exercise program on vertical jump performances and static balance in volleyball players with trunk instability. J Sports Med Phys Fitness 52: 606-615.

26. Matrangola SL, Madigan ML (2009) Relative effects of weight loss and strength training on balance recovery. Med Sci Sports Exerc 41: 1488-1493.

27. Laufer Y, Dar G, Kodesh E (2014) Does a Wii-based exercise program enhance balance control of independently functioning older adults? A systematic review. Clin Interv Aging 9: 1803-1813.

28. Yost TL, Taylor AG (2013) Qigong as a novel intervention for service members with mild traumatic brain injury. Explore (NY) 9: 142-149.

29. Lee MS, Ernst E (2009) Qigong for movement disorders: A systematic review. Mov Disord 24: 301-303.

30. Gallagher (2003) Tai chi chuan and qigong: physical and mental practice for functional mobility. Topics in Geriatric Rehabilitation 19: 172-182.

31. Jahnke R, Larkey L, Rogers C (2010) A comprehensive review of health benefits of qigong and tai chi. Am J Health Promot 24: e1-e25.

32. www.pedro.org.au/spanish/downloads/pedro-scale/

33. De Morton NA (2009) The PEDro scale is a valid measure of the methodological quality of clinical trials: A demographic study. Aust J Physiother 55: 129-133.

34. Fauci A (2012) Harrison's Principles of Internal Medicine. 18th edn, McGrawHill, New York, pp: 151-154.

18

Basic Studies on Chemopreventive Properties of Quercetin and Curcumin and Other Plant-origin Compounds in Ovarian Cancer Cells

Radosław Kujawski[1*], Justyna Baraniak[2], Marcin Ożarowski[2,3], Małgorzata Kujawska[4], Magdalena Borowska[1], Malgorzata Kania[2], Joanna Bartkowiak-Wieczorek[5], Agnieszka Sobczak[6], Agnieszka Gryszczyńska[2], Katarzyna Manikowska[1], Joanna Liberska[1], Joanna Cichocka[7], Michał Szulc[1] and Piotr Ruszkowski[1]

[1]*Department of Pharmacology, Poznan University of Medical Sciences, Poland*

[2]*Department of Pharmacology and Phytochemistry, Institute of Natural Fibers and Medicinal Plants, Poland*

[3]*Department of Pharmaceutical Botany and Plant Biotechnology, Poznan University of Medical Sciences, Poland*

[4]*Department of Toxicology, Poznan University of Medical Sciences, Poland*

[5]*Department of Clinical Pharmacy and Biopharmacy, Poznan University of Medical Sciences, Poland*

[6]*Department of Pharmaceutical Chemistry, Poznan University of Medical Sciences, Poland*

[7]*Wielkopolska Centre for Advanced Technologies (WCAT), Adam Mickiewicz University in Poznan, Poland*

*****Corresponding author:** Radosław Kujawski, Department of Pharmacology, Poznan University of Medical Science, Rokietnicka 5a Str., 60-806 Poznań, Poland, E-mail: radkuj@ump.edu.pl

Abstract

Despite the increasing number of studies on the molecular actions of quercetin and curcumin, their anticancer efficacy, safety and molecular aspects of chemopreventive action in the ovarian cancer prophylaxis or treatment and also their potential in the sensitization to cytostatics used in the clinical practice remains still not clearly understood.

Based on basic studies we have summarized evidences for inhibitory activities of several often studied plant-origin bio-active compounds (mostly quercetin and curcumin) against ovarian cancer cells proliferation, their mechanisms of action as well as their strong potential to sensitization of ovarian cancer cells to the presence of several platinum-based cytostatics - cisplatin and oxaliplatin. Up to date only several dietary, clinical (cohort and case–control) studies evaluating the association of some flavonoids (mostly nonisoflavones) and its subgroup components consumption and ovarian cancer risk were already performed. According to the researchers, there has been no association between ovarian cancer risk and total nonisoflavone flavonoids intake. There is a still an insufficient amount of data designed to explain the effect of quercetin or curcumin (alone or together) on ovarian cancer development and/or its chemotherapy. Obtained results provide limited support for an association between nonisoflavone flavonoids intake and ovarian cancer risk, therefore there is a need for further and more accurate studies to be confirmed. We are of the opinion that this paper will contribute to a better understanding of the molecular basis for positive interactions between concomitant usage of quercetin or curcumin with above-mentioned cytostatics and other bio-active agents. This work may also contribute to an increase in the number of preclinical studies or other clinical, dietary trials using these or other phenolic / alkaloid, plant-origin constituents in order to investigate efficiency and safety of pharmacotherapy of ovarian cancer patients.

Keywords: Ovarian cancer; Chemoprevention; Flavonoids; Quercetin; Curcumin; Cisplatin

Abbreviations: A2780 (wild - type): A2780 (cisR) (cisplatin-resistant) and A2780 (ZD0473R) (ZD0473-resistant)-Ovarian Cancer Cells; CAT: Catalase; CDDP: Cis-diammine Dichloro Platinum; CHOP: CCAAT/Enhancer-binding protein Homologous Protein; cyto-c: Cytochrome c; DNA-PK: DNA-dependent Protein Kinase; DR5: Cell Death Receptor; EFO-27: Ovarian Cancer Cell Line; ENDOG: Endonuclease G; ERS: Endoplasmic Reticulum-Stress; GPx: Glutathione Peroxidase; IP3: Inositol, 1,4,5-Trisphosphate; MMP-2 and MMP-9: Two Metallo Proteinases; MPEG-PCL: Nanoformulated Quercetin; OVCAR: Human Ovarian Carcinoma Cell Line; PI: 1-Phosphatidylinositol; PIP Kinase: 1-Phosphatidylinositol 4-Phosphate 5-Kinase; Q: Quercetin, 3,3',4',5-7-Pentahydroxyflavone; RF: Resistance Factor; ROS: Reactive Oxygen Species; SCOV-3-Human Ovary Cancer Cell Line; SOD 1: Superoxide Dismutase; TQ: Thymoquinone: TRAIL: Apoptosis-Inducing Ligand; Type II EBS: Type II Estrogen Binding Sites; UCP2: Uncoupling Protein 2

Introduction

Ovarian cancer is the most leading cause of death from gynecological cancer in the Western world [1-3]. This may be due to the absence of early symptoms which causes the disease. In approximately two-thirds of patients the disease spreads beyond the ovaries [4] resulting in poor prognosis of ovarian cancer stems mainly from the high percentage of cases diagnosed at an advanced stage. Although most patients with advanced ovarian cancer respond to first-line chemotherapy, 80% of the patients ultimately succumb to death due to recurrence [5].

New strategies to improve clinical response and to reduce toxicity of cancer therapy focus nowadays on chemoprevention, which hopes to identify substances that can suppress cancer transformation [6]. According to the current state of knowledge chemoprevention includes using agents that affect cell-cycle progression and apoptosis, signal transduction, oncogene activation, polyamine metabolism, angiogenesis, gap junctional intercellular communication, and more [6,7]. According to guidelines for cancer prevention published by the American Cancer Society Guidelines, one of the key lifestyle factors thought to modify cancer risk is a diet, especially that rich in plant-origin compounds [8-11]. Although nowadays natural therapies are being more and more often considered by physicians to be used even in cancer patients, together with targeted therapies, still little is known about their interaction with conventional chemotherapeutic agents. Numerous studies indicate that chemopreventive phytochemicals with phenolic structure, for example flavonoids or curcuminoids, possessing antiproliferative and antioxidant properties that can overcome problems of drug resistance and nonspecific toxicity towards normal cells, by reducing the side-effects that are associated with chemotherapy [10,12,13].

Flavonoids with several functions in pathological processes of cancer are polyphenolic compounds with a basic benzo-γ-pyrone structure being widely distributed in all foods of plant origin such as fruit, vegetable, tea and wine [9,14,15]. Some studies indicate that the observed pharmacological activities of flavonoids on ovarian cancer may depend on their structure [9,12]. Based on the range and structural complexity, flavonoids can be categorized into six major subclasses: flavones, isoflavones, flavonols, flavanones, anthocyanidins and flavan-3-ols [11,16], among which flavones, isoflavones and flavonols are reported in the highest amounts of consumption in the human diet and have biological activity in ovarian cancer [8,9,17,18].

One of the most abundant flavonol, identified in various types of vegetable [19-21], caper fruits [22], fruits [23], herbs (dill), some types of tea [24] and wine [25], being of the most extensively studied in this field is the quercetin [11,26-28]. Numerous studies have demonstrated that another plant-origin constituent-curcumin (a yellow substance belonging to the polyphenols superfamily; active component of turmeric, a common Indian spice, derived i.e. from the dried *Curcuma longa* rhizome) and its derivatives possess anti-oxidant, anti-inflammatory and anti-cancerous activities [29,30].

In this manuscript we aimed to summarized, based on basic studies, evidences of inhibitory activities against ovarian cancer cells proliferation of several plant-origin bio-active compounds, mainly quercetin and curcumin, described their cytotoxic potential when treated alone or with other phenolic or alkaloid substances, as well as their strong potential to sensitization of ovarian cancer cells to the presence of several cytostatics, mostly platinum-based ones. Only few experiments with quercetin and curcumin applied together on ovarian cancer cells were carried out so far.

Already published literature presents a number of experimental, pre-clinical results of *in-vitro, in-vivo* studies concerning the mechanism of action of quercetin and curcumin and their bio-active metabolites against ovarian cancer cells proliferation and/or *in vivo* tumor development. Although there have been published some reviews summarizing knowledge in this subject [31-34], in this paper we have presented more precise of dose-dependent in vitro, in vivo aspects of action of above mentioned plant origin bio-active compounds in relation to platinum-based cytostatics towards ovarian cancer.

Methods

We have done a review of *in vitro* and *in vivo* studies evaluating the correlation between the ability to inhibit ovarian cancer cells proliferation, defining the mechanisms of action of these bio-active compounds, administered alone, in combine treatment, in combination with other metabolites or two platinum-based cytostatics (cisplatin, oxaliplatin). For this purpose a systematic search for relevant publications was made using PubMed, Medline, Google Scholar databases. English and nonEnglish papers published up to February 2017 were screened using the following keywords "flavonoid", "quercetin", "curcumin", "ovarian cancer", "molecular", "platinum-based cytostatics", "cisplatin". Clinical (cohort or case–control studies) studies scanned based on their title, abstract, and their major aims, their full texts were excluded.

Results

The knowledge gained as a result of the above methodology is presented below.

Chemoprotective activities in ovarian cancer cells of quercetin, alone or with cytostatics or other plant compounds

Early in vitro study on OVCAR 433 ovarian cancer cell line demonstrated synergistic antiproliferative activity of quercetin (Q) with cisplatin (CDDP) acting through an interaction with type II estrogen binding sites (type II EBS). A dose-dependent growth inhibition (range of concentrations was 0.01 μM to 2.5 μM and 0.01 μg/ml to 2.5 μg/ml for Q and CDDP, respectively) when administered separately, while their combination resulted in a synergistic action. Two other studied flavonoids as rutin (3-rhamnosyl-glucoside of quercetin) and hesperidin (3'-5-3-hydroxy-4-methoxyflavone) were ineffective, both alone and in combination with CDDP [35]. Another experiment showed the capability of quercetin to reversible dose-dependent inhibition of cancer cells proliferation in the range of concentrations between 10 nM to 10 μM, without such effect of rutin and hesperidin [35]. Moreover, a synergistic, dose-dependent inhibition of colony formation of cells from 4 primary ovarian tumors expressing type II EBS and reduction of hyperthermia (42°C) effect in three out of four tumors analyzed was also observed in the case of quercetin (0.1 μM to 10 μM; max 10 μM), while rutin and hesperidin were ineffective in synergizing with hyperthermia [36]. Quercetin inhibited proliferation of human ovarian carcinoma OVCAR-5 cells (IC50 for growth inhibition=63 μM; LC50 for cytotoxicity=17 μM) via suppression of signal transduction activity by concentration-dependent declining in 1-phosphatidylinositol (PI) 4-kinase leading to an 80% decrease in PI kinase activity and a 65% decrease in the concentration of the second messenger, inositol 1,4,5-trisphosphate (IP3), closely correlated with its concentration change. PI-4 kinase is the first committed enzyme in the PI phosphorylation pathway of signal transduction leading to the production of the second messengers [37].

Studied flavonol acted synergistically also with one of the major soy isoflavones genistein, is a promising reagent for cancer chemoprevention and/or treatment [38-44] with minimal or no toxicity to nonmalignant human cells [45,46] in ovarian carcinoma OVCAR-5 cells causing i.e. arrests the cell cycle at G1 and S phase [37]. As the authors assumpted quercetin blocked the cell cycle at G1 and S phase boundary, while the second one attacked the cell cycle at G2 and/or early M phase. In another experiment [47] both metabolites, as in the case by Prajda et al. [37], blocked the phosphatidylinositol conversion to IP3 signal transduction pathway, mainly by the inhibition of PI kinase (EC 2.7.1.67) and another member of the signaling route-1-phosphatidylinositol 4-phosphate 5-kinase (PIP kinase, EC 2.7.1.68), respectively. For these experiment conditions the IC50 values for quercetin and genistein (mean ± SE) were as follows: 66 ± 3.0 and 32 ± 2.5 μM; in clonogenic assays they were 15 ± 1.2 and 5 ± 0.5 μM, respectively. When such flavone was added to the cultures of OVCAR-5 cells followed 8 h later by genistein, synergism was still observed in growth inhibition [47]. This flavonoid acted also synergistically with antiviral ribavirin in OVCAR-5 cells (as well as in human myeloma 8226 cell line). Additionally, quercetin inhibited of PI-4 kinase activity as well as the activity of another studied enzyme-PIP-5 kinase (EC 2.7.1.68) in cells. The observed IC50 and LC50 values in growth inhibition for ribavirin were of 35 and 23 μM, respectively. A synergistic antiproliferative action was observed when quercetin was added 24 h after ribavirin and in combined treatment of ribavirin with studied flavonol [48]. An inhibition of activity of PI kinase by quercetin in ovarian cancer cells was also observed by Weber et al. [49], as well as a dose-dependent inhibition of PIP kinase in the case of genistein, while tiazofurin lowered the guanosine tri-phosphorane (GTP) concentration required for phosphoinositide-specific phospholipase C (PLC) protein. Combinations of tiazofurin with quercetin, tiazofurin with genistein, and quercetin with genistein yielded a synergistic kill of ovarian cancer cells [49].

An *in vitro* (A2780 and A2780cisR ovarian cancer cell lines) time (sequence)-dependent synergistic mechanism of action of quercetin and other bio-active metabolite-thymoquinone (TQ) with cytostatics such as cisplatin and oxaliplatin, was observed by Nessa et al. [50]. TQ is known antioxidant from a variety of biological activities including chemoprevention and inhibition of tumor growth [51]. It was demonstrated that although the oxaliplatin was the most active from all used compounds, among plant-derived metabolites, thymoquinone was the most active, with higher activity in the resistant cell line than in the parent cell line. Although these two phytochemicals were less active than both platinum cytostatics, they had resistance factor (RF) higher than the platinum drugs. RF is defined as the ratio of the concentration of the drug required for 50% cell kill in the resistant cell line to that in the parent cell line. The greatest synergism was observed when the phytochemicals were added first followed by platinum drug 2 h later and the least synergism was observed when the two compounds were administered as a bolus. Authors hypothesized that the addition of the plant-origin compounds 2 h before platinum drug may sensitize cancer cells to platinum action, thus offering a means of overcoming drug resistance [51].

Results by Gao et al. [52] with a novel form of nano-formulation of quercetin yielded a promising *in vitro* and *in vivo* antiproliferative effects. Such form of quercetin inhibited the growth of A2780S ovarian cancer cells on a dose dependent manner. In this experiment quercetin treatment induced the apoptosis of A2780S cells associated with activation of proteases essential in programmed cell death development-caspase-3 and caspase-9. The profile of other molecular markers, Mcl-1 and Bcl-2 proteins, has also changed causing their down regulation, also Bax upregulation and mitochondrial transmembrane potential change, suggesting an induction of apoptosis through the mitochondrial apoptotic pathway. Furthermore, an intravenous administration of such nanoformulated quercetin (MPEG-PCL micelles) significantly suppressed the growth of established xenograft A2780S ovarian tumors through causing cancer cell apoptosis and inhibiting angiogenesis *in vivo* [52]. In another study [53] an analysis of cytotoxic potential of quercetin (with final concentrations: 0.1; 0.5; 1, 5, 10, 50, 100, 500 μM) in a set of ovarian cancer cells: SCOV-3, EFO27, OVCAR-3, A2780P revealed a significantly increase of sensitivity of some of them to cisplatin and paclitaxel. In this study a similar sensitivity of studied ovarian cancer cells for quercetin was obtained (with IC50 values for OVCAR-3 cells=42 μM; for EFO27 cells=59 μM; for A2780P cells=70 μM; SCOV-3 cells=90 μM). A treatment of cells with 1 and 5 μM quercetin with those two cytostatics (in three concentrations marked as: $K1=(10^{-1}) \times K2$; $K3=10 \times K2$) caused a significant increase of sensitivity of all three cell line to paclitaxel, especially on SCOV-3 cell line which before the supplementation with quercetin was resistant to this drug. Also the sensitivity to cisplatin of OVCAR-3 and A278OP cells increased. Hence, results from this study revealed also a potential of analyzed flavonoid to overcome the chemoresistance of ovarian cancer cells to some cytostatics [53].

Catanzaro et al. [54] showed that among studied fifteen plant polyphenols, quercetin (as well as rhein and capsaicin) (0.01 μM to 100 μM) was able to cause the arrest of the human ovarian carcinoma 2008 cells and their cisplatin (CDDP)-resistant subclones-C13 cells cycle, suggesting that such cell cycle regulatory proteins are possibly involved in their intracellular mechanism of action. This effect was more potent in C13 cisplatin (CDDP)-resistant cells. Furthermore, a dose-dependent (10 μM to 50 μM) cytotoxic effects and cell cycle modulation of the quercetin in SKOV3 cancer cells and in its cisplatin (CDDP)-resistant counterpart (SKOV3/CDDP) cells was also observed in another experiment by Catanzaro et al. [55]. In this study evident changes in the distribution of cell cycle phases in the CDDP-resistant SKOV3/CDDP ovarian cell line caused by the presence of studied flavonoid and the significant decrease of the cyclin D1 expression in SKOV3 cells (probably linked with the G1/S phase alteration) were proved, but not in SKOV3/CDDP cells. Quercetin influenced also the G2/M phase of cell cycle, however without affecting the cyclin B1 levels (required for G2/M phase) which indicates the involvement of other possible mechanisms [55].

Recently, an enhancement by quercetin (50 μM, 100 μM, 200 μM) of apoptotic death of human ovarian cancer SKOV-3, OVCAR-3 and TOV-21G cells to the presence of the tumor necrosis factor-related apoptosis-inducing ligand (TRAIL) (25 ng/ml) through activation of JNK cellular signal transduction kinase, upregulation of a transcription factor CCAAT enhancer-binding protein (C/EBP)) homologous protein (CHOP), induction of cell death receptor DR5, activated by TRAIL [56,57], was observed [58]. According to the authors, the combination of quercetin with TRAIL did not affected on DR5 receptor expression, ROS (important upstream signals required for the upregulation of death receptors; capable to induce CHOP expression) [59] mediated endoplasmic reticulum-stress (ERS) [58]. In this study a combined treatment of the cells with both TRAIL and quercetin showed significantly higher cell death compared to TRAIL or quercetin applied alone. The IC50 values for quercetin combined with or without TRAIL in ovarian cancer cells such as SKOV-3, OVCAR-3 and TOV-21G cells were found to be 222.1 ± 5.64 μM *vs.* 153.3 ± 4.03 μM, 217.2 ± 4.89 μM *vs.* 147.4 ± 3.86 μM, and 237.6 ± 6.07 μM vs. 159.4 ± 3.64 μM, respectively. However, 200 μM quercetin did not significantly affect cell viability in normal ovarian cells (HOSE cells). Apoptosis in these three cell lines was induced at 14.85 ± 2.93%, 11.99 ±2.33%, and 12.67 ± 2.61% by quercetin, at 9.42 ± 1.75%, 8.53 ± 1.21%, and 10.82 ± 2.01% by TRAIL, and at 36.42 ± 5.04%, 30.34 ± 4.54%, and 33.29 ± 5.28% by the combination of the two agents. In accordance with these results, activation of caspase-3, 8, and 9 and PARP cleavage were significantly increased when the SKOV-3 cells were exposed to both, quercetin and TRAIL. These observations clearly indicated that quercetin was able to increase TRAIL-induced apoptosis in studied ovarian cancer cells. Analyzed flavonoid significantly affected mitochondrial membrane potential in SCOV-3 cells significantly increased the intracellular ROS levels and decreased the levels of DΨm in SKOV-3 cells in a dose-dependent manner. Thus, results by Yi et al. [58] strongly emphasized the role of ROS in the up-regulating of CHOP and enhancing the effects of TRAIL-induced apoptosis by quercetin. Furthermore, quercetin enhancement TRAIL mediated inhibition of tumor growth of human SKOV-3 xenograft was associated with induction of apoptosis, activation of caspase-3, CHOP and DR5. According to the authors all obtained results suggest that quercetin could be an attractive candidate for combined chemotherapy against cancer.

Results concordant to those obtained by Yi et al. [58] were observed in a study by Ren et al. [59]. In this study a time (after 24 or 48 h of treatment) and a dose-dependent manner (0, 0.12, 0.23, 0.47, 0.94, 1.88, 3.75, 7.5, 15 or 30 mg/ml) inhibition of the proliferation of SKOV-3 cancer cells by quercetin occurred. Also an *in vitro* inhibition of cell cycle progression from G0/G1 to G2/M, cell apoptosis induction (analyzed by Hoechst staining and morphologically) and reduction of survivin protein level due the presence of this flavonol was also confirmed. In this study the strongest inhibitory effect on cell growth was observed following treatment with 30 mg/ml quercetin, when the inhibitory rate of cell proliferation reached peak value 58.72%. The total apoptosis rate of the SKOV3 cells treated with 15 mg/ml quercetin was significantly higher than that of the control cells (33.62 ± 1.17 *vs.* 7.13 ± 0.92%, n=6, P<0.01). When the cells were treated with 30 mg/ml quercetin, the total apoptosis rate was 69.12 ± 2.97%, which was significantly higher than that of the low dose (15 mg/ml) of quercetin group and the control (n=6, P<0.01). Further detailed analysis revealed that following treatment with quercetin the number of cells at G0/G1 phase was significantly increased, while the number of cells at S and G2/M phases was relatively decreased compared with the control group. It suggested therefore that quercetin can cause cell cycle arrest at the G1 phase for ovarian cancer SKOV3 cells, may prevent the cell cycle progression from G1 to S phase and can induce cell apoptosis. Thus, these results clearly indicated that cell cycle arrest may be one of the important mechanisms underlying the quercetininduced inhibition of ovarian cancer SKOV3 cell growth, as well as quercetininduced cell apoptosis [59].

Results from another study by Yang et al. [60], similar to those obtained by Maciejczyk et al. [53] or Yi et al. [58] showed that quercetin pretreatment at a low dose may augment drug-resistant ovarian cancer cells for cisplatin chemotherapy by involving the endoplasmic reticulum-stress (ERS) proces via alternation of STAT3 kinase signaling (phosphorylation), a key player involved in ovarian cancer [61,62], modulated by ERS [60]. In this study quercetin decreased the viability of both the C13* and P-ris cells in a dose-dependent manner, with an IC50 value of approximately 100 μM at 48 h; the growth of both cell types could only be significantly inhibited with quercetin concentrations >40 μM, with a negligible cytotoxicity in both cell types at a dose 20 μM. Furthermore, cisplatin treatment with quercetin pretreatment had the greatest inhibitory effect on cancer cell growth. Such pretreatment markedly potentiated the cytotoxicity of cisplatin in studied ovarian cancer cells, and the apoptotic behavior was due to the activation of caspase-9 and caspase-3 of the intrinsic pathway-it was observed that quercetin pretreatment rather than cisplatin alone significantly increased the levels of cleaved caspase-9, cleaved caspase-3 and PARP proteins. Studied plant metabolite at a dose higher than 20 μM had a greater impact on cisplatin cytotoxicity and this influence was dose dependent [60].

In a ovarian cancer xenograft mice quercetin (40 mg/kg; i.p.) enhanced the antitumor effect of cisplatin (3 mg/kg; i.p.). Tumors from mice treated with cisplatin in combination with quercetin pretreatment had repressed STAT3 kinase phosphorylation, lower BCL-2 protein and higher apoptosis levels. The weekly intraperitoneal administration of cisplatin for 4 weeks only modestly reduced the tumor growth by 44.2%, while its weekly treatment day after the 40 mg/kg quercetin treatment remarkably decreased tumor growth by 89.6%. Summarizing, Yang et al. [60] revealed a hitherto undescribed cellular response demonstrating that the quercetin pretreatment, involving the ERS process, may be a promising way to solve the systemic side effects and high incidence of resistance to cisplatin in ovarian cancer pharmacotherapy.

Although previous results indicating pro-apoptotic effect of mostly relatively high concentrations of quercetin (40 μM to 100 μM), *in vitro* (in human ovarian cancer C13* and SKOV3 cells) and *in vivo* results by Li et al. [63] have demonstrated that quercetin even at low concentrations may cause the attenuation of cisplatin and other anti-neoplastic agents (taxol, pirarubicin and 5-fluorouracil) therapeutic effects in ovarian cancer cells by reducing ROS damage. In this study the IC50 value in cisplatin-treated C13* cells was approximately 80 μM (IC50=78.8 μM, 95% CI: 72.9 μM to 85.1 μM). It was shown that low concentrations of analyzed flavonoid (20 μM), not high concentrations (80 μM), antagonized the cytotoxic effects of cisplatin in C13* cells. It was done by increasing cell resistance to cisplatin in varying degrees; decreasing in numbers of apoptotic cells treated with cisplatin and 20 μM of quercetin than with cisplatin alone. High concentrations of quercetin had an additive effect with cisplatin. Similar to those results, treatment using other neoplastic drug taxol (3 μM), pirarubicin (3 nM) and 5-Fu (5 μM) in combination with quercetin (in a series of increasing doses) resulted in more cell resistance than treatment with three drugs alone. Quercetin at the 20 μM concentration showed anti-apoptotic effects against these three drugs. Studied flavonol showed also a low-concentration-specific protecting effect to ovarian cancer cells treated with 5-Fu, similar to the results obtained with cisplatin. In combination with taxol or pirarubicin, however, it maintained the effect of promoting cells survival against anticancer drugs even at relatively high concentrations (80, 100 μM). Further detailed analysis of quercetin influence on the oxidative injury of ovarian cancer cells caused by cisplatin revealed that low concentrations of quercetin were observed to suppress ROS-induced injury, reduce intracellular ROS level. It was shown, for example, that the quantities of both ROS: cH2AX (a common marker of DNA damage) and 8-hydroxydeoxyguanosine (8-OHdG; a marker of oxidative DNA stress) were much lower in the treatment group of 80 μM cisplatin combined with the low concentration of quercetin (20 μM) than the group of 80 μM cytostatic alone. Contrary to this, 80 μM cisplatin with high concentration (60 μM; 100 μM) of analyzed plant metabolite increased the intensity of fluorescence. Combination treatment with quercetin (20 μM) had a more obvious decrease of 8-OHdG than that of cH2AX, compared to cisplatin treatment alone (36.40% and 19.33%, respectively). Moreover, comparing to cells treated with vehicle control or cisplatin alone, treatment with an additional 20 μM quercetin lead to a reduction in intracellular levels of ROS. Furthermore, low quercetin concentration caused increased expression of endogenous antioxidant enzymes transcripts (superoxide dismutase 1-SOD1, endonuclease G-ENDOG, cytochrome c-cyto-c, glutathione peroxidase-GPx, catalase-CAT and uncoupling protein 2-UCP2). Summarizing, obtained results suggested a ROS-mediated mechanism of action of quercetin attenuating anti-neoplastic drugs effects. Surprisingly, in an applied xenogeneic model (a nude mouse xenograft model injected with C13* cells), studied flavonol (40 mg/kg; i.p.; daily) led to a substantial reduction of therapeutic efficacy of cisplatin. For example, it was found out that tumors from mice treated with cisplatin in combination with quercetin were approximately 1.8 times larger at day 30 than those treated with cisplatin alone (P<0.001). Evenmore, tumors treated with combination of quercetin and cisplatin (72.53 ± 7.33 mg) were significantly heavier than that treated with cytostatic alone (41.47 ± 6.72 mg) (P<0.001). With this effect also an enhancement of the endogenous SOD1 enzyme expression and reduction of the ROS-induced damage in xenograft tumor tissue were observed. The SOD1 protein was highly overexpressed in tumors treated with quercetin or cisplatin with quercetin compared to tumors treated with vehicle or cisplatin alone [63]. Overall, data obtained by Li et al. indicated that administration of quercetin at low concentrations may antagonize the cytotoxic effects of anti-neoplastic drugs in studied ovarian cancer cells, and that this plant metabolite is able to decrease the levels of oxidative injury caused by cisplatin [63].

An induction of apoptosis of human ovarian carcinoma SKOV-3 and A2780 cells through activation of the extrinsic death receptors and intrinsic mitochondrial apoptotic pathways via modulation of expression levels of cleaved caspase-3 (as was shown in experiments by Yi et al. [58] or Yang et al. [60]) and induction of overexpression of miR-145 by quercetin was also confirmed by Zhou et al. [64]. These results are with the trend of studies indicating that some microRNAs, including the miR-145, are downregulated in ovarian cancer [65,66], and that cancer cells growth inhibition caused by quercetin may be correlated with the modulation of several miRs expression of [60, 63, 67,68].

Quercetin, among other eight studied compounds, was also able to inhibit OVCAR5, OVCAR3, TOV112D, CAOV3 ovarian cancer cells growth via induction of apoptosis and inhibition of the glycolytic pathway-by blocking five glycolysis pathway molecules-(glucose transporter 1 (GLUT1), hexokinase II (HKII), PFKFB3 (an isozyme; a component of fructose-2, 6-bisphosphate (Fru-2, 6-BP), an allosteric activator of 6-phosphofructo-1-kinase (PFK1) [69]), pyruvate dehydrogenase kinase 1 (PDHK1) and lactate dehydrogenase (LDH)) via an increased extracellular glucose and decreased lactate production, which was especially seen at low oxygen conditions. Variation in oxygen levels between 0.5% and 7% had a relatively small effect on the efficacy of the studied inhibitors. The IC50 values of quercetin for OVCAR5, TOV112D, OVCAR3, CAOV3 cells were 154, 94, 21, 240 μM, respectively [70]. The choice of glycolytic pathway enzymes analyzed in this study was due to the fact, that they are well substantiated and considered a 'hallmark' of advanced cancers [71]. The fact that cancer cells reduce their dependence on mitochondrial oxidative phosphorylation and are more reliant on glycolysis provides a wide range of potential targets for therapy. Targeting aerobic glycolysis is a promising strategy to preferentially kill cancer cells which are dependent on this pathway and in recent years multiple glycolytic inhibitors have been developed [72,73].

The above-described results were related so far to quercetin being a non-physically component of the plant extract. Wang et al. [74] demonstrated results of the influence of quercetin aglycone (and seven other flavonols: myricetin-3-galactoside, quercetin-3-galactoside, quercetin-3-glucoside, quercetin-3-xylopyranoside, quercetin-3-arabinopyranosdie, quercetin-3-arabinofuranoside, quercetin-3-rhamnopyranoside) as well as eleven member of A-type proanthocyanidins isolated from Vaccinium macrocarpon (American cranberry) against SKOV-3 and OVCAR-8 cancer cells. Two of them, quercetin aglycone and PAC DP-9, showed promising *in vitro* cytotoxic and anti-proliferative properties. Compared to quercetin glycosides, quercetin aglycone exhibited higher cytotoxicity against these cancer cell lines (IC50=83 and 61 μg/ml for SKOV-3 and OVCAR-8 cells, respectively).

Both compounds strongly induced apoptosis led to caspase-3 activation and PARP deactivation, and increased sensitivity to cisplatin (concentrations of: quercetin aglycone 10 μg/ml, cisplatin=15 μg/ml or 60 μg/ml; measurement after 12 h of cisplatin treatment). In addition, quercetin aglycone (and PAC DP-9) deactivated the MAPK-ERK kinases pathway, induced downregulation of: cyclin D1 kinase, DNA-dependent protein kinase (DNA-PK) and the phospho-histone H3 - proteins - often overexpressed in ovarian cancer cells.

Also this aglycone caused an upregulation of p21 protein, and the cell cycle progression arrest (G1/S-phase arrest in OVCAR-8 cells after the treatment for 24 and 48 h). In conclusion, according to Wang et al. the integration of quercetin (and/or PAC DP-9) in ovarian cancer chemotherapy may improve outcomes. Moreover, among studied compounds quercetin aglycone induced cellular apoptotic events including cell cycle arrest and suppression of DNA repair pathways highlighted their potential as dietarily available therapeutic agents [74]. The quercetininduced apoptotic cell death correlated with several kinases phosphorylation was also proved in the study by Kim et al. [75] but in a different cell line model. In this study the presence of quercetin, detected in Rubus coreanus Miquel (RCM) extract, or other phenolic compound - an ellagic acid, caused an apoptosis of the doxorubicinresistant NCI/ADRRES ovarian cancer cells induced the phosphorylation of JNK and AKT kinase. The same effect was observed in the case of RCM extract, however, without the synergism with doxorubicin in reduction of cells viability [75].

An inhibition of proliferation of ovarian cancer cells by quercetin (0, 2.5, 5 and 10 μg/ml; after 72 hours) was also observed by Choi et al. [76]. This study was performed not only on paclitaxel sensitive (SCOV-3) but also on SCOV-3/PAX (paclitaxel resistant) ovarian cancer cells as well. The action was compared to 80% methanolic extract of Rhus verniciflua Stokes (syn. *Toxicodendron vernicifluum* Stokes) (RVS) (50, 100, 200 and 500 μg/ml) in which quercetin was present. In this study quercetin dose-depedently (more potent than fisetin alone) reduced cell growth. Other activities of quercetin, observed in the case of another analyzed flavonoid-butein, such as strong activation of cleavage of caspase-9, -8, -3, and PARP, reduction of AKT phosphorylation or SKOV-3/PAX cells arrest in sub-G1 phase, were not further examined [76].

Recent study by Ediriweera et al. [77] demonstrated also a cytotoxic potential of quercetin (and other three compounds) isolated from the chloroform extract of *Mangifera zeylanica* Hook.f. bark in ovarian epithelial cancer (SKOV-3), as well as in three other cancer cell lines - triple negative breast cancer (MDA-MB-231), estrogen receptor positive breast cancer (MCF-7), and normal mammary epithelial (MCF-10A) cells. Quercetin was found to be cytotoxic to all three cancer cell lines examined in a dose dependent manner. IC50 values for quercetin at 24 h and 48 h for SKOV-3 cells were 170.18 ± 3.92, 109.9 ± 2.64 mM, respectively. Also a DPPH free radical scavenging activity (EC50=33.1 ± 0.59 mM) of quercetin was shown [77].

Studies by Liu et al. [78] on human ovarian cancer (OC) CAOV3 cells and on primary OC cells provided evidences for a novel role of endoplasmic reticulum (ER-responsible for protein translocation, protein folding, and protein post-translational modifications) stress (perturbations in ER function triggering the unfolded protein response (UPR), a tightly orchestrated collection of intracellular signal transduction reactions designed to restore protein homeostasis; triggering the apoptotic machinery ultimately leading to cell death under severe or chronic stress conditions) as, as authors described, a "double edge sword" participating in quercetin-induced apoptosis [78]. In this study quercetin (40 μM; 80 μM for 48 h) irreversibly evoked ER stress to involve in mitochondria apoptosis pathway via the p-STAT3/Bcl-2 axis in OC cell lines and in primary OC cells. The quercetin-induced ER stress activated protective autophagy concomitantly by activating the p-STAT3/Bcl-2 axis in this process. Moreover, the autophagy scavenger-3-methyladenine (3MA) was shown to enhance quercetin's anticancer effects in an ovarian cancer mice xenograft model (5×10^{-6}) of human ovarian cancer CAOV3 cells in 100 ul volume of PBS injected s.c. into the right supra scapula region of mice). For this purpose following *in vivo* experimental conditions were carried out: 5 days after tumor implantation the mice were treated i.p. with 80 mg/kg of quercetin twice a week; 30 mg/kg 3MA twice a week; a combination of 30 mg/kg 3 MA and 80 mg/kg of quercetin twice a week; or a vehicle control injected with the same volume of saline for 4 weeks [78]. The results of this study are consistent with the trend of predecessor studies [56,60,77] showing that quercetin has the potential to induce protective autophagy in cancer cells through AKT-mTOR and hypoxia-induced factor 1α signaling [79,80] and in this way to induce autophagy in ovarian cancer cells [81].

There is also a growing number of studies justifying the use of plant-derived bio-active metabolites, especially polyphenols, in cancerogenesis prevention/inhibition by applying them in combinations with other micronutrients for achieving pleiotropic effects [34,82-89]. This is especially interesting when one considers the fact of their poor bioavailability in the human body. In addition, their interactions with other natural compounds in a diet may hinder or complicate consistency of their efficacy [90]. According to the supporters of this strategy these compounds, which are abundant from dietary sources, show great promise in cancer treatment, especially considering their potential safe use. Due to their ability to modulate multiple biological mechanisms involved in cancer initiation/progression, they may offer more comprehensive therapeutic effects than single drugs [34]. It is believed that the bioavailability, as well as chemopreventive or even therapeutic properties of these nutrients, may be enhanced and expanded in combination therapies that include natural compounds of the same or different chemical class. Thus, a combinations of i.e. polyphenols with micronutrients essential for maintaining integrity and stability of extracellular matrix and therefore provides the opportunity to expand the preventive/therapeutic effect of their anti-cancer action. They include targeting complementary metabolic pathways important in curtailing cancer invasion and metastasis. Therefore, specifically designed combinations of several bio-active compounds, especially polyphenols or combinations of polyphenols with other natural agents aimed at defined biological targets will expand metabolic effects of constituents of such mixtures in controlled and reproducible ways. In addition, proper combinations of micronutrients enable use of lower doses of individual components without compromising their efficacy, rather than expanding the scope of cellular mechanisms affected. According to researchers this approach may open up a possibility of developing more effective anti-cancer strategies [34].

In the context of the above information such anti-cancer potential of quercetin with EGCG (at concentrations between 0 and 1000 μg/ml) and in combination with the micronutrient mixture against ovarian cancer using two different cell lines (ES-2 or A-2780) or in athymic female mice inoculated with ES-2 cells was demonstrated by Roomi et al. [82,91-93]. Studied micronutrient mixture EPQ (containing the following nutrients in the relative amounts indicated: vitamin C (as ascorbic acid and as Mg, Ca ascorbates, and ascorbyl palmitate) 700 mg; L-lysine 1000 mg; L-proline 750 mg; L-arginine 500 mg; N-acetyl cysteine 200 mg; standardized green tea extract (80% polyphenol) 1000 mg; quercetin as quercetin dihydrate, from Saphora japonica 50 mg; selenium 30 g; copper 2 mg; manganese 1 mg) was investigated and the proposed mechanism of action was via modulation of expression of two metalloproteinases ((MMP-2 and MMP-9) (these MMPs are prognostic for survival and metastatic potential in ovarian cancer [94-96]. Athymic female mice inoculated with ES-2 ovarian cancer cells showed that dietary intake of EPQ (0.5%, w/w) inhibited weight and burden of tumors by 59.2% ($p<0.0001$) and 59.7% ($p<0.0001$), respectively [91]. In a study with mice injected (i.p.) with A-2780 cancer cells, control mice developed large ovarian tumors, whereas five out of six mice in the EPQ group developed no tumors, and one, only a small tumor-tumor growth was suppressed by EPQ by 87% ($p<0.0001$) [92]. *In vitro* analyzes proved also the antiproliferative potential of EPQ. EPQ exhibited 35% toxicity over the control in ES-2 cells [91] and 80% in A-2780 cells [92] at 1000 g/mL concentration. ES-2 cells demonstrated only MMP-2, with and without PMA, which was inhibited by EPQ in a dose dependent fashion, with near total inhibition at 1000 g/ml [91]. A-2780 cells demonstrated only MMP-9 expression, which EPQ inhibited in a dose dependent fashion, with virtual total block at 250 g/mL concentration [92], while the migration of ES-2 cells were inhibited in a dose dependent manner with total block of invasion and migration at 500 g/ml [91]. However, it is difficult to indicate which compound of nutrient mixture examined the higher anticancer activity, a 1000 mg quercetin dihydrate concentration may suggest its crucial role in the EPQ action, however such hypothesis along with their putative action in a synergistic manner requires further evaluation [91,93]. Nevertheless, these studies clearly give credit for the usage of natural health compounds widely presented in human diet to prevent or inhibit ovaries carcinogenesis [91-93].

Studies on curcumin alone or with quercetin and other compounds in ovarian cancer cells

A potential of curcumin and quercetin for enhancing cisplatin sensitivity in two ovarian cancer cell lines: SKOV3 and CAOV3 (less susceptible to cisplatin, with a higher IL-6 protein production) was observed by Chan et al. [51]. Both compounds inhibited the growth of SKOV3 and CAOV3 cells in a dose-dependent and similar manner (quercetin at 10 μM to 20 μM; curcumin at 5 μM to 15 μM). Such inhibition was attained by day 2-3 after drug treatment and persisted thereafter (in max. 5 days experiment duration). They increased the sensitivity of CAOV3 and SKOV3 cells to cisplatin (2 μg/ml) (the concentrations of quercetin were as follows: 0; 5; 10; 15; 20 μM, while curcumin were as follows: 0; 2.5; 5. 10; 15 μM). This effect of sensitization was obtained when the compounds were added 24 h before or simultaneously with cisplatin. In an applied experimental model the high IL-6 protein producing CAOV3 cells were less susceptible to cisplatin-induced cytotoxicity than the low producer, SKOV3 cell line. The survival rate of CAOV3 cells at 2 days after treatment with 1 mg/ml of cisplatin was 87%, whereas that of SKOV3 was at 45% (IC50 values for the two cell lines were 6.1 mg/ml and 0.9 mg/ml, respectively). According to authors these difference resembles the levels of resistance seen in clinics (2-4-fold) and are more closely than laboratory-induced cisplatin resistant cell lines (which are in the order of 10-1000-fold) [97]. In this experiment curcumin inhibited the production of interleukin IL-6 in CAOV3 cells suggesting that one of the possible mechanisms for synergy between cisplatin and curcumin was related to decrease autologous production of IL-6. However, such synergy was also observed in the SKOV3 cell line (exerting low IL-6 expression) indicating that this action was most probably a result of multiple targeting [51].

A complex study by Montopoli et al. [98] confirmed curcumin cytotoxic activity in ovarian cancer cells and strongly revealed its synergistic action to cisplatin and a third generation platinum derivative drug, oxaliplatin-1R, 2R-diamnocycloexanoxalateplatinum (II) leading to an increase of cisplatin's and oxaliplatin's cytotoxicity in wild type human ovarian cancer cell line and C13 cisplatin-resistant ones when they were combined treated. It was shown that curcumin caused a concentration- and time-dependent inhibition of ovarian cancer cell viability. Its synergism with cisplatin and oxaliplatin in such action also occurred. In this study all compounds caused concentration-dependent inhibition (0.01 μM to 100 μM) of cell viability. The IC50 values for curcumin were 14.92 μM; 7.87 μM; 6.36 μM after 24 h, 48 h and 72 h, respectively; for cisplatin were as follows: 1.35 μM; 0.96 μM; 0.94 μM after 24 h, 48 h and 72 h, respectively. While for oxaliplatin following values were obtained in above-mentioned time periods: 5.62 μM; 2.52 μM; 3.58 μM, respectively. Montopoli et al. showed that curcumin was more effective in cisplatin-resistant than in cisplatin-sensitive ovarian cancer cells. Moreover, a synergistic inhibitory effect on cell viability of curcumin (0.1 μM to 1 μM) with platinum drugs (all at concentrations: 0.1 μM to 5 μM) in both, in wild type 2008 and C13 cells, was clearly visible. A curcumin alone (0.5 μM, 1.0 μM, 5.0 μM) significantly reduced the percentage of wild type 2008 cells in G2/M phase in a concentration-dependent fashion and caused apoptosis (sub-G0), whereas in C13 cells it significantly increased numbers of cells in G0/G1 phase and reduced cells in S and G2/M, in comparison with untreated cells (with similar results after all three studied experimental periods: 24 h, 48 h, 72 h). Compared to single-drug treatment, curcumin combined with cisplatin or oxaliplatin, at concentrations lower than IC50 (0.5 μM for all three), caused the best dose- and time-dependent increases in cell-cycle arrest and apoptosis. According to Montopoli et al. [98] these results suggested a crucial role for curcumin in alteration of cell-cycle parameters, when combined with platinum drugs. It was clearly indicated that concurrent treatment of curcumin with platinum drugs makes cisplatin-resistant ovarian carcinoma cells more susceptible to the action of the platinum drugs. It was also shown that in cisplatin-resistant cells (compared to cisplatin-sensitive cells), higher glutathione content may be parallel to lower ROS level (used as a markers of curcumin's antioxidative potential), and that curcumin is able to cause the concentration-dependent changes of ROS or glutathione after different time of incubation (an increase of ROS after 2 h incubation, but increase in glutathione after 24 h). Similarly, curcumin's early pro-oxidative effect (increased ROS and reduced glutathione) and late antioxidant effect (increased glutathione) have been shown by Weir et al. [99] in ovarian cancer cells and i.e. in human myeloid leukaemia cells [100]. Therefore, study by Montopoli et al. provided an evidence that curcumin is able to increase the glutathione level in both, cisplatin-sensitive and cisplatin-resistant, ovarian cancer cells, suggesting that the increased susceptibility of ovary cancer cell to combined treatment of curcumin with platinum drugs is not related to a glutathione elimination [98].

A synergism of actions between platinum drugs-cisplatin and oxaliplatin, applied in binary combination with the curcumin and anethole were also observed in three ovarian cancer cells: A2780 (wild - type), A2780 (cisR) (cisplatin-resistant) and A2780 (ZD0473R) (ZD0473 - resistant) in another experiment by Nessa et al. [101]. Both plant metabolites were able to increase intracellular levels of glutathione and glutathione-S-transferase, hence their possessed an antioxidative activity [102-104]. Although, in this study, oxaliplatin was found to be the most active and analyzed plant compound-anethole-had the lowest activity at all, it had a greater activity in the resistant cells (A2780 (cisR) and A2780 (ZD0473R)) than other compounds. The obtained results indicated that anethole was better able to induce programmed cell death i.e. apoptosis of the resistant cell lines than of the parent cell line. Moreover, applied 2/0 combinations of anethole with both cisplatin and oxaliplatin were found to be highly synergistic, indicating that pretreatment of ovarian cancer cells with the phytochemical serves to sensitize them to platinum (cisplatin and oxaliplatin) action. Similar effects were observed in the case of curcumin. The role of NF-κB as a potential molecular target in the action of studied plant-origin compounds was strongly postulated by authors and others [105]. The enhanced cell kill resulting from treatment of cancer cells with these two phytochemicals (applied 2/0 sequence of administration) may be related to the reduced expression of NF-κB and down-regulation of AKT kinase and cyclooxygenase-2 (COX2) protein pathways. It was therefore stated that bolus addition of platinum drugs and the selected phytochemicals leading to change from agonistic to antagonistic in action may suggest that concurrent administration of these two compounds in some cases may cause failure of sensitize the ovarian cancer cells to platinum action, perhaps due to less significant reduction in the expression of NF-κB [50]. Thus, the prior treatment of ovarian cancer cells with anethole and curcumin appeared to be the critical determinant in lowering the expression of NF-κB [101]. The observed action of anethole promoting cell survival at a lower concentration (0.2 μM) and promoting cell death at higher concentrations (25 μM) seemed to support such thesis [101].

Conclusions

Upon basic studies in this paper we have summarized available evidences of inhibitory activities of several often studied plant-origin bio-active compounds (mostly quercetin and curcumin) of ovarian cancer cells proliferation, their mechanisms of action (relying i.e. on suppression of signal transduction activity of several cellular kinases [37,47-49,60,75], induction of apoptosis [52,58], cell cycle arrest [37,55,59]) induction of ER stress activating protective autophagy via the p-STAT3/Bcl-2 axis [78], as well as their strong potential to sensitization of ovarian cancer cells to the presence of several platinum-based cytostatics (cisplatin and oxaliplatin) [75] and others.

Up to date several dietary, clinical (cohort and case–control) studies evaluating the association of some flavonoids (mostly nonisoflavones) and its subgroup components consumption and ovarian cancer risk were already performed (Mohammadi et al. [32], Parvaresh et al. [33], Hua et al. [6]). According to the researchers, there has been no association between ovarian cancer risk and total nonisoflavone flavonoids intake [32]. Although, some studies reported an inverse association between certain nonisoflavone flavonoids subclasses (flavonols) [106,107] or other individual flavonoids (i.e. kaempferol and luteolin [107] and apigenin [108]) and ovarian cancer risk, there is a still an insufficient amount of data designed to explain the effect of quercetin or curcumin (alone or together) on ovarian cancer development and/or its chemotherapy. According to Mohammadi et al. [32] these results provide limited support for an association between nonisoflavone flavonoids intake and ovarian cancer risk; therefore there is a need for further and more accurate researches to be confirmed. Thus, we are of the opinion that this paper will contribute to a better understanding of the molecular basis for positive interactions between concomitant usage of quercetin or curcumin with above-mentioned cytostatics and other bio-active agents. This work may also contribute to an increase in the number of preclinical studies or other clinical, dietary trials using these or other phenolic/alkaloid, plant-origin constituents in order to investigate efficiency and safety of pharmacotherapy of ovarian cancer patients. We hope that such point of view, presented in this paper, extended by actual state of knowledge will be helpful to find other connections between active substances like quercetin and curcumin and cytostatics depending on dose.

Acknowledgement

This publication is financed by funds allocated to the statutory activities of the Institute of Natural Fibers and Medicinal Plants and the various Departments of Poznan University of Medical Sciences.

References

1. Gallion HH, Pieretti M, DePriest PD, van Nagell JR Jr (1995) The molecular basis of ovarian cancer. Cancer 76: 1992-1997.
2. Poole EM, Konstantinopoulos PA, Terry KL (2016) Prognostic implications of reproductive and lifestyle factors in ovarian cancer. Gynecol Oncol 142: 574-587.
3. Stadel BV (1975) Letter: The etiology and prevention of ovarian cancer. Am J Obstet Gynecol 123: 772-774.
4. Schuijer M, Berns EM (2003) TP53 and ovarian cancer. Hum Mutat 21: 285-291.
5. Kim MK, Kim K, Han JY, Lim JM, Song YS (2011) Modulation of inflammatory signaling pathways by phytochemicals in ovarian cancer. Genes Nutr 6: 109-115.
6. Aggarwal BB, Shishodia S (2006) Molecular targets of dietary agents for prevention and therapy of cancer. Biochem Pharmacol 71: 1397-1421.
7. Hong WK, Sporn MB (1997) Recent advances in chemoprevention of cancer. Science 278: 1073-1077.
8. Crane TE, Khulpateea BR, Alberts DS, Basen-Engquist K, Thomson CA (2014) Dietary intake and ovarian cancer risk: a systematic review. Cancer Epidemiol Biomarkers Prev 23: 255-273.
9. Hua X, Yu L, You R, Yang Y, Liao J, et al. (2016) Association among dietary flavonoids, flavonoid subclasses and ovarian cancer risk: A Meta-Analysis. PLoS One 11: e0151134.
10. Key TJ, Schatzkin A, Willett WC, Allen NE, Spencer EA, et al. (2004) Diet, nutrition and the prevention of cancer. Public Health Nutr 7: 187-200.
11. Lewandowska H, Kalinowska M, Lewandowski W, St pkowski TM, Brazska K3 (2016) The role of natural polyphenols in cell signaling and cytoprotection against cancer development. J Nutr Biochem 32: 1-19.
12. Cassidy A, Huang T, Rice MS, Rimm EB, Tworoger SS (2014) Intake of dietary flavonoids and risk of epithelial ovarian cancer. Am J Clin Nutr 100: 1344-1351.
13. Kandaswami C, Lee LT, Lee PP, Hwang JJ, Ke FC, et al. (2005) The antitumor activities of flavonoids. In Vivo 19: 895-909.
14. Corcoran MP, McKay DL, Blumberg JB (2012) Flavonoid basics: Chemistry, sources, mechanisms of action, and safety. J Nutr Gerontol Geriatr 31: 176-189.
15. D'Archivio M, Filesi C, Di Benedetto R, Gargiulo R, Giovannini C, et al. (2007) Polyphenols, dietary sources and bioavailability. Ann Ist Super Sanita 43: 348-361.
16. U.S. Department of Agriculture (2003) USDA database for the flavonoid content of selected foods. Beltsville, Maryland 20705: 1-77.
17. Gates MA, Tworoger SS, Hecht JL, De Vivo I, Rosner B, et al. (2007) A prospective study of dietary flavonoid intake and incidence of epithelial ovarian cancer. Int J Cancer 121: 2225-2232.
18. McCann SE, Freudenheim JL, Marshall JR, Graham S (2003) Risk of human ovarian cancer is related to dietary intake of selected nutrients, phytochemicals and food groups. J Nutr 133: 1937-1942.
19. Ko EY, Nile SH, Sharma K, Li GH, Park SW (2015) Effect of different exposed lights on quercetin and quercetin glucoside content in onion (Allium cepa L.). Saudi J Biol Sci 22: 398-403.
20. Koh E, Wimalasiri K, Chassy A, Mitchell A (2009) Content of ascorbic acid, quercetin, kaempferol and total phenolics in commercial broccoli. J Food Comp Anal 22: 637-643.
21. Sun T, Xu Z, Wu CT, Janes M, Prinyawiwatkul W, et al. (2007) Antioxidant activities of different colored sweet bell peppers (Capsicum annuum L.). J Food Sci 72: S98-102.
22. Francesca N, Barbera M, Martorana A, Saiano F, Gaglio R, et al. (2016) Optimised method for the analysis of phenolic compounds from caper (Capparis spinosa L.) berries and monitoring of their changes during fermentation. Food Chem 196: 1172-1179.
23. Zielinski AAF, Alberti A, Braga CM, da Silva KM, Canteri MHG, et al. (2014) Effect of mash maceration and ripening stage of apples on phenolic compounds and antioxidant power of cloudy juices: A study using chemometrics. LWT-Food Sci Technol 57: 223-229.
24. Jeszka-Skowron M, Krawczyk M, Zgola-Grzeskowiak A (2015) Determination of antioxidant activity, rutin, quercetin, phenolic acids and trace elements in tea infusions: Influence of citric acid addition on extraction of metals. J Food Comp Anal 40: 70-77.
25. Martelo-Vidal MJ, Vázquez M (2014) Determination of polyphenolic compounds of red wines by UV-VIS-NIR spectroscopy and chemometrics tools. Food Chem 158: 28-34.
26. Kelly GS (2011) Quercetin. Monograph. Altern Med Rev 16: 172-194.
27. Maalik A, Khan FA, Mumtaz A, Mehmood A, Azhar S, et al. (2014) Pharmacological Applications of Quercetin and its Derivatives: A Short Review. Tropical J Pharmaceutical Res 13: 1561-1566.
28. Nam JS, Sharma AR, Nguyen LT, Chakraborty C, Sharma G, et al. (2016) Application of Bioactive Quercetin in Oncotherapy: From Nutrition to Nanomedicine. Molecules 21: E108.
29. Terlikowska KM, Witkowska AM, Zujko ME, Dobrzycka B, Terlikowski SJ, et al. (2014) Potential application of curcumin and its analogues in the treatment strategy of patients with primary epithelial ovarian cancer. Int J Mol Sci 15: 21703-21722.
30. Vallianou NG, Evangelopoulos A, Schizas N, Kazazis C (2015) Potential anticancer properties and mechanisms of action of curcumin. Anticancer Res 35: 645-651.
31. Chen SS, Michael A, Butler-Manuel SA (2012) Advances in the treatment of ovarian cancer: A potential role of antiinflammatory phytochemicals. Discov Med 13: 7-17.
32. Mohammadi V, Dehghani S, Larijani B, Azadbakht L (2016) Ovarian cancer risk and nonisoflavone flavonoids intake: A systematic review of epidemiological studies. J Res Med Sci 21: 123.
33. Parvaresh A, Razavi R, Rafie N, Ghiasvand R, Pourmasoumi M, et al. (2016) Quercetin and ovarian cancer: An evaluation based on a systematic review. J Res Med Sci 21: 34.
34. Niedzwiecki A, Roomi MW, Kalinovsky T, Rath M (2016) Anticancer Efficacy of Polyphenols and Their Combinations. Nutrients 8: E552.

35. Scambia G, Ranelletti FO, Panici BP, Bonanno G, De Vincenzo R, et al. (1990) Synergistic antiproliferative activity of quercetin and cisplatin on ovarian cancer cell growth. Anticancer Drugs 1: 45-48.
36. Scambia G, Ranelletti FO, Panici BP, Piantelli M, Bonanno G, et al. (1992) Inhibitory effect of quercetin on primary ovarian and endometrial cancers and synergistic activity with cis-diamminedichloroplatinum (II). Gynecol Oncol 45: 13-19.
37. Prajda N, Singhal RL, Yeh YA, Olah E, Look KY, et al. (1995) Linkage of reduction in 1-phosphatidylinositol 4-kinase activity and inositol, 5-trisphosphate concentration in human ovarian carcinoma cells treated with quercetin. Life Sci 56: 1587-1593.
38. Hedelin M, Lof M, Andersson TM, Adlercreutz H, Weiderpass E (2011) Dietary phytoestrogens and the risk of ovarian cancer in the women's lifestyle and health cohort study. Cancer Epidemiol, Biomarkers Prev 20: 308-317.
39. Lee JY, Kim HS, Song YS (2012) Genistein as a Potential Anticancer Agent against Ovarian Cancer. J Tradit Complement Med 2: 96-104.
40. Li Y, Mi C (2003) Proliferation inhibition and apoptosis onset in human ovarian carcinoma cell line SKOV3 induced by Genistein. Ai Zheng 22: 586-591.
41. Myung SK, Ju W, Choi HJ, Kim SC (2009) Soy intake and risk of endocrine-related gynaecological cancer: A meta-analysis. British J Obstet Gyn 116: 1697-1705.
42. Sarkar FH, Li Y (2003) Soy isoflavones and cancer prevention. Cancer Invest 21: 744-757.
43. Solomon LA, Ali S, Banerjee S, Munkarah AR, Morris RT, et al. (2008) Sensitization of ovarian cancer cells to cisplatin by genistein: The role of NF-kappaB. J Ovarian Res 1: 9.
44. Wang X, Xin XY, Huang YH (2006) Regulative effect of genistein on xenografted tumor of ovarian carcinoma cell on nude mice. Zhongguo Zhong Yao Za Zhi 31: 901-904.
45. Li Y, Che M, Bhagat S, Ellis KL, Kucuk O, et al. (2004) Regulation of gene expression and inhibition of experimental prostate cancer bone metastasis by dietary genistein. Neoplasia 6: 354-363.
46. Tatsuta M, Iishi H, Baba M, Yano H, Uehara H, et al. (1990) Attenuation by genistein of sodium-chloride-enhanced gastric carcinogenesis induced by N-methyl-N'-nitro-Nnitrosoguanidine in Wistar rats. Int J Cancer 80: 396-399.
47. Shen F, Weber G (1997) Synergistic action of quercetin and genistein in human ovarian carcinoma cells. Oncol Res 9: 597-602.
48. Li W, Shen F, Weber G (1999) Ribavirin and quercetin synergistically downregulate signal transduction and are cytotoxic in human ovarian carcinoma cells. Oncol Res 11: 243-247.
49. Weber G, Shen DF, Li W, Yang H, Look KY, et al. (2000) Signal transduction and biochemical targeting of ovarian carcinoma. Eur J Gynaecol Oncol 21: 231-236.
50. Nessa MU, Beale P, Chan C, Yu JQ, Huq F (2011) Synergism from combinations of cisplatin and oxaliplatin with quercetin and thymoquinone in human ovarian tumour models. Anticancer Res 31: 3789-3797.
51. Chan MM, Fong D, Soprano KJ, Holmes WF, Heverling H (2003) Inhibition of growth and sensitization to cisplatin-mediated killing of ovarian cancer cells by polyphenolic chemopreventive agents. J Cell Physiol 194: 63-70.
52. Gao X, Wang B, Wei X, Men K, Zheng F, et al. (2012) Anticancer effect and mechanism of polymer micelle-encapsulated quercetin on ovarian cancer. Nanoscale 4: 7021-7030.
53. Maciejczyk A, Surowiak P (2013) Quercetin inhibits proliferation and increases sensitivity of ovarian cancer cells to cisplatin and paclitaxel. Ginekol Pol 84: 590-595.
54. Catanzaro D, Vianello C, Ragazzi E, Caparrotta L, Montopoli M (2014) Cell cycle control by natural phenols in cisplatin-resistant cell lines. Nat Prod Commun 9: 1465-1468.
55. Catanzaro D, Ragazzi E, Vianello C, Caparrotta L, Montopoli M (2015) Effect of quercetin on cell cycle and cyclin expression in ovarian carcinoma and osteosarcoma cell lines. Nat Prod Commun 10: 1365-1368.
56. Kurbanov BM, Fecker LF, Geilen CC, Sterry W, Eberle J (2007) Resistance of melanoma cells to TRAIL does not result from upregulation of antiapoptotic proteins by NFkappaB but is related to downregulation of initiator caspases and DR4. Oncogene 26: 3364-3377.
57. van Geelen CM, Pennarun B, Le PT, de Vries EG, de Jong S (2011) Modulation of TRAIL resistance in colon carcinoma cells: Different contributions of DR4 and DR5. BMC Cancer 11: 39.
58. Yi L, Zongyuan Y, Cheng G, Lingyun Z, Guilian Y, et al. (2014) Quercetin enhances apoptotic effect of tumor necrosis factor-related apoptosis-inducing ligand (TRAIL) in ovarian cancer cells through reactive oxygen species (ROS) mediated CCAAT enhancer-binding protein homologous protein (CHOP)-death receptor 5 pathway. Cancer Sci 105: 520-527.
59. Ren MX, Deng XH, Ai F, Yuan GY, Song HY (2015) Effect of quercetin on the proliferation of the human ovarian cancer cell line SKOV-3 in vitro. Exp Ther Med 10: 579-583.
60. Yang Z, Liu Y, Liao J, Gong C, Sun C, et al. (2015) Quercetin induces endoplasmic reticulum stress to enhance cDDP cytotoxicity in ovarian cancer: involvement of STAT3 signaling. FEBS J 282: 1111-1125.
61. Michaud-Levesque J, Bousquet-Gagnon N, Beliveau R (2012) Quercetin abrogates IL-6/STAT3 signaling and inhibits glioblastoma cell line growth and migration. Exp Cell Res 318: 925-935.
62. Sheng WJ, Jiang H, Wu DL, Zheng JH. Early responses of the STAT3 pathway to platinum drugs are associated with cisplatin resistance in epithelial ovarian cancer. Braz J Med Biol Res 46: 650-658.
63. Li W, Liu M, Xu YF, Feng Y, Che JP, et al. (2014) Combination of quercetin and hyperoside has anticancer effects on renal cancer cells through inhibition of oncogenic microRNA-27a. Oncol Rep 31: 117-124.
64. Zhou J, Gong J, Ding C, Chen G (2015) Quercetin induces the apoptosis of human ovarian carcinoma cells by upregulating the expression of microRNA-145. Mol Med Rep 12: 3127-3131.
65. Wu H, Xiao Z, Wang K, Liu W, Hao Q (2013) MiR-145 is downregulated in human ovarian cancer and modulates cell growth and invasion by targeting p70S6K1 and MUC1. Biochem Biophys Res Commun 441: 693-700.
66. Zhang S, Lu Z, Unruh AK, Ivan C, Baggerly KA, et al. (2015) Clinically relevant microRNAs in ovarian cancer. Mol Cancer Res 13: 393-401.
67. Tao SF, He HF, Chen Q (2015) Quercetin inhibits proliferation and invasion acts by up-regulating miR-146a in human breast cancer cells. Mol Cell Biochem 402: 93-100.
68. Zhang X, Guo Q, Chen J, Chen Z (2015) Quercetin enhances cisplatin sensitivity of human osteosarcoma cells by modulating microRNA-217-KRAS axis. Mol Cells 38: 638-642.
69. Clem B, Telang S, Clem A, Yalcin A, Meier J, et al. (2008) Small-molecule inhibition of 6-phosphofructo-2-kinase activity suppresses glycolytic flux and tumor growth. Molecular Cancer Therapeutics 7: 110-120.
70. Xintaropoulou C, Ward C, Wise A, Marston H, Turnbull A, et al. (2015) A comparative analysis of inhibitors of the glycolysis pathway in breast and ovarian cancer cell line models. Oncotarget 6: 25677-25695.
71. Hanahan D, Weinberg RA (2011) Hallmarks of cancer: The next generation. Cell 144: 646-674.
72. Tennant DA, Durán RV, Gottlieb E (2010) Targeting metabolic transformation for cancer therapy. Nat Rev Cancer 10: 267-277.
73. Zhao Y, Butler EB, Tan M (2013) Targeting cellular metabolism to improve cancer therapeutics. Cell Death Dis 4: e532.
74. Wang Y, Han A, Chen E, Singh RK, Chichester CO, et al. (2015) The cranberry flavonoids PAC DP-9 and quercetin aglycone induce cytotoxicity and cell cycle arrest and increase cisplatin sensitivity in ovarian cancer cells. Int J Oncol 46: 1924-1934.
75. Kim MK, Choi HS, Cho SG, Shin YC, Ko SG (2016) Rubus coreanus Miquel extract causes apoptosis of doxorubicin-resistant NCI/ADR-RES ovarian cancer cells via JNK phosphorylation. Mol Med Rep 13: 4065-4072.

76. Choi HS, Kim MK, Choi YK, Shin YC, Cho SG, et al. (2016) Rhus verniciflua Stokes (RVS) and butein induce apoptosis of paclitaxel-resistant SKOV-3/PAX ovarian cancer cells through inhibition of AKT phosphorylation. BMC Complement Altern Med 16: 122.

77. Ediriweera MK, Tennekoon KH, Adhikari A, Samarakoon SR, Thabrew I, et al. (2016) New halogenated constituents from Mangifera zeylanica Hook.f. and their potential anti-cancer effects in breast and ovarian cancer cells. J Ethnopharmacol 189: 165-174.

78. Liu Y, Gong W, Yang ZY, Zhou XS, Gong C, et al. (2017) Quercetin induces protective autophagy and apoptosis through ER stress via the p-STAT3/Bcl-2 axis in ovarian cancer. Apoptosis 22: 544-557.

79. Zhou Y, Liang X, Chang H, Shu f, Wu Y, et al. (2014) Ampelopsin-induced autophagy protects breast cancer cells from apoptosis through Akt-mTOR pathway via endoplasmic reticulum stress. Cancer Sci 105: 1279-1287.

80. Wang K, Liu R, Li J, Mao J, Lei Y, et al. (2011) Quercetin induces protective autophagy in gastric cancer cells: involvement of Akt-mTOR and hypoxia-induced factor 1alpha-mediated signaling. Autophagy 7: 966-978.

81. De A, De A, Papasian C, Hentges S, Banerjee S, et al. (2013) Emblica officinalis extract induces autophagy and inhibits human ovarian cancer cell proliferation, angiogenesis, growth of mouse xenograft tumors. PLoS One 8: e72748.

82. Roomi MW, Ivanov V, Kalinovsky T, Niedzwiecki A, Rath M (2006) Inhibition of matrix metalloproteinase-2 and invasion of human ovarian cancer cell SK-OV-3 with lysine, proline, arginine, ascorbic acid and green tea extract. J Obstet Gynaecol Res 32: 148-154.

83. Ahmad KA, Harris NH, Johnson AD, Lindvall HC, Wang G, et al. (2007) Protein kinase CK2 modulates apoptosis induced by resveratrol and epigallocatechin gallate in prostate cancer cells. Mol Cancer Ther 6: 1006-1012.

84. Hsieh TC, Wu JM (2008) Suppression of cell proliferation and gene expression by combinatorial synergy of EGCG, resveratrol and gamma-tocotrienol in estrogen receptor-positive MCF-7 breast cancer cells. Int J Oncol 33: 851-859.

85. Hsieh TC, Wu JM (2009) Targeting CWR22Rv1 prostate cancer cell proliferation and gene expression by combinations of the phytochemicals EGCG, genistein and quercetin. Anticancer Res 29: 4025-4032.

86. Saha A, Kuzuhara T, Echigo N, Suganuma M, Fujiki H (2010) New role of (-)-epicatechin in enhancing the induction of growth inhibition and apoptosis in human lung cancer cells by curcumin. Cancer Prev Res (Phila) 3: 953-962.

87. Tang SN, Singh C, Nall D, Meeker D, Shankar S, et al. (2010) The dietary bioflavonoid quercetin synergizes with epigallocatechin gallate (EGCG) to inhibit prostate cancer stem cell characterstic, invasion migration and epithelial-mesenchymal transition. J Mol Signal 5: 14.

88. Niedzwiecki A, Roomi MW, Kalinovsky T, Rath M (2010) Micronutrient synergy--a new tool in effective control of metastasis and other key mechanisms of cancer. Cancer Metastasis Rev 29: 529-542.

89. Zhou DH, Wang X, Yang M, Shi X, Huang W, et al. (2013) Combination of low concentration of (-)epigallocatechin gallate (EGCG) and curcumin strongly suppresses the growth of non-small cell lung cancer in vitro and in vivo through causing cell cycle arrest. Int J Mol Sci 14: 12023-12036.

90. Williamson G, Manach C (2005) Bioavailability and bio efficacy of polyphenols in humans. II. Review of 93 intervention studies. Am J Clin Nutr 81: 243S-255S.

91. Roomi MW, Kalinovsky T, Rath M, Niedzwiecki A (2016) A nutrient mixture modulates ovarian ES-2 cancer progression by inhibiting xenograft tumor growth and cellular MMP secretion, migration and invasion. Int J Clin Exp Med 9: 814-822.

92. Roomi MW, Niedzwiecki A, Rath M (2016) Abstract 4053: A unique nutrient mixture suppresses ovarian cancer growth of A-2780 by inhibiting invasion and MMP-9 secretion. In Proceedings of the 107th Annual Meeting of the AACR, New Orleans, LA, USA.

93. Roomi MW, Kalinovsky T, Rath M, Niedzwiecki A (2017) A specific mixture of nutrients suppresses ovarian cancer a-2780 tumor incidence, growth, and metastasis to lungs. Nutrients 9: E303.

94. Davidson B, Goldberg I, Gotlieb WH, Kopolovic J, Ben-Baruch G, et al. (1999) High levels of MMP-, MMP-9, MT1-MMP and TIMP-2 mRNA correlate with poor survival in ovarian carcinoma. Clin Exp Metastasis 17: 799-808.

95. Davidson B, Goldberg I, Gotlieb WH, Kopolovic J, Ben-Baruch G, et al. (2002) The prognostic value of metalloproteinases and angiogenic factors in ovarian carcinoma. Mol Cell Endocrinol 187: 39-45.

96. Wu X, Li H, Kang L, Li L, Wang W, et al. (2002) Activated matrix metalloproteinase-2a potential marker of prognosis for epithelial ovarian cancer. Gynecol Oncol 84: 126-134.

97. Trimmer EE, Essigmann JM (1999) Cisplatin. Essays Biochem 34: 191-211.

98. Montopoli M, Ragazzi E, Froldi G, Caparrotta L (2009) Cell-cycle inhibition and apoptosis induced by curcumin and cisplatin or oxaliplatin in human ovarian carcinoma cells. Cell Prolif 42: 195-206.

99. Weir NM, Selvendiran K, Kutala VK, Tong L, Vishwanath S, et al. (2007) Curcumin induces G2/M arrest and apoptosis in cisplatin-resistant human ovarian cancer cells by modulating Akt and p38 MAPK. Cancer Biol Ther 6: 178-184.

100. Sandur SK, Ichikawa H, Pandey MK, Kunnumakkara AB, Sung B, et al. (2007) Role of pro-oxidants and antioxidants in the anti-inflammatory and apoptotic effects of curcumin (diferuloylmethane). Free Radic Biol Med 43: 568-580.

101. Nessa MU, Beale P, Chan C, Yu JQ, Huq F (2012) Studies on combination of platinum drugs cisplatin and oxaliplatin with phytochemicals anethole and curcumin in ovarian tumour models. Anticancer Res 32: 4843-4850.

102. Bouthillier L, Charbonneau M, Brodeur J (1996) Assessment of the role of glutathione conjugation in the protection afforded by anethol dithiolthione against hexachloro-,3-butadiene-induced nephrotoxicity. Toxicol Appl Pharmacol 139: 177-185.

103. Chen CH, deGraffenried LA (2012) Anethole suppressed cell survival and induced apoptosis in human breast cancer cells independent of estrogen receptor status. Phytomedicine 19: 763-767.

104. Drukarch B, Schepens E, Stoof JC, Langeveld CH (1997) Anethole dithiolethione prevents oxidative damage in glutathione-depleted astrocytes. Eur Pharmacol 329: 259-262.

105. Banerjee S, Padhye S, Azmi A, Wang Z, Philip PA, et al. (2010) Review on molecular and therapeutic potential of thymoquinone in cancer. Nutr Cancer 62: 938-946.

106. Rossi M, Bosetti C, Negri E, Lagiou P, La Vecchia C (2010) Flavonoids, proanthocyanidins, and cancer risk: a network of case-control studies from Italy. Nutr Cancer 62: 871-877.

107. Rossi M, Negri E, Lagiou P, Talamini R, Dal Maso L, et al. (2008) Flavonoids and ovarian cancer risk: A case-control study in Italy. Int J Cancer 123: 895-898.

108. Gates MA, Vitonis AF, Tworoger SS, Rosner B, Titus-Ernstoff L, et al. (2009) Flavonoid intake and ovarian cancer risk in a population-based case-control study. Int J Cancer 124: 1918-1925.

Nutraceuticals: Curative Integrative Cancer Treatment

Oroma B Nwanodi*

Department of Obstetrics and Gynecology, Locum Tenens, Salinas CA, USA

***Corresponding author:** Nwanodi OB, Department of Obstetrics and Gynecology Locum Tenens, Salinas, CA-93902-0059, USA. E-mail: o.nwanodi@juno.com

Abstract

Statement of Purpose: Although 75% of breast cancer patients may use integrative medicine, only 11.5% early-stage breast cancer patients believe integrative medicine has anticancer activity. The gap in users of and firm believers in integrative medicine indicates a need to increase awareness of integrative medicine's applicability to curative cancer treatment. As diet, nutraceuticals, and traditional Chinese medicine are used by up to 82% of cancer patients who use integrative medicine, this paper focuses on nutraceuticals. As female cancer patients are most likely to use integrative medicine, nutraceuticals specific to breast, cervical, endometrial, and ovarian cancer are reviewed.

Methods: PubMed searches in September 2016 and January 2017, and accompanying hand searches were performed for English language, free full text articles published from 2012 onwards. Search terms were combinations of the key words: Homeopathy, phytochemicals, breast cancer, cervical cancer, endometrial cancer, ovarian cancer, cancer, prevention, treatment. Curative nutraceutical treatments were taken from these searches. Supplemental hand searches were performed as needed.

Findings: Integrative nutraceutical therapies are based on biologic plausibility. Individual nutraceuticals are frequently comprised of numerous phytochemical types, and have multiple mechanisms of action. Agonist-antagonist mechanisms are not exclusive to phytoestrogens, complicating which derivative or whole nutraceutical to use. Research on breast and cervical cancer inhibitors has seemingly outpaced that for endometrial and ovarian cancer. Breast cancer inhibitors include terpenes, isoflavones, organosulphurs, organoselenium compounds, and withanolides.

Conclusion and Significance: Potential nutraceutical candidates for curative cancer treatment abound. Discerning which constituents, which extraction method, and which delivery method to use for an efficacious treatment is an essential, lengthy process. If nutraceuticals such as limonene and Kahalalide F move forward to Phase III trials a nutraceutical cancer treatment pipeline may be established. Withaferin-A and derivatives for breast and ovarian cancer appear to be the leading gynecologic cancer nutraceutical drug candidates.

Keywords: Cancer treatment; Integrative cancer treatment; Naturopathic medicine; Nutraceuticals; Phytochemicals; Phytonutrients; Traditional chinese medicine

Introduction

One-time integrative medicine use ranges from 42% in the United States to 75% in France [1]. Upon cancer diagnosis patients are interested in conventional and integrative therapies [2]. Post cancer diagnosis, 17% of Italian, 27% of Austrians, 35.9% of Europeans overall, 44% of German gynecologic cancer, 47.2% of Canadian, and 50% of German breast cancer patients use integrative medicine therapies [2-6]. Consistent with this, integrative gynecologic cancer treatment is regarded as reasonable by 44.5%, and practiced by 24.2% of 310 Hessian region ObGyns who responded to a survey at an educational meeting [7]. Nonetheless, extremes in integrative cancer treatment are evident. In one study, 75% of breast cancer patients used integrative medicine [8]. However, as few as 11.5% of early stage breast cancer patients may perceive integrative medicine as having anticancer activity [9]. Pediatric oncology integrative medicine ranges from 12% to 42% in Europe and 25% to 82% in the United States [1].

In Dutch pediatric oncology patients, female gender is predictive of integrative cancer use [10]. Similarly, a cross-sectional study of three Pennsylvanian oncology centers found that being female (p=0.005), having breast cancer (p=0.016), and being at 12 to 36 months post diagnosis (p=0.017) most associated with integrative cancer treatment [11]. Time from diagnosis had an n shaped association with integrative cancer treatment [11]. Herbal and traditional Chinese medicine (TCM; excluding acupuncture) are received by 74.5% of patients at European integrative oncology centers [6]. Among Italian cancer patients as few as 38.3% currently and as many as 84.2% previously used nutraceuticals comprised of diet, dietary supplements, and herbs [12].

Nutraceuticals

Nutraceuticals range from active constituent phytochemicals, minerals, and vitamins, through whole functional foods [13]. Integrative nutraceutical therapies are based on biologic plausibility and have played an historical role in the development of the prescription pharmaceutical industry [14]. Willow bark derived analgesic aspirin, Aspergillus terreus derived cholesterol-lowering lovastatin, *Camellia sinensis* (green tea) polyphenols derived sinecatechins for *Condyloma acuminata* (external genital wart [EGW]) treatment, Podophyllum species derived podophyllin for EGW and *Molluscum contagiosum*, as well as the chemotherapeutics taxol derived from *Taxus brevifolia* (Pacific yew tree), taxotere derived from *Taxus baccata* (European yew tree), topotecan derived from *Camptotheca acuminata*, and vincristine derived from *Catharanthus roseus* (Madagascar periwinkle), are just a few examples [15,16]. Thus historically, nutraceuticals have been a starting point of new pharmaceutical drug development.

Nutraceuticals may provide benefits in conservative serving sizes: A cup of appropriately prepared green tea can provide 300 to 1,000 mg of epigallocatechin-3-gallate (EGCG) [17]. Clinical trial EGCG dosing is based 10 mg/kg body weight, which can be achieved from green tea [18]. Pharmaceuticals may require enormous amounts of the biologic source: 1,520 *Taxus chinensis* (Chinese yew) trees, an endangered species, are used to produce 1 kg of paclitaxel [19]. Therefore, pharmaceuticals may require partially or totally synthetic manufacturing processes including plant cell suspension cultures to preclude extinction of their natural sources [19].

Most pharmaceuticals require a health care providers' prescription, whereas nutraceuticals, being food or dietary supplement products with health modifying effects do not require a prescription [20]. Thus, nutraceuticals lie in a gray zone between prescription pharmaceuticals and open market household items [13]. Nonetheless, nutraceutical agriculture and manufacturing may have to comply with good agricultural practices, good manufacturing practices, and standard operating procedures [21]. Nutraceuticals undergo *in vitro* and *in vivo* pharmacokinetic, pharmacologic, therapeutic, safety, and head-to-head comparative effectiveness studies as do pharmaceuticals [20]. Clinical pharmacology studies of nutraceuticals are essential for nutraceutical development and delineation [22]. Nutraceuticals' use as prophylaxis against and treatment of pharmaceuticals' adverse effects is the subject of a separate paper, which also addresses nutraceuticals' inherent adverse effects. This paper reviews nutraceuticals as curative (alternative) cancer treatment, focusing on gynecologic cancer treatment.

Methods

PubMed searches in September 2016 and January 2017, and hand searches in August 2016, January 2017, and March 2017 were performed for English language, free full text articles published from 2012 onwards. Search terms were combinations of the key words: Homeopathy, phytochemicals, breast cancer, cervical cancer, endometrial cancer, ovarian cancer, cancer, prevention, and treatment. Curative nutraceutical treatments were taken from these searches, as shown in Figure 1. Cytotoxic treatments and nutraceutical mechanisms of action were taken from these searches. These searches retrieved 184 articles, of which 127 articles were from the PubMed searches and 57 articles were from content driven hand searches. Of these, there were 14 duplicate articles, 16 redundant articles, and 55 extraneous articles, resulting in a total of 85 excluded and 99 included articles.

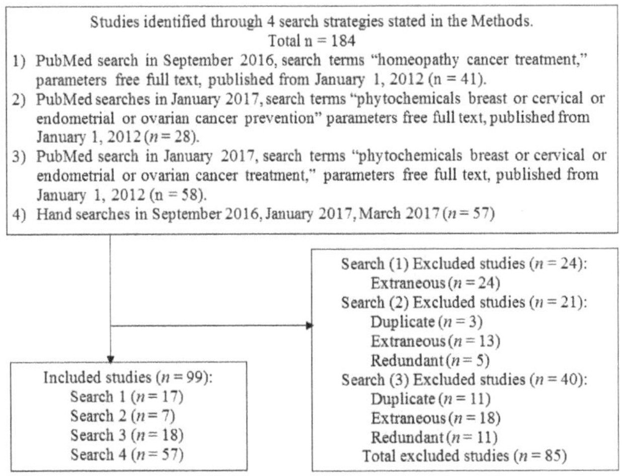

Figure 1: Literature selection flowchart.

Nutraceuticals by phytochemical classification

This study does not review vitamins and minerals per se. However, whole fruits and vegetables, and fruit and vegetable derived phytochemicals may be vitamin and mineral rich. Fruit and vegetable derived phytochemicals may be studied based on mechanism of action, pathologies treated, or biochemical classification. By mechanism of action, the Matrix MetalloProtease (MMP) inhibitors aqueous cinnamon extract, green tea extract, curcumin, fenugreek derived steroidal saponin, and marine compound derived chitooligosacharides would be grouped together. However, each of these nutraceuticals has multiple mechanisms of action. Therefore, nutraceuticals and cancer treatment capabilities are initially presented based on chemical classification. There are numerous biochemical nutraceutical categories including alkaloids, lipids, organic acids and polysaccharides, organosulphurs, phenols, phytic acids, phytosterols, and terpenes, as indicated in Figure 2. Functional foods and other nutraceuticals comprised of constituent compounds will have constituent compounds from multiple biochemical classifications. The encompassing groups of alkaloids, organic acids, and polysaccharides will be briefly mentioned. Nutraceuticals from the secondary and tertiary groups will be briefly mentioned. Then attention will turn to those nutraceuticals pertinent to breast, cervical, and ovarian cancer treatment.

Alkaloids

Alkaloids are physiologically active, vegetable-based, organic, nitrogen-containing ring compounds. Alkaloids may belong to additional biochemical phytonutrient groups based on further chemical structure definition and resultant activity. Alkaloids can be co-constituents of a functional food, as is the case with *Camellia sinensis* tea leaves, which also contain flavonoids, steroids, gallic tannins and catecholic tannins (flavanols) [23]. There are numerous alkaloid sub-classifications: Coffee derives aroma from trigonelline, a bitter alkaloid, and bitter taste from caffeine, a purine-like alkaloid [24]. Alkaloids include colchicine from *Colchicum autumnale* (autumn crocus or meadow saffron), scopolamine/hyoscine from *Hyoscyamus niger* (henbane or stinking nightshade), physostigmine from *Physostigma venenosum* (Calabar bean), reserpine from

Rauwolfia serpentine (Indian snakeroot or devil pepper), and taxol from *Taxus brevifolia* (Pacific yew) [24].

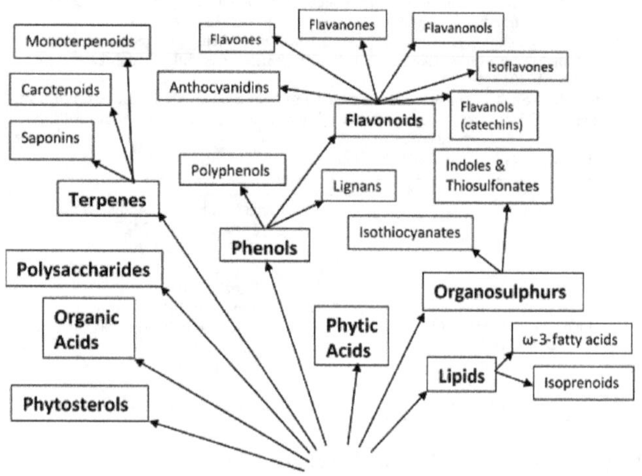

Figure 2: Nutraceuticals biochemical classification.

Organic acids and polysaccharides

Organic acids and polysaccharides are mentioned first as these are encompassing chemical composition groupings. Constituents thereof will belong to additional biochemical phytonutrient groups based on chemical structure and resultant activity. Organic acids are carbon containing acids. Polysaccharides are comprised of bonded sugar molecules.

Organic acids: Organic acids are inflammatory mediators with antioxidant, chemopreventive, and hepatoprotective properties [25]. Cinnamic acid in Aloe vera, ellagic acid (a polyphenol organic acid, found in berries, green tea, guava, pecans, and walnuts), ferulic acid in oats and rice, gallic acid in tea, oxalic acid in coffee, spinach, and tea, and salicylic acid in peppermint are a few examples [25]. Ellagic acid is a reactive epoxide scavenger that inhibits DNA methylation and DNA topoisomerase [26].

Polysaccharides: Mushrooms are immune boosting chemopreventive polysaccharides [25]. Fibrous polysaccharides also bind carcinogens, lower bile acids, and modulate estrogen metabolism [26]. Polysaccharides from the TCM adaptogen ginseng up regulates granzyme and perforin expression and increases the whole blood natural killer cell (NKC) concentration leading to increased NKC cytotoxicity and decreased radiation therapy adverse effects [27]. Perforin forms pores in target cells allowing serine protease granzyme to diffuse into target cells and initiate apoptosis.

Organosulphur compounds

Sulphur's pungent odor is a hallmark of the organosulphur compounds comprised of indoles, thiosulfonates, and isothiocyanates. Organosulphur compounds, which include indole-3-carbinol (I3C) and diindolylmethane (DIM), are commonly derived from cruciferous vegetables. Cephalosporins which were developed from *Acremonium fungi* and *penicillin* from *Penicillium fungi* are also organosulphurs.

Indoles and Thiosulfonates: Indoles and thiosulfonates result from the ingestion and digestion of some cruciferous vegetables [25,28]. Indoles induce and activate cytochrome P450 for phase I detoxification [25]. In A/J mice, I3C inhibits lung adenoma [28]. In BALB/c mice DIM inhibits lung metastasis [28]. While I3C is rapidly hydrolyzed in the stomach, hydro and lipo-phobic DIM requires combination with vitamin E and phosphatidylcholine for bioavailability [28].

Isothiocyanates: Allium compounds found in garlic induce glutathione s-transferase (GST) and microsomal monooxygenases [26]. Garlic, onion, and turnips are isothiocyanate sources. Cabbage, garden cress, and Indian cress derived benzyl isothiocyanate (BITC) and watercress derived phenethyl isothiocyanate (PEITC) may be less studied than the phenols, terpenes, and thiosulfonates that are also found in allium containing vegetables [29,30]. Nonetheless, BITC activates AP-1, caspase-3, MAPK, and NF-κβ while inhibiting other protein kinases [31]. BITC induces apoptosis, G2/M phase cell-cycle arrest, glutathione depletion, and reactive oxygen species (ROS) generation [31]. PEITC inhibits phase I enzymes but activates phase II enzymes [31].

Lipids

There are numerous lipid subgroups including fats, waxes, glycolipids, phospholipids, and polyprenyl compounds. Steroids, fat-soluble vitamins, and isoprenoids (terpenoids) are polyprenyl compounds. Omega-3- and omega-6-polyunsaturated fatty acids (PUFAs) are essential fatty acids [25].

Isoprenoids: Isoprenoids enhance antioxidative power by improving receptor functionality [25]. Farnesol (from floral essential oil) and geraniol (from citronella, geranium, lemon, palmarosa, and rose oils) have *in vivo* cytotoxicity against murine liver cancer, leukemia, and melanoma [32]. Cell membrane phospholipid bi-layers are protected from free radicals by isoprenoids [25]. Isoprenoids production by microorganisms including *Escherichia coli*, and *Saccharomyces cerevisiae* reduces the likelihood of supply limitations [33,34]. Therefore, it is biologically plausible and ecologically reasonable that isoprenoid-phospholipid conjugates be studied for potential medicinal purposes [32].

Omega-3-PUFAs: Omega-3-PUFAs are immune boosting, platelet aggregating, anti-inflammatories [25]. Omega-3-PUFAs are consumed as docosahexanoic acid (DHA) and eicosapentanoic acid (EPA) [35]. Omega-3-PUFAs reduce coronary heart disease risk; decrease triglycerides, blood pressure, and inflammatory markers; improve endothelial function; prevent some cardiac arrhythmias; reduce vasoconstriction; enhance fibrinolysis and reduce fibrin formation; and decrease the risk of microalbuminuria and sudden cardiac death [35]. Omega-3-PUFAs form resolvins and protectins, suppress COX-2, IL-β, and TNF-α [35]. Omega-3-PUFAs bind peroxisome proliferator receptor activator (PPAR) gamma, allowing omega-3-PUFAs to inhibit cell proliferation and induce cancer cell apoptosis [35]. DHA has greater dose dependent pro-apoptotic activity against DU145 prostate carcinoma cells than does EPA. DHA's pro-apoptotic activity is mediated *via* MAPK, NF-κβ, p53, and PI3K-Akt signaling pathways [36].

Phenols

Phenols which may be best known for the fruit and vegetable rainbow have a phenylalanine base. Coumarins, flavonoids, lignans, polyphenols, quinones, stilbenes, tannins, and xanthones, comprise the phenols category. Flavonoids in turn are comprised of anthocyanidins, flavones, flavanones, flavanonols, isoflavones, and flavanols. Each gram of *Camellia sinensis* leaf extract contains 700 mg of phenols, of which 14 mg are flavonoids [23].

Coumarins: Coumarins are fragrant benzopyrones. Coumarins are also found in *Artemisiascoparia* (yin-chen wormwood), *Citrus spp.* (orange), and *Glycyrrhiza uralensis* (licorice) [37]. Fungi convert coumarin from moldy *Melilotus spp.* (sweet clover) to 4-hydroxycoumarin that dimerizes to dicoumarol, a variant of which is warfarin [37]. Comparatively high coumarin content differentiates cassia cinnamon (*Cinnamomun cassia*) from true Ceylon cinnamon, *C. verum* that has minuscule coumarin content [38]. Coumarin's reduction of melanoma recurrence and inhibition of renal-cell carcinoma did not withstand corroborating trials [37]. Coumarin has dose dependent cytotoxicity against the Hep2 cell line [39]. Carbon-4 substituted coumarins are antiproliferative against breast and liver carcinomas [39]. Carbon-4 substituted coumarins inhibit aromatase, protein kinase, quinone reductase induction, sulphatase, 17β-HSD3, Cdc25, DNA intercalation, HDACs, Hsp90, microtubulin, NF-κβ, and TNF-α [40]. Carbon-4 substituted coumarins are also down regulating selective estrogen receptor modulators (SERMs) [40]. A synthetic coumarin with a 4-position methylene thiol linker to a 6-membered heteroaromatic ring (4-Hydrazinyl-2-{[(6-methyl-2-oxo-2H-chromen-4-yl) methyl]sulfanyl}-6-phenylpyrimidine-5-carbonitrile) is cytotoxic to MCF-7 breast cancer and HepG2 hepatocarcinoma cells, IC50 5.5 mg/ml and 6.9 mg/ml, respectively [39]. Potential cytotoxicity is indicated with IC50 of 4 μg/ml or 10 μM or less [41]. *Ferula narthex* Bioss (an Ayurvedic spice called "Raw") derived sesquiterpene (C15H24) cholorform soluble coumarin, C24H30O4 has an *in vitro* IC50 of 14.074 ± 0.414 μg/ml against PC3 cells [42]. Prediction of Activity Spectra achieved a probability to be active score of 0.303 with human histone acetyltransferase that should correlate with anti-pancreatic cancer activity [42].

Flavonoids: Flavonoids have a broad mechanism of action array. Flavonoids are antioxidants, anti-angiogenic, anti-proliferative, active oxygen species scavengers, electrophiles, metal chelators, hydrogen peroxide producers, nitrosation inhibitors, and phase I detoxification enzyme modulators [25,26,43]. Flavones, flavanones, flavonols, flavanonols, isoflavones, flavanols, anthocyanidins and anthocyanins comprise the flavonoid category. Flavonoids including apigenin, kaempferol, nobiletin, quercetin, and rutin are found in cocoa, edible fruits, leafy vegetables, herbs, spices, legumes, tea and red wine [25,26]. Rutin, a compound flavonol-disaccharide found in citrus fruits is the primary active ingredient of the homeopathic treatment *Ruta* [44]. Rice bran oil tricin arrests MDA MB 468 breast cancer cells in G2/M phase [45].

Anthocyanidins and anthocyanins: This group includes cyanidin, delphinidin, malvidin, peonidin, and petunidin, which are found in blueberries [43,46]. Carob fruit contains delphinidin, pelargonidin and cyanidin [47]. Delphinidin is an anthocyanidin that affects NF-κβ regulation [47]. Cyanidin-3-0-β-glucopyranoside (C3G) from pigmented oranges, berries, and grapes activates caspase-3 in DU145 cells, and induces p21 protein expression in LnCap cells, resulting in antiproliferative effects against DU145 and LnCap prostate cancer cell lines [48]. C3G is associated with increased concentration of P75NGFR tumor suppressor from normal-like cell phenotype [48]. C3G antioxidant effect may be specific to androgen-independent tumors [48]. C3G has dose dependent ROS activity, requiring 100 μM [48].

Flavanonol: Dihydrokaempferol has been isolated from the roots of *Smilax bockii* and from *S. glabra* (sarsaparilla) rhizomes [49]. Both *Smilax bockii* and *S. glabra* are used in TCM [49]. The leaves of *S. glycyphylla* (sweet sarsaparilla) contain (2R,3R)-dihydrokaempferol-3-O-β-D-glucopyranoside [49]. *S. china* yields dihydrokaempferol and dihydrokaempferol-3-O-α-L-rhamnoside, which are less apoptotic to MCF-7 and MDA-MB-231 than are resveratrol and oxyresveratrol [49]. Taxifolin (dihydroquercetin) is a constituent of milk thistle seeds' silymarin extract and *S. glabra* rhizome [49]. Taxifolin-3-O-glycoside is one of the major active constituents of the tuber of *S. china* [49]. Like dihydrokaempferol and dihydrokaempferol-3-O-α-L-rhamnoside, taxifolin is weakly cytotoxic [50].

Flavanones: The flavanones hesperetin and naringenin undergo transformation by neohesperidose and rutinose becoming flavanone glycosides hesperidin, neohesperidin, narirutin, and naringin [51]. Hesperetin is apoptotic to A431 epidermoid skin carcinoma via cyclin and MAPK regulation [51]. Naringenin is effective against A431, B16-F10 melanoma, and *in vivo* HepG2 cells [51]. In murine models, Naringenin dosed at 50 mg/kg body weight suppresses lung cancer [51]. Naringenin induces G0/G1 and G2/M phase cell cycle arrest, ROS generation, and down regulates TGF-β1 [51]. Naringenin induces mitochondrial apoptosis *via* Bax, Bcl-2, caspase-3, and p53 [51]. Naringenin modulates CYP1A1, NF-κβ and PCNA [51]. Hesperidin (IC50=150.43 μM), is more cytotoxic than naringin and neohesperidin against HepG2, and is also anti-proliferative and apoptotic against A549 lung cancer and NCI-H358 non-small cell lung cancer (NSCLC) cells [51]. Hesperidin activates Erk, MMPs, mitochondrial calcium overload, ROS production, and membrane potential loss, while modulating fibroblast growth factor and NF-κβ pathways [51]. Naringin activates caspase-8 and caspase-9 [51]. Naringin inhibits MAPK-AP1 and IKKs-IκB-NF-κβ pathways [51].

Flavones: Citrus fruit derived flavones include apigenin, chrysoeriol, diosmetin, and luteolin. Apigenin and luteolin have other sources, including celery and parsley [43]. Polymethoxyflavones (PMF) are unique to citrus species' peels, thus used in TCM [52]. Tangeretin, a tangerine derived PMF is anti-inflammatory in microglial cells, suppresses adipocyte storage of triglycerides, and induces G1 arrest or apoptosis in cancer cells [52]. Tangeretin and nobiletin (another PMF) are antiproliferative to A549, MCF-7 and MDA-MB-435 breast cancer, HT-29 colon cancer, and HL-60 leukemia cell lines [51,53,54]. Nobiletin decreases Bcl-2 and increases Bax, leading to G2/M phase cell cycle arrest and apoptosis [51]. Nobiletin modulates hypoxia-TGF-induced epithelial-mesenchymal transition, inhibits notch-1 and TGF-β1/Smad3 signaling, while promoting microRNA-200b re-expression [51]. *In vitro*, the tangeretin derivative 5-AcTMF is antiproliferative to MCF-7, the U226 myeloma and CL1-5 NSCLC cell lines [52]. The tangeretin derivative 5-demethyltangeretin is more cytotoxic than tangeretin against A549, H460, and HI299 cell lines, with 79, 57 and 56 fold lower IC50 respectively [51]. The nobiletin derivative 5-demethylnobiletin has demonstrated *in vivo* antiproliferative activity against human NSCLC [51].

Flavonols: Tea is the source of several flavanols: Epicatechin (EC), epigallocatechin (EGC), epicatechin-3-gallate (ECG), EGCG, galloyl polyphenol, thearubigin, and theaflavins [43]. Green tea derived galloyl polyphenol and EGCG decrease retinoblastoma protein (Rb) phosphorylation, arresting cells in G1 phase [55]. The green tea polyphenols reactivate tumor suppressor genes by demethylation [55]. Green tea has the most EGCG, then white tea, and least of all black tea. Black tea derived thearubigin and theaflavins are anti-angiogenic [43]. The constituent epicatechin of *Maytenus buchananii* (a small evergreen tree), a traditional Cameroonian anti-cancer treatment, has an excellent MIC of 32 to 128 μg/ml against Staphylococcus aureus [56].

Other flavonols include quercetin from apples, berries, and red onions, and kaempferol from citrus fruits [43]. Luteolin and quercetin induce apoptosis in TRAIL-resistant cancer cells. Kaempferol, luteolin, and quercetin have shown dose dependent reduction in OVCAR3 ovarian cancer growth and VEGF production [25]. Quercetin is cytotoxic to papillary urothelial carcinoma T24 cells, $p<0.05$ [57]. *M. buchananii* quercetin has an EC50 of 1.38 μg/ml and a TEAC of 89.69 μg/ml. *M. buchananii* quercetin-3-O-α-L-rhamnopyranoside has an EC50 of 1.56 μg/ml and TEAC of 90.93 μg/ml. *M. buchananii* quercetin-3-O-β-D-glucopyranoside has a MIC of 16 to 64 μg/ml against *S. aureus* which is significant as it is less than 100 μg/ml. Quercetin-3-O-β-D-glucopyranoside also has an EC50 of 1.42 μg/ml and a TEAC of 89.76 μg/ml [56]. *Maytenus* was initially studied for maytansine, an excessively cytotoxic antileukemic, single macrocyclic ring compound. Semisynthetic and natural two macrocyclic ring Maytansinoids are under development for colon cancer treatment [56].

Isoflavones: Like lignans, isoflavones are also phytoestrogens [43]. Daidzein, genistein, and kievitone have structural similarities to 17β-estradiol (E2). Daidzein, genistein, and kievitone elevate sex hormone-binding globulin (SHBG), are anti-oxidants, apoptotic, and inhibit angiogenesis, topoisomerase, tyrosine kinase, EGFR, IGFR-1 and NF-κB signaling pathways [26,43,58]. Genistein and other isoflavones preferentially bind the anti-proliferative estrogen receptor β (ER-β), functioning as SERMs, potentially balancing estrogen receptor α (ER-α)'s hyperproliferative effects in adipose tissue, the bone, breast, liver, ovarian thecal cells, prostate, and uterus [59].

Lignans: Lignans are also phytoestrogens. Lignans are derived from berries, flaxseed, sesame seed, whole grains [43]. Matairesinol and secoisolariciresinol are weak estrogen agonists, elevate SHBG, and inhibit aromatase [26]. Like the isoflavone phytoestrogen genistein, the lignin metabolite, enterolactone, is a dose dependent agonist-antagonist cancer specific modulator [43].

Polyphenols: Polyphenols are antioxidants. Polyphenols affect cancer by inhibiting cyclooxygenase, DNA topoisomerase, and DNA methylation, inducing phase II detoxification, and influencing cell signaling [25,26]. Polyphenols include cocoa, curcumin (found in turmeric), rice bran oil phenolics, caffeic acid, ferulic acid, and ferulic acid esters [45].

Quinones: Thymoquinone and dithymoquinone are derived from *Nigella sativa L.* seed (blackseed) [60]. *Nigella sativa* was the biblical and the prophet Mohammed's curative black cumin, Hippocrates and Doscorides' Melanthion [60,61]. *Nigella sativa* is also used in Ayurveda and TCM [61]. *Nigella sativa* seed methanolic extract inhibition of Erlich ascites carcinoma in mice led to patenting of thymoquinone and dithymoquinone for additional research [60]. Thymoquinone and dithymoquinone displayed *in vivo* cytotoxicity to multidrug resistant cells [60]. Thymoquinone has cytotoxic activity against MCF-7/Doxorubicin via PTEN, p53, and p21 upregulation; NF-κβ, PI3K-Akt, phase I enzymes, and PPAR inhibition, and phase II enzyme (GST and N-acetyl transferase) activation [61]. Thymoquinone induces caspace-3 apoptosis against Hep-2 cells, whereas caspace-3, -8, and -9 are activated against HL60 p53-myeloid leukemia [61]. Thymoquinone inhibits COX2, which affects breast, lung, stomach, and pancreatic cancers [61]. Thymoquinone inhibits MMPs and VEGF and induces apoptosis via Bak-Bax induction and Bcl-2 and Bcl-XL inhibition [61]. Thymoquinone is also active against bladder, colon, bone, and skin cancers [61].

The *Plumbago (leadwort), Drosera (sundews), Nepenthes* (monkey cups or tropical pitcher plants), and *Juglans nigra* (black walnut drupe) derived quinone plumbagin and the *Ardisia elliptica* (shoebutton ardisia) derived rapanone are under investigation as chemotherapeutics [41]. *In vitro*, plumbagin has an IC50 less than 10 μM against A549 (1.14 ± 0.02 μM), $Caco_2$ colorectal adenocarcinoma (0.07 ± 0.01 μM), DLD-1 human colon adenocarcinoma cells (0.98 ± 0.11 μM), HepG2, MCF-7 (0.06 ± 0.01 μM), and SPC212 mesothelioma cell lines (0.27 ± 0.01 μM) (Kuete et al., 2016) [41]. Of these, plumbagin shows greater cytotoxicity than doxorubicin against Caco-2 (0.72 ± 0.13 μM) and MCF-7 (0.35 ± 0.05 μM) [41]. Plumbagin had previously shown good cytotoxicity against Caski, Colo-38, HeLa, MiaPaCa-2, PF-382 leukemia T-cells, and U87MG glioblastoma-astrocytoma cell lines [41]. Rapanone achieved an IC50 of 2.27 ± 1.52 μM against SPC212 cells, 46.62 μM against DLD-1 cells [41].

Stilbenes: Resveratol, a berry, grape, and peanut derived polyphenol with stilbene derivates, upregulates cancer cell line wild-type p53 [43,62]. Rhapoantigenin, a synthetic stilbene derivative of resveratrol, which also degrades HIF-1α (thereby suppressing VEGF and MAPK), has shown greater anti-angiogensis effect than resveratrol [43]. Stilbenes also activate forkhead box (FOX) O apoptosis transcription factors, while inhibiting Akt, IGF1, the PI3K-Akt and Ras-MEK pathways [43].

Tannins: Fruits' astringency may derive from tannins [47]. Plant derived tannins are subdivided into hydrolysable tannins that are ellagic acid or gallic acid esters and condensed, non-hydrolysable tannins that are oligo- or polymeric proanthocyanidins [47]. Brown algae derived tannins are a separate class, phlorotannins. Tannins may have 12 or more hydroxyl groups and five or more phyenyl groups. Gallic acid and flavan-3-ols may be classified as pseudo tannins. Condensed, non-hydrolysable tannins, which include flavan-3-ols are also classified as flavanols, in which category catechins were mentioned above.

Hydrolysable or pyrogallol-type tannins: Punicalagin, ellagic acid, punicalin are ellagitannins, while gallagic acid is a gallotannin. Carob pods have 0.95 mg/gm of hydrolysable tannins, while carob fruit have 0.237 mg/gm to 1.647 mg/gm of gallic acids, which is the third highest gallic acid content after chestnuts and cloves [47]. Carob fruit fiber contains at least three sets of gallic acid based tannins: Epigallocatechin with four gallic acid units, hexose with two to five gallic acid units, and pentoses with two gallic acid units [47]. Carob fruit fiber also contains prodelphinidin dimer and trimer [47].

Syzygium cumini (Indian blackberry) or *Eugenia jambolana*, and *Phyllanthus emblica* or *Emblica officinalis* (Indian gooseberry, one of the three fruits from which Ayurvedic triphala is made) contain ellagic acid and gallic acid [63]. Indian gooseberry also contains the ellagitannins chebulagic acid, corilagin, emblicanin (also found in Amla), furosin, geraniin, isocorilagin (the α-anomer of corilagin), and pyrogallol (also found in chestnut and oak bark) [63]. Chebulagic, ellagic, and gallic acids, and corilagin inhibit NF-κβ [63]. Corilagin is apoptotic to SKOv3ip, Hey, and HO-8910PM ovarian cancer cell line by inducing G2/M phase arrest and TGF-β/Akt/Erk/Smad modulation [63]. Cdc2, Cdk2, Cdk4, Cdk6, cyclin B1 and E inhibition by gallic acid is pro-apoptotic [63].

Punicalagin, derived from *Punica granatum* (pomengranate) is metabolized to ellagic acid [64]. Pomengranate tannins have antiaromatase actitivity against MCF-7 cells that have been transfected with the aromatase gene [64]. Punicalagin, ellagic acid, and total pomengranate tannin are apoptotic to HT-29 cells [64]. Punicalagin and total pomengranate tannin inhibit NF-κβ response element binding and TNF-α mediated COX-2 expression [64]. Punicalagin is apoptotic to U87MG cells via PARP breakage and caspase-3 and -9 activation [64]. Punicalagin also triggers autophagy cell death in U87MG cells by increasing AMPK-p27 [64].

Condensed or Non-hydrolysable tannins: Proanthocyanidins including flavan-3-ol groups and their galloyl esters form 2.75 mg/gm of carob pods [47]. Litchi contains proanthocyanidins A1, A2, and A6, and procyanidins B2 and B4 [63]. Proanthocyanidins are polymeric tannins that are depolymerized to anthocyanidins.

Xanthones: Pericarps of *Garcinia mangostana* (Mangosteen Linn fruit) contain α-Mangostin and gartanin [65,66]. α-Mangostin has anticancer and chemosensitizing activity to melanoma and pancreatic cancer [66]. α-Mangostin has dose dependent anticancer activity against A549 cells via ROS-mediated apoptosis induction, but these effects are negated by N-acetyl cysteine [66]. α-Mangostin dose dependently increases the Bax/Bcl-2 ratio, inhibits A549 cell migration, down regulates A549 antioxidants - catalase, glutathione peroxidase, and GSH [66]. Gartanin is dose dependently anti-proliferative to T98G glioma cells via PI3K/Akt/mTOR signaling pathway autophagy modulated G1 cell cycle arrest [65]. Garatanin is anti-migratory to T98G cells via MAPK signaling pathway suppression of MMP-2 and -2 [65].

Phytic Acids: Phytic acids include defatted rice bran phytate and inositols [45]. Inositols include inositol phophates, inositol hexakisphosphate (InsP6), and myo-Inositol [67]. Cereals, legumes, and oilseeds yield InsP6, which is broken down to myo-Inositol and inositol phosphates [67]. Inositol hexaphosphate inhibits proliferation [26]. Inositols inhibit cell cycles by inhibiting pRB phosphorylation and increasing pRB/E2F complex formation [67]. Inositols reduce PI3K, disrupt FGF receptor binding and EGF-transduction, down regulate Akt and Erk, inhibit NF-κβ, and decrease COX2 and PGE2 expression [67]. Inositols impair β-catenin translocation, N-cadherin, Notch-1, SNAI1 release, and Wnt-activation [67]. Inositols inhibit MMPs and ROCK1/2 release, decrease cofilin and fascin, upregulate focal adhesion kinase (FAK) and e-cadherin, impairing invasiveness and contributing to cancer microenvironment alterations [67]. DU145 tumors are reduced almost 64% by InsP6 [67].

Phytosterols: Lettuce, nuts, capers, flaxseed, cucumbers, rice bran are phytosterol sources. Stigmasterol is a soy-lipid derived phytosterol, and campesterol is a saw palmetto derived phytosterol [45]. β-Sitosterol does not stimulate the endometrium, nor do plant stanols and stanol esters stimulate ER-positive MCF-7 [68]. β-Sitosterol may be most biologically active with liposomal delivery [68]. β-Sitosterol down regulates NF-κβ, thereby sensitizing cancer cells to TNF-α induced apoptosis [68]. β-Sitosterol reduces MDA-MB-231 triple negative breast cancer (TNBC) and MCF-7 tumors by 66% and 87% respectively, and low density lipoprotein by 8.8% [68]. β-Sitosterol's activity against MDA-MB-231 is significant as although TNBC comprises only 15% of breast cancer, TNBC is treatment resistant, being unresponsive to endocrine and other targeted treatments [69]. β-Sitosterol and lupeol are the main anticancer constituents of *Nardostachys jatamansi* DC, a traditional Himalayan medicine herb used for cancer treatment [70].

Terpenes: Terpenes are single or multiple hydrocarbon compounds, categorized as saponins, and mono- or higher terpenoids, including tetraterpenes, based on the number of carbon atoms and isoprene residues [25].

Saponins: Saponins are antioxidants, immune modulators, and cell proliferation regulators [25,26]. Saponins are found in legumes and ginseng [26].

Betulinic acid: Betulinic acid from *Betula alba* (birch) bark, a plant triterpenoid saponin is a known chemopreventive, antiviral, anti-inflammatory, and antioxidant [71]. Betulinic acid increases IL-2, TNF-α, and CD4+ lymphocyte subsets. Betulinic acid increases the CD4+:CD8+ ratio in a dose dependent manner. Betulinic acid dosed at 200 mg/kg decreased B-cell lymphoma 2 (Bcl-2) protein and cell proliferation marker (Ki-67) protein expression and increased caspase-8 protein expression more than did 25 mg/kg cyclophosphamide, $p<0.05$ [72].

Escin: Escin from *Aesculus hippocastanum* (horse chestnuts) inhibits extracellular signal regulated kinase (ERK) and p38 mitogen-activated protein kinase (MAPK) cell proliferation, motility, and apoptosis pathways for anti-angiogenic endothelial cell migration and motility inhibition [43]. Crude ethyl acetate and methanol extracts of *Mangifera pajang* (bambangan, a noncommercial mango) kernel, have strong to moderate cytotoxic activity against the HT-29 colon cancer cell line at IC50 of 10 μg/ml [72]. Crude petroleum ether and chloroform extracts of M. pajang stem bark have strong activity at 15 μg/ml [72]. A component flavonol glycoside, quercitrin had very strong cytotoxic activity against HT-29 at IC50 of 3.82 ± 0.91 μg/ml [72].

Tripterine: Tripterine, the major active component of *Trypterigium wilfordii* (thunder duke vine), should be anti-angiogenic and cytotoxic due to modulation of MMP-9, intercellular adhesion molecule (ICAM)-1, vascular endothelial growth factor (VEGF), cell survival inhibitor of apoptosis protein (IAP)-1, X-linked (X)-IAP, Bcl-2, Bcl-xL, flice inhibitory protein (cFLIP), survivin and cell proliferation molecules (cyclin D1, COX-2) in tumor cells [43]. At doses 500-fold higher than its anti-angiogenic activity, withaferin A from *Withania somnifera* (ashwagandha, Indian ginseng), has demonstrated direct anti-tumor activity in breast, pancreatic, and prostate cancers [43,73].

Monoterpenoids: Monoterpenoids induce apoptosis, cell differentiation, and phase I and II detoxification enzymes, including GST, affect cellular energy, and inhibit cell proliferation [25,26]. Monoterpenoids include limonene found in cardamom and Perillyl alcohol derived from the essential oils of lavandin, peppermint, spearmint, cherries and celery seeds. Ferula species derived umbelliprenin inhibits MMPs, but only has greater anti-tumor activity than cisplatin against M4Beu melanoma, and is ineffective against A549, DLD-1, MCF-7, PA1 paclitaxel-sensitive ovarian cancer, and PC3 prostate cancer cell lines [74]. Similarly, *F. gummosa* derived sesquiterpene coumarin feselol has anti-tumor activity against U937 but not M14, MCF-7, T98G, A549, Saos-2, and FRO cell lines [74].

Diterpenoids: In gallbladder cancer, the diterpenoid oridonin derived from anti-angiogenic *Rabdosia rubescens* (Dong Ling Cao), activates caspase-3 and 9 mitochondrial pathway apoptosis, activates PARP1 cleavage, increases the Bax/Bcl-2 ratio, and inhibits NF-κβ nuclear translocation [69,75]. In acute lymphoblastic leukemia, oridonin inhibits the Akt-mTOR and Raf-MEK-Erk pathways, but in *in vitro* human osteosarcoma cells shows Akt and MAPK inhibition [69]. Oridonin treated murine L929 fibrosarcoma cells indicate Erk-p53 activation leading to G2/M phase cell cycle arrest [69]. GSH induction by coffee-derived compounds including Kahweol palmitate, a diterpene ester, inhibits DMBA model breast cancer initiation [26].

Tetraterpenes: Carotenoids are anti-oxidant tetraterpenes [25]. β-carotene found in apricots, carrot, pumpkins, sweet potato is also antiangiogenic, antiproliferative, and induces cellular differentiation [26]. Astaxanthin, β-carotene, cryptoxanthin, lycopene, lutein, and zeaxanthin have breast cancer animal model anti-cancer activity [43]. Lycopene is found in tomatoes and watermelon, lutein and zeaxanthin are found in broccoli, cayenne and red pepper, corn, leafy greens (collard, kale, romaine lettuce, spinach, and turnip), paprika, and peas [76].

A Combination Herbal

Yangzheng xiaoji, a 16 herb TCM dose dependently inhibits adhesion of A549, MCF-7, HRT18 colorectal cancer cells, HGC27 gastric cancer cells, and MG-63 osteosarcoma cells via the P13K pathway and anti-angiogenesis [77]. The *Yangzheng xiaoji* extract DME25 inhibits cancer growth by inhibiting FAK pathway phosphorylation [77].

Whole Plant Nutraceuticals

Cardamon

In female Swiss albino mice, cardamom, garlic, and saffron are chemoprotective against DMBA induced skin cancer [28]. Cardamon stimulates phase II detoxification and anti-oxidation in female Swiss albino mice with DMBA treated skin and livers [28]. Cardamom contains numerous phytochemicals, some of which are mentioned below. Phase I trials of limonene, a major constituent of cardamom suggest breast, colorectal, and prostate cancer inhibition with minimal toxicity at doses up to 100 mg/kg [28]. D-Limonene is metabolized to perillyl alcohol, which inhibits G-protein isoprenylation [26]. D-Limonene inhibits gastric and lung cancers and leukemia [28]. 1,8-cineole inhibits and induces apoptosis in SK-MEL-28 human melanoma cells, B16-F1 murine melanoma cells, and Molt 4B and HL-60 human leukemia cells [28]. Linalool uses p53 upregulation against leukemia, and inhibits renal adenocarcinoma and amelanotic melanoma [28]. α-Pinene and α-Terpineol are anti-inflammatory to oral buccal cells [28]. Myrcene is chemoprotective against DMPA in rats, and apoptotic in human hepatoma cell lines. Trans-nerolidol is cytotoxic to A-549 human lung carcinoma cells and DLD-1 cells [28].

Artemisia capillaris (wormwood), which is known to inhibit CNE-2 nasopharyngeal carcinoma, DMBA induced breast cancer, SMMC-7721 human hepatoma, HL-60 leukemia, HepG2, Huh-7 human liver cells, HeLa cervical cancer, and mouse liver cells, contains borneol, which is also a constituent of cardamom [28,78]. Borneol is anti-oxidative, cytotoxic, DNA-damaging, and DNA-protective to Caco-2 and VH10 [28].

Marine compounds

Ecteinascidia turbinata, the source of the active ingredient of Trabectedin, approved for the treatment of platinum-sensitive ovarian cancer and tumor soft tissue sarcoma, displays *in vitro* and *in vivo* transcription factor inhibition [79]. *Elysia rufescens* derived *Kahalalide F,* is the basis for synthetic PM02734, which is in Phase II clinical trials for evaluation of H322 and A549 cell line apoptosis [79]. *Kahalalide F* inhibited breast, liver, and pancreatic cancer, as well as melanoma in Phase I trials. *Spisula polynyma* derived ES-285-HC1 has inhibited solid hepatocellular, prostate, and renal cancer *in vivo* [79]. *Dicathais orbita* containing the indole derivatives tyrindoleninone, tyrindolinone, 6-bromoisatin and 6,6′-dibromoindirubin, demonstrated *in vivo* apoptotic activity against azoxymethane exposed rat distal colon cells [79]. *Dicathais orbita* derived tyrindoleninone and 6-bromoisatin are twice as apoptotic to the KGN tumor-derived granulosa cell line than to normal primary human granulosa cells (HGC), 66% to 31%, respectively [79]. The biological plausibility of 6-bromoisatin containing compounds will be presented in a separate article on oncologic homeopathic remedies.

Effect on Breast, Cervical, and Ovarian Cancers

As known nutraceutical inhibition of endometrial cancer focuses on I3C, this section focuses on breast, cervical, and ovarian cancers [26].

Breast cancer

Breast cancer inhibitors include allium derivatives, β-carotene and other carotenoids, catechin, coumarin, curcumin, dithiolthiones, dried green coffee, fiber, glucosinolates and indoles (DIM and I3C), d-Limonene, isoflavones and lignans, glycirrhizic acid, kahweol palmitate, orange oil, protease inhibitors/Bowman-Birk inhibitor (BBI), rosemary extract, and selenium/organoselenium compounds [26,80]. Actual annual integrative cancer treatment costs for an early stage breast cancer patient are USD 1,594 [81]. An idealized integrative treatment program for stage 4 breast cancer that includes bromelain, coenzyme Q10, curcumin, green tea, intravenous artesunate and ascorbic acid, melatonin, mistletoe injections, *Trametes versicolor* mushroom, vitamin D3, and Wobenzyme TM digestive enzymes has an annual total cost of USD 27,137.16 [81].

In murine studies BITC has proven MCF7 and HBL-100 inhibition by p53-LKB1 and p73-LKB1 pathway activation, which enhances p53 signaling [82]. As LKB1 activation is associated with improved breast cancer outcomes this finding is significant [82]. BITC increases breast cancer cell p53, Erk, and cyclic adenine monophosphate-response-element-binding protein (CREB) phosphorylation, but decreases Akt phosphorylation [82]. *In vitro* studies against MDA-MB-231, MDA-MB-468, BT474, T47D, Hs578t, HCT116p53-/-, and HCT116p53+/+ cells show BITC induced p53-independent apoptosis [82].

Bitter gourd derived triterpenoids have demonstrated moderate cytotoxicity to MCF-7 and MDA-MB-231 breast cancer cells, IC50 of 19 and 23 M respectively at 72 hours [83]. Bitter gourd derived triterpenoids have several mechanisms of action. In some cases, caspase-dependent apoptosis occurs [83]. Akt-NF-κB signaling is down-regulated, p38 mitogen activated protein kinase and p53 are up-regulated, ROS generation and cytoprotective autophagy are increased, and histone deacetylases (HDACs) protein expression is decreased [83]. In other cases, apoptotic peroxisome proliferator-activated receptor (PPAR) γ-targeted gene products' modulation occurs [83].

Caffeic acid phenethyl ester from propolis, which is from floral resins of buds and sprouts of green trees that is collected by bees, has dose and time dependent strong cytotoxicity against MDA-MB-231, IC50 of 14.08 μM and excellent cytotoxicity against Hs578T, IC50 of 8.01 μM [84]. Caffeic acid phenethyl ester is caspase-3 dependent apoptotic and anti-proliferative by NF-κβ inhibition, which also increases the Bax: Bcl-2 ratio [84]. *Cephalotaxus griffithii Hook. F.* (Griffith's plum yew) needle derived flavonoids *via* petroleum ether extraction are moderately cytotoxic to ZR751 breast cancer cells, IC50 22.3 ± 3.9 μg/ml [85]. Curcumin and sulforaphane, also modulate HDACs for breast cancer antiproliferation [83]. The ML-1 lectin containing mistletoe extracts Iscador M special and Iscador Qu, dosed at 15 g/dl have strong cytotoxic activity to the MAXF-401-NL breast cancer line [80].

In murine studies, CYD-6-28, a synthetic analog of oridonin, a diterpenoid terpene, dosed at 5 mg/kg, inhibited TNBC cell lines HCC1806 and HCC1937 [69]. CYD-6-28 induces Erk, p21, caspase-3, -7, -8 and PARP cleavage, G2/M-phase cell cycle arrest, and death receptor 5 (DR5) mediated apoptosis [69]. CYD-6-28 inhibits Akt, cyclin D1, FLIPL, STAT3, and XIAP [69]. CYD-6-28's efficacy may be due to improved aqueous solubility and cell permeability from a thiazole ring at A-ring C-1 and C-2 [69].

Edible *Phaleria macrocarpa* (Scheff.) Boerl fruit (mahkota dewa) of Indonesian traditional medicine has flavonoid, flavonol, phenol, saponin, and terpenoid derivatives [86]. Ethyl acetate and methanol extracts have strong cytotoxicity comparable to standard gallic acid, with IC50 8.15 ± 0.02 g/ml in DPPH antioxidant assay [86]. Gallic acid is cytotoxic to brain, breast, cervix, colon, esophageal, and gastric cancer cell lines [86]. The chloroform extract has excellent cytotoxicity against MDA-MB-231 breast cancer cells, IC50 7.80 ± 1.57 μg/ml at 48 hours [86]. The *P. macrocarpa* hexane extract has excellent cytotoxicity against MDA-MB-231, IC50 4.6 ± 1.32 μg/ml at 48 hours, while the ethyl acetate extract has good cytotoxicity against MDA-MB231, IC50 6.4 ± 1.09 μg/ml at 48 hours [86]. Ethanolic mango seed extract may be apoptotic to MCF-7 cells via ROS induction [87]. Ethanolic kernel extract of *Mangifera indica L.* (waterlily mango) has dose dependent strong cytotoxicity to MCF-7, IC50 15.6 μg/ml, moderate cytotoxicity to MDA-MB-231, IC50 31.25 μg/ml, and insignificant cytotoxicity to MCF-10A, all at 72 hours [88].

In vitro and *in vivo* mouse studies showed that the flavone, chloroform extracted luteolin from *Eclipta alba* (Bhringraj) dose and time dependently selectively activates intrinsic apoptosis by releasing mitochondrial apoptogenic proteins into the cytosol, inhibiting caspase-9, up regulating pro-apoptotic molecular chaperone heat shock protein 60 (Hsp60) and down regulating anti-apoptotic protein XIAP in MCF-7 and MDA-MB-231 cells, but spares MCF-10A normal breast epithelial cells [89]. Luteolin was also found to be more active than the twice as available coumarin wedelolactone component of E. alba [89]. Chloroform extracted *E. alba* luteolin was effective at 50, 100, and 200 μg/ml. Future studies should explore the efficacy of lower concentrations.

Nobiletin and tangeretin are dose dependently antiproliferative to MCF-7 and MDA-MB-435 cells via G1 cell cycle phase arrest [51]. Naringin increases p21, modulates the β-catenin pathway, and induces G1 phase cell cycle arrest, resulting in TNBC apoptosis and anti-proliferation [51]. Hesperidin activates caspase-3 and p53 mediated apoptosis against MCF-7 cells [51]. Hesperetin is antiproliferative to MDA-MB-231 cells by GLUT1 and GLUT4 down regulation, and IR-β and Akt phosphorylation inhibition, which reduces basal and insulin-stimulated glucose uptake [51]. Naringenin inhibits MCF-7 basal and insulin-stimulated glucose uptake via PI3K and MEK inhibition [51]. Hesperetin suppresses *in vivo* aromatase expression; therefore, it is biologically plausible that hesperetin will be effective against ER+ breast cancers [51]. Hesperetin and naringenin have *in vitro* activity against HER2 positive cancers, which is biologically plausible as hesperetin and naringenin are HER2 tyrosine kinase inhibitors [51]. The quinones plumbellagiagin and rapanone induce caspase independent, ROS and MMP mediated MCF-7 cell apoptosis [41].

Crude ethyl acetate and methanol extracts of *M. pajang kernel*, and crude petroleum ether and chloroform extracts of the stem bark have strong cytotoxic activity against MCF-7 cells at IC50 of 10 μg/ml and 15 μg/ml, respectively [72]. The cycloartane triterpene component, 3β-hydroxy-cycloart-24-ene-26-oic acid had moderate cytotoxic activity towards MCF-7 at IC50 13.03 ± 0.81 μg/ml [72]. *Pseuduvaria monticola* leaf menthol extracts (6E,10E) isopolycerasoidol and (6E, 10E) isopolycerasoidol methyl ester are selectively anti-proliferative and cytotoxic to MCF-7 and MDA-MB-231 cells via ROS induced changes to mitochondrial membrane permeability, dose dependent caspase 3,7, and 9 activation, anti-apoptotic Bcl-2 down regulation, and nuclear accumulation of p38 MAPK [90]. At 48 hours, (6E,10E) isopolycerasoidol had IC50 59 ± 5.1 M against MCF-7 and IC50 76 ± 8.5 M against MDA-MB-231, while (6E,10E) isopolycerasoidol methyl ester is more potent at IC50 43 ± 2.4 against MCF-7 and IC50 58 ± 2.6 against MDA-MB-231 [90]. Normal human breast epithelial MCF-10A cells are comparatively spared with IC50 of 94 ± 5.9 M for (6E,10E) isopolycerasoidol, and IC50 90 ± 4.7 M for (6E,10E) isopolycerasoidol methyl ester [90].

Silibinin, the main active flavonoid component of Silymarin, derived from *Silibum marianum* (milk thistle) seeds, is anti-angiogenic by MMP-2 and capillary formation suppression, and inhibition of angiogenic signaling molecules [43,77]. Silibinin induces caspase cascade apoptosis in TRAIL-resistant cancers, down regulates Akt-mediated NF-κB1 [77]. Silibinin inhibits MDA-MB-231 breast cancer cell line metastases by inhibiting mRNA levels of GDP dissociation inhibitor (D4-GDI) expression and cell division cycle 42 [77].

Withaferin A has numerous mechanisms of action: Inactivation of Akt and NF-kB to achieve apoptosis, decrease in pro-survival protein B-cell lymphoma 2 (Bcl-2), gap-2/mitosis (G2/M) cell cycle arrest, generation of ROS, induction of protease-activated receptor-4 (Par-4), activation of caspase 3 and 9 activities, DNA damage, inhibition of molecular chaperone heat shock protein 90 (HSP90), regulation of forkhead box O 3a (FOXO3a) and Bcl-2 interacting mediator of cell death (Bim), and inhibition of Notch-1 [73,91,92]. For breast cancer inhibition, withaferin A activates the extracellular signal–regulated kinase (ERK)-ribosomal S6 kinase (RSK) and ETS-like transcription factor 1 (Elk1)-C-EBP homologous protein (CHOP) kinase pathways which upregulate DR5 transcription [92]. This mechanism also provides synergism with celecoxib, etoposide, and TRAIL [92].

Cervical Cancer

Betulinic acid dosed at 100 mg/kg and 200 mg/kg showed dose dependent *in vivo* anti-tumor activity in U14 cervical cancer bearing mice, which approximated to that of 25 mg/kg cyclophosphamide, $p < 0.05$ [71]. *Conium maculatum* (hemlock) ethanolic extract is dose and time dependent anti-proliferative via sub-G stage cell cycle arrest by 48 hours [93]. At 24 hours ROS generation is increased. By 48 hours MMP depolarization, phosphatidyl serine externalization, morphological changes, DNA damage, decreased Bcl-2:Bax, and caspase-3 dependent apoptosis occur in HeLa cells [93]. *C. maculatum* ethanolic extract is also effective against A375, A549, and HepG2 cell lines, with WRL68 normal liver cells surviving treatment better than PBMCs, indicating limited harm to normal tissue [93].

Crude ethyl acetate and methanol extracts of *M. pajang* kernel, and crude petroleum ether and chloroform extracts of the stem bark have strong cytotoxic activity against the HeLa cervical cancer cell line at IC50 of 10 μg/ml and 15 μg/ml, respectively [72]. 3β-hydroxy-cycloart-24-ene-26-oic acid had strong anti-cancer activity towards MCF-7 cells at IC50 6.27 ± 0.61 μg/ml [72]. Quercitrin had moderate to strong cytotoxic activity at 11.93 ± 0.63 μg/ml [72]. Oridonin inhibits the HeLa cell line P13K-Akt pathway [69].

Curcumin and emodin down regulate TGF-β receptor II, P-Smad3, and Smad4, which inhibits TGF- induced migration and invasion in HeLa and SiHa cervical cancer cell lines [94]. Curcumin and emodin up regulate the Bax:Bcl-2 ratio which inhibits p15, p16, p21, p27, CDK6, CyclinD1, and Pin1 expression, thereby inhibiting Wnt/β-catenin in HeLa cells [94]. SiHa cells were chosen for TGF-β resistance [94]. Curcumin and emodin are syngergistic. Curcumin and emodin were dosed at IC50: For curcumin, 15 μM in SiHa and 25 μM in HeLa cells, representing strong cytotoxicity. For emodin, 40 μM in SiHa and HeLa cells [94]. Curcumin and emodin may not be as good candidates for cervical cancer inhibition as *M. pajang* extracts, but, if tolerated, curcumin offers additional overall health benefits, such that curcumin and emodin for chemosensitization should not be overlooked.

The phenol, naringin modulates GM3 ganglioside, affecting EGFR signaling, resulting in HeLa suppression [51]. Taxifolin is synergistic with andrographolide (a diterpenoid lactone) against HeLa cells by reducing andrographolide induced protective autophagy, while increasing mitochondrial outer-membrane permeabilization, caspase dependent, and independent cell death [50].

In vivo athymic nude mice models show that withaferin A, dosed at 8 mg/kg intraperitoneally on alternate days, can reduce CaSki human papilloma virus (HPV) types 16 and 18 positive, cervical cancer cell line tumors by 70%, p<.01 at 6 weeks of treatment [73]. The withaferin A derivative, 3-azido Withaferin A (3-azidoWA), irreversibly inhibits MMP-2 via dose dependent pro-apoptotic extracellular par-4 secretion, resulting in suppressed motility and invasion of HeLa cervical and PC-3 prostate cancer cell lines (p<.01) [95]. *In vivo* mice studies indicate 3-azidoWA, dosed at 30 mg/kg/day intraperitoneally, dosed on day 8 or days 8 to 10, dose dependently activates capase-3 mediated apoptosis and is dose dependently anti-angiogenic [95]. Withaferin A down regulates human papilloma virus (HPV) E6 and E7 oncoproteins' expression, in turn reactivating p53-dependent tumor suppression [73,91].

Ovarian Cancer

The 71 and 87 percentage point survival advantages between Stage 1 and Stages IIIC and IV ovarian cancer respectively indicates a need for more effective treatment modalities for advanced stage ovarian cancer and mechanisms for ovarian cancer prevention [62]. However, a brief literature search suggests that much more could be done to find nutraceutical therapies targeted to ovarian cancer treatment.

The *P. macrocarpa* methanol extract has excellent cytotoxicity against SKOV-3 ovarian cancer cells, IC50 7.75 ± 2.56 μg/ml at 72 hours [86]. The *P. macrocarpa* hexane extracts have good cytotoxicity against SKOV-3, IC50 10.15 ± 2.71 μg/ml at 24 hours [86]. The P. macrocarpa ethyl acetate extracts have good cytotoxicity against SKOV-3, IC50 8.1 ± 1.81 μg/ml at 72 hours [86]. Withaferin A inhibits ovarian adenocarcinoma cell lines CaOV3 and SKOV3 by down regulating Notch1, Notch3, Cdc25C, total and phosphorylated Akt, and bcl-2 proteins, which in turn induces early apoptosis (p<0.05) and G2/M phase cell cycle arrest [96].

Future Research

Research is needed to determine which of the whole plant or organism, the natural phytochemical component, the semi-synthetic phytochemical, or the completely synthetic phytochemical, is the most efficacious form of a nutraceutical. Crude extracts can derive anti-cancer activity from phytochemical components that are removed with additional processing. This is the case with Ferula extracts that lose phenolic components when purified to terpenoid coumarins [74]. However, components of the whole plant or intact portions of the plant can have antagonistic effects, necessitating separation for maximal beneficial effect. For instance, quercitrin appears to antagonize *M. pajang* from which it is derived [72]. Trials of I3C should evaluate the concentration of the I3C metabolite DIM present following administration and metabolism of I3C [28]. Studies on cineole should determine the equivalence, if any, between 1,4-Cineole, the major phytochemical in cardamom, and 1,8-cineole, the most studied cineole [28]. Similarly, clarity is needed as to the activity of each isomer of limonene. All studies on isomeric phytochemicals should specify the isomer used for clarity, efficacy, and adverse effect ascertainment.

Similarly, delivery modality effectiveness for nutraceuticals displays enormous variation. Improving oral nutraceutical bioavailability is an emerging discipline [97]. While nano-encapsulated EGCG is 10-fold more efficacious than non-encapsulated EGCG, and berberine and curcumin act similarly, kaempferol is significantly less efficacious when encapsulated [43]. Nutraceutical microbial fermentation can improve bioavailability and antioxidant efficacy [45]. Therefore, the optimal delivery modality for each nutraceutical's optimal efficacy should be determined. In this light, quercetin is being studied as an enhancer for green tea polyphenol bioavailability and activity [98]. Pro-drug derivatives may need to be developed [52]. Similarly, with synthetic analogs, bioavailability enhancement may be possible without adverse effects as displayed by CYD-6-28 [69]. Then, the focus can shift to making manufacturers supply pharmaceutical grade nutraceuticals in the most efficacious delivery modality.

In vivo trials of withaferin A for ovarian adenocarcinoma treatment are a logical progression from successful *in vitro* CaOV3 and SKOV3 cell line studies [96]. Additional trials of *M. pajang* may indicate if a breast, cervix, or colon cancer treatment can be realistically pursued [72]. The *P. macrocarpa* extracts can be further studied for breast and ovarian cancer [86]. The main cytotoxic constituents of *M. indica L.'s* ethanolic kernel extract could be determined and studied *in vivo* [88]. *C. maculatum* ethanolic extract should undergo *in vivo* murine trials against A375, A549, HeLa, HepG2, and WRL68 cell lines, to assess efficacy and tolerability. Tangeretin, nobiletin and 5-AcTMF should be further trialed for breast, colon, leukemia, myeloma, and NSCLC treatment [52-54]. BITC should be further studied for breast cancer treatment [82].

Clinical trials of silibinin, *Ganoderma lucidum* polysaccharides and ganoderic acids, cordycepin from *Cordyceps millitaris*, EPA, γ-linolenic acid, *Yangzheng Xiaoji* and DME25 may lead to antimetastatic drug candidates [77]. Comparative effectiveness trials of EGCG, silibinin, curcumin, melatonin, oleanolic acid, resveratrol, withaferin A, enterolactone, kaempferol, and tripterine, listed from theoretically most anti-angiogenic activity to least anti-angiogenic activity, could determine which of these polyphenol nutraceuticals is the most anti-angiogenic for a given cancer [43]. These nutraceuticals can also be trialed with conventional chemoradiation to determine if synergism will permit chemoradiation dose reduction.

Nutraceutical treatment of TNBC is worthy of further investigation. β-Sitosterol, bitter gourd, caffeic acid phenethyl ester from propolis, chloroform extracted luteolin from *Eclipta alba, Phaleria macrocarpa chloroform* and hexane nobiletin extracts, *Pseuduvaria monticola* leaf menthol extracts (6E,10E) isopolycerasoidol and (6E,10E) isopolycerasoidol methyl ester, silibinin, and the tangeretin derivative 5-AcTMF may be potential drug candidates. Microenvironmental efficacy limitations of thymoquinone and its synthetic analogs should be performed to ascertain if microenvironmental effects limit thymoquinone's *in vivo* efficacy against bladder, bone, breast, lung, stomach, and pancreatic cancer cell lines, in addition to known limitations of thymoquinone in ID8-NGL mouse ovarian cancer [61,99].

Conclusion

Some nutraceuticals such as the Ferula species derived phytoestrogenic monoterpene umbelliprenin have very limited curative anti-cancer effects that can be limited to a single cancer. Other nutraceuticals, such as the natural MMP inhibitors, 3-azido WA, aqueous cinnamon extract, green tea extract, curcumin, fenugreek derived steroidal saponin, and marine compound derived chitooligosacharides should have a broader applicability. When the incidence and severity of a cancer, for example TNBC is considered, there is benefit in developing a nutraceutical that initially seems to be exclusively of single indication benefit. The breadth and depth of the nutraceutical clinical pharmacology literature suggests that an increased range of curative nutraceutical cancer treatments will become available. However, endometrial cancer treatment should be given as much consideration as have breast, cervical, and ovarian cancers.

References

1. Schütze T, Längler A, Zuzak TJ, Schmidt P, Zernikow B (2016) Use of complementary and alternative medicine by pediatric oncology patients during palliative care. Support Care Cancer 24: 2869-2875.
2. King N, Balneaves LG, Levin GT, Nguyen T, Nation JG, et al. (2015) Surveys of cancer patients and cancer health care providers regarding complementary therapy use, communication, and information needs. Integr Cancer Ther 14: 515-524.
3. Arora S, Aggarwal A, Singla P, Jyoti S, Tandon S (2013) Anti-proliferative effects of homeopathic medicines on human kidney, colon and breast cancer cells. Homeopathy 102: 274-282.
4. Frenkel M (2015) Is there a role for homeopathy in cancer care? Questions and challenges. Curr Oncol Rep 17: 43.
5. Klafke N, Mahler C, von Hagens C, Rochon J, Schneeweiss A, et al. (2015) A complex nursing intervention of complementary and alternative medicine (CAM) to increase quality of life in patients with breast and gynecologic cancer undergoing chemotherapy: Study protocol for a partially randomized patient preference trial. Trials 16: 1.
6. Rossi E, Vita A, Baccetti S, Di Stefano M, Voller F, et al. (2015) Complementary and alternative medicine for cancer patients: Results of the EPAAC survey on integrative oncology centres in Europe. Support Care Cancer 23: 1795-1806.
7. Münstedt K, Maisch M, Tinneberg HR, Hübner J (2014) Complementary and alternative medicine (CAM) in obstetrics and gynaecology: A survey of office-based obstetricians and gynaecologists regarding attitudes towards CAM, its provision and cooperation with other CAM providers in the state of Hesse, Germany. Arch of Gynecol Obstet 290: 1133-1139.
8. Wanchai A, Armer JM, Stewart BR (2010) Breast cancer survivors' perspectives of care practices in Western and alternative medicine. Oncol Nurs Forum 37: 494-500.
9. Saghatchian M, Bihan C, Chenailler C, Mazouni C, Dauchy S, et al. (2014) Exploring frontiers: Use of complementary and alternative medicine among patients with early-stage breast cancer. The Breast 23: 279-285.
10. Singendonk M, Kaspers GJ, Naafs-Wilstra M, Schouten-van Meeteren A, Loeffen J, et al. (2013) High prevalence of complementary and alternative medicine use in the Dutch pediatric oncology population: A multicenter survey. Eur J Pediatr 172: 31-37.
11. Garland SN, Valentine D, Desai K, Li S, Langer C, et al. (2013) Complementary and alternative medicine use and benefit finding among cancer patients. J Altern Complement Med 19: 876-881.
12. Bonacchi A, Fazzi L, Toccafondi A, Cantore M, Mambrini A, et al. (2014) Use and perceived benefits of complementary therapies by cancer patients receiving conventional treatment in Italy. J Pain Symptom Manage 47: 26-34.
13. Schmitt J, Ferro A (2013) Nutraceuticals: Is there good science behind the hype? Br J Clin Pharmacol 75: 585-587.
14. Friedel WE, Matthes H, Bock PR, Zänker KS (2009) Systematic evaluation of the protocols and long-term mistletoe application in nonmetastatic colorectal carcinoma: clinical effects of supportive mistletoe treatment within chemo and/or radiotherapy multicenter, controlled, observational cohort study. J Soc Integr Oncol 7: 137-145.
15. George DR, Edris W, Hanson R, Gilman F (2016) Medicinal plants the next generation. Lancet 387: 220-221.
16. Yuan H, Ma Q, Ye L, Piao G (2016) The traditional medicine and modern medicine from natural products. Molecules 21: 559.
17. Seppo (2017) Hack your tea-how to get 5 times more out of a cup of green tea. AcneEinstein.com.
18. Chen L, Mo H, Zhao L, Gao W, Wang S, et al. (2017) Therapeutic properties of green tea against environmental insults. J Nutr Biochem 40: 1-13.
19. Andrews GR, Roberts SC (2017) Bioprocess engineering of plant cell suspension cultures. Appl Bioeng 12: 5.
20. Bagchi D (2008) Nutraceutical and functional food regulations in the United States and around the world. Academic Press, Burlington.
21. Drake PM, Szeto TH, Paul MJ, Teh AY, Ma JK (2017) Recombinant biologic products versus nutraceuticals from plants–a regulatory choice? Br J Clin Pharmacol 83: 82-87.
22. Minuz P, Velo G, Violi F, Ferro A (2017) Are nutraceuticals the modern panacea? From myth to science. Br J Clin Pharmacol 83: 5-7.
23. Tariq AL, Reyaz AL (2012) Phytochemical analysis of Camellia sinensis Leaves. Int J Drug Dev & Res 4: 311-316.
24. Buckingham J, Baggaley KH, Roberts AD, Szabó LF (2010) Dictionary of alkaloids, 2nd edition. CRC Press, Taylor & Francis Group, Boca Raton, FL, USA.
25. Rais J, Jafri A, Siddiqui S, Tripathi M, Arshad M (2017) Phytochemicals in the treatment of ovarian cancer. Front Biosci (Elite Ed) 9: 67-75.
26. Cline JM, Hughes CL (1998) Phytochemicals for the prevention of breast and endometrial cancer. In Foon KA, Muss HB (eds), Biological and Hormonal Therapies of Cancer, Kluwer Academic Publishers Boston, USA.
27. Sun Y, Guo M, Feng Y, Zheng H, Lei P, et al. (2016) Effect of ginseng polysaccharides on NK cell cytotoxicity in immunosuppressed mice. Exp Ther Med 12: 3773-3777.
28. Acharya A, Das I, Singh S, Saha T (2010) Chemopreventive properties of indole-3-carbinol, diindolylmethane and other constituents of cardamom against carcinogensis. Recent Pat Food Nutr Agric 2: 166-177.
29. Arshad MS, Sohaib M, Nadeem M, Saeed F, Imran A, et al. (2017) Status and trends of nutraceuticals from onion and onion by-products: A critical review. Cogent Food Agric 3: 1280254.
30. Zeng Y, Li Y, Yang J, Pu X, Du J, et al. (2017) Therapeutic role of functional components in alliums for preventive chronic disease in human being. Evid Based Complement Alternat Med 2017: 9402849.

31. Zhong WL, Qin Y, Chen S, Sun T (2017) Antitumor effect of natural product molecules against lung cancer. In a global scientific vision-prevention, diagnosis, and treatment of lung cancer. InTech, Rijeka.

32. Gliszczynska A, Niezgoda N, Gladkowski W, Switalska M, Wietrzyk J (2017) Isoprenoid-phospholipid conjugates as potential therapeutic agents: Synthesis, characterization and antiproliferative studies. PloS ONE.12: e0172238.

33. Liu W, Xu X, Zhang R, Cheng T, Cao Y, et al. (2016) Engineering Escherichia coli for high-yield geraniol production with biotransformation of geranyl acetate to geraniol under fed-batch culture. Biotechnol Biofuels 9: 58.

34. Tippmann S, Ferreira R, Siewers V, Nielsen J, Chen Y (2017) Effects of acetoacetyl-CoA synthase expression on production of farnesene in Saccharomyces cerevisiae. J Ind Microbiol Biotechnol 9: 1-2.

35. Varker KA, Ansel A, Aukerman G, Carson WE (2012) Review of complementary and alternative medicine and selected nutraceuticals: Background for a pilot study on nutrigenomic intervention in patients with advanced cancer. Alternate Therapies Health Med, 18: 26-34.

36. Sun Y, Jia X, Hou L, Liu X, Gao Q (2017) Involvement of apoptotic pathways in docosahexaenoic acid-induced benefit in prostate cancer: Pathway-focused gene expression analysis using RT 2 Profile PCR Array System. Lipids Health Dis 16: 59.

37. Yarnell E, Abascal K (2009) Plant coumarins: Myths and realities. Alternative and Complementary Therapies 15: 24-30.

38. Wang YH, Avula B, Nanayakkara NP, Zhao J, Khan IA (2013) Cassia cinnamon as a source of coumarin in cinnamon-flavored food and food supplements in the United States. J Agric Food Chem 61: 4470-4476.

39. Morsy SA, Farahat AA, Nasr MNA, Tantawy AS (2017) Synthesis, molecular modeling and anticancer activity of new coumarin containing compounds. Saudi Pharm J In press.

40. Dandriyal J, Singla R, Kumar M, Jaitak V (2016) Recent developments of C-4 substituted coumarin derivatives as anticancer agents. Eur J Med Chem 119: 141-168.

41. Kuete V, Omosa LK, Tala VRS, Midiwo JO, Mbaveng AT, et al. (2016) Cytotoxicity of Plumbagin, Rapanone and 12 other naturally occurring Quinones from Kenyan Flora towards human carcinoma cells. BMC Pharmacol Toxicol 17: 60.

42. Alam M, Khan A, Wadoo A, Khan A, Bashir S, et al. (2016) Bioassay-guided isolation of sesquiterpene coumarins from ferula narthex bioss: A new anticancer agent. Front Pharmacol 7: 26.

43. Wang Z, Dabrosin C, Yin X, Fuster MM, Arreola A, et al. (2015) Broad targeting of angiogenesis for cancer prevention and therapy. Semin Cancer Biol: S224-S243.

44. Freyer G, You B, Villet S, Tartas S, Fournel-Federico C, et al. (2014) Open-label uncontrolled pilot study to evaluate complementary therapy with Ruta graveolens 9c in patients with advanced cancer. Homeopathy, 103: 232-238.

45. Henderson AJ, Ollila CA, Kumar A, Borresen EC, Raina K, et al. (2012) Chemopreventive properties of dietary rice bran: Current status and future prospects. Advanced Nutrition 3: 643-653.

46. Aiyer HS, Warri AM, Woode DR, Hilakivi-Clarke L, Clarke R (2012) Influence of berry-polyphenols on receptor signaling and cell-death pathways: Implications for breast cancer prevention. J Agric Food Chem 60: 5693-5708.

47. Goulas V, Stylos E, Chatziathanasiadou MV, Mavromoustakos T, Tzakos A (2016) Functional components of carob fruit: Linking the chemical and biological space. Int J Mol Sci 17: 1875.

48. Sorrenti V, Vanella L, Acquaviva R, Cardile V, Giofrè S, et al. (2015) Cyanidin induces apoptosis and differentiation in prostate cancer cells. Int J Oncol 47: 1303-1310.

49. Raúl SC, Beatriz HC, Joseoziel LG, Francenia SSN (2017) Phenolic compounds in genus Smilax (Sarsaparilla). In M Soto-Hernandez, M Palma-Tenango, M del Roasario Garcia-Mateos, Eds., Phenolic compounds – Natural sources, importance and applications. Intech, Rijeka.

50. Alzaharna M, Alqouqa I, Cheung HY (2017) Taxifolin synergizes Andrographolide-induced cell death by attenuation of autophagy and augmentation of caspase dependent and independent cell death in HeLa cells. PLoS One 12: e0171325.

51. Yi L, Ma S, Ren D (2017) Phytochemistry and bioactivity of Citrus flavonoids: a focus on antioxidant, anti-inflammatory, anticancer and cardiovascular protection activities. Phytochem Rev 2017: 1-33.

52. Li YR, Li S, Ho CT, Chang YH, Tan KT, et al. (2016) Tangeretin derivative, 5-acetyloxy-40-tetramethoxyflavone induces G2/M arrest, apoptosis and autophagy in human non-small cell lung cancer cells in vitro and in vivo. Cancer Biol Ther 17: 48-64.

53. Hirano T, Abe K, Gotoh M, Oka K (1995) Citrus flavone tangeretin inhibits leukaemic HL-60 cell growth partially through induction of apoptosis with less cytotoxicity on normal lymphocytes. Br J Cancer 72: 1380-1388.

54. Morley KL, Ferguson PJ, Koropatnick J (2007) Tangeretin and nobiletin induce G1 cell cycle arrest but not apoptosis in human breast and colon cancer cells. Cancer Lett 251: 168-178.

55. Amin ARM, Karpowicz PA, Carey TE, Arbiser J, Nahta R, et al. (2017) Evasion of anti-growth signaling: A key step in tumorigenesis and potential target for treatment and prophylaxis by natural compounds. Semin Cancer Biol 35: S55-S77.

56. Tebou PL, Tamokou JD, Ngnokam D, Voutquenne-Nazabadioko L, Kuiate JR, et al. (2017) Flavonoids from Maytenus buchananii as potential cholera chemotherapeutic agents. S Afr J Bot 109: 58-65.

57. Oršolic N, Karac I, Sirovina D, Kukolj M, Kunštic M, et al. (2016) Chemotherapeutic potential of quercetin on human bladder cancer cells. J Environ Sci Health A, 51: 776-781.

58. Li Y, Meeran SM, Patel SN, Chen H, Hardy TM, et al. (2013) Epigenetic reactivation of estrogen receptor-a (ERa) by genistein enhances hormonal therapy sensitivity in ERa-negative breast cancer. Mol Cancer 12: 1.

59. Paterni I, Bertini S, Granchi C, Macchia M, Minutolo F (2013) Estrogen receptor ligands: A patent review update. Expert Opin Ther Pat 23: 1247-1271.

60. Crooks PA, Worthen DR, Ghosheh OA (2001) Use of the naturally-occurring quinones thymoquinone and dithymoquinone as antineoplastic and cytotoxic agents. Pharmaceutical Sciences Faculty Patents 72.

61. Rahmani AH, Alzohairy MA, Khan MA, Aly SM (2014) Therapeutic implications of black seed and its constituent thymoquinone in the prevention of cancer through inactivation and activation of molecular pathways.

62. Chen SS, Michael A, Butler-Manuel S (2012) Advances in the treatment of ovarian cancer – a potential role of anti-inflammatory phytochemicals. Discovery Medicine 13: 7-17.

63. Majee SB, Khattry V, Agarwal V, Biswas GR (2016) Polyphenols derived from four indigenous Indian fruits for cancer chemoprevention and chemotherapy. J Med Plants Res 10: 838-847.

64. Panth N, Manandhar B, Paudel KR (2017) Anticancer Activity of Punica granatum (Pomegranate): A Review. Phytother Res 31: 568-578.

65. Luo M, Liu Q, He M, Yu Z, Pi Z, et al. (2017) Gartanin induces cell cycle arrest and autophagy and suppresses migration involving PI3K/Akt/mTOR and MAPK signalling pathway in human glioma cells. J Cell Mol Med 21: 46-57.

66. Zhang C, Yu G, Shen Y (2017) The naturally occurring xanthone a-mangostin induces ROS-mediated cytotoxicity in non-small scale lung cancer cells. Saudi J Biol Sci [In press].

67. Bizzarri M, Dinicola S, Bevilacqua A, Cucina A (2016) Broad Spectrum Anticancer Activity of Myo-Inositol and Inositol Hexakisphosphate. Int J Endocrinol 2016: 5616807.

68. Grattan BJ Jr (2013) Plant sterols as anticancer nutrients: evidence for their role in breast cancer. Nutrients 5: 359-387.

69. Wu J, Ding Y, Chen CH, Zhou Z, Ding C, et al. (2016) A new oridonin analog suppresses triple-negative breast cancer cells and tumor growth via the induction of death receptor 5. Cancer Lett 380: 393-402.

70. Chaudhary S, Chandrashekar KS, Pai KS, Setty MM, Devkar RA, et al. (2015) Evaluation of antioxidant and anticancer activity of extract and fractions of Nardostachys jatamansi DC in breast carcinoma. BMC Complement Altern Med 15: 50.
71. Wang P, Li Q, Li K, Zhang X, Han Z, et al. (2012) Betulinic acid exerts immunoregulation and anti-tumor effect on cervical carcinoma (U14) tumor-bearing mice. Pharmazie 67: 733-739.
72. Ahmad S, Sukari MA, Ismail N, Ismail IS, Abdul AB, et al. (2015) Phytochemicals from Mangifera pajang Kosterm and their biological activities. BMC Complement Altern Med 15: 83.
73. Munagala R, Kausar H, Munjal C, Gupta RC (2011) Withaferin A induces p53-dependent apoptosis by repression of HPV oncogenes and upregulation of tumor suppressor proteins in human cervical cancer cells. Carcinogenesis 32: 169-1705.
74. Valiahdi SM, Iranshahi M, Sahebkar A (2013) Cytotoxic activities of phytochemicals from Ferula species. Daru 21: 39.
75. Bao R, Shu Y, Wu X, Weng H, Ding Q, et al. (2014) Oridonin induces apoptosis and cell cycle arrest of gallbladder cancer cells via the mitochondrial pathway. BMC Cancer 14: 217.
76. United States Department of Agriculture (n.d.) Agriculture research service. USDA food composition databases.
77. Jiang WG, Sanders AJ, Katoh M, Ungefroren H, Gieseler F, et al. (2015) Tissue invasion and metastasis: Molecular, biological and clinical perspectives. Semin Cancer Biol 35: S244-S275.
78. Jang E, Kim BJ, Lee KT, Inn KS, Lee JH (2015) A survey of therapeutic effects of Artemisia capillaris in liver diseases. Evid Based Complement Alternat Med.
79. Edwards V, Benkendorff K, Young F (2012) Marine compounds selectively induce apoptosis in female reproductive cancer cells but not in primary-derived human reproductive granulosa cells. Marine Drugs, 10: 64-83.
80. Zarogoulidis P, Tsakiridis K, Karapantzou C, Lampaki S, Kioumis I, et al. (2015) Use of proteins as biomarkers and their role in carcinogenesis. J Cancer 6: 9-18.
81. Standish LJ, Dowd F, Sweet E, Dale L, Weaver M, et al. (2016) Breast cancer integrative oncology care and its costs. Integr Cancer Ther April-June: 1-11.
82. Xie B, Nagalingam A, Kuppusamy P, Muniraj N, Langford P, et al. (2017) Benzyl Isothiocyanate potentiates p53 signaling and antitumor effects against breast cancer through activation of p53-LKB1 and p73-LKB1 axes. Sci Rep 7: 40070.
83. Bai LY, Chiu CF (2016) A triterpenoid from wild bitter gourd inhibits breast cancer cells. Sci Rep 6: 22419.
84. Stojko RA, Dzik KA, Modzierz A, Kubina R, Wojtyczka RD, et al. (2015) Caffeic acid phenethyl ester and ethanol extract of propolis induce the complementary cytotoxic effect on triple-negative breast cancer cell lines. Molecules 20: 9242-9262.
85. Moirangthem DS, Laishram S, Borah JC, Kalita MC, Talukdar NC (2014) Cephalotaxus griffithii Hook f. needle extract induces cell cycle arrest, apoptosis and suppression of hTERT and hTR expression on human breast cancer cells. BMC Complement Altern Med 14: 305.
86. Lay MM, Karsani SA, Mohajer S, Malek SNA (2014) Phytochemical constituents, nutritional values, phenolics, flavonols, flavonoids, antioxidant and cytotoxicity studies on Phaleria macrocarpa (Scheff.) Boerl fruits. BMC Complement Altern Med 14: 152.
87. Abdullah AH, Mohammed AS, Abdullah R, Mirghani MES (2015) Oxidative stress-mediated apoptosis induced by ethanolic mango seed extract in cultured estrogen receptor positive breast cancer MCF-7 cells. Int J Mol Sci 16: 3528-3536.
88. Abdullah AH, Mohammed AS, Abdullah R, Mirghani MES, Al-Qubaisi M (2014) Cytotoxic effects of Mangifera indica L. kernel extract on human breast cancer (MCF-7 and MDA-MB-231 cell lines) and bioactive constituents in the crude extract. BMC Complement Altern Med 14: 199.
89. Arya RK, Singh A, Yadav NK, Cheruvu SH, Hossain Z, et al. (2015) Anti-breast tumor activity of Eclipta extract in-vitro and in-vivo: Novel evidence of endoplasmic reticulum specific localization of Hsp60 during apoptosis. Sci Rep 5: 18457.
90. Taha H, Looi CY, Arya A, Wong AA, Wong WF, et al. (2015) Benzopyran derivatives from Pseuduvaria monticola induce mitochondrial-mediated apoptosis in human breast adenocarcinoma cells. PLoS ONE 10: e0126126.
91. Kakar SS, Ratajczak MZ, Powell KS, Moghadamfalahi M, Miller DM, et al. (2014) Withaferin A alone and in combination with cisplatin suppresses growth and metastasis of ovarian cancer by targeting putative cancer stem cells. PLoS ONE 9: e 107596.
92. Nagalingam A, Kuppusamy P, Singh SV, Sharma D, Saxena NK (2014) Mechanistic elucidation of the antitumor properties of withaferin a in breast cancer. Cancer Res 74: 2617-2629.
93. Mondal J, Panigrahi AK, Khuda-Bukhsh AR (2014) Anticancer potential of Conium maculatum extract against cancer cells in vitro: Drug-DNA interaction and its ability to induce apoptosis through ROS generation. Pharmacogn Mag 10: S524-S533.
94. Thacker PC, Karunagaran D (2015) Curcumin and emodin down-regulate TGF-Î² signaling pathway in human cervical cancer cells. PLoS One 10: e0120045.
95. Rah B, Amin H, Yousuf K, Khan S, Jamwal G, et al. (2012) A novel MMP-2 inhibitor 3-azidowithaferin A (3-azidoWA) abrogates cancer cell invasion and angiogenesis by modulating extracellular Par-4. PlosONE 7: e44039.
96. Zhang X, Samadi AK, Roby KF, Timmermann B, Cohen MS (2012) Inhibition of cell growth and induction of apoptosis in ovarian carcinoma cell lines CaOV3 and SKOV3 by natural withanolide Withaferin A. Gynecol Oncol 124: 606-612.
97. Ting Y, Jiang Y, Ho CT, Huang Q (2014) Common delivery systems for enhancing in vivo bioavailability and biological efficacy of nutraceuticals. J Funct Foods 7: 112-128.
98. Henning SM (2012) Quercetin to enhance the bioavailability and activity of green tea polyphenols in vitro and in vivo. Food Funct 3: 635-642.
99. Wilson AJ, Saskowski J, Barham W, Khabele D, Yull F (2015) Microenvironmental effects limit efficacy of thymoquinone treatment in a mouse model of ovarian cancer. Mol Cancer 14: 192.

20

Regulation of Gene Expression in Downstream Signaling Molecules by Herbal Compound in Insulin Resistant Diabetic Rats

Aiman Abbas Jafri[1], Suman Bala Sharma[1*], Kalpana Luthra[2], Mohit Mehndiratta[1], Nikhil Khurana[1] and Usha Rani Singh[3]

[1]*Department of Biochemistry, University College of Medical Sciences (University of Delhi), Dilshad Garden, Delhi, India*

[2]*Department of Biochemistry, All India institute of Medical Sciences, Ansari Nagar, Delhi, India*

[3]*Department of Pathology, University College of Medical Sciences (University of Delhi), Dilshad Garden, Delhi, India*

***Corresponding author:** Suman Bala Sharma, Director Professor Department of Biochemistry, University College of Medical Sciences, Dilshad Garden Delhi, India, E-mail- drsbs08@hotmail.com

Abstract

Background: In previous studies, Sharma et al. has already isolated an anti-hyperglycemic compound from the fruit pulp of *Eugenia jambolana* using HPLC and other chromatographic techniques. However, the effect of anti-hyperglycemic compound (FIIc) on the expression of PPAR gamma, IRS-1 and IRS-2 in high sucrose diet induced type 2 diabetic rats has not been studied so far.

Methods: There were exactly 24 Male Wistar rats were taken and fed on High Sucrose Diet (HSD) for the development of type 2 diabetic animal for 30 weeks. Active compound FIIc was given to group C and Pioglitazone to group D at dose of 20 mg/kg of b.w. orally for 30 weeks respectively. Blood was drawn for the estimation of plasma glucose and serum insulin at week o and at week 30 from retro orbital plexus. At the end of the study animal were sacrificed and organs including pancreas and skeletal muscles were isolated and stored at -80°C. Total RNA was isolated by using Trizol method and expression of PPAR gamma, IRS-1 and IRS-2 was quantified and compared among the study groups by Real Time PCR.

Results: After treatment with FIIc for 30 weeks we found a significant reduction in post prandial blood glucose levels in group C rats compared to group B. Serum insulin was also reduced in group C rats compared to group B. In skeletal muscles the mRNA expression of PPAR γ and IRS-1 was found to be 2.48 fold and 2.56 fold increased respectively as compared to group B. Similarly the mRNA expression of IRS-2 in pancreas was found to be 2.69 folds increased as compared to group B.

Conclusion: FIIc treatment for 30 weeks improves glycemic control and insulin sensitivity by increasing the mRNA expression of PPAR γ, IRS-1 and IRS-2.

Keywords: *Eugenia jambolana*; Type 2 diabetes; PPAR γ; IRS-1; IRS-2; Pioglitazone; Insulin resistance

Abbreviations PPAR γ: Peroxisome Proliferator Activated Receptor Gamma; IRS: Insulin Receptor Substrate; HSD: High Sucrose Diet; IGF1: Insulin like Growth Factor-1; T2DM: Type 2 Diabetes Mellitus; b.w.: Body Weight, RXR: Retinoic X Receptor; PI3K: Phosphoinositide 3 kinase; HPLC: High Performance Liquid Chromatography; β cell: Beta cell.

Introduction

Insulin resistance and beta cell failure are the hallmarks of type 2 diabetes [1,2] which appear to be genetically determined [3]. Insulin resistance is the first symptom of pathogenesis of diabetes which precedes the development of glucose intolerance. Initially, the pancreas increases the insulin secretion and production to compensate for hyperglycemia, and in due course of time it leads to beta cell failure [2].

Insulin initiates a wide variety of growth and metabolic effects by binding to the insulin receptor and activating its intrinsic tyrosine kinase. It causes phosphorylation on tyrosine residues of various downstream signaling molecules including insulin receptor substrate (IRS) proteins [4]. IRS molecules are key mediators in insulin signaling and play a central role in maintaining basic cellular functions such as growth, survival, and metabolism. They act as docking proteins between the insulin receptor and a complex network of intracellular signaling molecules [5,6]. Studies have shown that mice lacking IRS-1 exhibit retardation in embryonic and postnatal growth [7,8] indicating that IRS-1 is important for growth-promoting effects of IGF-I. These mice also showed resistance to the glucose-lowering effects of insulin.

Similarly the *IRS-2* is also a critical element in insulin-signaling pathways, and T2DM mice with the *IRS-2* gene knocked out possess insulin resistance in the liver [9]. IRS-2 deficient mice became insulin resistant at 6 weeks, presumably because of insulin resistance in the liver and they progressively developed type 2 diabetes at 10 weeks [10]. Despite insulin resistance, the amount of beta cells was also found to be reduced to 83% of that of wild type mice, which was in marked contrast to the 85% increase in the amount of beta cells in IRS-1 deficient mice at 6 weeks. Thus, insulin resistance in liver combined with absence of compensatory beta cell hyperplasia caused type 2 diabetes in IRS-2 deficient mice [10]. These results suggest that IRS-1 and IRS-2 may play different roles in the regulation of beta cell mass and function of individual beta cells.

On the other hand, PPAR γ has been reported to be expressed in various tissues including adipose and skeletal muscles [11-13]. Studies have reported that PPAR γ is a master regulator in the formation of fat cells and it plays an important regulatory role in adipocyte differentiation and metabolism [13]. Owing to their unique functions in regulating glucose, lipid and cholesterol metabolism, PPARs have drawn special attention for developing drugs to treat type-2 diabetes. Increased serum levels of fatty acids and lipids have known to be associated with insulin resistance. The activation of PPAR γ causes the uptake of lipids and fatty acids in fat depots and improves glycemic control and insulin sensitivity in peripheral tissues [13]. With the glycemic advantages of the PPAR-γ agonists such as Thiazolidinediones (TZDs), the PPAR γ agonists approach can improve the metabolic effects and minimize the side effects caused by either agent alone. Hence it has become a promising strategy for designing effective drugs against type-2 diabetes.

Hence, this study was planned to establish a molecular mechanism of antihyperglycemic compound (FIIc) which was isolated from the fruit pulp of *Eugenia jambolana* in the previous studies by Sharma et al. [14] (US patent No. 6,428,825 August 2002; Indian Process patent no 188759 May 2003; Indian Product Patent no: 2, 30, 753 February 2009) by studying its effect on PPAR γ, IRS-1 and IRS-2 at mRNA level in HSD fed T2DM animal model. By determining its molecular mechanism we can predict its therapeutic targets and a novel approach for the treatment of diabetes.

Material and Methods

Experimental animal model

Male Wistar rats weighing ≈ 150-180 grams were used as animal models of diabetes for the present study. The animals were procured from the central animal house, University College of Medical Sciences (UCMS), Delhi. The rats were fed on a standard chow diet (Hindustan Lever Ltd., Mumbai, India) and water *ad libitum*. The rats were housed under standard conditions of temperature (22°C ± 2°C) and 12 hour light dark cycle. For sacrificing animals CO2 inhalation was used.

Induction of type 2 diabetes by feeding High Sucrose Diet

The HSD as prepared by Madhu et al. [15] was used. It was prepared by mixing 12 liters of distilled water, 5.6 kg of chow diet, 1.8 kg of table sugar, 560 ml of palm oil, 40 ml of Vimeral, 40 ml of calcium syrup and 160 grams of maize powder. The composition of high sucrose diet is carbohydrate 60% to 70% predominantly sucrose, fat 20% to 25% and protein 15% to 20%. The prepared diet was kept at 4°C.

Methodology

Exactly 24 Male Wistar rats were taken for the present study and given standard chow diet for 2 weeks. After 2 weeks of acclimatization, animals were randomized into 4 groups (6 rats per group).

- Group A: Healthy control given normal chow diet
- Group B: Diabetic control given HSD
- Group C: Diabetic treated with FIIc (20 mg/kg of body weight/day) given HSD
- Group D: Diabetic treated with Pioglitazone (20 mg/kg of body weight/day) given HSD

Animals in group A were fed on normal chow diet whereas animals in group B, C and D were fed on High Sucrose Diet and water *ad libitum* throughout the study. Purified active compound FIIc and Pioglitazone were given orally to group C and group D orally, at a dose of 20 mg/kg of b.w./day for 30 weeks respectively. This is the effective dose standardized in previous studies done by Sharma et al. [14]. An equal volume of normal saline were given orally to group A and group B rats.

At week 26 a mild dose of Streptozotocin at a dose of 15 mg/kg of body weight were given intraperitoneally to group B, group C and group D rats and were followed till week 30. Blood was drawn from retro orbital plexus from overnight fasted animals on day 1 and afterwards at week 30 of the study. Blood/serum was collected for the estimation of glucose and insulin respectively. Fasting blood glucose and 2 hour post prandial blood glucose were estimated for the confirmation of diabetes. 2 hour post prandial blood glucose was estimated after giving a glucose load at a dose of 2 gm/kg of body weight in overnight fasted rats. At the end of 30th week all the animals were sacrificed and their organs including skeletal muscles and pancreas were dissected out and stored at -80°C.

RNA extraction by Trizol method

The quantitative mRNA expression levels of PPAR γ, IRS-1 were measured in skeletal muscles and *IRS-2* was done in pancreatic tissues, depending upon their site of expression in the four study groups. At the end of the study, all the animals were sacrificed and the above mentioned tissues were dissected out and fixed in the Trizol reagent for extraction of RNA according to the manufacturer's protocols. 50 mg to 100 mg of tissue was taken and homogenized in 1 ml of Trizol reagent using a plastic pestle or a sonicator (Thermo Scientific, USA). Sample was centrifuged at 12,000 g at 4°C for 10 minutes using a cooling centrifuge (Remi CPR 24, India). Pellets obtained were discarded and supernatant was transferred into another aliquot.

It was incubated at room temperature for 5 minutes. 200 μl of biotechnology grade chloroform (Amresco, USA) was further added and incubated at room temperature for 15 mins. Again the sample was centrifuged at 12,000 g 15 mins at 4°C. The aqueous phase obtained after centrifugation was transferred in another aliquot and 0.5 ml of biotechnology grade pure isopropanol was added to the aqueous phase. Sample was mixed by inverting the aliquot and incubated at room temperature for 10 mins.

The sample was again centrifuged at 12,000 g at 4°C for 10 min. After centrifugation the supernatant was removed and pellets obtained was left intact. 1 ml of biotechnology grade 75% ethanol was added and mixed properly by inverting the aliquot. The sample was again centrifuged at 7,500 g at 4°C for 5 minutes. The supernatant obtained was discarded and the aliquot was incubated on a dry bath at 57°C for 10 minutes.

After incubation 50 μl of nuclease free water (Amresco, USA) was added and sample was put into -20°C deep freezer. The quality of isolated RNA was determined spectrophotometrically (260/280 nm, 260/230 nm) using a Nano Drop (Thermo Scientific, Wilmington, DE, USA). The yield of RNA obtained was high and varied between 5000 ng/μl to 6000 ng/μl.

cDNA preparation

The RNA obtained from the tissues was used for the preparation of cDNA by using a First Strand cDNA synthesis kit (Thermo Scientific, Waltham, USA). After thawing and mixing the components of the kit properly, 1 μl of sample RNA, 0.5 μl of oligo dt primer and 0.5 μl of random hexamer were mixed in 9 μl of nuclease free water to make up the volume to 11 μl and incubated on a dry bath at 65°C for 5 minutes. After incubation, 4 μl of 5X reaction buffer, 1 μl of RiboLock RNase inhibitor, 2 μl of 10 mM dNTP mix and 2 μl of M-MuLV reverse transcriptase enzyme were added.

The master mix obtained was briefly centrifuged to remove any air bubbles and to bring any sample adhering at the walls to the bottom. This reaction mix was put for cDNA synthesis (Eppendorf master cycler nexus gradient, Eppendorf, Germany). The programming used was 25°C for 5 minutes, 45°C for 60 minutes, 70°C for 5 minutes and the reaction was put to end by bringing the reaction at 4°C. The cDNA obtained was diluted by adding 60 μl of nuclease free water and was stored in a -80°C deep freezer.

Real Time PCR Quantification

The cDNA obtained was used as a sample for the determination of expression levels of PPAR γ, IRS-1 and IRS-2 by using Qiagen Thermal Cycler (Rotor-Gene Q 2plex+HRM System, Qiagen, USA) with Maxima SYBR Green/ROX qPCR Master mix (Thermo Scientific, USA). Alpha tubulin was used as an internal control gene.

- The primer sequences for PPAR γ, IRS-1, IRS-2 and alpha Tubulin were as follows
- PPAR γ Primer sequence- Fwd primer- 5'CCCTGGCAAAGCATTTGTAT 3', Rev Primer- 5'GGTGATTTGTCTGTTGTCTTTCC 3'
- IRS- 1 Primer sequence- Fwd Primer- 5' TCAACAGCAGTCCCTACCAC- 3', Rev Primer- 5'-GCTGTGATGTCCAGTTACGC- 3'
- IRS- 2 Primer sequence- Fwd Primer- 5'-TCCAGAACGGCCTCAACTAT- 3', Rev Primer- 5'-AGTGATGGGACAGGAAGTCG- 3'
- Alpha tubulin Primer sequence- Fwd primer- 5'TAGCAGAGATCACCAATGCC 3', Rev Primer- 5' GGCAGCAAGCCATGTATTTA 3'

Real time PCR was conducted in a final volume of 20 μl consisting of 10 μl Maxima SYBR Green, 1 μl forward primer (10 mM), 1 μl reverse primer (10 mM), 3 μl cDNA sample and 5 μl nuclease free water. The amplification parameters consisted of an initial activation at 95°C for 5 min followed by 40 cycles of a 3-step PCR (denaturation at 95°C for 15 sec, annealing at 52°C for 30 sec, and extension at 75°C for 30 sec). The PCR products formed was detected simultaneously and shown on the LCD display by measuring the increase in fluorescence caused by the binding of SYBR green dye into the major grooves of double helical DNA. The relative fold change in the mRNA expression levels of PPAR γ, IRS-1, IRS-2 and alpha Tubulin was calculated by the $2^{-\Delta\Delta Ct}$ method as described by Schmittgen et al. [16]. The results were normalized to the mRNA expression level of alpha tubulin.

Statistical analysis

The statistical analysis was carried out by using analysis of variance (ANOVA) followed by tukeys test.

Results

As shown in Table 1, we observed a significant decrease in post prandial blood glucose levels in group C and group D rats compared to group B at week 30 after treatment with FIIc and Pioglitazone. However, no significant difference in fasting blood glucose levels was observed at week 0 among the four study groups.

At week 30 fasting serum insulin levels were also found to be decreased in group C and group D rats as compared to group B after treatment with FIIc and Pioglitazone. However this decrease is statistically not significant.

Parameters	Time Points	Group A	Group B	Group C	Group D	p Value
FBG (mg/dl)	0 Weeks	86.5	85.5	84	84.33	a=0.0167
	30 Weeks	89.66	102.16a	93.16b	98.16c	b=0.1783 c=0.5471
PPBG (mg/dl)	0 Weeks	122.66	124.83	123.33	126.33	a=0.0001
	30 Weeks	136.83	236.83a	190.50b	183.33c	b=0.0007 c=0.0001
Insulin (pmol)	0 Weeks	13.16	14.66	14.75	14.32	a=0.0030
	30 Weeks	15.71	29.71a	23.88b	21.88c	b=0.1411 c=0.0631

a=Healthy control *vs.* diabetic control, b=Diabetic control *vs.* diabetic treated with FIlc, c=Diabetic control *vs.* diabetic treated with Pioglitazone

Table 1: Showing Fasting blood glucose, post prandial blood glucose and serum Insulin levels at week 0 and at week 30 after treatment with FIIc and Pioglitazone.

In Figure 1, 2.4 and 3.53-fold increases in PPAR r mRNA expression levels in skeletal muscles of groups C and D respectively were observed, when compared to group B after treatment with active herbal compound FIIc and Pioglitazone for 30 weeks.

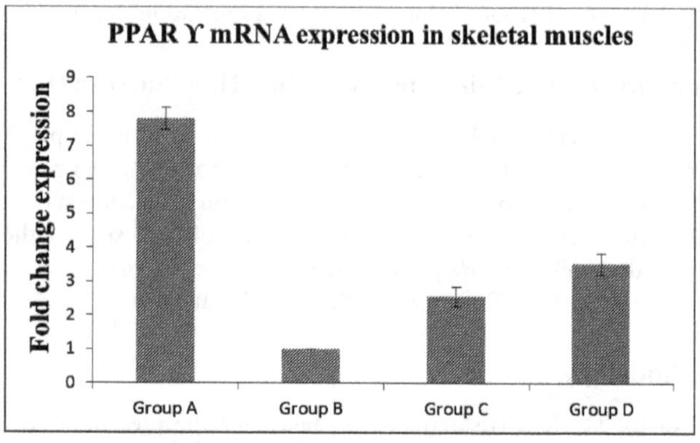

Figure 1: Showing PPAR γ mRNA expression level in skeletal muscles at week 30 after treatments with FIIc and Pioglitazone.

In Figure 2, a 2.56 and 2.81 folds increase in IRS-1 mRNA expression level in skeletal muscles of group C and group D respectively was observed, when compared to group B after treatment with active herbal compound FIIc and Pioglitazone for 30 weeks.

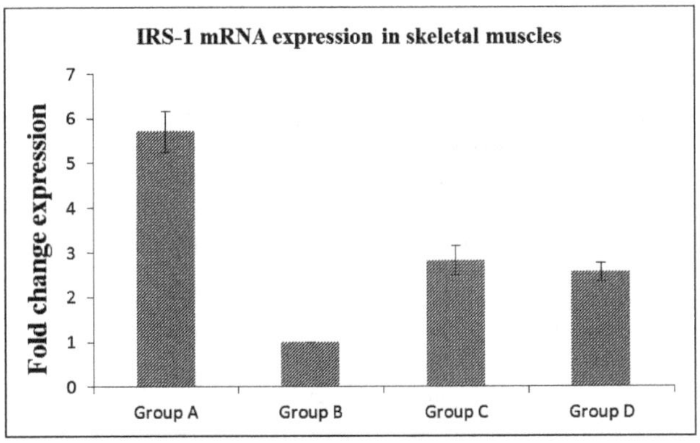

Figure 2: IRS-1 mRNA expression level after treatment with FIIc and Pioglitazone in skeletal muscles at week 30.

In Figure 3, a 2.69 and 2.05 folds increase in IRS-2 mRNA expression level in pancreas of group C and Group D respectively was observed, as compared to group B after treatment with active herbal compound FIIc and Pioglitazone for 30 weeks

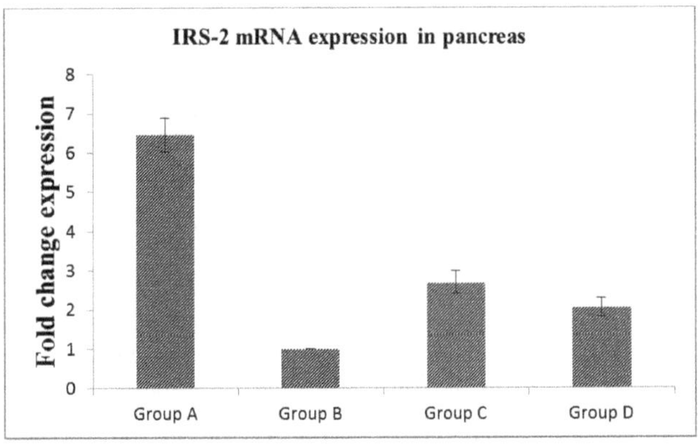

Figure 3: IRS-2 mRNA expression level after treatment with FIIc and Pioglitazone in pancreas at week 30.

Discussion

This study was conducted in HSD fed type 2 diabetic rats to study the effect of herbal anti-hyperglycemic compound (FIIc) on peripheral insulin sensitivity by measuring the mRNA expression levels of PPAR γ, IRS-1 and IRS-2. After treatment with FIIc at week 30, we observed a 2.48 and 2.56 folds increase in PPAR γ and IRS-1 mRNA expression level in skeletal muscles of group C as compared to group B. Similarly, a 2.69 folds increase in IRS-2 mRNA expression level in pancreas of group C was observed, as compared to group B. A significant fall in post prandial blood glucose levels was also observed in group C and Group D rats as compared to group B. serum insulin was also found to be reduced in group C as compared to group B as an indicator of reduced insulin resistance upon treatment with FIIc for 30 weeks.

Insulin resistance is a characteristic feature of type 2 diabetes in which a higher than normal levels of insulin is required for maintaining normal glucose levels. Various studies have reported that PPAR γ is down regulated in type 2 diabetes and insulin resistant states and up regulation of PPAR γ upon binding of the synthetic PPAR γ ligands in T2DM results in a marked improvement in whole body insulin sensitivity and improved glycaemic control [13,17-19]. Similarly, studies have also reported that IRS-1 is an important element in insulin signaling pathways and defect in the *IRS-1* gene has been reported to be associated in the generation of T2DM [20,21]. Literature survey has also reported a significantly reduced IRS-1 mRNA levels in obese subjects and insulin resistant subjects compared with healthy lean and insulin sensitive subjects [22]. Hence, above studies showed that IRS-1 plays an important role in the susceptibility to type 2 diabetes. Similarly IRS-2 is also an important player in insulin-signaling pathways. Genetic studies have also reported that IRS-2 knockout resulted in the development of insulin resistance in the liver and type 2 diabetes [9-10,23-24].

When insulin binds to cell surface receptors it initiates a cascade of events by activating the intra cellular tyrosine kinase domain of β subunit which leads to a rapid auto phosphorylation of downstream signaling molecules such as IRS-1, IRS-2 and several Shc proteins which in turn activates further intracellular signaling intermediates [25] hence leads to uptake of glucose, lipids and other metabolites. We strongly suggested that cause of insulin resistance lies at the post receptor level of insulin signaling. Thus, various studies in the past failed to explain a normal or slightly reduced insulin receptor tyrosine kinase activity in insulin resistance subjects, in spite for a substantial reductionin insulin action [26].

In a recent study it has been reported that upon treatment with a Chinese herbal traditional medicine (a partial PPAR γ agonist) prevented hyperglycaemia and weight gain *in vivo* [27]. Studies have also reported that herbal drugs were found to be useful in improving the mRNA expression of IRS-1 [28,29] and IRS-2 in type 2 diabetes [30,31]. The possible mechanism of FIIc through which it improves the PPAR γ mRNA expression is through the binding of retinoic X receptor (RXR) present on the DNA. Upon binding it causes co-repressor release and co-activator binding and resulting in increased affinity for the specific PPAR response element, which modulates gene transcription.

Similarly, In a recent study it has been reported that upon treatment with herbal traditional Chinese medicine in T2DM, resulted in significantly increased expression of IRS-1, PI3K and other downstream signaling molecules suggesting an effective herbal therapy for insulin resistance by regulating the PI3K/Akt signaling pathway in adipose tissues [32]. During insulin signaling pathway, the activation of PI3K phosphorylates Akt, which further activates the downstream signaling molecules and mediates glucose uptake and intracellular glycogen synthesis in skeletal muscle. In our study we also observed a similar finding suggesting that this might be the possible mechanism of action of our herbal active compound FIIc.

Animal studies have also reported that down regulation of IRS-2 causes peripheral insulin resistance leading to β cell failure and T2DM [9,10,34] and up-regulation of IRS-2 in β cells leads to improved glucose tolerance and prevents diabetes in IRS-2 deficient and obese mice [33]. Increased serum insulin and IGF1 levels activates Akt pathway is also an important factor for the up regulation of IRS-2. In our study we have observed decreased serum insulin levels and increased mRNA expression levels of IRS-2 at week 30 of the study. Hence our results are in accordance with the previous studies and this might be the possible mechanism of action of FIIc in regulation of insulin signaling mechanism in improving glycemic control.

Acknowledgements

The authors acknowledge Indian Council of Medical Research, Ansari Nagar, New Delhi for their financial support.

References

1. Marlon EC (2013) Beta cell dysfunction and insulin resistance. Front Endocrinol (Lausanne) 4: 37.
2. Sesti G, Federici M, Hribal ML, Lauro D, Sbraccia P, et al. (2001) Defects of the insulin receptor substrate (IRS) system in human metabolic disorders. Faseb J 15: 2099-2111.
3. De Fronzo RA (1997) Pathogenesis of Type 2 diabetes: Metabolic and molecular implications for identifying diabetes genes. Diabetes Rev 5: 177-269.
4. White MF (1997) The insulin signaling system and the IRS proteins. Diabetologia. 40: S2-S17.
5. Rondinone CM, Wang LM, Lonnroth P, Wesslau C, Pierce JH, et al. (1997) Insulin receptor substrate (IRS) 1 is reduced and IRS-2 is the main docking protein for phosphatidylinositol 3-kinase in adipocytes from subjects with non-insulin-dependent diabetes mellitus. Proc Natl Acad Sci 94: 4171-4175.
6. Bunner AE, Chandrasekera PC, Barnard ND (2014) Knockout mouse models of insulin signaling: Relevance past and future. World J Diabetes. 5:146-159.
7. Araki E, Lipes MA, Patti ME, Brüning JC, Haag B, et al. (1994) Alternative pathways of insulin signaling in mice with targeted disruption of the IRS-1 gene. Nature 372: 186-190.
8. Tamemoto H, Kadowaki T, Tobe K, Yagi T, Sakura H, et al. (1994) Insulin resistance and growth retardation in mice lacking insulin receptor substrate-1. Nature 372: 182-186.
9. Withers DJ, Gutierrez JS, Towery H, Burks DJ, Ren JM, et al. (1998) Disruption of IRS-2 causes type 2 diabetes in mice. Nature. 391: 900-904.
10. Kubota N, Tobe K, Terauchi Y, Eto K, Yamauchi T, et al. (2000) Disruption of insulin receptor substrate 2 causes type 2 diabetes because of liver insulin resistance and lack of compensatory beta-cell hyperplasia. Diabetes. 49: 1880-1889.
11. Grygiel-Górniak B (2014) Peroxisome proliferator-activated receptors and their ligands: nutritional and clinical implications-a review. Nutr J 14: 13:17.
12. Ji S, Yang R, Lu C, Qiu Z, Yan C, et al. (2014) Differential expression of PPAR γ, FASN, and ACADM genes in various adipose tissues and longissimusdorsi muscle from yanbian yellow cattle and yan yellow cattle. Asian-Australas J Anim Sci 27: 10-18.
13. Wang YX. PPARs (2010) Diverse regulators in energy metabolism and metabolic diseases. Cell Res 20: 124-137.
14. Tanwar RS, Sharma SB, Singh UR, Prabhu KM (2011) Antiatherosclerotic potential of active principle isolated from Eugenia jambolana in streptozotocin-induced diabetic rats. Evid Based Complement Alternat Med 2011: 127641.
15. Madhu SV, Aslam M, Galav V, Bhattacharya SK, Aiman AJ (2014) Atorvastatin prevents type 2 diabetes mellitus- an experimental study. Eur J Pharmacol. 728: 135-140.
16. Schmittgen TD, Livak KJ (2008) Analyzing real-time PCR data by the comparative CT method. Nature Protocols. 3: 1101-1108
17. Bermúdez V, Finol F, Parra N, Parra M, Pérez A, et al. (2010) PPAR-γ agonists and their role in type 2 diabetes mellitus management. Am J Ther 17: 274-283.
18. Lecarpentier Y, Claes V, Vallée A, Hébert JL (2017) Interactions between PPAR gamma and the Canonical Wnt/Beta-Catenin pathway in type 2 diabetes and colon cancer. PPAR Res 5879090.
19. Larsen TM, Toubro S, Astrup A (2003) PPAR γ agonists in the treatment of type II diabetes: Is increased fatness commensurate with long-term efficacy ? IntJ Obes Relat Metab Disord 27: 147-161.
20. Carvalho E, Jansson PA, Axelsen M, Eriksson JW, Huang X, et al. (1999) Low cellular IRS 1 gene and protein expression predict insulin resistance and NIDDM. FASEB J. 13: 2173-2178.
21. Aytug S, Reich D, Sapiro LE, Bernstein D, Begum N (2003) Impaired IRS-1/PI3-kinase signaling in patients with HCV: A mechanism for increased prevalence of type 2 diabetes. Hepatology 38: 1384-1392.
22. Kovacs P, Hanson RL, Lee YH, Yang X, Kobes S, et al. (2003) The role of insulin receptor substrate-1 gene (IRS1) in type 2 diabetes in Pima Indians. Diabetes. 52: 3005-3009.
23. Brady MJ (2004) IRS2 takes center stage in the development of type 2 diabetes. J Clin Invest 114: 886-888.
24. Taniguchi CM, Ueki K, Kahn CR (2016) Complementary roles of IRS-1 and IRS-2 in the hepatic regulation of metabolism. J Clin Invest 126: 4387.
25. Boucher J, Kleinridders A, Kahn RC (2014) Insulin Receptor Signaling in Normal and Insulin-Resistant States. Cold Spring Harb Perspect Biol. 6: a009191.
26. Draznin B (2006) Molecular mechanisms of insulin resistance: serine phosphorylation of insulin receptor substrate-1 and increased expression of p85alpha: The two sides of a coin. Diabetes. 55: 2392-2397.
27. Atanasov AG, Wang JN, Gu SP, Bu J, Kramer MP, et al. (2013) Honokiol: A non-adipogenic PPAR γ agonist from nature. Biochim Biophys Acta 1830: 4813-4319.
28. Hu X, Wang M, Bei W, Han Z, Guo J (2014) The Chinese herbal medicine FTZ attenuates insulin resistance via IRS1 and PI3K in vitro and in rats with metabolic syndrome. J Transl Med 12: 47.
29. Yang L, Wang Z, Jiang L, Sun W, Fan Q, et. al. (2017) Total flavonoids extracted from oxytropisfalcata bunge improve insulin resistance through regulation on the ikkβ/nf-κb inflammatory pathway. Evid Based Complement Alternat Med 2405124.
30. Kuznetsova A, Yu Y, Hollister-Lock J, Opare-Addo L, Rozzo A, et al. (2016) Trimeprazine increases IRS2 in human islets and promotes pancreatic β cell growth and function in mice. JCI Insight 1: e80749.
31. Hennige AM, Burks DJ, Ozcan U, Kulkarni RN, Ye J, et al. (2003) Up regulation of insulin receptor substrate-2 in pancreatic beta cells prevents diabetes. J Clin Invest 112: 1521-1532.
32. Lin X, Taguchi A, Park S, Kushner JA, Li F, et al. (2004) Dysregulation of insulin receptor substrate 2 in beta cells and brain causes obesity and diabetes. J Clin Invest 114: 908-916.
33. Hennique AM, burks DJ, Ozcan U, Kulkarni RN, Park S, et al. (2003) Up regulation of insulin receptor substrate-2 in pancreatic beta cells prevents diabetes. J Clin Invest. 112: 1521-1532

21

Ionic Detoxification Reduces Obesity and Fatty Liver in Rats Fed a High-Fat Diet

Hsien-Tsung Yao*

Department of Nutrition, China Medical University, 91, Hsueh-Shih Road, Taichung, 404, Taiwan

Abstract

Background: Ionic detoxification (ID) or ionic water bath treatment is a simple alternative method to improve health but lacks scientific evidence. It is hypothesized that regular ID treatment can increase the excretion of toxic molecules from the body and improve metabolic disorders including obesity.

Methods: To investigate the effect of ID treatment on high-fat diet-induced obesity and fatty liver, male Wistar rats were fed a low-fat control diet, a high-fat (HF) diet, or a HF diet with ID treatment (3 times/week) for 11 weeks. Triglyceride contents and fatty acid metabolic genes in perirenal adipose tissue and liver were determined.

Results: Rats fed the HF diet had significantly higher body weight, liver weight, and adipose tissue (perirenal and epididymal) weight than did animals fed the low-fat diet. ID treatment significantly reduced body weight and perirenal adipose tissue weight induced by the HF diet. In addition, ID treatment reduced hepatic cholesterol and triglyceride contents. In liver, ID treatment reduced fatty acid synthesis (acetyl-CoA carboxylase and fatty acid synthase mRNA) more significantly than fatty acid oxidation (carnitine palmitoyl-transferase 1 and acyl CoA oxidase mRNA). In perirenal adipose tissue, ID treatment increased the lipolysis rate and reduced the triglyceride level. However, ID treatment had no significant effects on lipogenesis gene expression or adipose size in perirenal adipose tissue.

Conclusions: The results of this study suggest that regular ID treatment may have beneficial effects on reducing obesity and fatty liver.

Keywords: Ionic detoxification; Ionic water bath; Obesity; Fatty liver; High-fat diet; Rats

Abbreviations: ACC: Acetyl-CoA Carboxylase; ACOX: Acyl CoA Oxidase; ALT: Alanine Aminotransferase; CPT-1: Carnitine Palmitoyl-Transferase 1; FAS: Fatty Acid Synthase; HOMA: Homeostasis Model Assessment; ID: Ionic Detoxification; ORP: Oxidation Reduction Potential; PPAR-α: Peroxisome Proliferator-Activated Receptor α; SREBP-1: Sterol Regulatory Element-Binding Transcription Factor 1

Introduction

Humans are now regularly exposed to electromagnetic pollution from indoor electrical equipment and outdoor electrical appliances. Studies suggest that exposure of the human body to electromagnetic pollution can lead to electrical imbalances and the production of electrostatic forces in the body and may be responsible for reducing physical activity, oxygen uptake, and immune system function and potentially increasing stress and some degenerative illnesses [1]. Recent evidence suggests that exposure to electromagnetic fields (e.g., high-frequency voltage transients, dirty electricity) is contributing to the worldwide epidemics of obesity and diabetes [2]. Also, excess accumulation of small positively or negatively charged particles (or molecules) in the body derived from exogenous electromagnetic stimulation or endogenous electrostatic forces may attract charged molecules in some tissues, resulting in the development and progression of diseases such as cardiovascular disease [3]. The electron charge in the body may remain until it can be reduced by means of an electrical current or electrical discharge.

Ionic detoxification (ID), also called ionic water bath treatment, is bathed the local or whole body in warm water with electrolysis of water and considered to be a simple way to improve health in many countries, but rigorous scientific evidence is lacking. The hands, feet, or body are bathed in warm water while an ion generator (a stainless steel spring) produces a stream of positive (H+) and negative (OH-) ions from the cathode and anode, respectively. The ion streams may attract oppositely small charged molecules to the ion generator and thus balance electricity in the body. Therefore, by continuously transmitting a microcurrent through the entire body for a period a time, ID treatment may reduce the accumulation of excessively small charged molecules in the body. After ID treatment, the amount of precipitates (neutralized molecules) can be observed in the water as various colors and unfavorable flavors from different individuals. However, it is still unclear what kinds of molecules are excreted from the body during ID treatment.

In addition to oxygen gas, abundant hydrogen gas is produced in the water (hydrogen-rich water) during electrolysis and lowers the oxidation-reduction potential (ORP). The hydrogen-rich water bath may provide electricity to the body and lower the body's electric potential similar to the action of grounding. Grounding is known to reduce the alternating current electric potential at the surface of the body and lower perturbations in electric charges of molecules inside the body [4]. Grounding can normalize the function of all body systems and improve sleep, relieve chronic pain, increase the respiratory rate and blood oxygenation, and reduce blood glucose, red blood cell aggregation, and inflammation [4,5].

***Corresponding author:** Hsien-Tsung Yao, Department of Nutrition, China Medical University, 91 Hsueh-Shih Road, Taichung 404, Taiwan. E-mail: htyao@mail.cmu.edu.tw

We hypothesized that ID treatment may normalize cell function by reducing electrical potential and electrical imbalances in the body, which may increase cell detoxification and improve metabolic disorders. In this study, we investigated the possible anti-obesity effect of ID treatment in a diet-induced obesity model, which mimics the pathogenesis of human obesity [6].

Materials and Methods

Ionic detoxification (ID)

The ID system, which included a main engine and a stainless steel spring array (ion generator), was purchased from Health and Medical Sales, Inc (USA). The salt (NaCl) concentration in the water bath was 0.04%. The microcurrent was approximately at 1 A. The temperature of the water bath was set at 32°C. For this study, rats were fixed in a plastic bag and each rat tail was bathed in the ID system for 8 min, as plotted in Figure 1. The concentration of dissolved molecular hydrogen in the water bath during electrolysis was measured with an ENH-1000 electrode (TRUSTLEX Inc, Osaka, Japan). The ORP value was determined by use of an MP-103 electrode (Gondo Electronic Co., Ltd. Taipei, Taiwan). The concentration of molecular hydrogen and the ORP value in water bath during electrolysis were monitored with gentle stirring.

Animals and treatment

Ten-week-old male Wistar rats (BioLASCO Taiwan Co., Ltd., Ilan, Taiwan) were randomly divided into three groups: (a) the control group (Control), which was fed a standard laboratory rodent diet; (b) the high-fat diet group (HF), which was fed a high-fat diet; and (c) the high-fat diet group with ionic detoxification (HF+ID), which was fed the high-fat diet and underwent ID treatment. The high-fat diet contained 17% lard, 2% soybean oil, 0.5% cholesterol, 0.05% cholic acid, and 80.45% standard laboratory rodent diet. For ID treatment, rats were fixed in a plastic bag and each rat tail was bathed in warm water in the ID apparatus for 8 min (at 15:00 pm). The same treatment was conducted three times (Monday, Wednesday, Friday) weekly. After ID treatment, the ammonia concentration in bathed water was measured (Randox Laboratories, Crumlin, UK), and then the bathed water was heated in an oven at 100°C to remove the moisture. The residue was extracted with ethanol and the resulting extract was vacuumed dry as the lipid content of residue.

The rats were housed in plastic cages in a room kept at a temperature of 23 ± 1°C and relative humidity of 60 ± 5% with a 12 h light-dark cycle. Food and drinking water were available ad libitum for 11 weeks. Body weight was measured once per week. At the end of the 11 week experimental period, food intake was measured and feces were collected for 2 days. Rats were fasted for 12 h before being sacrificed (at 8:00 AM). The rats were sacrificed by exsanguination via the abdominal aorta while under carbon dioxide (70%/30%, CO_2/O_2) anesthesia. Heparin was used as the anticoagulant. Plasma was separated from the blood by centrifugation (1750 xg) at 4°C for 20 min. The liver and adipose tissues (epididymal and perirenal) from each animal were excised and weighed. In this study, we found that perirenal fat pads were reduced by ID treatment more significantly than epididymal adipose tissue weight. Therefore, epididymal adipose tissue was used for further histological and biochemical examinations. Parts of the liver and perirenal fat pads were excised and fixed in 10% neutral formalin followed by dehydration in ascending grades of alcohol, clearing in xylene, and embedding in paraffin wax. Liver sections and perirenal fat pads were stained with hematoxylin and eosin (H&E) for the histological examination [7]. The other parts of liver and adipose tissues were immediately stored and frozen at -80°C.

This study was approved by the Animal Center Management Committee of China Medical University. The animals were maintained in accordance with the guidelines for the care and use of laboratory animals as issued by the Animal Center of the Ministry of Science and Technology, Taiwan.

Determination of plasma biochemical parameters

Plasma concentrations of glucose, total cholesterol, and triglyceride were determined by enzymatic methods with kits purchased from Audit Diagnostics (Cork, Ireland). Plasma insulin was determined by using a rat insulin enzyme-linked immunosorbent assay (ELISA) kit purchased from Mercodia (Uppsala, Sweden). High-density lipoprotein (HDL) cholesterol was measured after the removal of very-low-density lipoprotein and low-density lipoprotein cholesterol by heparin-manganese precipitation (Randox Laboratories, Crumlin, UK). Plasma alanine aminotransferase (ALT) activity was determined by using a commercial kit purchased from Randox Laboratories (Antrim, UK).

The homeostasis model assessment (HOMA) was used as an index of insulin resistance [8]. It was calculated by the formula

HOMA=fasting glucose [mmol/L] ×fasting insulin [μU/mL]/22.5.

Determination of liver, adipose tissue, and fecal lipid contents

Total lipids from liver, adipose tissue (perirenal), and feces were extracted with chloroform/methanol solution (v/v, 2:1) according to the method of Folch et al. [9]. Triglyceride and cholesterol in the solvent extract were emulsified by the addition of Triton X-100 [10] and their contents were determined by use of commercial enzymatic kits (Randox Ltd, Antrim, UK).

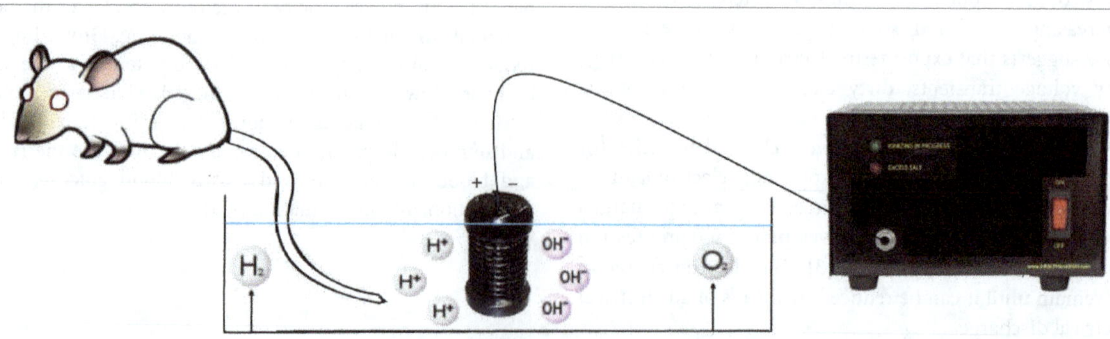

Figure 1: Rat was bathed in ID system with electrolysis of water.

Determination of fatty acid metabolic genes

Total RNA was extracted from homogenized liver tissue by using TRIZOL reagent (Invitrogen, Carlsbad, CA, USA) according to the manufacturer's instructions. Total RNA (1 μg) was reverse-transcribed into first-strand cDNA by using 200 units of MMLV-RT (Promega) in a total volume of 20 μl. For real-time PCR, a SYBR system with self-designed primers and 12.5 ng cDNA was used. The self-designed primers were as follows: peroxisome proliferator-activated receptor ([PPAR-α] forward: GGCTCGGAGGGCTCTGTCATC; reverse: ACATGCACTGGCAGCAGTGGA), acyl CoA oxidase ([ACOX] forward: GGATAACGGCTACCTGAAGATG; reverse: GAACAAGGTCGACAGAGGTTTAG), carnitine palmitoyl-transferase 1 ([CPT-1] forward: TATGTGAGGATGCTGCTTCC; reverse: CTCGGAGCTAAGCTTGTC), acetyl-CoA carboxylase ([ACC] forward: ACCGGCTGAGTGATGGTGG; reverse: GGGAGCGCATTACAGACGG), fatty acid synthase ([FAS] forward: GCGGCTTCTGTGCCTGTTG; reverse: TCGGCAGCCCAGGCTAAGG), and sterol regulatory element-binding transcription factor 1 ([SREBP-1] forward: ACGAGCTACCCTTCGGTGA; reverse: TGTGTCTCCTGTCTCACCCC). Amplification using 40 cycles of 2 steps (95°C for 15 s and 60°C for 1 min) was performed on an ABI Prism 7900HT sequence detection system (Foster City, CA, USA).

Determination of lipolysis rate in adipose tissues

The lipolysis rate was analyzed according to the procedure of Berger and Barnard [11]. Glycerol release from adipose tissue was expressed as the lipolysis rate. Perirenal adipose tissue was rinsed in a 0.85% NaCl solution, patted dry, and weighed. A total of 0.2 g of adipose tissue was added to 1.0 ml of prewarmed TES [N-tris (hydroxymethyl) methyl-2-aminoethanesulfonic acid] buffer (containing 1 mM isoproterenol) and incubated at 37°C for 1 hour. After incubation at 70°C for 10 minutes, the reaction mixture was centrifuged at 100 xg at room temperature for 30 s. The resulting supernatant was used to determine the glycerol concentration (Randox Diagnostic, Crumlin, UK). The lipolysis rate is expressed as μmol glycerol/g/h.

Statistical evaluation

Statistical differences among the groups were calculated by using one-way ANOVA (SAS Institute, Cary, NC, USA) and were considered to be significant at $p<0.05$, as determined by Duncan's new multiple-range test.

Results

As shown in Figure 2, during electrolysis of water, the concentration of molecular hydrogen in water bath increased with time. The concentration reached up to 1041 ppb at 8 min (Figure 2A). In contrast, the ORP value in water bath decreased with time (Figure 2B). The ORP value at 8 min was -237 mv.

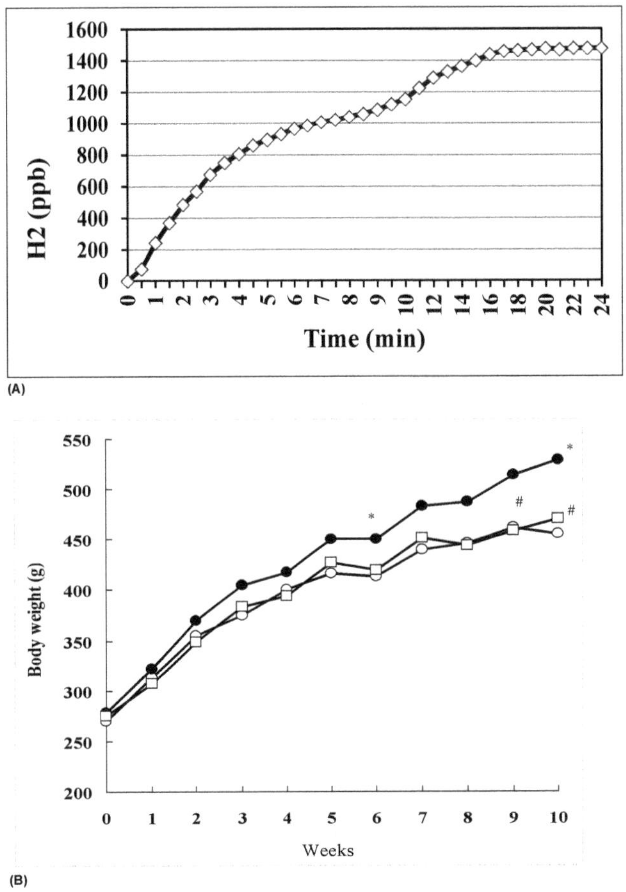

Figure 2: Changes in molecular hydrogen (H2) (A) and oxidation-reduction potential (ORP) (B) in water during electrolysis. Results are expressed as the mean of 3 determinations. The detection method is described in the Methods.

As shown in Figure 3, body weight increased in rats fed the high-fat diet compared with that in rats fed the low-fat control diet after 10 weeks of feeding ($p<0.05$). At the end of the study (11 weeks), daily food intake was lower and relative liver weight and relative epididymal and perirenal adipose tissue weights were higher in rats fed the high-fat diet than in rats fed the low-fat control diet ($p<0.05$; Table 1). ID treatment reduced ($p<0.05$) body weight and relative perirenal adipose tissue weight in rats fed the high-fat diet. There was no significant difference ($p>0.05$) in relative liver weight between the HF and HF+ID groups.

Table 2 show the plasma biochemical parameters, including glucose, insulin, total cholesterol (TC), triglyceride, HDL-cholesterol, TC/HDL-C, ALT, and HOMA values, in rats among the groups. The plasma insulin concentration and HOMA, an index of insulin resistance, were significantly higher ($p<0.05$) in the HF group than in the control group. These results indicated that rats fed the high-fat diet developed insulin resistance. However, there were no significant differences ($p>0.05$) in glucose, insulin, or HOMA values between the HF and HF+ID groups. No significant changes in plasma lipids (total cholesterol, HDL-cholesterol, triglyceride) or ALT were observed among the groups.

Figure 4 shows the histological examination of liver with H&E staining and hepatic triglyceride and cholesterol contents in rats. Rats fed the high-fat diet had significantly higher numbers of oil droplets (Figure 4B) and increased cholesterol (Figure 4D) and triglyceride (Figure 4E) contents ($p<0.05$) in liver than did animals fed the control diet. ID treatment reduced oil droplet numbers (Figure 4C) and triglyceride and cholesterol contents in rats fed the high-fat diet ($p<0.05$).

Table 3 shows the fecal excretions of cholesterol and triglyceride in rats. Rats fed the high-fat diet had significantly higher fecal cholesterol and triglyceride levels than did rats fed the low-fat control diet ($p<0.05$). There were no significant differences in fecal triglyceride and cholesterol levels between the HF and HF+ID groups ($p>0.05$).

The gene expression of *PPAR-α SREBP-1, ACOX, CPT-1, ACC*, and

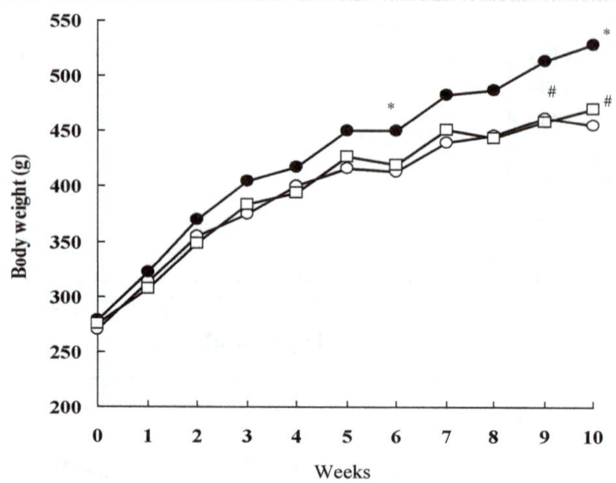

Figure 3: Effects of ID treatment on body weight gain in rats. *Significantly different from the control group at p<0.05. #Significantly different from the HF group at p<0.05. Control: normal control diet group (○); HF: high-fat diet group (●); HF+ID: high-fat diet + ID treatment group (□).

Group[b]	Control (n=4)	HF (n=6)	HF+ID (n=6)
Initial body weight (g)	270.0 ± 10.4	279.1 ± 15.1	275.8 ± 10.4
Final body weight (g)	442.0 ± 47.8	521.8 ± 51.5*	457.6 ± 32.4#
Food intake (g/day)	25.6 ± 0.2	21.1 ±0.5*	20.5 ± 0.6
Liver weight			
(g)	11.9± 1.4	18.2 ± 1.7*	15.7 ± 0.6#
(g /100 g b.w.)	2.7 ± 0.1	3.5 ± 0.1*	3.4 ± 0.2
Epididymal adipose tissue			
(g)	5.5 ± 1.9	9.1 ± 1.7*	7.4 ± 1.4#
(g /100 g b.w.)	1.2± 0.4	1.7 ± 0.2*	1.6 ± 0.3
Perirenal adipose tissue			
(g)	3.8 ± 1. 7	11.2 ± 2.8*	6.9 ± 1.9#
(g /100 g b.w.)	0.8 ± 0.3	2.1 ± 0.5*	1.5 ± 0.3#
Total adipose tissues			
(g)	9.3 ± 3.5	20.3 ± 4.1*	14.3 ± 3.0#
(g /100 g b.w.)	2.1 ± 0.7	3.9 ± 0.6*	3.1 ± 0.5#

[a] Values are mean SD of 4 to 6 rats; [b] Control: control group; HF: high-fat diet group; ID: high-fat diet with ID treatment group; * Significantly different from the Control group at *p*<0.05; # Significantly different from the HF group at *p*<0.05

Table 1: Body weight, tissue weight, and food intake in rats fed the control diet, the high-fat diet, or the high-fat diet with ID treatment[a].

Group[b]	Control (n=4)	HF (n=6)	HF+ID (n=6)
Glucose (mg/dL)	158.0 12.6	186.2 ± 51.0	172.8 ± 41.9
Insulin (µg/L)	0.2 ± 0.0	0.5 ± 0.2*	0.5 ± 0.2
Total cholesterol (mg/dL)	61.5 ± 14.4	73.0 19.0	63.5 ± 18.5
Triglyceride (mg/dL)	72.2 ± 27.4	70.2 ± 22.1	77.8 ± 21.8
HDL-cholesterol (mg/dL)	26.5 ± 2.5	23.3 ± 6.7	22.2 ± 5.1
TC/HDL-C	2.3 ± 0.3	3.2 ± 0.8	2.8 ± 0.7
ALT (U/L)	52.3 ± 6.2	48.8 ± 13.4	48.3 ± 12.1
HOMA	15.3 ± 2.9	38.3 ± 14.7*	44.3 ± 19.5

[a] Values are mean ± SD of 4 to 6 rats; [b] Control: control group; HF: high-fat diet group; HF+ID: high-fat diet with ID treatment group; * Significantly different from the Control group at *p*<0.05.

Table 2: Plasma parameters in rats fed the control diet, the high-fat diet, or the high-fat diet with ID treatment[a].

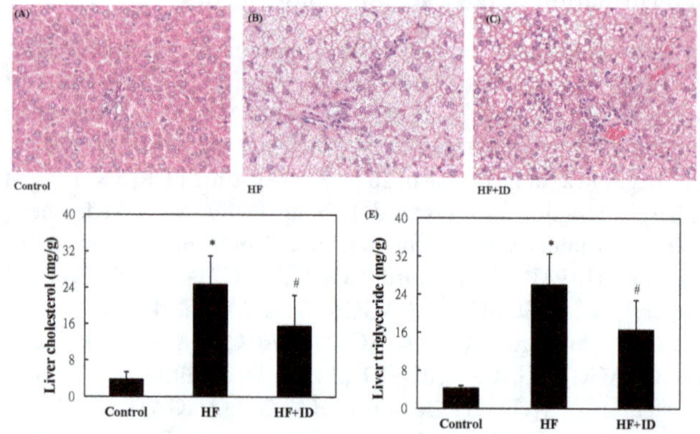

Figure 4: Histopathological alterations (A-C) and cholesterol (D) and triglyceride (E) contents in livers of rats after ID treatment. (A-C) H&E stain, 400X. (D,E) Results are expressed as mean ± SD for 4 to 6 rats. *Significantly different from the control group at p<0.05. #Significantly different from the HF group at p<0.05. Control: normal control diet group (n=4); HF: high-fat diet group (n=6); HF+ID: high-fat diet + ID treatment group (n=6).

Group[b]	Control (n=4)	HF (n=6)	HF+ ID (n=6)
Cholesterol			
(mg/g)	5.5 ± 0.2	10.4 ± 0.3*	10.4 ± 0.2
(mg/day)	51.0 ± 1.4	143.0 ± 3.5*	140.7 ± 2.6
Triglyceride			
(mg/g)	3.9 ± 0.1	5.8 ± 0.1*	5.9 ± 0.1
(mg/day)	18.1 ± 0.3	37.6 ± 1.2*	36.6 ±1.0

[a] Values are mean ± SD of 4 to 6 rats in each group; [b] Control: control group; HF: high-fat diet group; HF+ID: high-fat diet with ID treatment group; * Significantly different from the Control group at *p*<0.05.

Table 3: Fecal lipids levels in rats fed the control diet, the high-fat diet, or the high-fat diet with ID treatment[a].

FAS in liver is shown in Figure 5. In liver, FAS gene expression was significantly reduced in the HF group compared with the control group (p<0.05; Figure 5F). ID treatment further reduced (p<0.05) ACC and FAS gene expression (Figures 5E and 5F). Also, ACOX and CPT-1 gene expression was significantly reduced (p<0.05) in rats after ID treatment (Figures 5C and 5D).

Figure 6 shows the histological examination of perirenal adipose tissue with H&E staining and ACC and FAS gene expression in perirenal adipose tissue. No significant change in fat size was found among the groups (Figures 6A-6C). There were no significant differences in ACC or FAS mRNA levels (Figures 6D and 6E) between the HF and HF+ID groups (p>0.05). A higher triglyceride content and lower lipolysis rate in perirenal adipose tissue was found in rats fed the high-fat diet (p<0.05; Figures 6F and 6G). Notably, ID treatment reduced the triglyceride content and increased the lipolysis rate in perirenal adipose tissue (p<0.05).

Discussion

In this study, ID treatment was shown to reduce body weight, adiposity, and lipid accumulation in the liver of rats fed a high-fat diet. Our results also suggested that ID treatment reduced fatty acid synthesis (ACC and FAS gene expression) more significantly than fatty acid oxidation (CPT-1 and ACOX gene expression) in liver, resulting in a lower triglyceride content. A higher lipolysis rate and a lower triglyceride content were observed in perirenal adipose tissue after ID treatment, which might, at least in part, explain the anti-obesity effect.

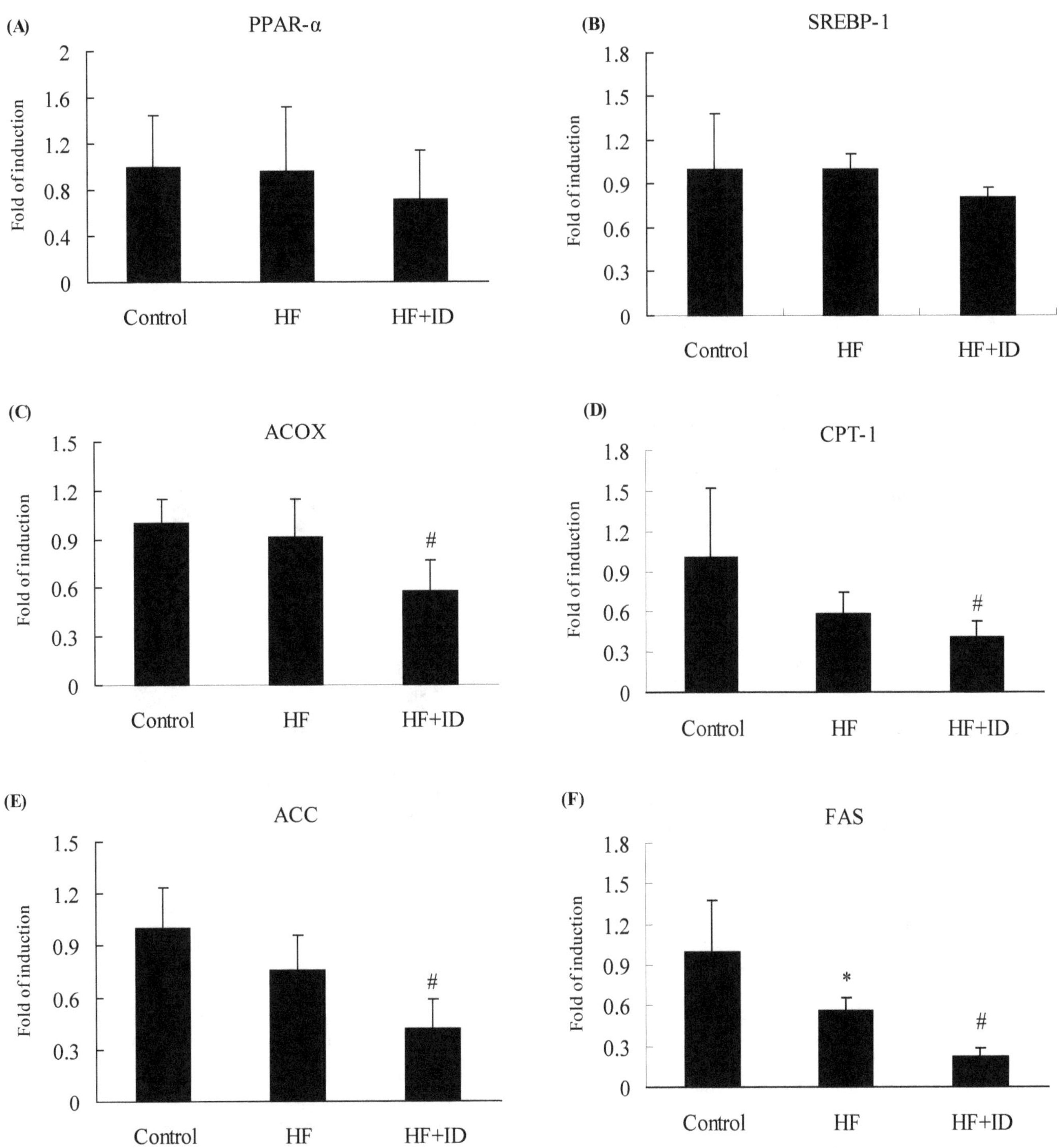

Figure 5: Changes in PPAR-α (A), SREBP-1 (B), ACOX (C), CPT-1 (D), ACC (E), and FAS (F) gene expression in rats. Results are expressed as mean ± SD for 4 to 6 rats. *Significantly different from the control group at $p<0.05$. #Significantly different from the HF group at $p<0.05$. Control: normal control diet group (n=4); HF: high-fat diet group (n=6); HF+ID: high-fat diet + ID treatment group (n=6).

In this study, regular ID treatment (3 times/week) for 11 weeks reduced the accumulation of relative adipose tissue (epididymal+perirenal; -20.1%) and body weight (-12.3%) induced by the high-fat diet. However, ID treatment had no significant effect on plasma biochemical parameters including plasma lipids, glucose, insulin resistance (HOMA), and ALT. These results indicated that ID treatment can reduce adiposity without affecting other plasma biochemical parameters in this model. In addition, daily food intake and fecal lipid excretion were not changed after ID treatment, indicating that energy intake was not affected by ID treatment. In this study, ID

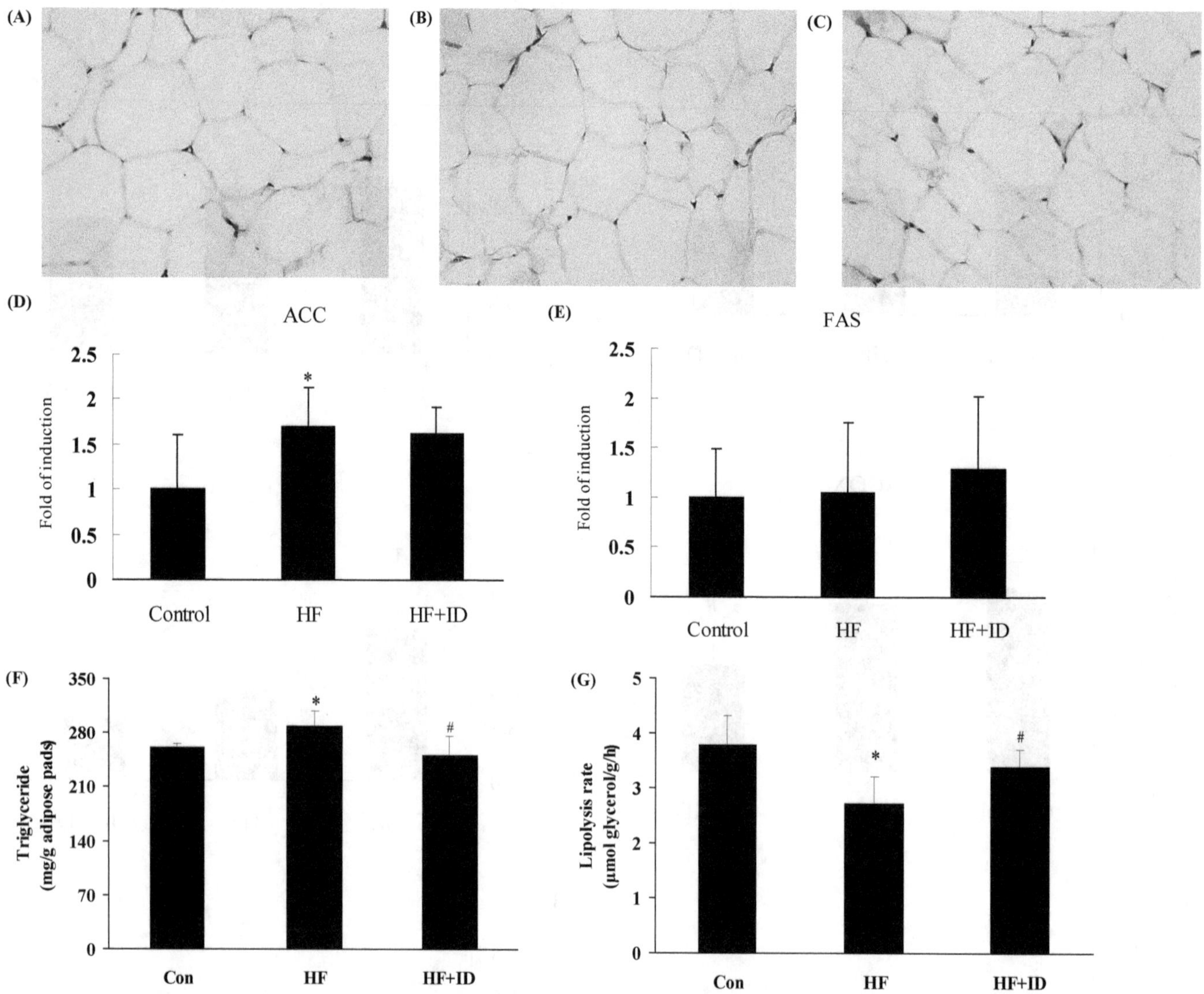

Figure 6: Histopathological examination with H&E staining (A-C), ACC and FAS gene expression (D,E), triglyceride content (F), and lipolysis rate (G) in perirenal fat pads in rats. Results are expressed as mean ± SD for 4 to 6 rats. *Significantly different from the control group at p<0.05. #Significantly different from the HF group at p<0.05. Control: normal control diet group (n=4); HF: high-fat diet group (n=6); HF+ID: high-fat diet + ID treatment group (n=6). H&E stain, 400X.

treatment had no effect on lipogenesis in perirenal adipose tissue as indicated by no change in ACC and FAS gene expression. It is therefore suggested that the reduced adiposity after ID treatment may be due to an increased lipolysis rate in perirenal adipose tissue, resulting in lower triglyceride content.

Notably, a lower hepatic triglyceride and cholesterol level were observed after ID treatment. This result indicated that ID treatment could reduce fatty liver. Geelen et al. [12] indicated that de novo fatty acid synthesis in liver could be reduced after high-fat diet feeding. In this study, rats fed the high-fat diet had reduced ACC and FAS gene expression with no changes in ACOX and CPT-1 gene expression in liver. ID treatment reduced ACC (-44.7%), FAS (-60.7%), CPT-1 (-29.3%), and ACOX (-36.2%) gene expression, indicating that ID treatment might suppress both the fatty acid synthesis and the fatty acid oxidation pathways. However, ID treatment appeared to reduce fatty acid synthesis more significantly than fatty acid oxidation. This result may explain why ID treatment can lower hepatic triglyceride content.

The human body is a conductor of electricity. In our hypothesis, during ID treatment, small positively or negatively charged molecules in the body can be moved by means of continuously transmitted microcurrents through the entire body and be attracted by the ion generator. These actions may result in a lower level of exogenous or endogenous charged molecules, thus balancing them and increasing cell detoxification. In this study, we found unknown lipids (50 mg/rat) and ammonia (0.67 mg/rat) in the bathed water after ID treatment. It is thus suggested that parts of charged molecules excreted from the body are lipophilic molecules. At physiological pH, most of the ammonia molecules are protonated (NH_4^+). Therefore, ID treatment may increase detoxification by removing small charged molecules attracted by the ion generator. Finally, the neutralized molecules were precipitated or dissolved in water with unfavorable flavors and colors (particularly in black in this study). Similar observations are also found in humans after ID treatment. Our results suggest that ID treatment may enhance cell detoxification by removing ammonia and small lipophilic charged molecules from the body. The other route of elimination of small toxic molecules during ID treatment may be possibly through forward (direct) osmosis from the microvasculature of the skin into warm water bath. Indeed, we recently found that ID treatment (bathing the rat abdominal region) reduced the hepatic activity of CYP1A1/1B1 (unpublished data), the enzyme that can be induced by various carcinogens [13]. Therefore, ID treatment may improve some metabolic disorders such as obesity and fatty liver after elimination of toxic molecules.

The other explanation for reducing adiposity and fatty liver by ID treatment may be related to the production of hydrogen-rich water (containing abundant molecular hydrogen) during the process of electrolysis (Figure 2). Hydrogen-rich water has a negative ORP value that can provide electricity to the body and lower the body's electrical potential similar to the action of grounding [4]. Molecular hydrogen is known to be the smallest molecule that can rapidly penetrate biomembranes into cells and displays antioxidant and anti-inflammation activities [14,15]. Even at low concentrations locally or throughout the whole body, molecular hydrogen can act as a signal to regulate cell function [14,16]. It has been shown that drinking hydrogen water can reduce obesity by enhanced fatty acid and glucose expenditure and stimulated energy metabolism [16]. Taking a hydrogen-rich water bath can also incorporate molecular hydrogen into the skin and distribute it throughout the body via blood flow within only 10 min [14]. Taken together, these data suggest that the reduced adiposity and fatty liver caused by regular ID treatment may be partially due to lower body electrical potential and increased molecular hydrogen uptake from the hydrogen-rich water bath.

In summary, our results showed that ID treatment may have beneficial effects on reducing adiposity through an increased lipolysis rate in adipose tissue. In addition, ID treatment may lower fatty acid synthesis and reduce fatty liver. These results may be attributed to the ability to increase the excretion of toxic or charged molecules, lower electric potential, and increase molecular hydrogen uptake during ID treatment. Further study is needed to investigate the beneficial effects of ID treatment on detoxification and metabolic disorders and the clinical applications of ID.

Acknowledgments

We are thankful for Buddha's full support. This study was financially supported by grant aid (MOST 106-2320-B-039-041-MY3) from the Ministry of Science and Technology, Taiwan.

References

1. Jamieson KS, ApSimon HM, Jamieson SS, Bell JNB, Yost MG (2007) The effects of electric fields on charged molecules and particles in individual microenvironments. Atmos Environ 41: 5224-5235.
2. Milham S (2014) Evidence that dirty electricity is causing the worldwide epidemics of obesity and diabetes. Electromagn Biol Med 33: 75-78.
3. Zheng BW, Ho WC (2013) Electromagnetic principles in cardiovascular disease development. Taiwan Crit Care Med 14: 57-60.
4. Chevalier G, Sinatra ST, Oschman JL, Sokal K, Sokal P (2012) Earthing: Health implications of reconnecting the human body to the Earth's surface electrons. J Environ Public Health 2012: 291541.
5. Oschman JL, Chevalier G, Brown R (2015) The effects of grounding (earthing) on inflammation, the immune response, wound healing, and prevention and treatment of chronic inflammatory and autoimmune diseases. J Inflamm Res 8: 83-96.
6. Ghibaudi L, Cook J, Farley C, van Heek M, Hwa JJ (2002) Fat intake affects adiposity, comorbidity factors, and energy metabolism of Sprague-Dawley rats. Obes Res 10: 956-963.
7. Drury AR, Wallington EA (1980) Carleton's Histological Techniques. 5th ed., Oxford University Press, London, UK.
8. Matthews DR, Hosker JP, Rudenski AS, Naylor BA, Treacher DF, et al. (1985) Homeostasis model assessment: Insulin resistance and beta-cell function from fasting plasma glucose and insulin concentrations in man. Diabetologia 28: 412-419.
9. Folch J, Lees M, Sloane-Stanley GM (1957) A purification of total lipid from animal tissue. J Biol Chem 226: 497-509.
10. Carlson SE, Goldfarb S (1977) A sensitive enzymatic method for determination of free and esterified tissue cholesterol. Clin Chim Acta 79: 575-582.
11. Berger JJ, Barnard RJ (1999) Effect of diet on fat cell size and hormone-sensitive lipase activity. J Appl Physiol 87: 227-232.
12. Geelen SN, Blázquez C, Geelen MJ, Sloet van Oldruitenborgh-Oosterbaan MM, Beynen AC (2008) High fat intake lowers hepatic fatty acid synthesis and raises fatty acid oxidation in aerobic muscle in Shetland ponies. Br J Nutr 86: 31-36.
13. Shimada T, Oda Y, Gillam EM, Guengerich FP, Inoue K (2001) Metabolic activation of polycyclic aromatic hydrocarbons and other procarcinogens by cytochromes P450 1A1 and P450 1B1 allelic variants and other human cytochromes P450 in Salmonella typhimurium NM2009. Drug Metab Dispos 29: 1176-1182.
14. Ichihara M, Sobue S, Ito M, Ito M, Hirayama M, et al. (2015) Beneficial biological effects and the underlying mechanisms of molecular hydrogen-comprehensive review of 321 original articles. Med Gas Res 5: 12.
15. Ohta S (2012) Molecular hydrogen is a novel antioxidant to efficiently reduce oxidative stress with potential for the improvement of mitochondrial diseases. Biochim Biophys Acta 1820: 586-594.
16. Kamimura N, Nishimaki K, Ohsawa I, Ohta S (2011) Molecular hydrogen improves obesity and diabetes by inducing hepatic FGF21 and stimulating energy metabolism in db/db mice. Obesity (Silver Spring) 19: 1396-1403.

22

Meteorosensitivity in a Group of Patients Affected by Multiple Sclerosis and Hospitalized in a Rehabilitation Facility

Lorenzo Freti[1], Vincenzo Condemi[1*], Marianna Mazza[2], Marco Di Nicola[2], Luigi Janiri[2], Andrea Antonietti[3], Massimo Gestro[1] and Umberto Solimene[1]

[1]*Department of Biomedical Sciences for Health-State University of Milan; Via Mangiagalli 31, Milan, Italy*
[2]*Istitute of Psychiatry and Clinical Psychology, Catholic University of Sacred Heart, Largo A. Gemelli 8, Rome, Italy*
[3]*Fondazione Don Gnocchi Onlus, IRCCS Santa Maria Nascente Centre; Via Alfonso Capecelatro 66, Milan, Italy*

Abstract

Background: In the recent decades, the relationship between psycho-physical disorders and weather conditions has taken on an increased scientific solidity. Furthermore, it is known to every clinician that healthcare practice has an important role in the management of psycho-physical disorders of patients affected by multiple sclerosis. Given that meteorosensitivity is related to the psycho-physical feebleness, this study is an attempt to clarify if treatments in a non-acute care rehabilitation centre can reduce the meteorosensitivity in patients with multiple sclerosis.

Methods: In the spring 2014, 42 patients with MS, at Fondazione Don Gnocchi Santa Maria Nascente Centre (Milan, Italy), were observed by two evaluations (initial and final). The initial evaluation was the administration of METEO-Q, a questionnaire able to quantify the meteorosensitivity degree of the subjects, and Beck Depression Inventory-II, mainly. For each patient, passed one month, the final evaluation was carried out with the same modalities.

Results: A statistically significant difference was found between initial and final meteorosensitivity degree (P=0.01), with better scores in final evaluations for most of the subjects. The correlation between Beck Depression Inventory-II and meteorosensitivity degree resulted significant and positive (R=0.377; P=0.001) and it confirms the link between psycho-physical feebleness and meteorosensitivity. Finally, no significant correlation emerged between initial meteorosensitivity degree and body mass index (R=0.187; P=0.236).

Conclusions: This study confirms the possibility of improving meteorosensitivity, probably by rehabilitation too. Future studies could clarify the effects of health care practice on meteorosensitivity.

Keywords: Multiple sclerosis; Rehabilitation; Biometeorology; Complementary therapies; Depression

Abbreviations: MS: Multiple Sclerosis; MTS: Meteorosensitivity or Meteorosensitive; MD: Meteorosensitivity Degree; SR: Daily Average Solar Radiation; T: Daily Average Temperature; RH: Daily Average Relative Humidity; QS: METEO-Q Scores, Δ: Variation (final value - initial value).

Introduction

Multiple sclerosis (MS) is a demyelinating, chronic, inflammatory and autoimmune disease, with progressive course. It affects the white matter, and less the grey matter, in the Central Nervous System [1]. In the world, it has an incidence of 7:100.000 cases/year, each person has 1:400 chances to get it over lifetime and its onset occurs typically between 20 and 40 years old [2].

In patients with MS, a cellular and humoral immunity disorder produces disseminated injuries of nervous tissue, known as demyelinating plaques. They generally happen during critical episodes, defined as exacerbations. During an exacerbation phase, a worsening of neurological clinical picture usually occurs. In most of patients, it can regress with different degrees (remission phase) and tend to repeat over the next years. Often, remissions become smaller than exacerbations, until the worsening of neurological picture become constant [3]. It could cause different symptoms such as motor, sensory, or visual impairment, fatigue, bowel, bladder, and sexual dysfunctions [4]. MS can also determine the onset of cognitive impairments [5] and psychiatric symptoms, mainly depression [6]. For these reasons, patients with MS can be psycho-physically feeble.

Nowadays, meteorosensitivity (MTS) is no longer considered as a suggestion derived from popular myths, but it is studied by medical biometeorology. It is defined as the susceptibility of the subject to the action of one or more meteorological phenomena. They can cause physical and psychic upsets or exacerbations of preexisting symptoms. Therefore, meteorosensitive subjects reveal some difficulties to solve physical and psychic perturbations generated by physical energy of meteorological events. For these reasons, MTS can be considered as a "general adaptation syndrome", because it is linked to the daily stress management. The action of meteorological factors and other stressor events can make difficult to maintain the physiological variables balanced. When the limits of homeostatic compensation are overstepped, several somatoform disorders can develop. Therefore, the ability to manage stress represents an important prognostic factor. In fact, psycho-physical reactivity can reach a compensation state in order to successfully face meteorological stressor events [7].

Amongst the weather factors able to influence psyche, brightness is the most studied. It influences the vivacity of psycho-physical reactions by conditioning specific neuroendocrine mechanisms

***Corresponding author:** Vincenzo Condemi, Department of Biomedical Sciences for Health-State University of Milan; Via Mangiagalli 31, 20133-Milan, Italy, E-mail: vincenzo.condemi@unimi.it

involved in circadian and circannual rhythms. The two last editions of the Diagnostic and Statistical Manual of Mental Disorders recognize a disorder in which people become depressed in a certain period of the year, such as winter and summer, the Seasonal Affective Disorder (SAD) [8]. SAD seems to be related to latitude [9], in fact one of the causes of SAD is the variation in hours of daily sunshine [10]. Moreover, several trials show an efficacy of bright light on depressive symptomatology in non-seasonal depression [11]. Weather factors seem to be related also to both attempted and completed suicides with a non-seasonal pattern [12]. Other conditions, such as anxiety [13], concentration reductions [14] and aggressions [15] seem to show a significant meteorotropism.

The other strongest evidences regard the combined action of high and low temperatures and humidity on cardiovascular and musculoskeletal systems [16,17].

Therefore, it is appropriate to consider patients with MS as particularly meteorosensitive subjects and to choose MS for the study of MTS.

Patients affected by MS are susceptible especially to relatively high temperature. This condition is known as Uhthoff's phenomenon. It is a disorder of neurological functions that is stereotyped, short in duration (less than 24 hours), reversible and related to recurrent fluctuations in axonal conduction properties. These acute changes can be linked to various antecedent triggering factors, all of which are associated in some way with an increase in core body temperature. The main causal factors are high environmental temperature, fever, physical exercise, hot baths or showers, increase of psychological stress and perimenstrual period [18].

Medical Biometeorology's approach to disease is the same as Eastern medicine [19]. As explained previously, right mental behaviours can avoid a psycho-physical imbalance, reach a compensation state in order to successfully face stressor events and consequently avoid physical disease. That is why psychological assistance and/or meditation are essential for the eradication of meteorosensitivity. Some symptomatological therapies are also possible and already adopted. They are physical and bioenergetics techniques; Reiki, acupuncture, homeopathy and phytotherapy are peculiar examples. In different ways, they act by stimulating the physiological organic reactions [20].

Moreover, climatotherapy, that uses the positive action exercised by the climate of specific places, could represent an option to be investigated better.

Finally, healthcare practice has also an important role in the management of psycho-physical disorders of patients [21]. Therefore, it is logical to wonder whether the clinical-rehabilitation practice can represent a symptomatological care for meteorosensitivity. The main purpose of this study is to provide some clarifications of this issue, taking in exam a sample of patients affected by multiple sclerosis.

Material and Methods

Subjects

Patients with MS flocking to Fondazione Don Gnocchi, Santa Maria Nascente Centre (Milan-Italy) were selected according to specific inclusion/exclusion criteria. After the inclusion/exclusion procedures, 42 patients (female=28% to 67.7%; male=14% to 33.3%) were observed. In this rehabilitation centre, generally people are recovered with no exacerbation of disease in course. Therefore, their permanence in the structure could be also a temporary interruption of their chaotic race of everyday life, because they receive assistance from the health workers and socialize with other people with MS.

Inclusion/exclusion criteria

The following patients with MS were included in the study:

a) with no current exacerbation, for assessing only people with a stable clinical condition;

b) regardless the clinical picture (Kurtzke's EDSS and MS type), because, given the study protocol and methods, they were not considered as important elements;

c) with a normal adjusted score (≥ 24) of Mini Mental State Examination (MMSE), Measso et al. version (22), for selecting only people able to answer suitably to questionnaires;

d) whose treatment cycle lasted for at least a month;

e) that finished the previous rehabilitation cycle for more than one month before the initial evaluation. Thus, this period can be compared with the observation month.

Evaluation scales

For patient inclusion and exclusion, MMSE, Measso et al. [22] version was employed.

For patient evaluation, the following scales were employed:

a) Beck Depression Inventory-II (BDI-II), for the evaluation of depressive symptoms and behavioural characteristics of depression [23,24].

b) METEO-Q questionnaire, for establishing the meteorosensitivity degree (MD) of the subject (Questionnaire 1). It is a self-assessment questionnaire recently developed and validated with an excellent internal consistency: Cronbach's α (items 1-5) = 0,81 and Cronbach's α (items 6-11) = 0,87 [25]. It is composed of two groups of items (1-5 and 6-11) and one checklist. Each group of items, independently from the other, allows determining the MD of the subject. The only other available statistic about METEO-Q is an accuracy of 0,73 in a sample of bipolar subjects and 0,68 in a sample of healthy subjects [26]. The METEO-Q questionnaire analyses all the main symptoms usually correlated to weather/climatic conditions. In fact, this study does not examine a specific symptom, even if patients with MS usually refer some typical upsets.

Study protocol

In the spring 2014, each admitted patient was included/excluded according to the inclusion/exclusion criteria. On the day of his entry, each patient was evaluated (initial evaluation). The initial evaluation was:

a) Administration of BDI-II;

b) Administration of METEO-Q;

c) Registration of subjects' height and weight, used for the body mass index (BMI) calculation.

After one month from initial evaluation, the final one was carried out with the same modalities. About the administration modalities of METEO-Q, some clarifications (specific of this case) need to be done. In METEO-Q instructions, there are not specific indications about a temporal parameter to which patient should refer to during the answers. Therefore, a time frame of 1 month was chosen: patients

METEO-Q questionnaire

(Mazza M., Di Nicola M., Janiri L.)

Name…………………. Date of Birth………….. Date of Evaluation…………………..

For every item attribute a score as the following legend:
0 = absent, 1 = light, 2 = moderate, 3 = considerable, 4 = serious.

1) Variations of mood in relation to the change of latitude, the geographic zone, the jet leg. [ ]
Specify induced modifications………………………………………………………

2) Variations of mood in relation to atmospheric changes (ex.: when it begins or when it stops raining, when it is cloudy, when it is sunny or when the sun suddenly goes down, when humidity increases). [ ]
Specify induced modifications………………………………………………………

3) Variations of mood in relation to the brightness of the sky (when days are more or less luminous or when days "grow tall" or "they are shortened" according to the seasons). [ ]
Specify induced modifications………………………………………………………

4) Variations of mood caused by the temperature changes (warmer or colder days). [ ]
Specify induced modifications………………………………………………………

5) Mood changes caused by the seasons changing. [ ]
Specify induced modifications………………………………………………………

6) Indicate the degree of relation between the set in symptomatology and the climatic or atmospheric change. [ ]

7) Tendency of these disturbs to minimize or disappear when the triggering condition stops or when an opposite environmental condition comes up. [ ]

8) Eventual coincidence of these disturbs with other cyclical phenomena (ex.: menstrual cycle). [ ]

9) Presence of prodromical symptoms few days before the climatic modifications (irritability, weariness…). [ ]

10) Interference with daily activities due to disturbs induced by climatic changes. [ ]

11) Uneasiness feelings induced by climatic changes. [ ]

Metereopathy Checklist

Indicate the disturbs related to meteorological changes that you mostly frequently experience.
For every voice mark: absent = 0, light = 1, moderate = 2, considerable = 3, severe = 4.

- lability of mood; (oscillations of mood within a day or few more days)	0 1 2 3 4
- extreme reactivity to external events;	0 1 2 3 4
- depression;	0 1 2 3 4
- anxiety;	0 1 2 3 4
- asthenia;	0 1 2 3 4
- lack of appetite, anhedonia;	0 1 2 3 4
- irritability, nervousness;	0 1 2 3 4
- indefinite feeling of malaise;	0 1 2 3 4
- vague pain, articular pain, muscular pain ;	0 1 2 3 4
- vertigos;	0 1 2 3 4
- headache;	0 1 2 3 4
- nausea;	0 1 2 3 4
- alterations of the cardiac rhythm (tachycardia);	0 1 2 3 4
- difficulty with concentration;	0 1 2 3 4
- insomnia;	0 1 2 3 4
- excessive sleepiness;	0 1 2 3 4
- lack of appetite;	0 1 2 3 4
- excessive appetite;	0 1 2 3 4
- digestion's disfunctions; (meteorism, belches, acidity, flatulence, irritable colon)	0 1 2 3 4
- alterations of sexuality; (lack of desire or on the contrary hyperactivity)	0 1 2 3 4
- weakness during working activities.	0 1 2 3 4
Other:………………………………………………………...	0 1 2 3 4

TOTAL SCORE ITEMS 1-5: x =

TOTAL SCORE ITEMS 6-11: x =

CUT-OFF SCORES

Male

	Low sensitivity	Medium sensitivity	High sensitivity	Meteoropathy
Items 1-5	x<2	3<x<5	6<x<8	x>9
Items 6-11	x<2	3<x<4	5<x<7	x>8

Female

	Low sensitivity	Medium sensitivity	High sensitivity	Meteoropathy
Items 1-5	x<4	5<x<7	8<x<10	x>11
Items 6-11	x<3	4<x<6	7<x<10	x>11

Questionnaire 1: METEO-Q questionnaire and its instructions and cut-off scores.

were asked to refer to their condition of the previous month. This has the aim of making the initial and final METEO-Q scores comparable. Furthermore:

a. Items 1-5 were not administered, because they are related to conditions considered unchangeable during the interval between initial and final evaluations;

b. As explained previously, items 6-11 are sufficient for assessing MTS;

c. Patients tried to evaluate especially air temperature, solar radiation and humidity influences. This choice is explained in the following paragraph.

During initial and final evaluations, patient's treatments were not influenced.

Once collected all data, the necessary statistical calculations were performed (see "Statistical methods").

Because initial evaluations were not carried out all on the same day, the subjects have not been exposed precisely to the same weather factors and this is a methodological problem. This point was partially engaged by considering some meteorological data (revealed by the State University of Milan's meteorological station) in the statistical methodology.

Climatological database and geo-demographic characteristics

The climatological database was released by State University of Milan from February to June 2014. The following meteorological parameters were considered: solar radiation (SR), daily average temperature (T) and relative humidity (RH), because they are the only ones that can influence also the indoor environment of the structure that is devoid of air conditioning.

Milan (45°27′50.98″N 9°11′25.21″E), the second-most populous city in Italy, serves as the capital of Lombardy. Milan's climate is similar to much of northern Italy's inland plains, where hot, sunny summers and moderately cold, wet and foggy winters prevail. The spring season (March-May) is characterized by strong weather variability: in March it may happen some snow, while in May temperatures >30°C are possible.

Statistical methods

Preliminarily, the Shapiro-Wilk test was applied with the aim of verifying the normality of distributions. After having pointed out the non-normality of data distributions, non-parametric tests were chosen to verify if:

a. a significant difference between initial and final MD was present (intra-group difference);

b. a significant correlation between BDI-II scores and MD was present;

c. a significant correlation between initial MD and BMI was present.

The answer to question (a) represents the main purpose of this study.

Questions (b) and (c) were engaged with the aim of providing some additional data on MTS study.

To answer question (a), Wilcoxon signed-ranked test was applied. In this case the comparison was made between initial and final METEO-Q scores (QS). To answer questions (b) and (c), Spearman's rank correlation coefficient was applied. For question (b) the Spearman's rank correlation coefficient application was carried out without discerning between initial and final evaluation. Instead, for question (c) it was carried out between initial QS and the BMI of each patient.

The same test was employed for engaging the meteorological matter previously described in "Study protocol". Through Spearman's rank correlation coefficient, the MD variation (Δ=final score-initial score) was compared with ΔT and ΔSR. In so doing, it is possible to obtain a clue about if ΔMD is due to the health care practice, rather than the passage to a more favourable meteorological condition. RH was not considered in statistical methodology, because it has not an approximately linear trend over time (see "4. Discussion").

All statistical significance levels were posed to p=0.05 and all confidence intervals to 95%.

For Shapiro-Wilk test application the statistical software R was employed. Descriptive statistics calculations and the several non-parametric tests were carried out through the statistical software SPSS.

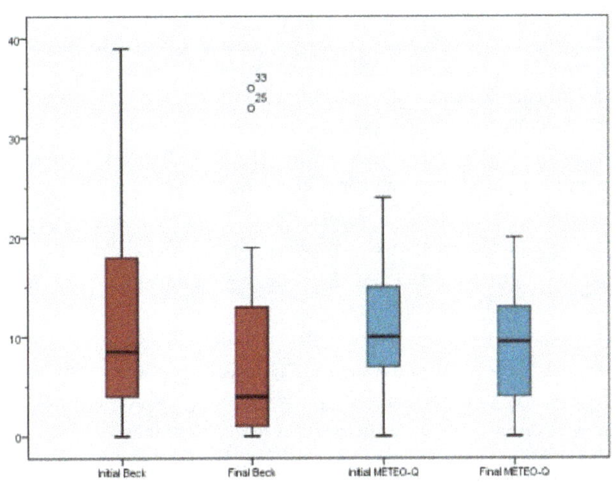

Figure 1: Boxplots constructed with raw data, both initial and final, obtained by the administration of the evaluation scales to the patients.

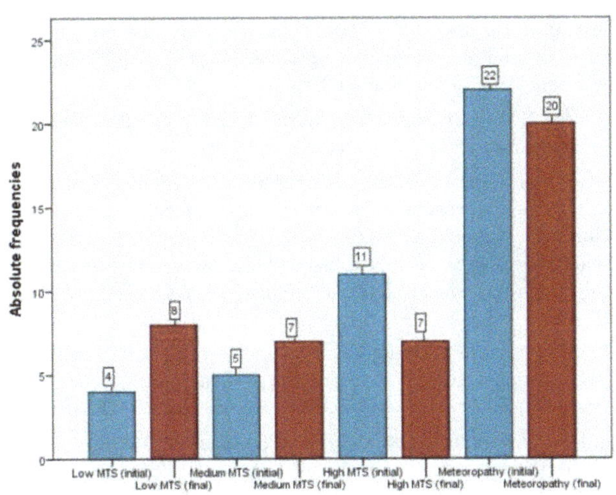

Figure 2: Absolute frequencies of the several METEO-Q cut off scores. The blue bars represent initial evaluations, while the red bars the final ones.

Results

According to the position and distribution measures and to the analysis of frequencies, it is possible to assert that a general decrease of all evaluation scores occurred. Graphic visualization of data distributions is possible by observing Figure 1. How data frequencies related to METEO-Q varied passing from initial to final evaluation is represented in Figure 2. After Wilcoxon signed-ranked test application, a statistically significant difference was observed (p=0.01).

Through Spearman's rank correlation coefficient, the only statistically significant correlation observed was between BDI-II and MD (R=0.377; p=0.001). Instead, as shown in Table 1, the other correlations were not statistically significant. Finally, Figure 3 shows the trend of daily T and SR passing from 1st February to 30th June 2014. In this figure RH was not considered because it has constant daily variation.

Comparisons	R	p
MD and BDI-II	0.377	0.001**
MD and B.M.I.	0.187	0.236
ΔMD and ΔT	-0.155	0.327
ΔMD and ΔSR	0.063	0.693

*: correlation is significant to level 0.05 (two tails); **: correlation is significant to level 0.01 (two tails)

Table 1: Rho correlation coefficients (R) and p-values (p) resulted from the comparisons between the variables considered.

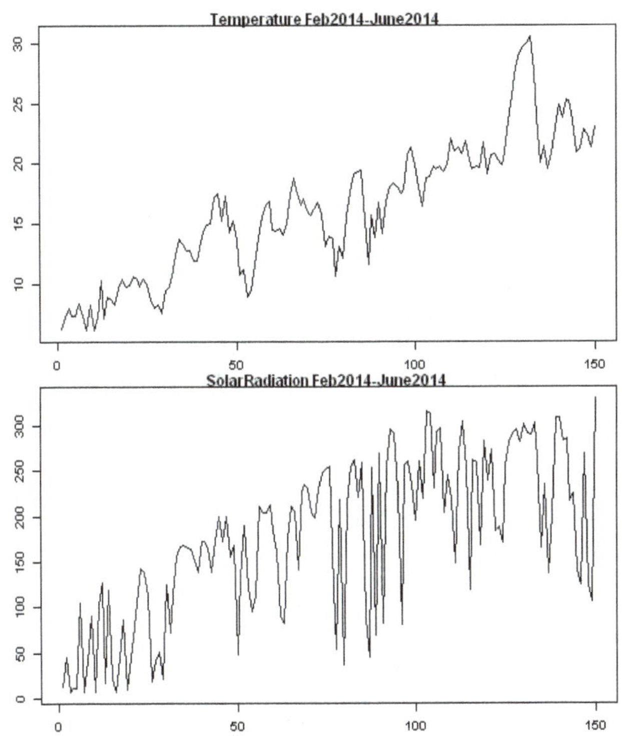

Figure 3: The trend of daily T and SR passing from 1st February to 30th June 2014.

Discussion

The observed decrease of BDI-II scores is an index of depression improvement in most of the patients. Final QS also were resulted generally lower than the initial ones. In fact, the correlation between BDI-II scores and MD was resulted positive (R>0) and statistically significant. It means these variables are related: according to this result, considering MTS in conjunction with psycho-physical feebleness seems to be suitable.

The main question of this study is the first one posed. The difference between initial and final QS was resulted statistically significant. It means that MTS improvement was not due to chance. However, it is not possible to precisely establish to what factor/s it is imputable to, because of the absence of a control group in the statistical methodology and the difficulty to exclude that it is due to the passage to a more favorable meteorological condition. Given that no significant correlation about the meteorological issue resulted, there is a tendency to think that, in this specific case, the influence on MD is due more to health care practice. However, the control group is essential for more suitable results. This thought can be extended with more certainty only to T and SR, whose values increased nearly linearly passing from March to May in Milan (Figure 3).

The last comparison was not resulted statistically significant. Considering this sample, BMI does not seem to be related to MD. More studies are necessary; in fact the excessive or insufficient BMI indicates a psycho-physical feebleness and therefore MTS.

These are reflections on results obtained in a study for which some methodological limits are present. They are due to the impossibility:

a. to perform a blind or a double-blind study;

b. to consider patient's memory and perceptions surely reliable;

c. to consider bigger samples of patients;

d. to consider daily variation of meteorological variables;

e. to consider the micro-climate indoor conditions (even if air conditioning was not present).

Conclusions

The present study demonstrates that MTS is a modifiable condition, maybe through health care practice.

For this practice the approach to patient is crucial too. The official medicine tends to consider the human being in his physical part and it gives no relevance to his psychic and moral aspects. This vision could not be enough in treating several pathologies, such as some psychosomatic diseases or MTS itself. They need a different approach, which considers also the action of the psyche on the human body. In order to ensure a more complete attention to the patient, our suggestion to health professionals, although into the limit of own professional competences and complementarily to the traditional cares, is to educate patients to acquire more correct mental approaches towards several life situations. In other words, our suggestion is to abide by bio-psycho-social model, based as much as possible on collaborative care. The health care professional should be more aware about the connections between mind and body and became a guide for those patients who want to find their road to a life of wealth. This approach should be adopted in future studies on MTS, for which this study could represent a starting point. Considering the methodological limits previously cited, further studies are necessary with the aim of clarifying the effects of health care practice on MTS, for example taking in exam some bigger groups of patient and a control group not subject to any treatment.

Acknowledgments

We thank Fondazione Don Gnocchi, Santa Maria Nascente Center, especially Dr. Angelo Montesano's Service of Outpatient Rehabilitation and Dr. Marco Rovaris's Unit of Neuromotor Rehabilitation and Multiple Sclerosis Centre, for the availability and support they shown us. For the same reasons we also thank the participants involved in this study.

References

1. Compston A, Coles A (2002) Multiple sclerosis. Lancet 359: 1221-1231.
2. Weinshenker BG, Bass B, Rise GP, Noseworthy J, Carriere W, et al. (1989) The natural history of multiple sclerosis: a geographically based study, 2. Predictive value of the early clinical course. Brain 112: 1419-1428.
3. Confavreux C, Vukusic S, Moreau T, Adeleine P (2000) Relapses and progression of disability in multiple sclerosis. New Engl J Med 343: 1430-1438.
4. Nomjooyan F, Ghanavati R, Majdinasab N, Jokari S, Janbozorgi M (2014) Uses of complementary and alternative medicine in multiple sclerosis. J Tradit Complement Med 4: 145-152.
5. Schoonheim MM, Meijer KA, Geurts JJ (2015) Network collapse and cognitive impairment in multiple sclerosis. Front Neurol 6: 82.
6. Sarısoy G, Terzi M, Gümüş K, Pazvantoğlu O (2013) Psychiatric symptoms in patients with multiple sclerosis. Gen Hosp Psychiat 35: 134-140.
7. Solimene U, Brugnoli A (2000) Meteorologia e climatologia medica. Tempo, clima e salute. Mediamed, Rome.
8. American Psychiatric Association (2013) Diagnostic and Statistical Manual of Mental Disorders (5thedn) American Psychiatric Association, Washington.
9. Kegel M, Dam H, Ali F, Bjerregaard P (2009) The prevalence of seasonal affective disorder (SAD) in Greenland is related to latitude. Nord J Psychiat 63: 331-335.
10. McWilliams S, Kinsella A, O'Callaghan E (2014) Daily weather variables and affective disorder admissions to psychiatric hospitals. Int J Biometeorol 58: 2045-2057.
11. Martiny K (2004) Adjunctive bright light in non-seasonal major depression. Acta Psychiat Scand 425: 7-28.
12. Deisenhammer EA (2003) Weather and suicide: The present state of knowledge on the association of meteorological factors with suicidal behaviour. Acta Psychiat Scand 108: 402-409.
13. Bulbena A, Pailhez G, Aceña R, Cunillera J, Rius A, et al. (2005) Panic anxiety, under the weather? Int J Biometeorol 49: 238-243.
14. Pelagatti MM, Fuà D, Galliani C, Condemi V (2006) Statistical investigation on the relation between car accidents and warm katabatic winds. Nuovo Cimento C 29: 229-235.
15. Butke P, Sheridan SC (2010) An analysis of the relationship between weather and aggressive crime in Cleveland, Ohio. Weather, Climate, and Society 2: 127-139.
16. Yu W, Mengersen K, Wang X, Ye X, Guo Y, et al. (2012) Daily average temperature and mortality among the elderly: A meta-analysis and systematic review of epidemiological evidence. Int J Biometeorol 56: 569-581.
17. Strusberg I, Mendelberg RC, Serra HA, Strusberg AM (2002) Influence of weather conditions on rheumatic pain. J Rheumatol 29: 335-338.
18. Frohman TC, Davis LS, Beh S, Greenberg MB, Remington G, et al. (2013) Uhthoff's phenomena in MS-clinical features and pathophysiology. Nat Rev Neurol 9: 535-540.

19. Cheng YC (2015) Opportunities for traditional Chinese medicine to address unmet challenges in modern healthcare. J Tradit Complement Med 7: 2-4.

20. Solimene U, Brugnoli A, Minelli E (2002) Meteoropatie. Le condizioni atmosferiche che influiscono sulla salute e sull'umore. Red edizioni, Novara.

21. Van der Ploeg HP, Streppel KR, van der Beek AJ, van der Woude LH, van Harten WH, et al. (2008) Underlying mechanisms of improving physical activity behavior after rehabilitation. Int J Behav Med 15: 101-108.

22. Measso G, Cavarzeran F, Zappalà G, Barry DL, Thomas HC, et al. (1993) The mini mental state examination: Normative study of an Italian random sample. Dev Neuropsychol 9: 77-85.

23. Beck AT, Brown GK, Steer RA (1996) Manual for the Beck Depression Inventory-II. The Psychological Corporation, San Antonio.

24. http://www.rehabmeasures.org/Lists/RehabMeasures/PrintView.aspx?ID=904

25. Mazza M, Di Nicola M, Catalano V, Callea A, Martinotti G, et al. (2012) Description and validation of a questionnaire for the detection of meteoropathy and meteorosensitivity: The METEO-Q. Compr Psychiat 53: 103-106.

26. Janiri L, Spinetti G, Mazza M, Di Nicola M (2009) Meteoropathy. A new disease. In: Christodoulou G, Jorge M, Mezzich J, editors. Advances in Psychiatry. Beta Medical Publishers, Athens, p. 45-52.

Study of Patient Satisfaction with Persian Medicine in Referrals to *Behesht* Persian Medicine Clinic of Iran University of Medical Sciences in 2016

Hoorieh Mohammadi Kenari[1], Maryam Taqavi Shirazi[1], Rozita Jafari[2] and Maryam Moghimi[3*]

[1]*Research Institute for Islamic and Complementary Medicine, Iran University of Medical Sciences, Tehran, Iran*

[2]*School of Health Management and Information Sciences, Iran University of Medical Sciences, Tehran, Iran*

[3]*Persian Medicine Offices of Ministry of Health and Medical Education, Tehran, Iran*

Abstract

Background: Today, complementary and alternative medicine and a variety of traditional medicine, along with conventional medicine, are used to prevent and treat diseases. In Iran, Persian medicine is taught academically and its services are being provided to patients. The aim of this study is to evaluate the patient satisfaction with Persian medicine and the reasons for follow up or non-follow-up of treatment by patients referred to *Behesht* Persian medicine clinic of Iran university of Medical Sciences.

Methods: 394 cases were selected among patients who were treated by Persian medicine in the *Behesht* clinic in 2016. After extracting the data, a semi structured questionnaire regarding the degree of satisfaction with the treatment and the reasons for follow up or non-follow up of the patients was completed by making phone calls with participants. Data were then analyzed using software (Microsoft Excel 2016).

Results: Women were referred to the Persian medicine clinic more than men (72.5% versus 27.5%). The most common causes of referral were gastrointestinal diseases (15.1%) and musculoskeletal disorders (13.5%). 35% of the patients referred only once and did not follow the treatment. The most common causes of non-referral were the patient's own lack of attention to taking medication and follow-up (24.2%), disease recovery (23%), lack of appropriate response to treatment (20.8%) and relocation of the therapist (11.6%). 91.4% of participants did not mention any complications and 95.84% were satisfied with the behavior of doctors. Overall, 82.6% of patients had a tendency to recurrent referral to the clinic.

Conclusion: Despite the problems with referral of patients to the Persian medicine clinic, there is a high inclining rate that reflects the satisfaction of the treatment. Therefore, planning to solve existing problems and facilitating the referral of patients can increase the satisfaction rate of Persian medicine. More studies are needed in other Persian medicine centers to evaluate patients' satisfaction.

Keywords: Persian medicine; Patient satisfaction; Referral; Treatment

Introduction

Today, complementary and alternative medicine and a variety of traditional medicine, along with conventional medicine, are used to treat and restore health to sick people and prevent disease in healthy people or to enhance the quality of life, which is evidence of a promising future in this area [1,2]. Given that conventional therapies are based on traditional methods in health care systems, there is an increasing need to study and evaluate the effectiveness of these treatments [3]. On the other hand, since traditional medicine, complementary or alternative therapies have been formed in different cultures and different regions, their standards and methods of assessment, both at the national and international levels; have not been sufficiently developed [4].

Persian Medicine consists of the sum total of all the knowledge and practices used in diagnosis, prevention and elimination of diseases in Persia from ancient times to present. It seems that Persian scholars first conceived the theory of humors and then it became a world wild theme of medicine later. This theory was based on four humors including blood, phlegm, black bile and yellow bile which were the basis of diagnosis and treatment in that time [5]. Persian medicine is now provided in Iran by physicians who have passed the course of conventional medicine and can approach to the patient after considering his/her attitude and consent about the treatment method. Dealing with conventional medicine, Persian medicine can solve many health and medical problems, due to the history of several hundred years and high capacity of prevention and treatment [6].

In Persian medicine, in addition to abundant books containing valuable experiences of Iranian scholars that has been transmitted and used from generation to generation, in many references, examples of case reports or case series are available [7-9]. However, the important point in health systems is evidence gathering in certain frameworks and preferably randomized clinical trial studies. Unfortunately, the effects and responses to treatment in many cases of Persian medicine are not well understood in these frameworks, and research on their therapeutic effects is under development. Also, the limitations of the research method, such as low sample size, inappropriate control and

***Corresponding author:** Maryam Moghimi, Persian Medicine Office of Ministry of Health and Medical Education, Tehran, Iran, E-mail: mmoghimi60@yahoo.com

non-specific interventions, prevent the extension of the results [10-12]. Critics of complementary medicine also insist on the lack of evidence to support these therapies [13,14].

In Iran, in recent years, there have been many studies about the impact and effectiveness of Persian medicine fundamentals and treatments, some of which have led to confirmation, and some have rejected these outlooks [15-32].

Since Persian medicine is nowadays academic in Iran, it is essential to validate, assess and evaluate what is presented. Since it has not been a long time that this course entered the university, research in this field requires guidance and prioritization for a variety of topics. Also, despite the significant development of the use of traditional medicine around the world, measuring the efficiency and benefits of traditional therapies is important for health care providers and health policymakers. In this article, which can initiate the next extensive studies, the patient satisfaction with Persian medicine and the reasons for follow up or non-follow-up of treatment by patients referred to *Behesht* Persian medicine clinic of Iran university of Medical Sciences is discussed.

Materials and Methods

This study was conducted at *Behesht* Persian Medicine clinic of Iran University of Medical Sciences in Tehran.

394 cases were randomly examined from patients who were visited in *Behesht* clinic in 2016. The first visit documents were reviewed for each patient and the following data were extracted:

- Demographic characteristics
- The patient's chief complaint
- Therapeutic protocols (including dietary, medication, lifestyle modification and manual treatments)

Then, a semi structured questionnaire prepared by using the articles and previous experiences of Iranian professors, was fulfilled. Questions were asked from patients by telephone. Anyone who was not able to answer or was not available was excluded from the study. The questions were asked from the patient him/herself.

Each patient was followed up at least 6 months after the first visit. Causes of referral or non-referral of patients to the clinic for the second visit were asked by telephone. Then the collected data was analyzed using inferential statistics and Microsoft Excel 2016 software.

Results

In general, 393 cases of 5325 patients visited at *Behesht* Clinic in 2016 were randomly selected and studied. 317 of them were called by phone. In spite of repeated attempts to call with 76 patients, it was not possible. Of these, the mobile set of 20 patients were off, 30 of them did not cooperate with the researcher and did not answer the questions, the phone numbers of 15 were not registered in the file, and 11 had wrong phone numbers. The mean age of patients was 40.7% of which 27.5% were male and 72.5% were female (Table 1).

Of the 317 cases reviewed, 114 were new patients who had only one visit, 72 were visited twice, and 81 had three visits. Also, 50 participants were visited more than 3 times (Table 2).

In general, the patients presented various reasons for their lack of recurrence, the most common ones were the patient's own lack of attention to taking medication and follow-up (24.2%), disease recovery (23%), lack of appropriate response to treatment (20.8%), relocation of the therapist (11.6%), the intention of the patient to referral due to satisfaction with the treatment (10.09%), residence in a distant city from the clinic (3.1%) and treatment complications (2.2%) (Table 3). Chart 1 represents the most common causes of non-referral of patients to the clinic and chart 2 shows all of the factors reported by patients as the cause of non-referral.

In a survey of a total of 317 cases, the main complaint that led to referral to the Persian medicine clinic was digestive diseases (48 cases), musculoskeletal disorders (46 cases) and skin diseases (42 cases).

Of course, some complaints such as overweight or excessive weight loss or systemic diseases, such as diabetes and hypertension, etc. which was also categorized as general disorders, were the most common complaints with a total of 56 cases. Also, 10 cases were referred for cupping or massage therapy, as well as determination of the temperament which were categorized as miscellaneous diseases. Table 4 explains the patient complaints based on organ involvement.

Among the digestive disorders, flatulence with 73 cases and constipation with 66 cases were the most common complaints of patients (Figures 1 and 2). Among musculoskeletal diseases, various

Participants	Amplitude	Percent
Male	87	27.5
Female	230	72.5
Total	317	100

Table 1: Frequency of participants by gender.

Visit time	Frequency	Percent
Once	114	35
Twice	72	Jul-22
3 times	81	May-25
More than 3 times	50	Jul-15

Table 2: Frequency of visit times of patients.

	Cause of non-referral	Percent
1	patient's own lack of attention to taking medication and follow-up	24.2
2	disease recovery	23
3	lack of appropriate response to treatment	20.8
4	relocation of the therapist	11.6
5	satisfaction with the treatment (the patient intends to be visited again)	10.09
6	Residence in a distant city from the clinic	3.1
7	Treatment complications	2.2

Table 3: The most common causes of non-referral of patients to the clinic.

Chief complaint of the participants	Number	Percent
Skin, hair and nail diseases	42	13.2
Eye diseases	2	0.6
Ear, nose and throat (ENT) diseases	14	4.4
Neurologic diseases	22	6.9
Psychiatric diseases	20	6.3
Heart diseases	4	1.2
Disease of respiratory system	11	3.4
Digestive diseases	48	15.1
Urogenital diseases	8	2.5
Musculoskeletal disorders	44	13.8
Gynecologic diseases	36	11.3
General disorders	56	17.6
Miscellaneous diseases	10	3.1

Table 4: Frequency of complaints of patients referring to the clinic.

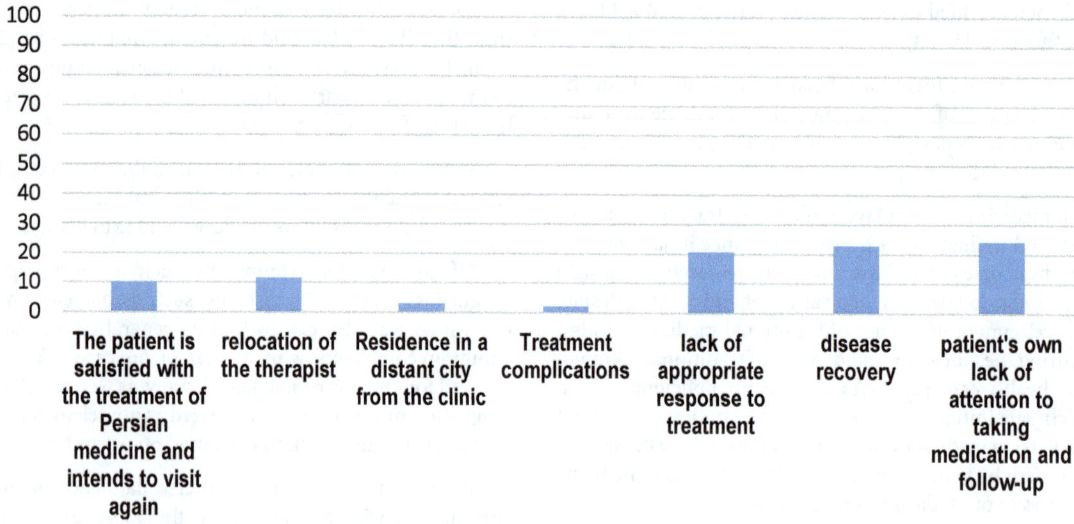

Figure 1: The columnar chart of the most common causes of non-referral of patients to the clinic.

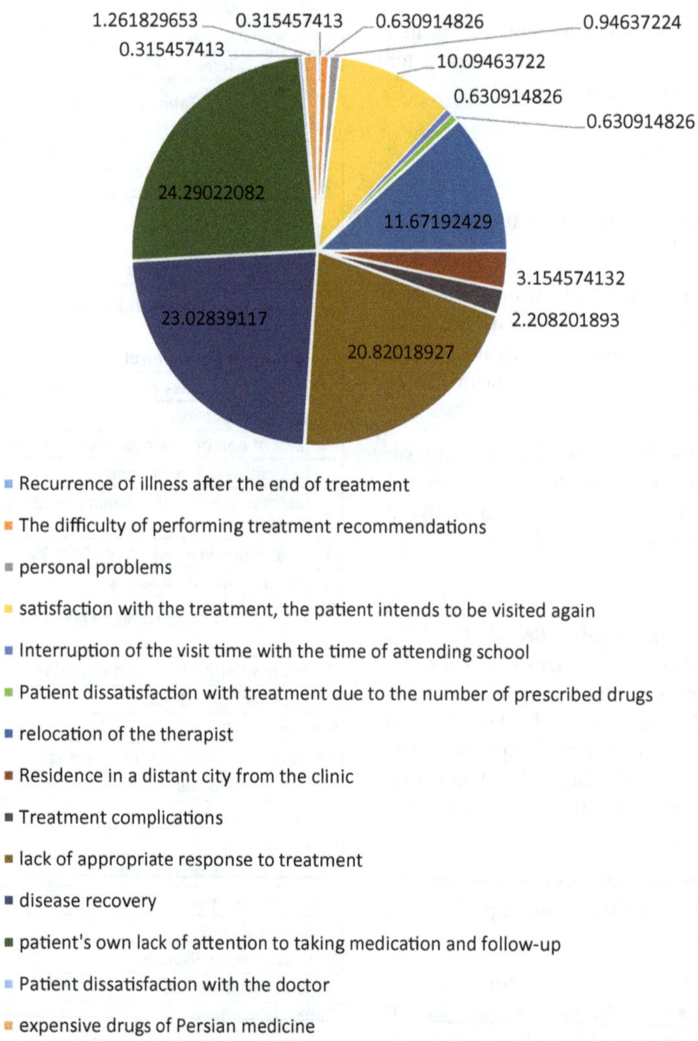

Figure 2: The pie chart of all factors reported by patients as the cause of non-referral.

joint pains with 38 cases and muscle spasm with 12 cases were the most common complaints. The most prevalent complaints in skin diseases were skin dryness with 18 cases, itching and hair loss with 7 cases. Headache with 29 cases and stress disorders with 35 cases were the most common complaints among neurological and psychiatric diseases. Some of the most prevalent complaints related to each organ are listed in Table 5.

It was found out about compliance with the recommendations that 69 patients had better observance of lifestyle modification and dietary measures, 215 had a tendency to use drugs, 20 had better performed manual treatments, and 13 did not comply with any of the treatments (Table 6).

In reviewing the possible complications caused by measures and medications, no complication of lifestyle modification was reported. 24 participants believed that they had drug complications however the type of complication did not be revealed. 3 cases also believed that they were affected by the complications of cupping therapy or other manual treatments and 290 reported no complications (Table 7).

Patients were also asked about satisfaction with the manner and behavior of physicians. 2 patients were dissatisfied with that while 11 reported tolerable behavior of physicians. The rest of the participants were satisfied with the manner of the physicians (Table 8).

System	chief complaint	Frequency
nervous system	Headache	29
	Memory disorders	9
	Dizziness and true vertigo	5
Psychiatry	Stress disorders	35
	Depression	8
	Obsessive compulsive disorder	6
Cardiovascular system	Palpitation	17
	Chest pain	3
Digestive system	Flatulence	73
	Constipation	66
	Stomach ache	11
	Regurgitation	10
	Excessive thirst	13
	Nausea	12
Musculoskeletal system	Arthralgia	38
	Muscle spasm	12
	Leg pain	7
Gynecology	Menstrual disorders	11
	Ovarian cyst	7
	Uterine fibroids	7
Urogenital system	Urine frequency	9
	Dysuria	4
Skin and hair	Skin dryness	18
	Itching	7
	Hair drop	7
	Acne	6
Respiratory system	Allergy	5
	Cough	3
ENT	Post nasal discharge (PND)	50
	Sinusitis	6
Eye	Low vision	1
	Xerophthalmia	1
General	Chronic fatigue	26
	Diabetes mellitus	9
	Anemia	12

Table 5: Frequency of the most common complaints related to each system.

Measures	Frequency	Percent
Lifestyle modification	69	21.7
Drug therapy	215	67.8
manual treatments	20	6.3
Failure to observe any measures	13	4.1

Table 6: Frequency of observance of therapeutic recommendations by patients.

complication	frequency	Percent
No complications	290	91.4
Drug complications	24	7.5
Manual treatment complications	3	0.9

Table 7: Frequency of complications caused by Persian medicine treatments.

Manner of physician	frequency	Percent
Too bad	1	0.3
Bad	1	0.3
Tolerable	11	3.4
Good	288	90.8
Very good	16	5.04

Table 8: Frequency of patient satisfaction with the manner and behavior of physicians.

Patient tendency	Frequency	Percent
Yes	262	82.6
No	52	16.4
abstainer	3	0.9

Table 9: Frequency of patient tendency to referral to the clinic.

Patients were asked about the tendency to referral to the clinic and follow-up treatment of which 262 participants tended to referral, 52 were uninterested and 3 did not answer this question (Table 9).

Discussion

In this study, 26.5% of participants were male and 72.5% were female which indicates that women are more likely to go to the Persian medicine clinic than men. Of course, this is not necessarily due to more incidence of disease in women or their more interest in Persian medicine, but since this study included reviewing the patient records of morning shift of the clinic, the educational shift, the referral of employed people to the clinic was less frequent at this time. The evidence is that several patients reported interruptions in the time of attendance at the clinic by working hours or school hours as a reason for not referring.

Regarding the frequency of visits, it should be noted that in Persian medicine, it is necessary for the patient to see his/her doctor several times. The purpose of those recurrent visits is to perform more diagnostic examinations and follow-up treatment. It means that sometimes, in the first visit, there are several distinct diagnoses requiring laboratory tests and medical imaging to achieve a definite diagnosis. Therefore, this should be considered in recurrent referrals. In many cases, it is necessary for the physician to assess the response to treatment within a certain period of time and based on this, he/she will make the necessary changes in approach to the patient. Therefore, in multi-stage therapies or in order to complete the logical follow-up of the treatment, referral is necessary and recommended. In these cases, recurrent referrals also increase the validity of treatment, however if the patient avoid referral to the doctor, misdiagnosis or incomplete treatment may occur which will lead to wasting of the cost and time of the patient, the doctor and the clinic, and unwanted complications may happen during this time. On the other hand, recurrent referrals may indicate that the patient has not been treated thoroughly and correctly.

In fact, there would be an error, a mistake or a problem in the treatment of the patient. Considering that the purpose of any medical activity is to reduce the incidence of disease and increase the outcome to the benefit of the patient, this kind of recapitulated referral means that capital, manpower, and equipment in the process of these activities are wasted without proper result. In addition, the patient will use the facilities that are considered for another patient when referring again [33]. Therefore, referral of patients should be targeted, *i.e.,* useful and necessary referrals should be increased and referrals that are due to errors or mistakes or other problems should be reduced. Preventive factors should be identified to reduce the number of unwanted visits. Instead, we need to increase the number of referrals that are needed to follow-up and complete the treatment. In this study, 114 patients had only one visit, 21 of whom had been treated, and the rest were dissatisfied with the continuation of treatment for various reasons, which could lead to waste of time and energy for physicians and patients themselves. Therefore, recommendation and emphasis on referral by the doctor can be a useful way to encourage patients to continue their treatment. Other patients who did not have recurrence indicated various reasons such as lack of attention to taking medication, relocation of the physician, the cost of treatment, dissatisfaction with the type of treatment offered and long distance of clinic from the home, as a cause of non-attendance.

In general, the most prevalent chief complaints reported in this study were digestive problems and musculoskeletal disorders. In the study of Mohammadian et al. [6] in Isfahan, the most common cause for referral is low back pain and fatigue. In a study in Sweden, musculoskeletal disorders are the first cause of referral, followed by respiratory, cardiovascular and digestive disorders [34]. Therefore, it seems that the majority of patients referring to traditional medicine clinics in different regions are patients with musculoskeletal disorders as well as gastrointestinal problems. Perhaps one of the reasons of why gastrointestinal diseases are more common in traditional medicine clinics is the therapists' emphasized attention to these problems and getting a more accurate digestive history. After gastrointestinal diseases, musculoskeletal disorders were just the most common complaints of patients that were consistent with the findings of conventional medicine. Arthritis is the second complaint of outpatient complaints in conventional medicine, and affects about 10% of the total human population as a result of chronic pain and inflammation of the joints [35-37]. Although this disease is not fatal, most patients, if left untreated, would suffer from chronic pain and complicated problems until the end of their life [24]. The most important remedy for this disease is prevention and lifestyle changes. Considering that there is currently no definitive treatment for this condition in conventional medicine and the pyramid of the population is also indicative of population aging, it seems that the use of preventive and therapeutic methods of Persian medicine are helpful for reducing the rate and severity of pain and symptoms of patients. This issue should be further investigated in future studies. Appropriate diet and healthy lifestyle are needed for every individual at any time of life. In this study, despite the fact that nobody had any problem or complication from the lifestyle modification, the rate of welcoming patients was lower and they tended to take drugs and pills. Because compliance with diet and lifestyle measures was difficult for patients due to the widespread of invalid lifestyle and even some who fully complied with the orders complained about it. Therefore, it is better to emphasize the patients that their current lifestyle is harmful to the health, and they need to change their lifestyle habits forever. In this case, patients will be less likely to complain of the difficulty of observing the measures.

The reason that some patients reported adverse drug reactions without knowing the type of complication was a defect in our questionnaire. Because from the Persian medicine point of view, the complications noted by patients can sometimes be part of the effects of the drug and is not a complication, such as disposal of waste substance through the intestines as diarrhea that patients mistakenly interpret it as a drug side effect. Such a defect must be corrected in future questionnaires.

In this study, it was found that satisfaction with the behavior of physicians was also desirable.

The following results are found from the review of various articles about patients' satisfaction with traditional and complementary therapies:

In a study conducted in Italy, the satisfaction of those who used the complementary method was evaluated and it was shown that the most of referrals are middle-aged women with higher education and social status and the most satisfaction is seen in this group [38]. In evaluating the satisfaction of referrals to traditional Chinese medicine in Switzerland, the satisfaction of those who used both conventional medicine and complementary therapies is higher than those who used only conventional medicine. This difference is due to fewer side effects of traditional Chinese medicine, better doctor-patient relationship, longer care times, and a variety of patient-facing therapies [39]. In a study in Isfahan, the satisfaction of patients with acupuncture is also good [40]. In the study of Rossi et al. the effectiveness of complementary therapies on cluster headaches was observed, and satisfactory patient satisfaction is observed with complementary therapies and treatment costs [41]. A study in Germany reported that complementary medicine has been effective in preventing many diseases, including cardiovascular disorders, migraine and Alzheimer [42]. A review article by Furlan et al. [43] about the effectiveness of complementary medicine on neck and low back pain has confirmed its real impact. Of course, complementary medicine and alternative medicine did not reduce the relative disability compared to the control group. In our study, the majority of patients tended to refer to the clinic and follow up treatment, which indicates the satisfactory patient satisfaction with Persian therapies in the *Behesht* Clinic.

As previously stated, long distance of the clinic from the patient's residence was one of the reasons for not referring patients to the clinic, which could lead to a lack of re-prescription of the drug and discontinuing the treatment. Therefore, development of Persian medicine clinics and the fair distribution of drugs in the city or even at the national level is necessary. Reliable and extensive research on Persian medicine drugs will validate these drugs and pharmacies will be more likely to sell them. Also, the number of people who are reluctant to use Persian therapies due to uncertainty about them will be reduced.

Another problem that some people complained about was the high cost of treatment. Especially those who fully complied with the treatments were dissatisfied with the cost of providing medications. Therefore, given the long duration of treatment in Persian medicine, it is imperative that policy makers of the health system and Persian medical managers provide certain solutions to insure the Persian medicine services and herbal drugs.

Because of dissimilarity of the treatments, evaluation of the treatment efficacy could not be verified, which should be investigated in subsequent studies in specialized and categorized groups.

References

1. Goldbeck-Wood S, Dorozynski A, Lie LG (1996) Complementary medicine is booming worldwide. BMJ 313: 131-133.
2. WHO Traditional Medicine (2003) Report by the Secretariat. Fifty-sixth world health assembly A56/18, Provisional agenda item 14.10.
3. Ardakani SM, Farjadmand F (2006) General guidelines for methodology in the field of traditional medicine research. Traditional Medicine research center of Shahid Beheshti University of Medical Sciences. Tehran.
4. Moradi lakeh M, Goosheh Gir A, Amini M (2008) Tendency to the topic of complementary /alternative traditional medicine in dissertation research (1370-1385). Payesh quarterly journal 7: 33-44.
5. Larijani B, Esfahani MM, Moghimi M, Ardakani SM, Keshavarz M, et al. (2015) Common types of diabetic dosage forms in medieval Persia. Pharm Hist (Lond) 45: 96-99.
6. Mahmoodian A, Golshiri P, Rezaee G, Akbari M (2012) Investigating the causes of referral and satisfaction of the traditional medicine users in Isfahan. Journal of Isfahan University of Medical Sciences 30:1550-1558.
7. Razes (2001) Al Havi [Liber Continent]. Ehyaol Toras al-Arabi Press. Beiruot.
8. Ahvazi A (2008) Kamel-al-Sanaat Al Tebiyah. Natural Medicine revival institute. Tehran.
9. Baha Al-dolah Razi (2009) Kholasat Al-Tajarob. Tehran University of medical sciences press. Tehran.
10. Rains JC, Penzien DB (2005) Behavioral research and the double-blind placebo controlled methodology: Challenges in applying the biomedical standard to behavioral headache research. Headache 45: 479-486.
11. Rains JC, Penzien DB, Mc Crory DC, Gray RN (2005) Behavioral headache treatment: History, review of the empirical literature, and methodological critique. Headache 45: S92-S109.
12. Bloom BS, Retbi A, Dahan S, Jonsson E (2000) Evaluation of randomized controlled trials on complementary and alternative medicine. Int J Technol Assess Health Care 16: 13-21.
13. Marcus DM (2002) Alternative medicine and the Arthritis. Foundation. Arthritis Rheum 47: 5-7.
14. Fitzcharles MA (2002) Is it time for rheumatologists to rethink the use of manual therapies? J Rheumatol 29: 1117-1120.
15. Mozafari Khosravi H, Jalali B, Afkhami M (2008) The Effect of Sour Tea on Glucose, lipid Profile and Lipoproteins in diabetic patients. J Endocrinol Metab 10: 589-597.
16. Asgari S, Rahimi P, Madani H, Mahzooni P, Kabiri N (2008) Effect of Juglans regia hydroalcoholic extract on the prevention of type 1 diabetes in adult male rats. Iranian J Diabet Lipid 7: 363-370.
17. Zadeh NH, Safari M, Khoshnevisan F (2005) Study of the Effect of Herbal Medicines on Neonatal Hyperbilirubinemia: In vitro. Iranian Children's Dis J 15: 133-138.
18. Kalantari Z, Jafari H (2006) Survey of Extract of White Cabbage in Prevention and Treatment of Peptic Ulcer Caused by aspirin in rats. Jour Guilan Uni Med Sci 15: 89-94.
19. Avijgan M, Saadat M, Zadeh NM, Hafizi M (2006) Antifungal Effect of Echinophora platyloba extract on Several Common Dermatophytes. Med Herb Quart J 5: 10-16.
20. Izadi j, Sharif M, Khalilian A, Jaribi ZHH, Azad Bakht M, et al. (2003) Evaluation of anti-parasite effects of Achillea Millefolium on mouse ocxir parasites. J Mazandaran Uni Med Sci 13: 27-35.
21. Bandegi AR (2002) Evaluation of the effect of manna of Alhaji on blood bilirubin in mice with experimental Hyperbilirubinemia. J Semnan Uni Med Sci 2: 161-166.
22. Ghotbi F, Nahidi S, Zangi M (2006) Effect of Clay Milk on Neonatal Jaundice Reduction. J Shahid Beheshti University of Medical Sciences 31: 347-352.
23. Kenari MH, Arabshahi SK, Bigdeli S, Ardakani SM (2011) Explaining the concept of citation of evidence in Persian medicine from the point of view of the experts of this field. J Trad Med Islam and Iran 2: 203-214.
24. Mehdi Barzi D, Naseri M, Zadeh FS, Nejad KM, Bahrami M (2008) Double-blind clinical trial of Marham e Mafasel with placebo control in patients with knee osteoarthritis. Daneshvar Journal 16: 1-2.
25. Fani A, Ghasedi M, Lion A, Alizadeh B (2010) The effect of turmeric on improving the clinical symptoms of patients with irritable bowel syndrome. J Arak Uni Med Sci 13: 109-115.
26. Akhondzadeh S, Noroozian M, Mohammadi M, Ohadinia S, Jamshidi AH, et al. (2003) Salvia officinalis extract in the treatment of patients with mild to moderate Alzheimer's disease: a double blind, randomized and placebocontrolled trial. J Clin Pharm Ther 28: 53-59.
27. Abed A, Minaiyan M, Ghannadi A, Mahzouni P, Babavalian MR (2012) Effect of Echium amoenum Fisch. Et Mey a Traditional Iranian Herbal Remedy in an Experimental Model of Acute Pancreatitis. ISRN Gastroenterol 14158.
28. Bonjar S (2004) Evaluation of antibacterial properties of some medicinal plants used in Iran. J Ethnopharmacol 94: 301-305.
29. Ahmadi A, Schwebel DC, Rezaei M (2008) The Efficacy of Wet-Cupping in the Treatment of Tension and Migraine Headache, Am J Chin Med 36: 37-44.
30. Taavoni S, Dorsareh F, Joolaee S, Haghani H (2012) The effect of massage therapy on physical signs of menopause 2: 21-28.
31. Siroos A, Khaki M, Goodarzi D (2007) Investigating the effect of capsule made from internal layer of chicken gizzard in treatment of urinary stones. J Arak Uni Med Sci 10: 12-17.
32. Jozi M, Amini R, Noorbakhsh V (2009) The Effect of Massage Therapy on Blood Pressure in Patients with 19: 261-265.
33. Khoshkam M (1994) Investigating the Causes of Patients' Referral to General Hospitals Affiliated to Iran University of Medical Sciences and Health Services. Thesis of Master for medical records, Iran University of Medical Sciences. Tehran.
34. Al-Windi A (2004) Determinants of complementary alternative medicine (CAM) use. Complement Ther Med 12: 99-111.
35. Koopman WJ (2001) Arthritis & allied Conditions. Lippincott William's and Wilkin Press, Philadelphia, USA.
36. Chapman MW (2001) Chapman's orthopaedic Surgery. Lippincott William's & Wilkins Press, Philadelphia, USA.
37. Klippel J, Dieppe P (1995) Practical Rheumatology. Mosby Press, USA.
38. Barbadoro P, Chiatti C, D'Errico MM, Minelli A, Pennacchietti L, et al. (2011) Complementary and alternative medicine (CAM) among adults in Italy Use and related satisfaction. Eur J Integr Med 13: e325-e332.
39. Michlig M, Ausfeld-Hafter B, Busato A (2008) Patient satisfaction with primary care: a comparison between conventional care and traditional Chinese medicine. Complement Ther Med 16: 350-358.
40. Mahmoodian SA, Babaee EM, Jafari M (2011) Referral causes and satisfaction of users of Acupuncture in Isfahan. Journal of Isfahan University of Medical Sciences 29: 2280-2288.
41. Rossi P, Torelli P, Di LC, Sances G, Manzoni GC, et al. (2008) Use of complementary and alternative medicine by patients with cluster headache: results of a multi-centre headache clinic survey. Complement Ther Med 16: 220-227.
42. Kraft K (2009) Complementary/Alternative Medicine in the context of prevention of disease and maintenance of health. Prev Med 49: 88-92.
43. Furlan AD, Yazdi F, Tsertsvadze A, Gross A, van Tulder M, et al. (2012) A systematic review and meta-analysis of efficacy, costeffectiveness, and safety of selected complementary and alternative medicine for neck and low back pain. Evid Based Complement Alternat Med 953139.

24

Complementary Medicine and Integrative Health Module for Undergraduate Medical Students, KSA

Ahmed T. El-Olemy[1,2*]

Department of Public Health and Community Medicine, Faculty of Medicine, Tanta University, Egypt
Department of Academic Affairs and Training Unit, National Center for Complementary and Alternative Medicine, Ministry of Health, Riyadh, Saudi Arabia

1
2

Abstract

Background: Medical education has undergone major transformation along with the change in concept of health and disease.

Objective: Increasing awareness, improving knowledge and acquiring skills of complementary medicine and integrative health for undergraduate medical students.

Methods: Complementary medicine and integrative health module was introduced during the year 2016-2017, for fourth year medical students at Dar Al Uloom University, Riyadh, KSA. The Methods of teaching and learning include interactive lectures, seminars, practical sessions, assignments, field visits, simulation, learning by doing (hands on training), case studies, problem based learning and self-directed learning. Topics covered during the course include; Introduction and overview of Complementary and Alternative Medicine (CAM), Epidemiology of CAM practices, Characteristics and comparison of CAM *vs.* Conventional Medicine, Integrative Medicine, Research models in CAM, Evidence based CAM, Medical ethics of CAM, Frauds and misconceptions related to CAM practices and products, Health education and communication in CAM, Manipulative and body based practices, Biological-based practices, Mind-body medicine, Energy based therapies, Whole medical systems; Traditional Chinese Medicine (TCM), Unani, Arabic or Hakim Medicine, Prophetic Medicine and Local traditional CAM therapies (Hijamah as a model), Acupuncture, Herbal Medicine, Naturopathy, Nutrition and food supplements, Apitherapy and Homeopathy.

Assessment of the module: The course comprises two types of assessments; continuous and final assessment. Continuous assessments toke place throughout the course. They are mostly based on course work as follows; Seminar (10%), Assignments (10%), Field visit report (10%) and Mid-term exam (20%). A proportion of 50% were taken in the final assessment. A student who scored 60 or more deemed to have passed this course.

Conclusion: The feedback received was most supportive of the module and appreciative of the teachers, the information provided and skills gained and the way in which it was delivered.

Keywords: Complementary medicine; Integrative health; Teaching; Medical students, KSA

Introduction

Many Saudis more than 70% use health care approaches developed outside of mainstream western or conventional medicine. When describing these approaches, people often use "alternative" and "complementary" interchangeably or integrative medicine. CAM is a group of diverse medical and health care systems, practices, and products that are not presently considered to be part of conventional medicine. Integrative medicine is a term that refers to combining, "treatments from conventional medicine and CAM for which there is some high-quality evidence of safety and effectiveness. Integrative medicine is an approach to care that puts the patient at the center and addresses the full range of physical, emotional, mental, social, spiritual and environmental influences that affect a person's health [1]. Integrative health care, involve bringing conventional and complementary approaches together in a coordinated way. The use of integrative approaches to health and wellness has grown within care settings across the United States. Researchers are currently exploring the potential benefits of integrative health in a variety of situations, including pain management for military personnel and veterans, relief of symptoms in cancer patients and survivors, and programs to promote healthy behaviors [2].

There it claims that non-mainstream practitioners and practices make can sound promising. However, researchers do not know how safe many of these treatments are or how well they work. Studies are underway to determine the safety and usefulness of many of these practices. To minimize the health risks of a non-mainstream treatment you should discuss it with your doctor. It might have side effects or interact with other medicines. Find out what the research says about it. Choose practitioners carefully. And tell all of your doctors and practitioners about all of the different types of treatments you use [3].

CAM therapies need to be evaluated with the same long and careful research process used to evaluate standard treatments. CAM therapies include a wide variety of botanicals and nutritional products, such as dietary supplements, herbal supplements, and vitamins. Many of these "natural" products are considered to be safe because they are present in, or produced by, nature. However, that is not true in all cases. In addition, some may affect how well other medicines work in the body. Herbal supplements may be harmful when taken by themselves, with other substances, or in large doses [4].

***Corresponding author:** Ahmed T El-Olemy, Department of Academic Affairs and Training Unit, National Center for Complementary and Alternative Medicine, Ministry of Health, Riyadh, Saudi Arabia, 11662 E-mail: a_elolemy@yahoo.com

Yet, despite increased CAM use by the patients, allopathic health care providers often lack sufficient knowledge of CAM therapies and products and their role in health and healing. They are unaware about the safety and effectiveness of CAM therapies. They lack the requisite expertise to collaborate with CAM practitioners to provide patients with an integrated approach to care [5,6]. CAM therapies have been associated with serious and even life-threatening adverse events [7]. Thus, conventional health care providers need to understand the safety and efficacy issues pertinent to widely-used CAM therapies, incorporate assessment of CAM use into their history and physical examinations of their patients, and collaborate with CAM practitioners to provide safe and integrated approach to care [8].

Medical education has undergone major transformation along with the change in concept of health and disease. It is becoming increasingly community oriented, learner-centered, self-learning, and self-peer assessing process [9]. Educational institutions, particularly those in developing countries such as Saudi Arabia face sorts of challenges in the implementation of change via the introduction of new systems and procedures. This is the more common type of organizational change they will encounter, as they become more global in their perspectives and face performance-based assessments such as accreditation [10-16].

Overall Aims and Objectives

Upon successful completion of the course, students should be able to

a) Define what is Traditional Medicine, Complementary Medicine, Integrative Health, other names and related terminologies, and how do they differ from each other and from that of conventional medicine.

b) Acquire a good knowledge about classifications of CAM modalities and therapies.

c) Discuss the concepts and principles of CAM modalities.

d) Identify the common local Traditional CAM practices in the Kingdom of Saudi Arabia with emphasis on Arabic and Islamic traditional healing practices and their prevalence.

e) Assess evidence of safety, efficacy, cost effectiveness and mechanism of action of different CAM modalities.

f) Access and search the literature and critically evaluate different types of CAM researches.

g) Decide who, why, where, and when people use CAM and which medical conditions are most suitable for CAM modalities.

h) Adopt medical ethics related to CAM.

i) Take a positive attitude towards evidence based CAM practices.

j) Identify common frauds and misconceptions related to CAM practices and products.

k) Acquire skills related to common, licensed and high prevalent local CAM practices.

l) Clarify the role of the National Center for Complementary and Alternative Medicine (NCCAM) in KSA as a national reference for all CAM concerns including regulations, licensing and accreditation.

m) Introduce health education message for common CAM users about evidence based CAM practices as well as frauds and misconceptions related to CAM use.

n) Communicate effectively with patients about their use of CAM practices.

Intended Learning Outcome of the Course (Ilos)

Knowledge and understanding

Upon successful completion of the course, students should be able to A-1) Describe the characteristics of Complementary and Integrative Medicine. A-2) Learn about safety, efficacy, cost effectiveness and mechanism of action of different CAM modalities. A-3) Learn about the history of herbal medicine, Prophetic medicine, TCM, tc. A-4) Enumerate side effects and complications of different CAM modalities. A-5) Describe the uses, indications and contraindications of the selected CAM practices. A-6) Learn about evidence based CAM practices. A-7) Enumerate and describe local traditional CAM practices. And A-8) Judge medical ethics related to CAM practice.

Intellectual skills

Upon successful completion of the course, students should be able to B-1) Suggest the right Complementary therapies for a particular health problem. B-2) Summarize common diseases where CAM therapies can be included in the management plan. B-3) Design suitable plan for management of particular cases using CAM modalities. B-4) Communicate efficiently with patient seeking CAM. B-5) Suggest health education message regarding proper use of CAM. And B-6) Deal with misconceptions of CAM modalities.

Professional and practical skills

At the end of the course, students should be able to C-1) Discuss the assignments of different cases in the practical notes concerning the complementary medicine practice used, theories, side effects and contraindications and suggest the disease(s) that can be managed using CAM based on evidence based medicine. C-2) Do interpretation of a research project including different cases treated by the use of CAM therapy, effectiveness and recommendations. C-3) Differentiate between the theories, concepts and principles of Allopathic Medicine and Traditional, complementary, alternative and integrative medicine. C-4) Acquire practical skills related to some practices such as Hijamah, Acupuncture, Herbal medicine, etc.

General and transferrable skills

At the end of the course, students should be able to D-1) Communicate within the team work. D-2) Plan and conduct a research task. D-3) Acquire presentation skills. D-4) Basic information/ health technology literacy.

Course Description

Topics to be covered

Topics to be covered during the course include 1) Introduction and overview of CAM. 2) Epidemiology of CAM practices. 3) Characteristics and comparison of CAM *vs.* Conventional Medicine. 4) Integrative Medicine. 5) Research models in CAM. 6) Evidence based CAM. 7) Medical ethics of CAM. 8) Frauds and misconceptions related to CAM practices and products. 9) Health education and communication in CAM. 10) Manipulative and body based practices. 11) Biological-based practices. 12) Mind-body medicine. 13) Energy based therapies. 14) Whole medical systems. 15) Traditional Chinese Medicine (TCM). 16) Unani, Arabic or Hakim Medicine. 17) Prophetic Medicine. 18) Local traditional CAM therapies (Hijamah as a model).

19) Acupuncture. 20) Herbal Medicine. 21) Naturopathy. 22) Nutrition and food supplements. 23) Apitherapy. And 24) Homeopathy.

Methods of teaching and learning

1. Interactive lectures.
2. Seminars.
3. Case studies.
4. Problem based learning.
5. Self-directed learning.
6. Practical sessions.
7. Simulation.
8. Learning by doing (hands on training).
9. Assignments.
10. Field visits

Interactive lectures: Interactive lectures will involve the students in active discussion, and may provide brief learning activities during the lecture to achieve the learning objectives stated under each topic.

Introduction and overview of CAM: At the end of the lecture, student should be able to define what is Traditional Medicine, Complementary Medicine, Integrative Health and other names and related terminologies, and how do they differ from each other and from that of conventional medicine. Discuss history of CAM, different classifications of CAM modalities and therapies describe the common CAM practices worldwide and in KSA, describe communication between patients and CAM practitioners and define National Center for Complementary and Alternative Medicine.

Epidemiology of CAM practices: At the end of the lecture, student should be able to describe the epidemiology of CAM in relation to time, place and person, the prevalence of CAM use in developed and developing countries and give examples, describe distribution of CAM practices in Saudi Arabia, impact of CAM worldwide and in KSA, determinants of CAM use, determine why and when are CAM used? Describe where do ill people go seeking for health? Answer the question does physician discuss with their patients use of traditional and complementary medicine? And does traditional and complementary medicine educated in different schools?

Characteristics and comparison of CAM vs. conventional medicine: At the end of the lecture, student should be able to describe different specifications and characteristics of CAM, differentiate between conventional and unconventional medicine, discuss difficulties in CAM research as compared to conventional medicine, explain causes of lack training in CAM and describe the difference between evidence based CAM and evidence based conventional medicine.

Integrative medicine: At the end of the lecture, student should be able to define integrative medicine, describe principles of integration, different models of integration and discuss the benefits and advantages of integration.

Research models in CAM: At the end of the lecture, student should be able to describe research methods as applied to CAM, demonstrate advantages and disadvantages of different CAM research models, describe pragmatic clinical trials, understand the role of placebo and therapeutic encounter in CAM research, explain how to design comparative effectiveness study and discuss how to define study outcomes and identify the role of research in the integration of CAM in health care system.

Evidence based CAM: At the end of the lecture, student should be able to define and explore evidence based medicine (EBM), discuss EBM pyramid, differentiate between evidence based CAM and conventional medicine, demonstrate primary and secondary sources of evidence and classify CAM practices according to evidence.

Medical ethics of CAM: At the end of the lecture, the student should be able to discuss the ethical issues of CAM; ethics of CAM practitioner towards patients, himself, the public and his colleagues and towards his job and discuss ethics of CAM practitioner towards advertisement of CAM practices and products.

Frauds and misconceptions related to CAM practices and products: At the end of the lecture, the student should be able to define frauds and misconceptions, explore frauds and misconceptions related to CAM practitioners and to CAM products and discuss examples of CAM misconceptions and frauds.

Health education and communication in CAM: At the end of the lecture, the student should be able to discuss how to communicate properly with patients seeking for CAM, how to deal properly with misconceptions about CAM, explore proper methods of health education and communication related to CAM and describe common health education messages for CAM users.

Mind-body medicine: (Hypnotherapy, Meditation, visualization, Prayer, Yoga, etc.): At the end of the lecture, student should be able to describe mind-body medicine, discuss how the mind-body medicine works in health and disease, the fundamentals and principles of mind-body medicine, discuss application of various mind-body therapies, describe evidence base regarding safety and efficacy of mind-body medicine and discuss different mind-body medicine practices in prevention and treatment of diseases.

Energy medicine: At the end of the lecture, student should be able to define different Energy medicine modalities, explain principals and mechanism of action of energy medicine, discuss evidence based safety and effectiveness of energy based medicine and describes various applications of the energy medicine in treatment.

Herbal medicine: At the end of the lecture, student should be able to define herbal medicine, discuss the history of herbal medicine, sources of information for herbal medical products, describe some important herbs in various geographic areas, scientific names and its botanical features related to medicinal importance with examples, describe how extractions and preparations of herbs are made, give examples of four medical local herbs; indications with high scientific evidence and discuss education, licensing and regulation of herbal medicine.

Apitherapy: At the end of the lecture, student should be able to define Apitherapy and its uses, describe composition and uses of Beeswax, propolis, Royal Jelly, Bee Pollen and Bee Venom, discuss possible side effects, and complications of Apitherapy and decide evidence based safety and effectiveness of Apitherapy.

Local traditional practices in KSA: At the end of the lecture, the student should be able to list and define different local traditional CAM practices in KSA, identify the prevalence of traditional CAM practices in the Kingdom of Saudi Arabia, discuss the advantages and disadvantages of local traditional CAM practices, describe the philosophical basis and principles of local traditional CAM practices, explain the difference between current trend of modern medicine and those practices and discuss evidence of safety and effectiveness of those practices.

Whole medical system (TCM): At the end of the lecture, the students should be able to define different components of Traditional Chinese Medicine (TCM), discuss philosophical background of TCM, describe models of the body and concept of disease in TCM and discuss the conditions that TCM may be useful.

Whole medical system (Naturopathy): At the end of the lecture, the students should be able to describe the history and ideology of naturopathy, describe the practice and practitioners of naturopathy, discuss regulations of naturopathy in different areas of the world and describe evidence based safety and efficacy of naturopathy.

Student led seminars

Guidelines for students seminar: Literature search of reliable sources and data basis must be done. Five seminars are scheduled during the module. Duration of each seminar is 2 hours. A staff member will be assigned as a Seminar Supervisor. The Seminar Supervisor will guide the group to coordinate with the group leader in assigning students for providing the presentation, assigning topics of seminars in coordination with the group leader, directly helping and advising students during preparation of the presentations, leading and supervising the seminars in terms of secure convenient venue, managing time for each presentation and keeping order during seminars sessions, facilitate group discussion after each presentation and assessing students (those who give presentations and who do not give presentations).

Students are divided into five groups. The seminar should be addressing the following: Introduction, methods, findings, critical appraisal of evidence, take home messages and references. The groups should work as a team to prepare the seminar. The work is divided such that every student should participate in preparation of the presentation. The presentation should be formatted by Microsoft office Power Point program. At least 10 to 15 slides are required for each presentation. The contribution of the sub groups should be compiled in one presentation and every student should have active participation in the presentation. Time should be managed in such a way that presentation is completed within the allocated time. Ten minutes are devoted for the tutor to give feedback and comments at the end of the seminar.

Other students (not giving presentations) have prepared properly for active collaboration and discussion by reading topics related to seminars prior to attending. All students should consider that they are assessed by the assigned tutor (Not only presenters of the seminar). Topics discussed during seminars are included in the module written exams.

Manipulative and body based practices: At the end of the seminar, student should be able to define Manipulative-based medicine, list the main types of manipulative therapy, explain the use of different manipulative therapies globally, describe different techniques of manipulative therapy, describe education, licensing and regulation of manipulative therapies, the safety and efficacy of manipulative based therapies and describe different models of integration of manipulative therapies.

Biological based practices: At the end of the seminar, student should be able to define and enumerate types of Biological based medicine, explain the philosophy and principles of Biological based practices, describe mechanism, effects and interaction of different Biological based practices, describe the evidence base regarding safety and efficacy of Biological based practices and discuss the rationale behind the use of Biological based practices.

Whole medical system (Homeopathy): At the end of the seminar, student should be able to discuss the history and definition of homeopathic medicine, describe mechanism of action and "the law of similar", identify evidence base, safety and efficacy of Homeopathic medicine, describe various applications of the Homeopathic remedy in treatment and describe education, licensing and regulation of homeopathy.

Whole medical system (Unani Medicine, Arabic or Hakim Medicine): At the end of the seminar, student should be able to define different components of Unani medicine, identify philosophical background of Unani medicine, describe models of the body and concept of disease in Unani medicine and discuss cases that Unani medicine may be useful in.

Nutritional therapy: At the end of the seminar, that student should be able to discuss background of nutritional therapy, enumerate types and best sources of macronutrients, enumerate types and best sources of micronutrients, discuss healthy eating, balanced diet and food pyramid, discuss examples of nutritional therapy (Mediterranean Diet and macrobiotic) and learn how to read Nutritional facts on Food label.

Practical sessions

Selected CAM therapies to be demonstrated by CAM therapists as a model include Prophetic Medicine, Acupuncture, and Cupping (Hijama) ***Location:*** NCCAM for practical session of prophetic medicine and Dar Al Uloom Faculty of Medicine for practical session of Acupuncture, and cupping (Hijama).

Local traditional CAM practices (Hijama): At the end of the session student should be able to define Al-Hijamah and discuss history of cupping, explain different types of cupping and cupping sets, discuss how to deal with patient before, during and after cupping, discuss indications, contraindications and precautions of cupping, describe different side effects related to cupping, Explain safe cupping techniques and infection control measures, discuss rules of choosing points of cupping according to research evidence, Simulation in cupping training (use of artificial skin), hands on training on volunteers, Adopt evidence based cupping and explain regulation of cupping in KSA.

Alternative CAM practices (Acupuncture): At the end of the session student should be able to define prevalence of acupuncture worldwide, discuss principles and theories of acupuncture, explain meridians and points of acupuncture, discuss indications, contraindications and precautions of acupuncture, describe different side effects related to acupuncture and how to avoid them, discuss rules of choosing points of acupuncture according to TCM and research evidence, adopt evidence based acupuncture and explain regulation of acupuncture worldwide and in KSA. Simulation was used in the practical sessions before application on human skin. This is followed by hands on training on volunteers.

Prophetic medicine: At the end of the session student should be able to define Prophetic Medicine and identify its principles and components, describe various aspects and types of Prophetic Medicine, discuss some examples of Prophetic Medicine in detail (Cupping, Cautery, Ruqia, Bees products and honey, camel milk and urine, herbal medicine, Zamzam water, zikr, dates AlMadena, etc.) discuss methods for integrating Prophetic Medicine by Muslim doctors and discuss examples of research studies done in prophetic medicine regarding safety and efficacy.

Assignments

CAM from evidence to integration: It includes criticism of one published clinical trial in CAM to identify the (PICO) question and to comment on the quality of the study. Each student should submit a report within one week from the lectures (Integrative Medicine and Evidence Based CAM).

Report on local traditional medicine therapies: Each student should submit (within one week after the lecture on local traditional practices) a report about one of the following local traditional medicine therapies (Hijamah, Cautery, Bone setting, Ruqia, Bees products and Honey) short essay.

Field visits

Guidelines for field visits: Students should follow instructions given to them prior to the visit. Students are encouraged to use transportation arranged and secured by the collage administration. Students are expected to behave as future doctors. At the end of the field visit, students are requested to give their feedback regarding fulfillment of the objectives of the visit and clarify any comments and suggestions they may have. Field visit report (written report should be submitted by each student within one week after the field visit about results of the field visit including what objectives has been achieved.

Objectives of field visit to the nearby community: Explore local traditional CAM practices in their community. Explain how the practitioner and practices be delivered. Assis quality of CAM practices and products provided. Assis and discuss skills of dealing with the patient. Give recommendations and future considerations of Local traditional CAM practices.

Assessment of the Module

The course comprises two types of assessment:

Continuous assessment

These assessments will take place throughout the course. They are mostly based on course work as follows; Seminar (10%), Assignments (10%), Field visit report (10%) and Mid-term exam (20%).

Final assessment

A proportion of 50% will be taken in the final assessment. This is the end of the course assessment, and will be conducted under formal examination conditions. The eligibility criteria for sitting the final examination will be the attainment of 75% of the attendance. This is based on (MCQs and SEQs). A student who score 60 or more will be deemed to have passed this course.

Quality Assurance and Evaluation Process

Any new course needs constant reviewing and monitoring to ensure that it meets the demands placed on it by the overall curriculum. This curriculum is no exception. Hence, there will be a number of evaluation strategies employed by the module. They are 1) Student feedback at the end of the module, seeking student comments on both teaching and learning, and assessment, along with the student views on the general course organization and implementation. 2) Student feedback on a sample of teaching and learning activities, obtained at the end of each activity. 3) Tutor feedback. 4) Examiner feedback. 5) Peer evaluation, where a staff member may visit a particular teaching and learning activity and provide formative feedback about its conduct. 6) Analysis of the students' examination results. 7) External reviews.

Discussion

The Complementary Medicine and Integrative Health Module were planned and implemented for increasing awareness, improving knowledge and acquiring skills of complementary medicine and integrative health for undergraduate fourth year medical students. The module covers one month of teaching in Dar AlUloom University, Riyadh, KSA. It located in the north part of Riyadh city, the capital of Saudi Arabia. It is a private University serving many specialties; medical, Pharmacy, dentistry, administration ...etc.

Study of the status of CAM education in health colleges in Saudi Arabia [17], revealed that there is no CAM specialized track or postgraduate education in any health college in Saudi Arabia and only Eleven (12.2%) colleges are teaching CAM courses in their curricula. Also, studying the knowledge and attitude of health professionals in the Riyadh region, Saudi Arabia, toward CAM (2012) recommended that Health educational organizations have to play a greater role by being the source of evidence-based knowledge of CAM. It reported that mass media represented 60.1% of sources of the knowledge of CAM followed by family, relatives, and friends (29.08%) and health educational organizations (14.71%) [18]. Hence the importance of introducing this module for teaching complementary medicine and integrative health for undergraduate medical students.

We try to cover most of topics related to CAM and integrative health. The National Center for Complementary Medicine and Integrative Health in USA classify CAM modalities into five main groups namely; Manipulative and body based practices, Biological-based practices, Mind-body medicine, Energy based therapies and whole medical systems [2]. The most common, evidence based CAM modalities were covered in the course. Also, practical skills related to acupuncture therapy, and cupping therapy (Hijama) was acquired. Students see, observe and criticize CAM practitioners during their work through field visit. They have opportunity to compare the ideal work according to knowledge gained and skills acquired versus the actual field work. They have active communication with patients in clinic. They acquired skills of searching data basis for evidence based CAM modalities. They share as a team work in preparing and presenting power point presentation of CAM topics.

Use a lot of methods of teaching and learning included; interactive lectures, seminars, practical sessions, assignments, field visits, simulation, learning by doing (hands on training), case studies problem based learning and self-directed learning helped learners to gain knowledge and acquire skills. This in accordance with many authors who stated that they have a great impact on knowledge and skills retention [19-21].

All students attended the course passed the exam. They highly satisfied with learning methods used, knowledge gained and skills acquired through self-assessment of the course at the end of the module. The feedback received was most supportive of the module and appreciative of the teachers, the information provided and skills gained and the way in which it was delivered. This learners' satisfaction with the course may have a good impact on retention. This is in agreement with El-Olemy et al. [22] who recorded health professional satisfaction with training on cupping therapy using the same methods of teaching. Notably, most of medical students expressed that CAM course needs to be integrated into their medical school curriculum, and this trend is consistent with other studies [23-25]. The long-term implications of this finding are many, including CAM capacity building in relation to clinical practice, research, teaching, and training [26].

Medical students tend to collect information on CAM from multiple sources as revealed in the study of Al-Mansour et al. [27] Accordingly, medical students reported that their most important sources of CAM information were peers, scientific journals, media, and Internet. Predictably, this CAM info-source scenario would change in future when CAM course will be integrated into main curriculum of all medical schools in KSA. Physicians with vast medical knowledge and multiple skills could discuss with the patient a variety of disease-related issues and put forward more than one option to be accepted, the best one, by the patient, that would fit into patient-centered approach currently in vogue in CAM/IM [28-30].

According to many studies, there are many barriers against integration of CAM curriculum and use of CAM therapies exist across the world. [31-33] In the context of western medical settings, lack of evidence for practices, lack of staff training, lack of reimbursement, legal issues raised by medical schools and institutions, relative lack of competent CAM providers, lack of appropriate equipment, and CAM therapies being too time consuming, were the main barriers (Tables 1 and 2) [31,32,34].

Limitations

This is a survey of fourth-year medical students in one university, and hence, its results may not generalizable to medical students in other universities in KSA. Similarly, the results may not be applicable to other health professionals such as nursing or dental students and first, or second or third or even fifth year students as their KAP tend to differ from fourth year students [23,35,36].

<table>
<tr><th>No</th><th>Topic</th><th colspan="2">Teaching and learning method</th><th>Hours</th></tr>
<tr><td>1</td><td>Introduction and overview of CAM</td><td colspan="2">Interactive lecture</td><td>2</td></tr>
<tr><td>2</td><td>Epidemiology of CAM practices</td><td colspan="2">Interactive lecture</td><td>2</td></tr>
<tr><td>3</td><td>Characteristics and comparison of CAM vs. Conventional Medicine</td><td colspan="2">Interactive lecture</td><td>2</td></tr>
<tr><td>4</td><td>Integrative Medicine</td><td colspan="2">Interactive lecture</td><td>2</td></tr>
<tr><td>5</td><td>Research models in CAM</td><td colspan="2">Interactive lecture</td><td>2</td></tr>
<tr><td>6</td><td>Evidence based CAM</td><td colspan="2">Interactive lecture</td><td>2</td></tr>
<tr><td>7</td><td>Medical ethics of CAM</td><td colspan="2">Interactive lecture</td><td>2</td></tr>
<tr><td>8</td><td>Frauds and misconceptions related to CAM practices and products</td><td colspan="2">Interactive lecture</td><td>2</td></tr>
<tr><td>9</td><td>Health education and communication in CAM</td><td colspan="2">Interactive lecture</td><td>2</td></tr>
<tr><td>10</td><td>Mind body medicine</td><td colspan="2">Interactive lecture</td><td>2</td></tr>
<tr><td>11</td><td>Energy medicine</td><td colspan="2">Interactive lecture</td><td>2</td></tr>
<tr><td>12</td><td>Local traditional practices in KSA</td><td colspan="2">Interactive lecture</td><td>2</td></tr>
<tr><td>13</td><td>Herbal medicine</td><td colspan="2">Interactive lecture</td><td>2</td></tr>
<tr><td>14</td><td>Apitherapy</td><td colspan="2">Interactive lecture</td><td>2</td></tr>
<tr><td>15</td><td>Whole medical system (TCM)</td><td colspan="2">Interactive lecture</td><td>2</td></tr>
<tr><td>16</td><td>Whole medical system (Naturopathy)</td><td colspan="2">Interactive lecture</td><td>2</td></tr>
<tr><td>Seminar 1</td><td>Manipulative and body based practices</td><td colspan="2">Student led seminar</td><td>2</td></tr>
<tr><td>Seminar 2</td><td>Biological based practices</td><td colspan="2">Student led seminar</td><td>2</td></tr>
<tr><td>Seminar 3</td><td>Whole medical system (Homeopathy)</td><td colspan="2">Student led seminar</td><td>2</td></tr>
<tr><td>Seminar 4</td><td>Whole medical system (Unani Medicine, Arabic or Hakim Medicine)</td><td colspan="2">Student led seminar</td><td>2</td></tr>
<tr><td>Seminar 5</td><td>Nutritional therapy</td><td colspan="2">Student led seminar</td><td>2</td></tr>
<tr><td>Practical session 1</td><td>Local traditional CAM practices (Hijama)</td><td colspan="2">Demonstration & simulation</td><td>12</td></tr>
<tr><td>Practical session 2</td><td>Alternative CAM practices (Acupuncture)</td><td colspan="2">Demonstration & simulation</td><td>12</td></tr>
<tr><td>Practical session 3</td><td>Prophetic medicine</td><td colspan="2">Demonstration & simulation</td><td>6</td></tr>
<tr><td>Field visit</td><td>field visit to the nearby community</td><td colspan="2">Field visit</td><td>6</td></tr>
<tr><td rowspan="4">SUBTOTAL</td><td>Interactive lectures</td><td>16 x 2 hours</td><td>32</td><td rowspan="4">78</td></tr>
<tr><td>Seminars</td><td>5 x 2 hours</td><td>10</td></tr>
<tr><td>Practical session</td><td>5 x 6 hours</td><td>30</td></tr>
<tr><td>Field visit</td><td>1 x 6 hours</td><td>6</td></tr>
<tr><td rowspan="7">GRAND TOTAL DURATION INCLUDING EXAMINATION</td><td>Interactive lectures</td><td colspan="2">32 hours</td><td rowspan="7">82</td></tr>
<tr><td>Seminars</td><td colspan="2">10 hours</td></tr>
<tr><td>Practical session</td><td colspan="2">30 hours</td></tr>
<tr><td>Field visit</td><td colspan="2">6 hours</td></tr>
<tr><td>Mid-term exam</td><td colspan="2">2 hours</td></tr>
<tr><td>Final exam</td><td colspan="2">2 hours</td></tr>
<tr><td>TOTAL hours available</td><td colspan="2">82 hours</td></tr>
</table>

Table 1: Details of teaching schedule.

No	Topic	ILOs	Teaching and learning methods	Student assessment method
1	Introduction and overview of CAM	A1, A7, C1, D1	lecture	MCQs & SEQs
2	Epidemiology of CAM practices	A1, A4, A5, A7, B6, C1, D1	lecture	MCQs & SEQs
3	Characteristics and comparison of CAM vs Conventional Medicine	A1, A2, A4, A5, A6, A7, A8, B4, B6, D1, D2	lecture	MCQs & SEQs
4	WHO strategy for TM/CM 2014-2023	A1, A2, A6, A7, A8, B4, B5, C1, D1, D2, D4	lecture	MCQs & SEQs
5	Integrative Medicine	A1, A2, A5, A6, B1, B2, B4	lecture	MCQs & SEQs
6	Research models in CAM	A6, A8, B1, B2, B4, C1, C2, C3, D2	lecture	MCQs & SEQs
7	Evidence based CAM	A6, A8, B1, B2, B4, C1, C2, C3, D2	lecture	MCQs & SEQs
8	CAM resources	B2, B3, C2, D4	lecture	MCQs & SEQs
9	Regulatory framework governing CAM	A7, A8, B4, B5, D1	lecture	MCQs & SEQs
10	Medical ethics of CAM	A8, C2, D1, D4	lecture	MCQs & SEQs
11	Frauds and misconceptions related to CAM practices and products	A1, A2, A7, B6	lecture	MCQs & SEQs
12	Health education and communication in CAM	A1, A2, A7, B6	lecture	MCQs & SEQs
13	Energy medicine	A2, A4, A5, B1, B2, B4, C1, C2, D1, D2, D3, D4	lecture	MCQs & SEQs
14	Local traditional practices in KSA	A2, A4, A5, A7, B1, B2, B4, C1, C2, D1, D2, D3, D4	lecture	MCQs & SEQs
15	Herbal medicine	A2, A4, A5, B1, B2, B4, C1, C2, D1, D2, D3, D4	lecture	MCQs & SEQs
16	Massage therapy	A2, A4, A5, B1, B2, B4, C1, C2, D1, D2, D3, D4	lecture	MCQs & SEQs
17	Reflexology	A2, A4, A5, B1, B2, B4, C1, C2, D1, D2, D3, D4	lecture	MCQs & SEQs
18	Apitherapy	A2, A4, A5, B1, B2, B4, C1, C2, D1, D2, D3, D4	lecture	MCQs & SEQs
19	Mind body medicine	A2, A4, A5, B1, B2, B4, C1, C2, D1, D2, D3, D4	lecture	MCQs & SEQs
20	Prophetic medicine	A2, A4, A5, A7, B1, B2, B4, C1, C2, D1, D2, D3, D4	lecture	MCQs & SEQs
21	Whole medical system (TCM)	A2, A4, A5, B1, B2, B4, C1, C2, D1, D2, D3, D4	lecture	MCQs & SEQs
22	Whole medical system (Naturopathy)	A2, A4, A5, B1, B2, B4, C1, C2, D1, D2, D3, D4	lecture	MCQs & SEQs
23	Nutritional therapy	A2, A4, A5, B1, B2, B4, C1, C2, D1, D2, D4	seminar	MCQs & SEQs
24	Biological based practices	A2, A4, A5, B1, B2, B4, C1, C2, D1, D2, D3, D4	seminar	MCQs & SEQs
25	Manipulative and body based practices	A2, A4, A5, B2, B3, C1, C2, D1, D2, D3, D4	seminar	MCQs & SEQs
26	Whole medical system (Homeopathy)	A2, A4, A5, B1, B2, B4, C1, C2, D1, D2, D3, D4	seminar	MCQs & SEQs
27	Whole medical system (Unani Medicine, Arabic or Hakim Medicine)	A2, A4, A5, B1, B2, B4, C1, C2, D1, D2, D3, D4	seminar	MCQs & SEQs
28	Local traditional CAM practices (Hijama)	A2, A4, A5, B1, B2, B4, C1, C2, C4, D1, D2, D3, D4	Demonstration	MCQs & SEQs
29	Alternative CAM practices (Acupuncture)	A2, A4, A5, B1, B2, B4, C1, C2, C4, D1, D2, D3, D4	Demonstration	MCQs & SEQs
30	Critical appraisal	A6, A8, B4, B6, C1, C2, C3, D1, D2, D3, D4	Demonstration	MCQs & SEQs
31	Prophetic medicine	A2, A4, A5, B1, B2, B4, C1, C2, D1, D2, D3, D4	Demonstration	MCQs & SEQs
32	field visit to the nearby community	A2, A4, A5, B1, B2, B4, C1, C2, D1, D2, D3, D4	Field visit	MCQs & SEQs

Table 2: Course ILOs Matrix-Teaching and learning strategy and student assessment.

Summary and Conclusion

Complementary Medicine and Integrative Health Module has been planned and implemented during the year 2016-2017 for fourth year medical students at Dar Al Uloom University, Riyadh, KSA. The Methods of teaching and learning included interactive lectures, seminars, practical sessions, assignments, field visits, simulation, learning by doing, case studies, problem based learning and self-directed learning. Topics covered during the course included; Introduction and overview of Complementary and Alternative Medicine (CAM), Epidemiology of CAM practices, Characteristics and comparison of CAM *vs.* Conventional Medicine, Integrative Medicine, Research models in CAM, Evidence based CAM, Medical ethics of CAM, Frauds and misconceptions related to CAM practices and products, Health education and communication in CAM, Manipulative and body based practices, Biological-based practices, Mind-body medicine, Energy based therapies, Whole medical systems; Traditional Chinese Medicine (TCM), Unani, Arabic or Hakim Medicine, Prophetic Medicine and Local traditional CAM therapies (Hijamah as a model), Acupuncture, Herbal Medicine, Naturopathy, Nutrition and food supplements, Apitherapy and Homeopathy. At the end of the module, two types of assessments; continuous and final assessments were done. Continuous assessments toke place throughout the course. They were mostly based on course work as follows; Seminar (10%), Assignments (10%), Field visit report (10%) and Mid-term exam (20%). A proportion of 50% had taken in the final assessment. A student who scored 60 or more deemed to have passed this course. The feedback received was most supportive of the module and appreciative of the teachers, the information provided and skills gained and the way in which it was delivered.

Acknowledgment

The author is grateful to all the staff at the college of medicine, Dar AlUloom University, Riyadh, KSA and staff members of National Center for Complementary and Alternative Medicine who has participated in the delivery of the module, assessment and final evaluation of the students.

References

1. Duke Integrative Medicine, 3475 Erwin Road, Durham, North Carolina, 27705, USA.
2. NCCIH, National Center for Complementary and Integrative Health (NCCIH), Complementary, Alternative, or Integrative Health: What's In a Name?

3. U.S National Library of Medicine. 8600 Rockville Pike, Bethesda, MD 20894. U.S. Department of Health and Human Services National Institutes of Health. Accessed at 12-11-2017.
4. U.S Department of Health and Human Services, National Institutes of Health, National Cancer Institute, USA.
5. Brown J, Cooper E, Frankton L, Steeves WM, Gillis RJ, et al. (2007) Complementary and alternative therapies: Survey of knowledge and attitudes of health professionals at a tertiary pediatric/women's care facility. Complem Thera Clini Pract. 13: 194-200.
6. Kemper KJ, O'Connor KG (2004) Pediatricians' recommendations for complementary and alternative medical (CAM) therapies. Ambula Pediat.4: 482-487.
7. Basila D, Yuan CS (2005) Effects of dietary supplements on coagulation and platelet function. Thrombo Resea 117: 49-53.
8. Barbara S, Janice MZ, Joyce KK, Sharon CF, Angela J (2012) Case-Based Online Modules to Teach Graduate Level Nursing Students About Complementary and Alternative Medical Therapies. J Prof Nurs 28: 125-129.
9. Sidrah N, Sadia J, Tauqir A, Asif Zia A (2010) Assessment of improvement in knowledge and skills amongst trainees of workshop on "labour and partograph". J Pak Med Assoc 60: 844-848.
10. Vicki W (2009) Summit on Integrative Medicine & The Health of the Public: Issue Background and Overview. Washington, DC: Institute of Medicine. Retrieval 2011-1-18.
11. Catherine Z, Andrew JV, Janet R (2008) ABC of Complementary Medicine. 2nd edtn. BMJ Books, ISBN: 978-1-4051-3657-0.
12. Lyn W, Freeman (2008) Mosby's complementary and alternative medicine: A research based approach. 3rd edtn, ISBN-13: 978-0323053464.
13. Mark SM (2014) Fundamental of Complementary and Alternative Medicine. 5th edtn. Elsevier Health Sciences. ISBN: 9780323298940.
14. Richard Liebowietz, Linda Smith, Tracy Gaudet (2006) The Duke Encyclopedia of New Medicine: Conventional and Alternative Medicine for All Ages. The Duke Center for Integrative Medicine. Rodale Books, USA.
15. Al-Jauziyah IIQ (1999) Healing with the medicine of the prophet. Dar-us-Salam Publications, Riyadh, Saudi Arabia.
16. Center for Integrative Medicine at the University of Arizona, USA.
17. Al-Rukban MO, AlBedah AM, Khalil MK, El-Olemy AT, Khalil AA, et al. (2012) Status of complementary and alternative medicine in the curricula of health colleges in Saudi Arabia. Complement Ther Med 20: 334-339.
18. AlBeda AM, El-Olem AT, Khalil MK (2012) Knowledge and attitude of health professionals in the Riyadh region, Saudi Arabia, toward complementary and alternative medicine. J Family Community Med 19: 93-99.
19. Morgan RL, Whorton J E, Gunsalus C (2000) A Comparison of Short Term and Long Term Retention: Lecture Combined with Discussion Versus Cooperative Learning. J Instruc Psy 27: 53-57.
20. Wood EJ (2004) Problem-Based Learning: Exploiting knowledge of how people learn to promote effective learning. Bioscience Education e-joiinmt 3: 3-13.
21. Jacobsen PA, Eggen P, Kauchak D (2005) Methods for Teaching: Promoting Student Learning in K-12 Classrooms (7 ed.). Boston: Prentice Hall.
22. El-Olemy AT, Al-Bedah AM, El-Olemy MA, Hussein AA, Elsubai IS, et al. (2017) Trainees' Feedback for the Assessment of Cupping (Al-Hijamah) Training Programs Directed towards Healthcare Professionals, Kingdom of Saudi Arabia. J Edu Soc Behav Sci 23: 1-11.
23. Akan H, Izbirak G, Kaspar EC, Kaya CA, Aydin S, et al. (2012) Knowledge and attitudes towards complementary and alternative medicine among medical students in Turkey. BMC Complement Altern Med. 12:115.
24. Yildirim Y, Parlar S, Eyigor S, Sertoz OO, Eyigor C, et al. (2010) An analysis of nursing and medical students' attitudes towards and knowledge of complementary and alternative medicine (CAM). J Clin Nurs 19: 1157-1166.
25. Alis O, Ganime S, Nuran B, Mumtaz MM, Nazan B, et al. (2007) An analysis of nursing and medical students' attitudes towards and knowledge of complementary and alternative medicine (CAM). J Altern Complement Med. 13: 1007-1010.
26. Al-Bedah AM, Aboushanab TS, Alqaed MS, Qureshi NA, Al-subai I, et al. (2017) Assessing the Effectiveness of Using Simulation in Cupping Therapy Training Course for Undergraduate Medical Students: A Study in Riyadh, KSA. J Adv Med Pharm Sci 13: 1-7.
27. Al Mansour MA, Al-Bedah AM, AlRukban MO, Elsubai IS, Mohamed EY, et al. (2015) Medical students' knowledge, attitude, and practice of complementary and alternative medicine: A pre- and post-exposure survey in Majmaah University, Saudi Arabia. Adv Med Educ Pract. 6: 407-420.
28. Scholl I, Zill JM, Harter M, Dirmaier J (2014) An integrative model of patient-centeredness - A systematic review and concept analysis. PLoS One. 9: e107828.
29. Saunders PA, Tractenberg RE, Chaterji R, Amri H, Harazduk N, et al. (2007) Promoting self-awareness and reflection through an experiential mind-body skills course for first year medical students. Med Teach. 29: 778-784.
30. Elder W, Rakel D, Heitkemper M, Hustedde C, Harazduk N, et al. (2007) Using complementary and alternative medicine curricular elements to foster medical student self-awareness. Acad Med. 82: 951-955.
31. Sierpina VS, Schneeweiss R, Frenkel MA, Bulik R, Maypole J (2007) Barriers, strategies, and lessons learned from complementary and alternative medicine curricular initiatives. Acad Med 82: 946-950.
32. Frenkel M, Arye EB (2001) The growing need to teach about complementary and alternative medicine: Questions and challenges. Acad Med 76: 251-254.
33. Fonfa AE (2007) Patient perspectives: Barriers to complementary and alternative medicine therapies create problems for patients and survivors. Integr Cancer Ther 6: 297-300.
34. Yeo AS, Yeo JC, Yeo C, Lee CH, Lim LF, et al. (2005) Perceptions of complementary and alternative medicine amongst medical students in Singapore-A survey. Acupunct Med. 23:19-26.
35. Furnham A, McGill C (2003) Medical students' attitudes about complementary and alternative medicine. J Altern Complement Med 9: 275-284.
36. DeSylvia D, Stuber M, Fung CC, Bazargan-Hejazi S, Cooper E (2011) The knowledge, attitudes and usage of complementary and alternative medicine of medical students. Evid Based Complement Altern Med 728902.

Stability and Efficacy of Anti-dermatophyte Creams From Extract of *Kigelia africana* Leaves

Fawehinmi AB[1*] and Oyedeji FO[2]

[1]*Nigeria Natural Medicine Development Agency Lagos, Nigeria*
[2]*Department of Chemistry, University of Ibadan, Nigeria*

Abstract

Dermatophytosis are skin infections caused by dermatophytes which can be pathogenic for humans and animals by infecting the stratum corneum, nails, claws or hair and which now affect more than 20%-25% of the world populations especially in the developing countries. Drug resistance and toxicity associated with long-term treatment with existing antifungal drugs necessitate the search for new drugs to treat dermatophytosis. The juice of *Kigelia africana* leaves has been used by the natives to treat dermatophytosis. The leaves were extracted with water, ethanol and petroleum ether. Phytochemical analyses of the extracts were carried out. Agar disc discussion method was used to determine the antifungal activities against clinical isolates of *Microsporum audouinii, Epidermophyton floccosum, Trichophyton mentagrophytes* and *Malassezia furfur.* Herbal creams formulated with 0.5, 1.0 and 2.0 g w/w of the extract were subjected to stability tests using standard methods. FTIR was used to determine if there were new functional groups formed during production of the herbal creams. Sensitivity and efficacy of the products were determined using animal model experiment.

The percentage yields of extracts are petroleum ether 6.3%, aqueous 6.5%, and ethanol 7.2%. Percentage ethanol phytochemical composition indicated that for Alkaloid (4.67%), saponins (2.48%), flavonoids (0.81%) and tannins (1.05%). The emulsion produced was an oil-in-water emulsion and had a white colour with pH of 7.02 spread of emulsion, rubbing-in effect and stability to centrifugation was very high. The antifungal results showed that the petroleum ether and aqueous extracts had 10 mm zones of inhibition, while ethanol extract had 15 mm at 10,000 μg/ml against *Trichophyton mentagrophytes.* Against *Microsporum audouinii,* the results are petroleum ether and aqueous extracts (10 mm) and ethanol extract (14 mm). Against *Epidermophyton floccosum,* the results are petroleum ether and aqueous extracts (10 mm) while ethanol was 13 mm. The zones of inhibition recorded by the extracts against *Malassezia furfur* are aqueous 4 mm, petroleum ether 12 mm and ethanol 15 mm respectively. The results for FTIR showed a spectrum of C-N stretch which peaks at 1019.00 cm^{-1} for Ka cream. Also, an O-H stretch peak was observed at 3254.00 cm^{-1}. Temperature stability tests carried out indicated increasing stability in the order Ka.water cream <Ka.pet. Ether cream <Ka.ethanol cream. Centrifuge testing indicated that there was no separation of the creams. Light testing indicated no change in the colour and odour of the products. There was no change observed in all the test samples during the freeze-thaw testing. Moisture loss on drying indicated Ka.W(6.37%) <Ka.E(6.79%) <Ka.Pet(6.40%). Animal studies evaluation of the ethanolic formulations of the cream indicated that their efficacy against the dermatophytes is concentration dependent and the efficacy is in the order *E. floccosum* (30.53 μm) < *M. audouinii* (31.37 μm) <*M. furfur* (36.22 μm) <*T. mentagrophyte* (37.01 μm).

The results showed that *Kigelia africana* ethanol extract can be used in herbal cream formulations for the management of dermatophytosis.

Keywords: Dermatophytosis; Keratinization; *Kigelia africana*; Alkaloid; *Malassezia furfur*

Introduction

Dermatophytosis is a skin infection caused by dermatophytes and is treated through the use of synthetic chemical derivatives which have been reported to succumb to resistance by the dermatophytes with prolonged usage on the skin [1]. It is principally cosmetic in the initial stages. Some of these chemicals include derivate of azoles, naphthoquinones, aminosterol and morpholine. Moghimipour et al. [2] reported that non availability and high cost of new generation antibiotics and antifungals due to low purchasing power of developing countries contributes to resistance by the pathogens. He also reported toxicity associated with long-term treatment with antifungal drugs but natural products found in plants seem to avoid these side effects Babayi et al. [3] reported compatibility of medicinal plant metabolites with human systems. Scherrer et al. [4] said that the efficacy of synergistic effects of active medicinal plants metabolites in eradication of human pathogens cannot be over emphasized. Aghel et al. also reported the resistance of many pathogens to synthetic drug therapies.

Dermatophytes such as *Trichopyhton mentagrophytes, Microsporium audouinii, Epidermophyton floccosum* and *Malassezia furfur* are fungi that require keratin for growth. These fungi can cause superficial infections of the skin, hair, and nails. Dermatophytes are spread by direct contact from other people (anthropophilic organisms), animals (zoophilic organisms) and soil (geophilic organisms) [5]. Fungal infections of the skin and nail form the most numerous and widespread group of mycosis. The prevalence of superficial mycotic infections has risen to such a level in the last decade that skin mycosis now affect

***Corresponding author:** AB Fawehinmi, Nigeria Natural Medicine Development Agency Lagos, Nigeria, E-mail: akinnbank@yahoo.com

more than 20%-25% of the world's population [6]. Dermatophytes thrive at surface temperatures of 25˚C-28˚C and the skin infection are encouraged by warm and humid conditions. Therefore, superficial fungal infections are common in tropical countries and further exuberated by wearing thick clothing. Some other factors that encourage proliferation of dermatophytosis include crowded living conditions and very low socioeconomic status with skin to skin contact. Dermatophytosis can also increase due to the absence or poor medicare and a weakened immune system (e.g., those infected with HIV or taking immunosuppressive drugs).

The leaves of *Kigelia africana* called pandoro (West Nigeria) is used by the Yorubas for the treatment of skin diseases [7]. It belongs to the family Bignoniaceae, and is widely distributed in the south, central and West Africa [8]. Oyedeji and Bankole-Ojo [9] carried out Quantitative evaluation of the anti-psoriatic activity of sausage tree (*Kigelia africana*) using methanol and hexane extracts of the stem, bark, leaves and fruit of the plant. The results of their studies showed that the topical application of *K. africana* exhibited an important anti-psoriatic activity with *K. africana* stem methanol extracts exhibiting the highest anti-psoriatic activity with little irritation potential. Agyare et al. investigated the antimicrobial and antioxidant properties of methanol leaf and stem bark extracts of *Kigelia africana* and methanol leaf and root extracts of *Strophanthus hispidus* and also determined the wound healing properties of the extracts. The antimicrobial activities of the methanol extracts were determined against two gram-positive and two gram-negative bacteria and a fungus using agar diffusion and micro-dilution methods. *K. africana* extracts (7.5% w/w) showed significant wound contraction at day 7 with 72% of wound closure whiles significant wound contractions were observed on day 11 for stem bark of *K. africana*, leaf and root extracts of *S. hispidus*. They also found out that wound tissues treated with the extracts showed improved collagenation, re-epitheliazition and rapid granulation formation compared with untreated wound tissues. The extracts were found to contain alkaloids, saponins, tannins, flavonoids, carbohydrates, and sapogenetic glycosides.

Materials and Methods

Plant materials

Leaves of *K. africana* were collected at the botanical gardens of the University of Ibadan. It was identified by the taxonomist and samples deposited at medicinal plants of Nigeria Herbarium of NNMDA. The plants were air dried in the shade and pulverized to fine-sized particles for solvent extraction processes.

Preparation of plant extracts

200 g of the pulverized plant sample was extracted with ethanol and petroleum ether using soxhlet extraction method. Rotary evaporator was used to recover the solvent from the mixture at the boiling point of the solvents. Aqueous extract of the sample was obtained by placing 200 g of the pulverized sample in a blender and 1 litre of hot distilled water added to it. The mixture was then thoroughly blended for five minutes and then filtered using a Whatman filter paper grade 1. Excess water was removed using a rotary evaporator set at 100˚C.

Determination of the phytochemical constituents

The extract was evaluated for the presence of tannins, flavonoids, saponins and alkaloids using simple qualitative and quantitative methods of Trease and Evans (1989) and Sofowora (1993).

Micro-organisms: Clinical isolates of *Microsporium aoudininn, Epidermophyton floccosum, Trychophyton mentagrophyte and Malassezia furfur* were obtained from Spectralab medical and diagnostic services, Sagamu, Ogun State.

Microbiological assay: Zones of inhibition was determined using the method as described by Irobi and Daramola (1994). 0.2 g of weighed extracts and 2.0 mL of mixture of DMSO and N-Hexane were used in preparing each stock of 10000 µg/mL. The stocks were then serially diluted to obtain 1000 µg/mL, 100 µg/mL and 10 µg/mL respectively. The zone of inhibition were measured in mm and recorded. The zones of inhibition produced by the solvents alone were subtracted from those of the extracts and solvents in order to obtain the zones of inhibition due to the extracts alone.

Materials for emulsion formulation : Cosmetic grade stearic acid, cetyl alcohol, parafin oil and triethanolamine were all obtained from Akilapa market in Ibadan while de-ionize water was obtained from International Institute of Tropical Agriculture (IITA) Ibadan, Oyo State. All oil soluble substances were placed in a stainless steel container and heated to between 70˚C-75˚C. All water-soluble substances were placed in another stainless steel container and heated to the same temperature. The oil phase was then added to the aqueous phase slowly with stirring. Heating was continued at the same temperature for about 10-15 minutes. The coarse emulsions formed were then cooled to about 35˚C gradually. The emulsions were allowed to stay at room temperature for twelve hours and then homogenized with the aid of a mechanical stirrer. The samples were then poured into labeled containers. Four emulsions were formulated based on four different formularies and labeled A-D. Emulsions containing 0.5%, 1% and 2%, of *Kigelia africana* ethanolic extracts were produced. The prepared herbal emulsions were then vigorously homogenized (Table 1).

Stability tests for the formulated emulsion: Stability tests were carried out on the emulsions following the methods as described by cannel whereby the temperature variation tests include storing the samples at -10˚C, 4˚C, 30˚C, 37˚C and 45˚C were carried out. All observations including pH, colour and odour were noted and recorded (Table 2). The creams were made to pass through freeze thaw cycles testing which involves making the samples pass through three cycles of temperature testing by placing the samples at -10˚C for 24 hours and then at room temperature for 24 hours (Table 3). The creams were made to pass through centrifuge testing whereby the samples were heated to 50˚C and they were then centrifuged for thirty minutes at 2000, 2500, 3000 and 4000 rpm (Table 4). They were then inspected for signs to determine if the dispersed phase of the emulsion has separated and risen to the top. The creams were made to pass through light testing whereby they were placed in test tubes and also in the actual package. They were then put in the window where direct sun rays fell on them. This method is used to determine the sensitivity of the emulsions to the ultra violet radiation (Table 5). Moisture loss on drying/residue content of the creams were determined by weighing 2.0 g of the cosmetic emulsion into a dried petri dish and kept in the oven at 105˚C for 2 hours after which they were taken out and cooled in a desiccator and weighed to a constant weight.

In vivo anti-dermatophytic activity

Ethical statement: The experimental procedures carried out in this study were in compliance with University of Ibadan ethics committee for the care and use of laboratory animals in line with approval number UI-ACUREC/App/12/2016/06.

Medicinal plants	Alkaloid (%)	Saponin (%)	Flavonoid (%)	Tannin (%)
K. africana	4.67 ± 0.11	2.48 ± 0.31	0.81 ± 0.62	1.05 ± 0.08
Each value in the table is the average ± standard deviation of triplicate experiments				

Table 1: The percentage phytochemical composition of the ethanol extract.

Concentration in µg/mL	10	100	1000	10000
T. mentagrophytes	5	7	10	10
M. audouinii	-	6	9	10
E. floccossum	4	5	8	10
M. furfur	4	5	9	10

Table 2: Zones of Inhibition (mm) of aqueous extract on microorganisms.

Concentration in µg/mL	10	100	1000	10000
T. mentagrophytes	9	10	14	15
M. audouinii	-	10	12	14
E. floccossum	8	10	11	13
M. furfur	7	8	12	15

Table 3: Zones of Inhibition (mm) of ethanol extract on microorganisms.

Concentration in µg/mL	10	100	1000	10000
T. mentagrophytes	4	7	10	10
M. audouinii	-	7	10	10
E. floccossum	4	8	10	10
M. furfur	3	5	11	12

Table 4: Zones of Inhibition (mm) of petroleum ether extract on microorganisms.

Product	Day 1			2 weeks			4 weeks			8 weeks			12 weeks			16 weeks		
	pH	Colour	odour	pH	colour	odour	PH	colour	odour	pH	colour	odour	pH	colour	odour	pH	colour	odour
Control	7.02	NCC	NCIO	7.02	NCC	NCIO	7.02	NCC	NCIO	7.02	NCC	NCIO	7.02	NCC	NCIO	7.02	NCC	NCIO
Ka.W	7.21	NCC	NCIO	7.21	NCC	NCIO	7.21	NCC	NCIO	7.21	NCC	NCIO	7.21	NCC	NCIO	7.21	NCC	NCIO
Ka.E	7.25	NCC	NCIO	7.25	NCC	NCIO	7.25	NCC	NCIO	7.25	NCC	NCIO	7.25	NCC	NCIO	7.25	NCC	NCIO
Ka.Pet	7.19	NCC	NCIO	7.19	NCC	NCIO	7.19	NCC	NCIO	7.19	NCC	NCIO	7.19	NCC	NCIO	7.19	NCC	NCIO

Table 5: Effect of temperature (-10°C) on cream samples after production.

Laboratory animals: Albino rats weighing between 150-200 g were obtained from the experimental animal unit of the faculty of Veterinary medicine of the University of Ibadan. They were kept in well ventilated rat cages with free access to water and feed and were left in this environment for two (2) weeks to acclimatize.

Selection and grouping of animals: The animals were randomly allocated to six (6) groups (5 rats/group) such that the difference in average weight did not exceed 5 g. Each animal was used once in the experiment. The rats were then inoculated with the dermatophytes. One week after inoculation of the animals with the dermatophytes, the inoculated skin area of 2 cm^2 were treated with the plants extracts and the formulated emulsions with plants extracts for seven days. At the end of seven days, the animals were euthanized by cervical dislocation.

Forty five (45) animals were required per batch and were grouped into 6 groups of 5 rats in a group.

- Group 1: Animals without any treatment-Negative control.
- Group 2: Animals treated with cream containing 1% Clotrimazole (Standard drug)-Positive control.
- Group 3: Animals treated with placebo (Emulsion without any medicinal plants)-Positive control.
- Group 4a: Animals treated with 0.5% medicinal plant extract alone.
- Group 4b: Animals treated with emulsion containing 0.5% medicinal plant extract.
- Group 5a: Animals treated with 1% medicinal plant extract alone.
- Group 5b: Animals treated with emulsion containing 1% medicinal plant extract.
- Group 6a: Animals treated with 2% medicinal plant extract alone.
- Group 6b: Animals treated with emulsion containing 2% medicinal plant extract.

Histopathological studies: 2 cm^2 skin areas were cut and put in 10% formalin for histo-pathological analysis. Skin biopsy samples were examined for presence of fungal hyphae, hair follicles, sebaceous gland, inflammation and tissue destruction using light microscope. (Culling CFA. Hand book of histo-pathological and histo-chemical techniques 1979; III edition).

Statistical analysis of data: Statistical analysis of data was carried out by one way ANOVA comparing all test groups *vs* control followed by tukeys post hoc analysis. Data is reported as mean ± SEM. P ≤ 0.05 was considered significant. Also epidermal thickness and keratin layer were obtained with the aid of calibrated Toupview® software.

FTIR analysis: The oil sample and the products were qualitatively characterized by the FT-IR technique. These were obtained on a Perkin

Elmer Fourier transform infrared spectrometer. The spectra were recorded between 4000-350 cm^{-1} using KBr discs.

Results and Discussion

The percentage yield of extracts by the solvents are in the order petroleum ether (6.3%) <aqueous (6.5%) <ethanol (7.2%).

The percentage phytochemical composition of the ethanol extract is listed in Table 1.

Antimicrobial Screening

Effect of aqueous extracts of *K. africana* against the microorganisms

At 10000 μg/mL, the activities of the extract were the same against three of the dermatophytes namely *T. mentagrophytes, M. aoudinin* and *E. floccossum* with zones of inhibition of 10 mm while it was 4 mm for *M. furfur*. At 1000 μg/mL, the zones of inhibition were in the range 5-10 mm with effect on *M. furfur* <*E. floccossum* <*M. audouinii* <*T. mentagrophytes*. Activities were noticed for the extract against the dermatophytes at 100 μg/mL in the order *E. floccossum* < *M. audouinii* <*T. mentagrophytes* <*M. furfur*. At 10 μg/mL, there was no activity of the extract against *M. audouinii*, but the activity against the other microorganisms were in the order *M. furfur*=*E. floccossum* <*T. mentagrophytes* (Table 2). The result shows that the extract was active against *T. mentagrophytes, E. floccossum* and *M. furfur* at all the concentrations though the activity is concentration dependent. The extract however has no activity against *M. audouinii* at 10 μg/mL. Owolabi et al. [10] reported that the aqueous extract of *Kigelia africana* water extract exhibited no antibacterial or antifungal activity at low concentrations, but the low activity observed here could be attributed to the conclusion by Arti and Kanika who observed that phytochemicals in little quantities have definite physiological action on the human body to fight antimicrobials.

Effect of ethanol extracts of *K. africana* against the microorganisms

The activities of ethanol extract of the plant at 10000 μg/mL range from 13-15 mm (Table 3). The zones of inhibition against the dermatophytes are in the order *E. floccossum* <*M. audouinii* <*T. mentagrophytes*=*M. furfur*. There was noticeable reduction in activities of the extract as the concentration reduced to 1000 μg/mL with zones of inhibition in the range 11-14 mm with activity against the organisms in the order *E. floccossum* <*M. audouinii* =*M. furfur* <*T. mentagrophytes*. At 100 μg/mL, the activities were in the order *T. mentagrophytes*=*M. audouinii* =*E. floccossum* <*M. furfur*. However no activity of the extract was recorded against *M. audouinii* at 10 μg/mL, but it was active against the other dermatophytes in the order *M. furfur* <*E. floccossum* <*T. mentagrophytes*. Previous study by Okafor et al. against the pathogens seems to agree with was observed in this study.

Effect of petroleum ether extracts of *K. africana* against the microorganisms

The activities of petroleum ether extracts of *K. africana* against the dermatophytes at 10000 μg/mL range from 10-12 mm (Table 4) with effect on *T. mentagrophytes*=*M. audouinii E. floccossum* <*M. furfur*. At 1000 μg/mL, there was no noticeable change in the activity compared to 10000 μg/mL. However, the activity against the dermatophytes reduced at 100 μg/mL which ranges from 5-8 mm with effect on *M. furfur* <*T. mentagrophytes*=*M. audouinii* <*E. floccossum*. It was observed that at 10 μg/mL, the extract had no effect on *M. audouinii* while the zones of inhibition on *T. mentagrophytes* and *E. floccossum* were 4 mm and 3 mm on *M. furfur*. Though there has not been much work carried out on the petroleum ether extracts of the plant to enable us compare, but the results obtained are very close to what was obtained for the aqueous extract of the plant.

Temperature stability testing

The results of changes in colour, odour and pH from date of production through 2, 4, 8, 12 and 16th week of production and stored at -10°C and 4°C are presented in Tables 5 and 6. At production through 4, 8, 12 and 16th week, the colour, odour and pH of the creams remain stable. This indicated that the temperature did not allow movement or dissociation of ions. At 30°C, there was no change in colour and odour of all the samples throughout the weeks of test. However, the pH of control dropped from 7.02 to 7.00 after 2 weeks of production and remained stable till 4th week. At 8th week, the pH further dropped by 0.01 to 6.99 and remained stable till 16th week. pH of 7.25 was measured for Ka.E sample on the day of production. However, after 2 weeks of production, the pH increased to 7.27 and remains stable till 16th week of test (Table 7). pH of 7.19 was measured for Ka.Pet sample on the day of production. However, after 4 weeks of production, the pH inceased to 7.20 and remain stable till 16th week of test. The same observation was made for pH of Ka.Pet sample which increased from 7.19 at production to 7.23 after 16 weeks of production. Same goes for Ka.W with increase in pH from 7.21 at the day of production to 7.26 at 16th week of production. The results of changes in colour, odour and pH from date of production through 2, 4, 8, 12 and 16th week of production and stored at 37°C is presented in Table 8. No noticeable changes in colour and odour were observed for all the samples. The same observation was made for pH of Ka.E sample which increased from 7.25 at production to 7.30 after 16 weeks of production. The same observation was made for pH of Ka.Pet, sample which increased from 7.19 at production to 7.23 after 16 weeks of production.

The results of changes in colour, odour and pH from date of production through 2, 4, 8, 12 and 16th week of production and stored at 45°C is presented in Table 9. No noticeable changes in colour and odour were observed for all the samples. The pH of Ka.W sample increased from 7.21 at production to 7.26 after 16 weeks of production. The same observation was made for pH of Ka.E sample which increased from 7.25 at production to 7.32 after 16 weeks of production and pH of Ka.Pet too increased from 7.19 to 7.25.

product	Day 1			2 weeks			4 weeks			8 weeks			12 weeks			16 weeks		
	pH	Colour	odour	pH	colour	odour	PH	colour	odour	pH	colour	odour	pH	colour	odour	pH	colour	odour
Control	7.02	NCC	NCIO	7.02	NCC	NCIO	7.02	NCC	NCIO	7.02	NCC	NCIO	7.02	NCC	NCIO	7.02	NCC	NCIO
Ka.W	7.21	NCC	NCIO	7.21	NCC	NCIO	7.21	NCC	NCIO	7.22	NCC	NCIO	7.22	NCC	NCIO	7.23	NCC	NCIO
Ka.E	7.25	NCC	NCIO	7.25	NCC	NCIO	7.25	NCC	NCIO	7.25	NCC	NCIO	7.25	NCC	NCIO	7.25	NCC	NCIO
Ka.Pet	7.19	NCC	NCIO	7.19	NCC	NCIO	7.19	NCC	NCIO	7.19	NCC	NCIO	7.19	NCC	NCIO	7.19	NCC	NCIO
NCC=No change in colour , CC=Change in colour, NCIO=No change in odour, CIO=Change in odour																		

Table 6: Effect of temperature (4°C) on cream samples after production.

product	Day 1			2 weeks			4 weeks			8 weeks			12 weeks			16 weeks		
	pH	Colour	odour	pH	colour	odour	PH	colour	odour	pH	colour	odour	pH	colour	odour	pH	colour	odour
Control	7.02	NCC	NCIO	7.00	NCC	NCIO	6.99	NCC	NCIO	6.98	NCC	1	6.98	1	1	6.98	1	1
Ka.W	7.21	NCC	NCIO	7.22	NCC	NCIO	7.24	NCC	NCIO	7.24	1	1	7.25	1	1	7.26	1	1
Ka.E	7.25	NCC	NCIO	7.25	NCC	NCIO	7.27	NCC	NCIO	7.27	1	1	7.27	1	1	7.27	1	1
Ka.Pet	7.19	NCC	NCIO	7.19	NCC	NCIO	7.19	NCC	NCIO	7.20	1	1	7.20	1	1	7.20	1	1
NCC=No change in colour , CC=Change in colour, NCIO=No change in odour, CIO=Change in odour																		

Table 7: Effect of temperature (30°C) on cream samples after production.

product	Day 1			2 weeks			4 weeks			8 weeks			12 weeks			16 weeks		
	pH	Colour	odour	pH	colour	odour	PH	colour	odour	pH	colour	odour	pH	colour	odour	pH	colour	odour
Control	7.02	NCC	NCIO	7.02	NCC	NCIO	7.02	NCC	NCIO	7.02	NCC	NCIO	7.02	NCC	NCIO	7.02	NCC	NCIO
Ka.W	7.21	NCC	NCIO	7.22	NCC	NCIO	7.24	NCIO	NCIO	7.24	NCIO	NCIO	7.25	NCC	NCIO	7.26	NCC	NCIO
Ka.E	7.25	NCC	NCIO	7.27	NCC	NCIO	7.27	NCC	NCIO	7.27	NCC	NCIO	7.30	NCC	NCIO	7.30	NCC	NCIO
Ka.Pet	7.19	NCC	NCIO	7.20	NCC	NCIO	7.22	NCC	NCIO	7.22	NCC	NCIO	7.23	NCC	NCIO	7.23	NCC	NCIO
NCC=No change in colour , CC=Change in colour, NCIO=No change in odour, CIO=Change in odour																		

Table 8: Effect of temperature (37°C) on cream samples after production.

product	Day 1			2 weeks			4 weeks			8 weeks			12 weeks			16 weeks		
	pH	Colour	odour	pH	colour	odour	PH	colour	odour	pH	colour	odour	pH	colour	odour	pH	colour	odour
Control	7.02	NCC	NCIO	7.02	NCC	NCIO	7.02	NCC	NCIO	7.02	NCC	NCIO	7.02	NCC	NCIO	7.02	NCC	NCIO
Ka.W	7.21	NCC	NCIO	7.23	NCC	NCIO	7.23	NCC	NCIO	7.25	NCC	NCIO	7.25	NCC	NCIO	7.26	NCC	NCIO
Ka.E	7.25	NCC	NCIO	7.29	NCC	NCIO	7.29	NCC	NCIO	7.29	NCC	NCIO	7.32	NCC	NCIO	7.32	NCC	NCIO
Ka.Pet	7.19	NCC	NCIO	7.21	NCC	NCIO	7.21	NCC	NCIO	7.24	NCC	NCIO	7.24	NCC	NCIO	7.25	NCC	NCIO
NCC=No change in colour, CC=Change in colour, NCIO=No change in odour, CIO=Change in odour																		

Table 9: Effect of temperature (45°C) on cream samples after production.

Centrifuge testing

No phase separation was detected in all the test samples at 2000, 2500, 3000 and 4,000 rpm as indicated in Table 10. This shows that the disperse phase is well particulated in the continuous phase thereby stable to centrifugation.

Light testing

As shown in Table 11, no changes were noticed for all the samples which indicated that they were not sensitive to ultra violet light.

Freeze-thaw testing

There was no change observed in all the test samples during the cycle testing (Table 12).

Table 13 shows the results for moisture loss on drying/residue content which suggest that the formulations may be stable to microbial attack because of the moisture content which falls within the acceptable limits.

Fourier transform infra-red spectrocopy analysis

Results of FTIR spectroscopic studies revealed the presence of various functional groups in the cream and the test sample (Figures 1 and 2). The spectrum of the placebo (cream alone) shows strong O-H stretch at 3373.00 cm^{-1} of amines. N=H bending at 1640.00 cm^{-1} indicated that the placebo contains an unsaturated amide group. O-H bending of phenyl group at 1409.00 cm^{-1} indicated the presence of carboxylic acid group in the sample, S=O stretch at 1040.00 cm^{-1} indicated presence of sulphoxide. There is a spectrum of C-N stretch which peaks at 1019.00 cm^{-1} for Ka cream, this peak serves as good evidence for the homo-polymerization reaction. Also, an O-H stretch peak was observed at 3254.00 cm^{-1}. Some of these functional groups found in the herbal cream formulations which are not in the cream base maybe responsible for the plants effectiveness in the management of dermatophytosis.

Sample	2000 rpm	2500 rpm	3000 rpm	4000 rpm
control	NPS	NPS	NPS	NPS
Ka.W	NPS	NPS	NPS	NPS
Ka.E	NPS	NPS	NPS	NPS
Ka.Pet	NPS	NPS	NPS	NPS
NPS=No phase separation, PS=phase separation				

Table 10: Centrifuge testing for the samples.

Control	NNC
Ka.w	NCC
Ka.E	NCC
Ka.et	NCC
NCC=No colour change, CC=colour change	

Table 11: Light testing.

Control	NPS
Ka.w	NPS
Ka.E	NPS
Ka.et	NPS
NPS=No Phase separation, PS=Phase separation	

Table 12: Freeze thaw testing.

Cream	Moisture loss on drying (%)	Residue content (%)
Kigelia africana aqueous	6.37	93.63
Kigelia africana ethanol	6.39	93.61
Kigelia africana pet.ether	6.40	93.60

Table 13: Determination of moisture loss on drying/residue content of medicinal plants extracts emulsions.

In vivo Anti-dermatophytic Activity

Efficacy of *Kigelia africana* ethanol cream formulations against *Microsporum audouinii*

Marked inflammation of the skin and foci of discontinuity of the

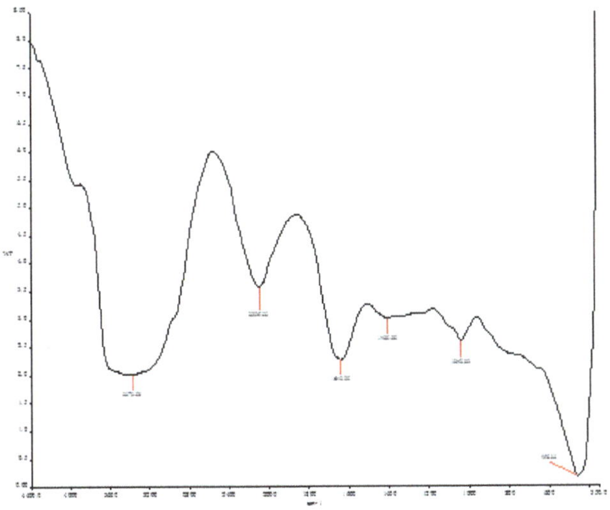

Figure 1: FTIR spectrum of emulsion alone (placebo).

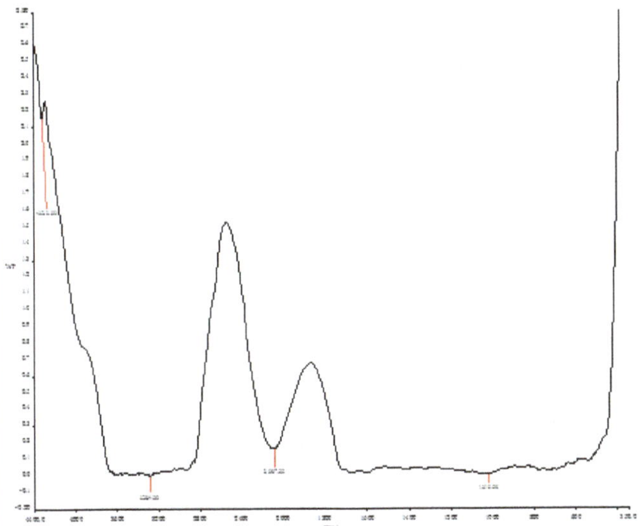

Figure 2: FTIR spectrum of *Kigelia africana* cosmeutical.

epidermis were observed in the untreated group (group 1) which confirms successful infection (Table 14). There was marked presence of fungal hyphae as shown in Figure 3. There were few hair follicles enmeshed within the sparse connective tissue in the dermis which indicated that the dermatophyte is feeding on the follicles (Figure 3). Very few sebaceous glands were seen showing that the oil in the sebaceous gland have been used up by the dermatophytes. Marked tissue destruction was observed. In the group treated with emulsion alone (group 3), Inflammation and tissue destruction of the skin were moderate in the group. There was marked presence of fungal hyphae which indicated that the cream alone has no medicinal effect on the dermatophyte infection and reduction of numbers of hair follicles also occurred as the dermatophye was able to attack unhindered. However the group has moderate number of sebaceous glands in the dermis showing the content of the emulsion provided alternative source for the dermatophyte thus reducing the effect on the glands.

In group 4a (0.5% plant extract alone), Inflammation and tissue destruction of the skin were moderate in the group (Table 14). Presence

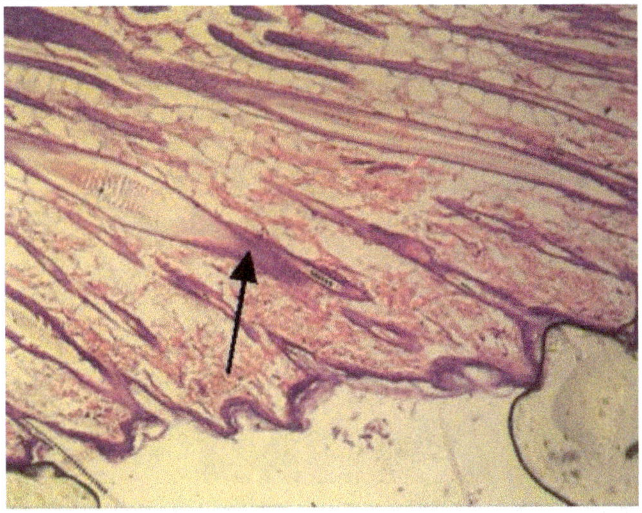

Figure 3: Fungal hyphae in the untreated control H&E stain, 100X.

Group	Fungal hyphae	Hair follicles	Sebaceous gland	Inflammation	Continuity/Tissue destruction
1	+++	+	+	+++	+++
2	-	+++	+++	-	-
3	+++	+	++	++	++
4a	++	+	++	++	++
4b	++	+	++	++	++
5a	+	++	++	+	+
5b	+	++	++	+	+
6a	-	++	++	-	+
6b	-	++	+++	-	+
Absent =-, Mild=+, Moderate=++, Marked=+++					

Table 14: Mycological efficacy of *Kigelia africana* formulations on *Microsporum audouinii.*

of fungal hyphae was also moderate while there was moderate number of hair follicles enmeshed within the sparse connective tissue in the dermis. There are moderate numbers of sebaceous glands in the dermis. Presence of fungal hyphae was moderate in group 4b (0.5% plant extract in emulsion). There are moderate hair follicles enmeshed within the sparse connective tissue in the dermis. There were also moderate numbers of sebaceous glands in the dermis. Inflammation and tissue destruction of the skin were also moderate in the group (Table 14). In groups 5a (1% plant extract alone), the inflammation and tissue destruction of the skin were moderate and same observation were recorded for 5b (1% plant extract in emulsion). Few numbers of fungal hyphae were seen with moderate amount of hair follicle and sebaceous gland. In group 6a (2% plant extract alone), no inflammation of the skin was seen but mild tissue destruction was however observed in the group. No fungal hyphae were seen which indicated that the extract was able to prevent the growth of the hyphae by the dermatophyte (Figure 4). There were moderate hair follicles in the dermis and also moderate amount of sebaceous glands. This may be as a result of the bio-actives in the extracts not been able to stop the growth of the fungal hyphae until after several applications. Same observation was made for group 6b (2% plant extract in emulsion) except for the abundance of sebaceous glands in the dermis which may have been on account of the fat in the emulsion been available as alternative to the oil in the sebaceous glands. This shows that 2% plant extract alone and 2% plant extract in emulsion are significantly effective as the standard drug in preventing the secretion

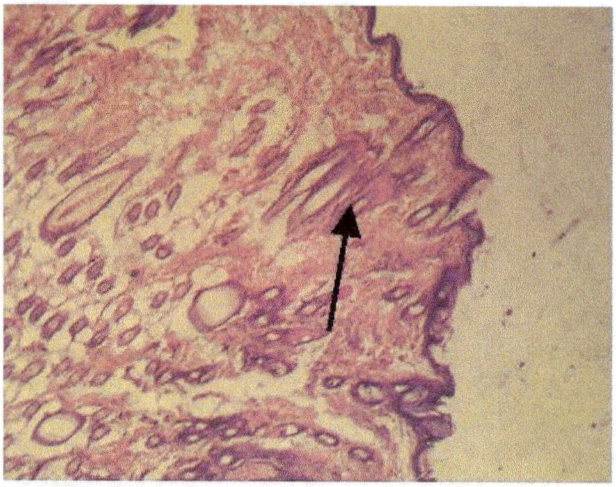

Figure 4: Shows the structure of intact skin from treated control with 1% clotrimazole H&E stain, 100X.

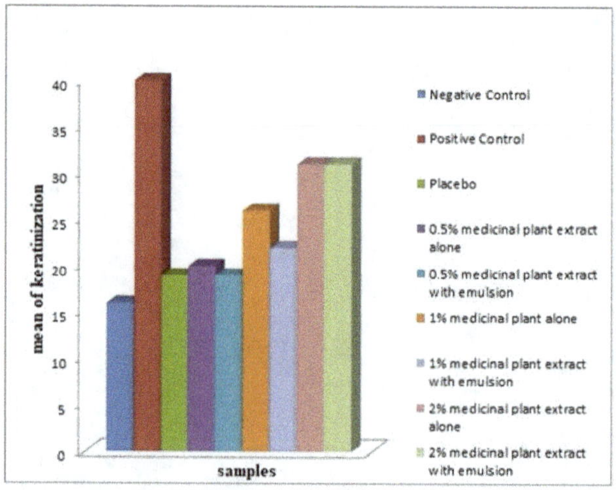

Figure 5: Effect of *Kigelia africana* extracts on keratinization in *Microsporium aoudinin* infected skin.

of keratinase which plays a vital role in the process of infection by *Microsporum audouinii*. From the results above, there is clear indication that efficacy of the formulations is concentration dependent.

Figure 5 shows the effect of the formulations on de-keratinization. Higher scores indicated improved efficacy. The untreated group 1 with the value 16.20 ± 0.76 µm indicated significant de-keratinization. Group 2 which is the standard drug (1% clotrimazole cream) showed high efficacy (39.45 ± 0.82 µm) indicating that it was able to reduce de-keratinization significantly by the dermatophyte. Emulsion alone (placebo), 0.5% *Kigelia africana* extract and 0.5% *Kigelia africana* extract emulsion cannot be said to be mycologically effective compared to the values obtained for the other formulations. However, 1% *Kigelia africana* extract alone and 1% *Kigelia africana* extract emulsion showed slight efficacy, but not as effective as the 2% *Kigelia africana* extract alone and 2% *Kigelia africana* extract emulsions which showed comparative efficacy with the standard drug.

Epidermal thickness of the skin biopsies ranged from 41.62 ± 0.58-92.37 ± 1.76 µm (Figure 6). Higher value indicates significant infection of the dermis with attendance inflammation of the skin and tissue destruction. The untreated group 1 with the value of 92.37 ± 1.76 µm indicated significant infection. Group 2 which is the standard drug (1% clotrimazole cream) showed that the drug was able to reduce the epidermal thickness significantly (36.52 ± 0.54 µm). The values obtained for emulsion alone (89.38 ± 0.56 µm) was not different from the untreated group. However, the efficacy of 0.5% *Kigelia africana* extract, 0.5% *Kigelia africana* extract emulsion, 1% *Kigelia africana* extract and 1% *Kigelia africana* emulsion in reducing the epidermal thickness is not significant compared with the untreated control. In contrast, there was significant efficacy of 2% *Kigelia africana* extract and 2% Kigelia africana emulsion compared with the values obtained for the standard drug.

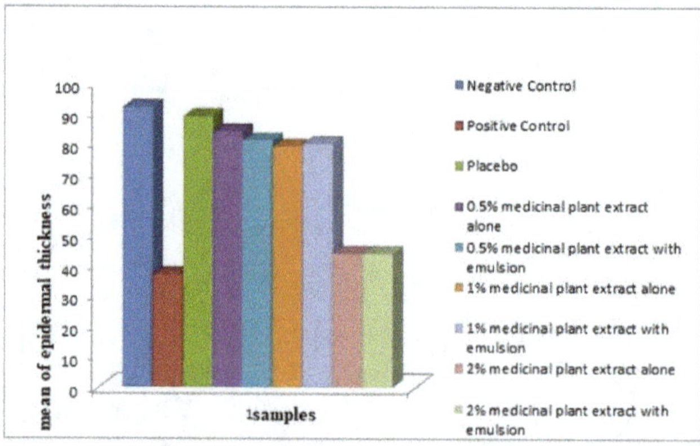

Figure 6: Effect of *Kigelia africana* extracts on epidermal thickness in *Microsporium aoudinin* infected skin.

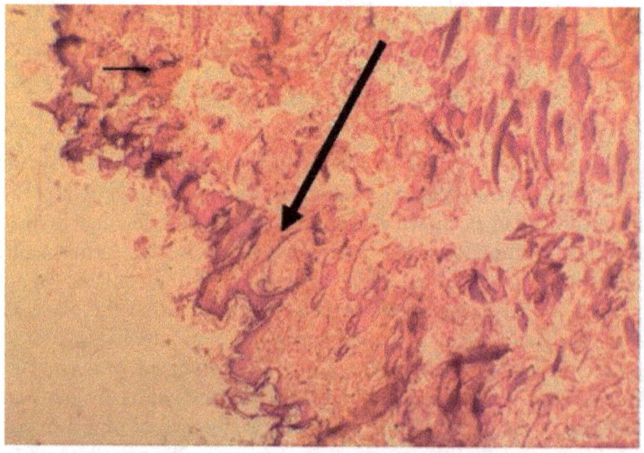

Figure 7: Inflammation of the skin tissue, H&E stain, 100X.

Efficacy of *Kigelia africana ethanol cream* formulations against *Epidermophyton floccosum*

Group 1 animals which are the untreated infected group showed marked inflammation of the skin and foci of discontinuity of the epidermis (Figure 7). Marked tissue destruction was also observed in the group compared to the other groups which were treated with various formulations. There was marked presence of fungal hyphae which implies successful infection by the dermatophyte. No hair follicles were seen this implies that the dermatophyte fed on the follicles. There were very few sebaceous glands. No inflammation and tissue destruction was observed in the group treated with 1% clotrimazole (group 2) showing that the drug was able to prevent the growth of the hyphae by the dermatophyte. No fungal hyphae were seen in the group. There were numerous hair follicles in the dermis and also moderate amount of sebaceous glands. Group 3 animals were treated with emulsion alone. Skin inflammation was marked while tissue destruction of the skin was moderate (Table 15). There was marked presence of fungal hyphae which indicated that the cream alone has no medicinal effect on the dermatophyte infection which a reduction of numbers in hair follicles. However there are few sebaceous glands in the dermis (Figure 8).

In group 4a, the animals were treated with 0.5% plant extract alone. Inflammation and tissue destruction of the skin were moderate in the group (Table 15). Presence of fungal hyphae was moderate while there were few hair follicles enmeshed within the sparse connective tissue in the dermis. There were few sebaceous glands in the dermis. Skin inflammation was moderate and tissue destruction of the skin were also mild (Table 15) in group 4b (0.5% plant extract in emulsion). Presence of fungal hyphae was few. There were few hair follicles enmeshed within the sparse connective tissue in the dermis. There are also few sebaceous glands in the dermis. In group 5a (1% plant extract alone), the inflammation and tissue destruction of the skin were mild. Few amounts of fungal hyphae were seen with few amounts of hair follicle and sebaceous gland. Same observation were recorded for group 5b (1% plant extract in emulsion).

No inflammation of the skin and tissue destruction was seen in group 6a (2% plant extract alone) which indicated that the extract was able to prevent the growth of the dermatophyte hyphae. No fungal hyphae were seen. There were moderate hair follicles in the dermis

Group	Fungal hyphae	Hair follicles	Sebaceous gland	Inflammation	Continuity/Tissue destruction
1	+++	-	+	+++	+++
2	-	+++	++	-	-
3	+++	+	+	+++	++
4a	++	+	+	++	++
4b	+	+	+	++	+
5a	+	+	+	+	+
5b	+	+	+	+	+
6a	-	++	++	-	-
6b	-	++	++	-	-
Absent =-, Mild=+, Moderate=++, Marked=+++					

Table 15: Mycological efficacy of *Kigelia africana* formulations on *Epidermophyton floccosum* infected skin.

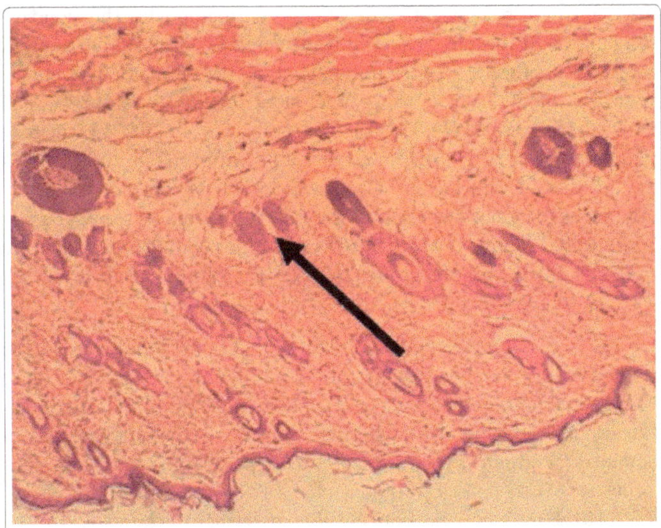

Figure 8: The inoculums of microconidia in follicular openings H&E stain 100X.

and also moderate amount of sebaceous glands. Same observation was made for group 6b (2% plant extract in emulsion). This indicated that 2% plant extract alone and 2% plant extract in emulsion are significantly effective as the standard drug.

Figure 9 shows the effect of the formulations on the keratin layer of the hair. The untreated control with the value 13.37 ± 0.39 indicated that the hairs were heavily infected with the dermatophyte. The effectiveness of 1% clotrimazole cream (39.86 ± 0.21 μm) in preventing attack by the dermatophyte on the keratin layer of the hair is demonstrated by the high value recorded. However, the group treated with the emulsion alone (15.30 ± 0.22 μm) and the group treated with 0.5% *Kigelia africana* extract emulsion (15.25 ± 0.28 μm) was not too different from the untreated group. 0.5% *Kigelia africana* extract, 1% *Kigelia africana* extract alone and 1% *Kigelia africana* emulsion showed slight efficacy compared to the untreated control. Comparatively, 2% *Kigelia africana* extract alone (30.94 ± 0.38 μm) and 2% *Kigelia africana* extract emulsion (30.53 ± 0.25 μm) showed mycological efficacy to other formulations.

Figure 10 showed the untreated group 1 with the value of 92.37 ± 1.76 μm which indicated significant infection. Group 2 which is the standard drug (1% clotrimazole cream) showed that the drug was able to reduce the epidermal thickness significantly (36.52 ± 0.54 μm). The values obtained for emulsion alone (89.38 ± 0.56 μm) was not statistically different from the untreated group. However, the efficacy of 0.5% *Kigelia africana* extract, 0.5% *Kigelia africana* extract emulsion, 1% *Kigelia africana* extract and 1% *Kigelia africana* emulsion in reducing the epidermal thickness is not significant compared with the untreated control. In contrast, there was significant efficacy of 2% *Kigelia africana* extract and 2% *Kigelia africana* emulsion compared with the values obtained for the standard drug.

Efficacy of *Kigelia africana ethanol cream* formulations against *Trichophyton mentagrophytes*

There was marked inflammation of the skin and foci of discontinuity of the epidermis in group 1 (Table 16). Marked presence of fungal hyphae shows successful infection. There were no hair follicles seen and few sebaceous glands were found. Marked tissue destruction was also

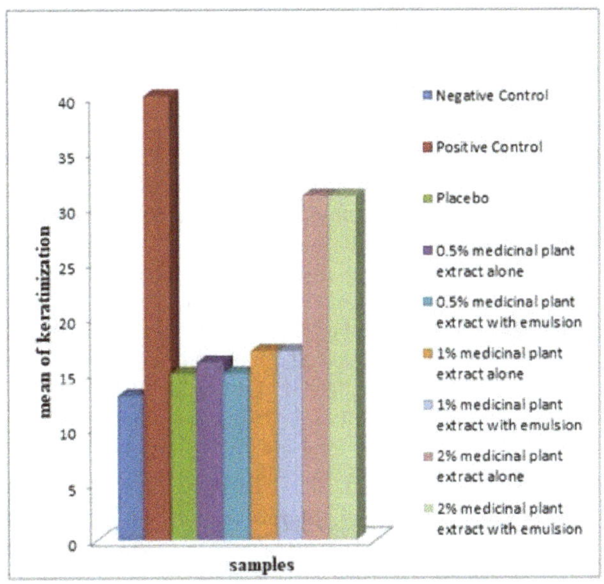

Figure 9: Effect of *Kigelia africana* extracts on keratinization levels in *Epidermophyton floccosum* infected skin.

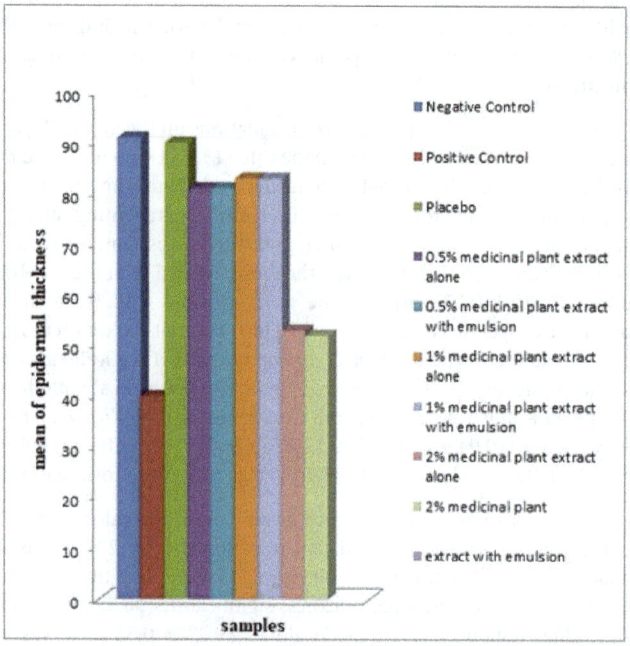

Figure 10: Effect of *Kigelia africana* extracts on epidermal thickess in *Epidermophyton floccosum* infected skin.

Group	Fungal hyphae	Hair follicles	Sebaceous gland	Inflammation	Continuity/ Tissue destruction
1	+++	-	+	+++	+++
2	-	+++	+++	-	-
3	++	+	+	++	++
4a	+	++	+	++	++
4b	+	++	+	++	++
5a	+	++	++	+	+
5b	+	++	++	+	+
6a	-	+++	++	+	+
6b	-	++	++	+	+
Absent =-, Mild=+, Moderate=++, Marked=+++					

Table 16: Mycological efficacy of *Kigelia africana* ethanol formulations against *Trichophyton mentagrophytes.*

observed in the group compared to the other groups which were treated with various formulations (Figure 11). No inflammation and tissue destruction was observed in group 2 (Table 16). There was absence of fungal hyphae indicating that the drug was able to prevent the infection by the dermatophyte. Numerous hair follicles and sebaceous glands were seen in the dermis. Group 3 animals treated with emulsion alone had moderate Inflammation and tissue destruction of the skin. There were few presences of fungal hyphae and also few hair follicles. Few sebaceous glands were also seen in the dermis (Figure 12). There was little presence of fungal hyphae in group 4a. Moderate amount of hair follicles enmeshed within the sparse connective tissue in the dermis were seen. There are few sebaceous glands in the dermis. Same observations made for group 4a were also seen in group 4b.

The inflammation and tissue destruction of the skin were also mild in group 5a (1% plant extract alone) (Table 16). Few amounts of fungal hyphae were seen with moderate amount of hair follicle and sebaceous gland. Same observation were recorded for 5b (1% plant extract in emulsion). In group 6a (2% plant extract alone), mild inflammation of

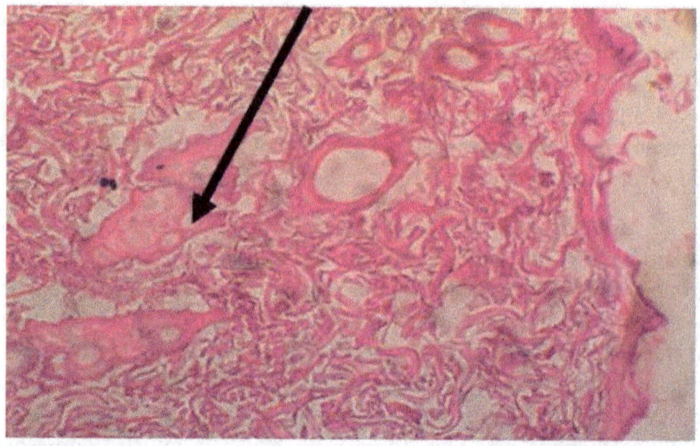

Figure 11: Hyperkeratosis, telogen follicles and absence of sebaceous gland, H&E stain, 100X.

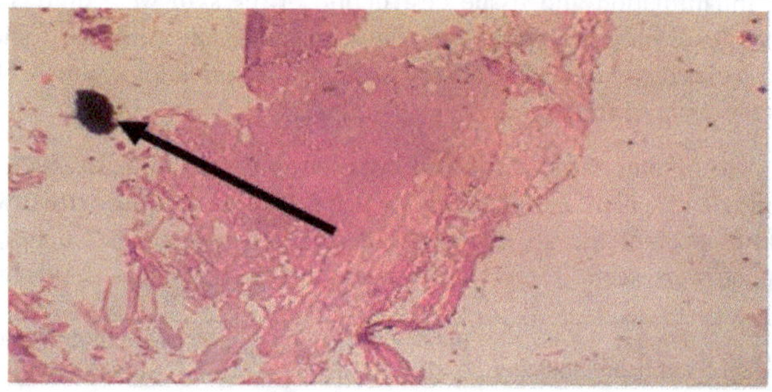

Figure 12: Tissue destruction of the skin tissues, H&E stain, 100X.

the skin and tissue destruction was seen. No fungal hyphae were seen which indicated that the extract was able to prevent the growth of the dermatophyte hyphae. There were numerous hair follicles in the dermis and also moderate amount of sebaceous glands. Same observation was made for group 6b (2% plant extract in emulsion). This shows that 2% plant extract alone and 2% plant extract in emulsion are closely effective as the standard drug.

The efficacy of the formulations on the keratin layer of the hair compared with the infected untreated control is shown in Figure 13. The untreated control group 1, with the value 11.37 ± 0.18 μm indicated that the hairs were heavily infected with the dermatophyte. The standard drug (1% clotrimazole cream) with the value 42.83 ± 0.33 μm showed mycological efficacy in preventing attack by the dermatophyte on the keratin layer of the hair. However, the values obtained for group 3 (18.82 ± 0.22 μm), group 4a (21.50 ± 0.44 μm) and group 4b (20.87 ± 0.60 μm) indicated that their efficacies were not different from one another. This implies that though infected by the dematophytes but not as heavily infected as the untreated control. The values obtained for groups 5a and 5b indicated slight efficacy by the formulations. Comparatively, group 6a (38.84 ± 0.52 μm) and group 6b (37.01 ± 0.39 μm) had close efficacy with the standard drug.

There was significant infection (74.01 ± 0.68 μm) as indicated by the result obtained for the epidermal thickness of untreated group (Figure 14). The values obtained for group 2 (40.41 ± 0.42 μm) indicated high efficacy by reducing the epidermal thickness. However, the values obtained for group 3 (61.81 ± 0.77 μm), group 4a (62.45 ± 0.86 μm), group 4b (62.45 ± 0.60 μm), group 5a (60.72 ± 0.58 μm) and group 5b (60.01 ± 0.42 μm) in reducing the epidermal thickness cannot be said to be significant compared with the untreated control. The values

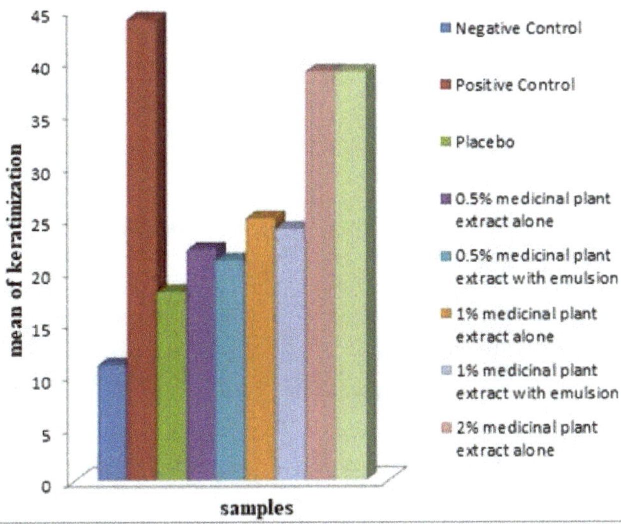

Figure 13: Effect of *Kigelia africana* extracts on keratinization in *Trichophyton mentagrophyte* infected skin.

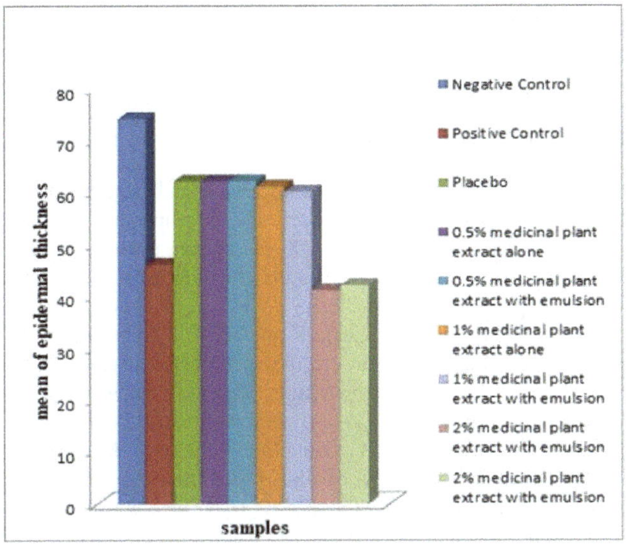

Figure 14: Effect of *Kigelia africana* extracts on epidermal thickness in *Trichophyton mentagrophyte* infected skin.

obtained for group 6a (41.33 ± 0.69 µm) and group 6b (41.72 ± 0.76 µm) compared favorably with the value for the standard drug.

Efficacy of *Kigelia africana* ethanol cream **formulations against *Malassezia furfur***

In the untreated group (group 1), moderate inflammation of the skin and foci of discontinuity of the epidermis were observed (Table 17). There was moderate presence of fungal hyphae which further indicated successful infection. Moderate tissue destruction was also observed in the group. There were few hair follicles enmeshed within the sparse connective tissue in the dermis which indicated that the dermatophyte is feeding on the follicles (Figure 15). Very few sebaceous glands were seen. No inflammation and tissue destruction was observed in the group treated with 1% clotrimazole (group 2) this is an indication that the drug was able to prevent the growth of the

Group	Fungal hyphae	Hair follicles	Sebaceous gland	Inflammation	Continuity/Tissue destruction
1	++	+	+	++	++
2	-	+++	++	-	-
3	++	+	+	++	++
4a	+	+	+	++	++
4b	+	+	+	++	++
5a	+	+	++	++	++
5b	+	+	++	++	++
6a	+	+	++	++	++
6b	+	+	++	++	++
Absent =-, Mild=+, Moderate=++, Marked=+++					

Table 17: Mycological efficacy of *Kigelia africana* ethanol formulations against *Malassezia furfur.*

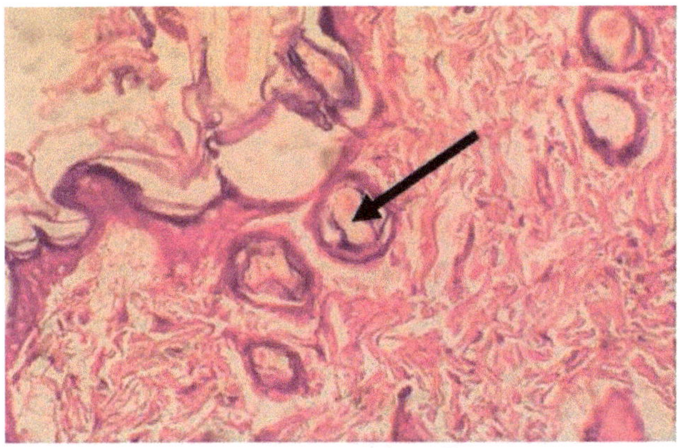

Figure 15: Isthmus lymphocytic mural folliculitis, H&E stain, 100X.

hyphae by the dermatophyte. There were numerous hair follicles in the dermis and also moderate amount sebaceous glands. Inflammation and tissue destruction of the skin were moderate in the group treated with emulsion alone (group 3). There was moderate presence of fungal hyphae. There were few numbers of hair follicles and sebaceous glands in the dermis (Figure 16). In group 4a (0.5% plant extract alone) and group 4b (0.5% plant extract in emulsion), inflammation and tissue destruction of the skin were moderate in the group (Table 17). There were few presences of fungal hyphae, hair follicles and sebaceous glands in the dermis. However, in groups 5a (1% plant extract alone) and 5b (1% plant extract in emulsion), few amount of fungal hyphae and hair follicle were seen with moderate amount of sebaceous gland. The inflammation and tissue destruction of the skin were also moderate (Table 17). Same observation were recorded for groups 6a (2% plant extract alone) and 6b (2% plant extract in emulsion).

The efficacy of the formulations on the keratin layer of the hair compared with the infected untreated control is shown in Figure 17. The value obtained (26.03 ± 0.30 µm) for the untreated control group 1 indicated that there was moderate infection of the hairs by the dermatophyte. The value obtained for the standard drug, 1% clotrimazole cream (48.18 ± 0.50 µm) indicated that there is significant prevention of attack by the dermatophyte on the keratin layer of the hair. The observation made for the group treated with the emulsion alone (28.73 ± 0.36 µm) indicated that the infection is gradually moving from moderate to mild. The results obtained for the other groups indicated that the moderate infection has been reduced to mild infection as can be seen in the groups treated with 0.5% *Kigelia africana* extract alone (30.17 ± 0.24 µm), the group treated with 0.5% *Kigelia africana* extract

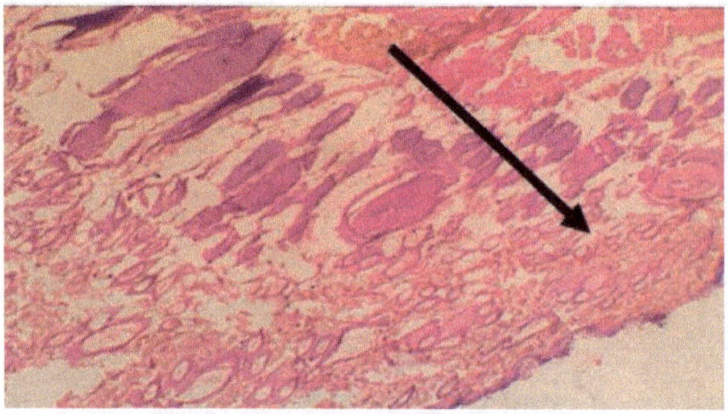

Figure 16: Infiltration of lymphosites, H&E stain, 100X.

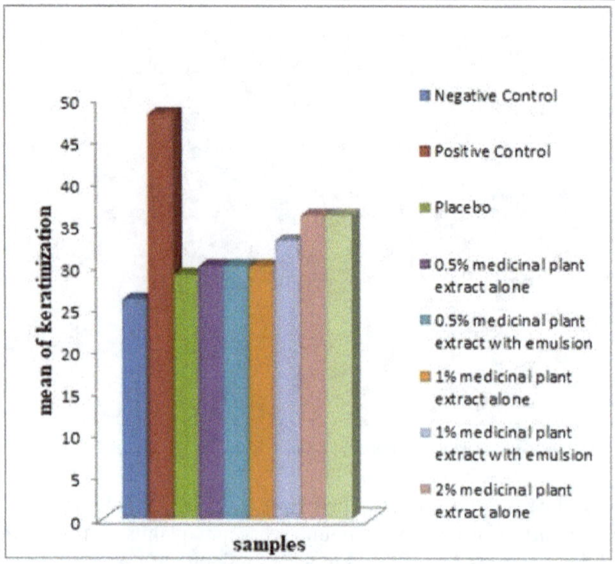

Figure 17: Effect of *Kigelia africana* extracts on keratinisation in *Malassezia furfur* infected skin.

emulsion (30.14 ± 0.14 μm), 1% *Kigelia africana* extract alone (31.22 ± 0.79 μm) and 1% *Kigelia africana* emulsion (31.66 ± 0.65 μm) which were not different from one another. This implies that there is slight efficacy by the formulations. However, 2% *Kigelia africana* extract alone (36.14 ± 0.45 μm) and 2% *Kigelia africana* extract emulsion (36.22 ± 0.36 μm) showed higher mycological efficacy compared to the other formulations.

The result obtained for the epidermal thickness of the untreated group indicated that there was significant infection (62.21 ± 0.97 μm). However, the values obtained for the standard drug (43.71 ± 0.53 μm) can be said to effectively reduce the epidermal thickness thereby indicating high efficacy against the dermatophyte (Figure 18). The values obtained for emulsion alone (62.14 ± 0.76 μm), 0.5% *Kigelia africana* extract (60.75 ± 0.93 μm), 0.5% *Kigelia africana* extract emulsion (60.37 ± 0.63 μm), 1% *Kigelia africana* extract (59.92 ± 0.34 μm), 1% *Kigelia africana* emulsion (58.00 ± 0.82 μm), 2% *Kigelia africana* extract alone (57.89 ± 0.76 μm) and 2% *Kigelia africana* emulsion with extract (56.91 ± 0.85 μm) in reducing the epidermal thickness cannot be said to be significant compared with the untreated control.

Comparative efficacy of the formulations against the dermatophytes

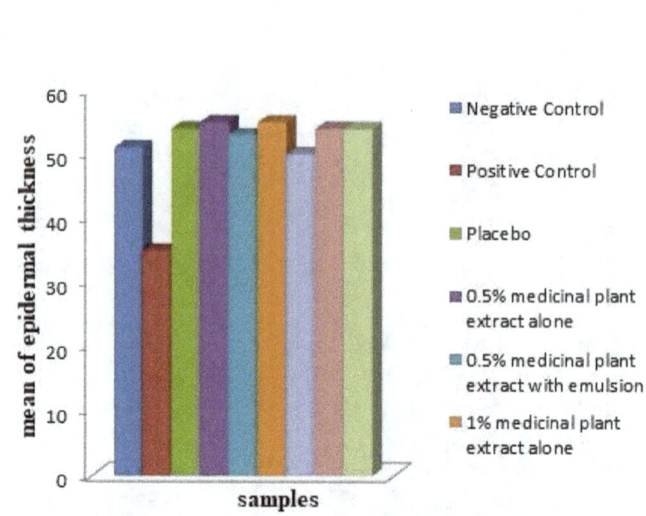

Figure 18: Effect of *Kigelia africana* extracts on epidermal thickness in *Malassezia furfur* infected skin.

Dermatophyte	Keratin layer (μm)	Epidermal thickness (μm)
Control (Uninfected rat)	55.46 ± 0.5	31.24 ± 0.21
M. audouinii	31.37 ± 0.53	44.11 ± 0.03
T. mentagrophyte	37.01 ± 0.39	41.72 ± 0.76
E. floccosum	30.53 ± 0.25	52.41 ± 0.12
M. furfur	36.22 ± 0.36	56.91 ± 0.85

Table 18: Comparative efficacy of the formulations against the dermatophytes.

Evaluation of the formulations tested indicated that their efficacy against the dermatophytes is concentration dependent (Table 18). Emulsion containing 2% of extracts possess significant mycological efficacy against dermatophytic infection caused by all the dermatophytes. The high efficacy could be explained on the basis of pharmacokinetics of the extracts on the skin. Data obtained for keratinization indicated that the cream was most statistically significant ($P<0.05$) with 37.01 ± 0.39 μm against *Trychophyton mentagrophyte* >*Malassezia furfur* (36.22 ± 0.36 μm) > *Microsporum audouinii* (31.37 ± 0.53 μm) >*Epidermophyton floccosum* (30.53 ± 0.25 μm). Also the cream was able to reduce epithermal thickness with the value (41.72 ± 0.76 μm) which is significant ($P<0.05$) against *Trychophyton mentagrophyte* > *Microsporum audouinii* (44.11 ± 0.03 μm) >*Epidermophyton floccosum* (52.41 ± 0.12 μm) >*Malassezia furfur* (56.91 ± 0.85 μm). The result obtained agrees with the works carried out on *Kigelia africana* by Jeyachandran and Mahesh [11-16] who in their study showed that the medicinal plant is medicinal for a managing a number of diseases. Similarly, previous data obtained during the *in vitro* antifungal tests we carried out on *Kigelia africana* further support the efficacy of the formulations. Various scientific studies indicated the usefulness of developing drugs from plants extract for treating skin ailments and it has been previously by Oyedeji and Bankole [9,17-20] that formulation of *Kigelia africana* extract as topical cream may lead to enhancement of stability and acceptability of the active ingredient. We can therefore conclude that the topical preparation is highly effective against skin damage caused by various dermatophytes [21-24].

Acknowledgement

We sincerely acknowledge the support of Dr. A Raheem of Spectralab Medical and Diagnostic Services, Sagamu, Ogun State.

References

1. Phillips RM, Rosen T (2013) Topical antifungal agents. In Wolverton SE. Comprehens Dermatol Ther 3: 460-472.
2. Moghimipour E, Ameri A, Saudatzadeh A, Salimi A, Siahpoosh A (2009) Formulation of an anti-dermatophyte cream from hydro-alcoholic extract of eucalyptus camaldulensis leaves. Jundishapur J Natur Pharma Prod 4: 32-40.
3. Babayi H, Kolo I, Okogun JI, Ijah UJ (2004) The antimicrobial activities of methanolic extracts of Eucalyptus camaldulensis and Terminalia catappa against some pathogenic microorganisms. Biokemistri; 16: 106-111.
4. Scherrer AM, Motti R, Weckerle CS (2005) Traditional plant use in the areas of Monte Vesole and Ascea, Cilento National park. J Ethnopharmacol 97: 129-143.
5. Kyle AA, Dahl MV (2004) Topical therapy for fungal infections. Am J Clin Dermatol 5: 443-451.
6. Havlickova B, Czaika VA, Friedrich M (2008) Epidemiological trends in skin mycoses worldwide. Mycoses 51: 2-15.
7. Aiyelola AA, Bello OA (2006) Ethnobotanical potentials of common herbs in Nigeria: A case study of Enugu state. Edu Res Rep 1: 16-22.
8. Olatunji AG, Atolani O (2009) Comprehensive scientific demystification of Kigelia africana: A review. African J Pure Appl Chem 3: 158-164.
9. Oyedeji OF, Bankole-Ojo OS (2012) Quantitative evaluation of the antipsoriatic activity of sausage tree (Kigelia africana). African J Pure Appl Chem 6: 214-218.
10. Owolabi OJ, Omogbai EKI, Obasuyi O (2007) Antifungal and antibacterial activities of the ethanolic and aqueous extract of Kigelia africana (Bignoniaceae) stem bark. African J Biotechnol 6:14.
11. Jeyachandran R, Mahesh A (2007) Antimicrobial evaluation of Kigelia africana (Lam). Res J Microbiol 2: 645-649.
12. Abubacker MN, Ramanathan R, Kumar ST (2008) Natural product radiance 7: 6-9.
13. Acharya D, Shrivastava A (2008) Indigenous herbal medicines: Tribal formulations and traditional herbal practices, Aavishkar Publishers, India, 1-44.
14. Akinyemi KO, Olukayode O, Okwara EC, Ibe CC, Fasuro KA (2005) Screening of crude extracts of six medicinal plants used in south-west Nigerian unorthodox medicine for anti-methicillin resistant Staphylococcus aureus activity. BMC Complement Altern Med 5: 6.
15. De-Benedetto A (2009) Atopic dermatitis: A disease caused by innate immune defects? J Invest Dermatol 129: 14-30.
16. Eleazu CO, Eleazu KC, Awa E, Chukwuma SC (2012) Comparative study of the phytochemical composition of the leaves of five Nigerian medicinal plants. J Biotechnol Pharma Res 3: 42-46.
17. Ghannoum M, Isham N, Verma A, Plaum S, Fleischer A, et al. (2013) In vitro antifungal activity of naftifine hydrochloride against dermatophytes. Antimicro Agents Chemother 57: 4369-4372.
18. Grace OM, Light ME, Lindsey KL, Mulholland DA, Van Staden J, et al. (2002) Antibacterial activity and isolation of active compounds from fruit of the traditional African medicinal tree Kigelia africana. South African J Botany 68: 220-222.
19. Hosseininejad M, Ebrahimi A, Hosseini F (2009) Isolation of Epidermophyton floccosum from a persian squirrel (Sciurusanomalus). Compar Clinic Pathol 19: 215-216.
20. Kumar R, Kumar T, Kamboj V, Chander H (2012) Pharmacological evaluation of ethanolic extract of Kigelia pinnata fruit against ethylene glycol induced urolithiasis in rats. Asian J Plant Sci Res 2: 63-72.
21. Lawal HO, Etatuvie SO, Fawehinmi AB (2012) Ethnomedicinal and pharmacological properties of Morinda lucida. J Natur Prod 5: 93-99.
22. Marks JG, Miller J (2006) Lookingbill and marks' principles of dermatology, 4th edtn, Elsevier, USA.
23. Meduri NB, Travis V, Heather R, Heidi J (2007) Phototherapy in the management of atopic dermatitis: A systematic review. Photodermatol Photoimmunol Photomed 23: 106-112.
24. Tadros T (2004) Application of rheology for assessment and prediction of the long-term physical stability of emulsions. Adv Colloid Interface Sci 108-109: 227-258.

Contamination of Bacteria and Associated Factors among Food Handlers Working in the Student Cafeterias of Jimma University Main Campus, Jimma, South West Ethiopia

Tsegaye Assefa[1], Haymanot Tasew[1], Beyene Wondafrash[2] and Jemal Beker[1*]

[1]*Department of Medical Laboratory Sciences and Pathology College of Public Health and Medical Sciences, Jimma University, Ethiopia*

[2]*Department of Nursing, College of Public Health and Medical Sciences, Jimma University, Ethiopia*

[*]**Corresponding author**: Beker J, Department of Nursing, College of Public Health and Medical Sciences, Jimma University, Ethiopia, E-mail: jemalbeker@yahoo.com

Abstract

Background: Food borne diseases continue to be a major global health problem and are the leading causes of morbidity and mortality in developing countries. Food handlers play a major role in the transmission of food borne pathogens via hands. This study aimed to assess the bacterial hand contamination and associated factors among food handlers working in the student cafeterias of Jimma University main campus.

Methods and materials: A cross-sectional study was conducted from May 2012 to April 2013 among food handlers working in the student cafeterias of Jimma University main campus. The data was collected by using structured questionnaire and observational checklist. Hand rinse samples was collected from participants and microbiologically examined for the presence of potential food borne bacterial contaminants using standard laboratory methods. The data was entered into a computer and analyzed using SPSS version-16.0 software.

Result: Among 230 food handlers, 114(49.6%) were tested positive for one or more potential food borne bacterial contaminants, and 73(31.7%) were tested positive for enteric pathogens. A total of 171 bacterial hand contaminants were isolated. *S. aureus* 54(23.5%), *Klebsiella spp.* 37(16.1%), *E. coli* 25 (10.9%), *Enterobacter spp.* 21(9.1%), *Citrobacter spp.* 10(4.3%), *Serratia marcescens* 6 (2.6%), *Pseudomonas aeruginosa* 8(3.5%), *Proteus spp.* 5(2.2%), *Providencia rettegri* 3(1.3%), and *salmonella spp.* 2(0.9%) were isolated with their corresponding prevalence rate. Bacterial hand contamination rate have significant association with service years (Chi-square=13.732, DF=4, P=0.008), age (χ^2=11.308, P=0.010) and cleanness of outer garments (χ^2=7.653, P=0.006).

Conclusion: The findings of this study emphasized the importance of food handlers' hands as a potential vector for potential food borne bacterial contaminants which could constitute a potential risk to food borne outbreaks. New employees and young and inexperienced food handlers should be well trained on personal hygienic practices pointing out on the importance of hand hygiene and appropriate hand washing techniques.

Keywords: Food handlers; Food borne bacterial contaminants; Isolation rate; Hand rinse

Introduction

Foodborne diseases can be defined as diseases commonly transmitted through food. Foodborne diseases comprise a broad group of illnesses caused by microbial pathogens, parasites, chemical contaminants and bio toxins. The burden of disease can be defined as the incidence and prevalence of morbidity, disability, and mortality associated with acute and chronic manifestations of diseases [1-3]. The Centers for Disease Control and Prevention has identified more than 400 food-related illnesses. About two thirds of all outbreaks involve bacteria. The illnesses are caused either by the microorganisms themselves or by the toxins they release [4]. The consumption of foods contaminated by foodborne pathogenic microorganisms and toxins produced by them cause's deaths, illnesses, hospitalization, and economic losses. Due to their widespread nature, foodborne diseases, in particular gastro-intestinal infections, represent a very large group of pathologies with a strong negative impact on public health [5].

Many food-borne disease incidents are reported every year in Africa. Numerous factors, contribute to this high number of incidents [6-9]. However, it is extremely important to note that most cases of food-borne disease in the region are not reported, so the true extent of the problem is unknown. In most countries of the region, the surveillance infrastructure for food-borne diseases of both microbiological and chemical etiology is weak or non-existent. This absence of reliable data on the burden of food-borne disease impedes understanding about its public health importance and prevents the development of risk based solutions to its management [2].

More aggravated situations and challenges prevail in Ethiopia where food safety issues are not well understood and have received little attention. In Ethiopia, according to the Ministry of Health annual report of 2011, dysentery and gastroenteritis were among the top ten diseases of outpatient visits although the report did not include all regions activity [10]. Food-borne diseases represent a persistent global health burden, and food handlers play a major role in their transmission [11]. Even though the sources of food contamination are diverse, food handlers serve as important source of food contamination either as carriers of pathogens or through poor hygienic practices [12]. The mishandling of food and the disregard of hygienic measures enable pathogens to come into contact with food and, in some cases, to survive and multiply in sufficient numbers to cause illness in consumers. Personal hygiene and environmental sanitation are among the key factors in the transmission of food borne diseases [13].

Several food-borne disease outbreaks are associated with poor personal hygiene of people handling foodstuffs. CDC reported that approximately 20% of food-related infections are due to food handlers [14]. Another study conducted in Malaysia also showed that approximately 10-20% of food-borne disease outbreaks are due to contamination by the food handlers [13]. Food workers may transmit pathogens to food coming from a contaminated surface of another food, or from hands contaminated with organisms from their gastrointestinal tract. This is also supported by report in which about 89% of outbreaks caused by food contamination by food workers, pathogens were transferred to food by workers' hands by Michaels et al. [15].

Food handlers are the most important sources for the transfer of microbial pathogens to food either from their hair, skin, hand, digestive systems, respiratory tracts, or from contaminated food prepared and served by them [16,17]. The hands are the last line of defence against exposure to pathogens which can occur either directly from the hand to the mouth, eye, nose, or other area of the skin, or indirectly by "handling" of food or water. The hands are particularly important since they are the last line of defence in the chain of transmission of gastrointestinal pathogens, either directly from hand-to-mouth, or indirectly by "handling" of food or water [18]. The hands of food handlers can be the vector to spread harmful microorganism through cross contamination, and during or after they experience gastrointestinal infection. An employee might contaminate his hands when using toilet, or bacteria might be spread from raw foods, from contaminated equipment, and environment [19]. Thus, these contaminated hands can transfer intestinal microbes to foods, equipment, and other workers in the food storage and preparation areas unless correct personal hygiene and adequate hand washing procedures are followed [20,21]. Some of the bacteria that can colonize the hands of food handlers are Escherichia coli and Staphylococcus aureus [22].

WHO emphasizes that "outbreaks of food-borne diseases can be reduced if both professional and domestic food-handlers understand the importance of correct hygienic food practices [12]. Food handlers should not smoke, sneeze, spit, cough, eat, handle money or engage in any act that could contaminate the food during the performance of their activities [23]. The role of the hands in disease transmission and the importance of hand hygiene in controlling infection in the food establishment are well established. Hand washing has been identified as the single most important means of preventing the spread of infection and if poorly or improperly implemented, can lead to foodborne illness outbreaks [23,24]. Food handlers in bigger eating establishments cater to a larger number of people, they are epidemiologically more important than domestic food handlers in spreading of food borne disease [11]. Nonetheless, bacterial hand contamination of food-handlers, may pose a real threat to those who are more susceptible to infection. Studying the hands microbial flora among the food handlers could have paramount importance to understand the hygienic practices of food handlers. The presence or absence of bacteria in the hands of food handlers can be used as a quantitative indicator of their behavior regarding food-related and personal hygiene [25,26]. There are few related studies in Ethiopia and specifically to this study area. Therefore, this study aimed at assessing the bacterial hand contamination among food handlers working in the student cafeterias of JU main campus.

Materials and Methods

Study area and period

The study was conducted at student cafeterias in Jimma University main campus, Jimma town, located at 355km southwest Ethiopia from May 2012 to April 2013. Its geographical coordinates are: 07039' Latitude and 36050' Longitude, at an altitude of 1700-1750 m above sea level. Jimma University is organized into six colleges, out of which four of them are located in the Jimma University main campus. Around 500 food handlers are currently working in the student cafeterias of Jimma University main campus.

Study design

Descriptive cross-sectional study design was used

Source population

All food handlers working in the student cafeterias of Jimma University main campus

Study population

Selected food handlers working in the student cafeterias of Jimma University main campus

Inclusion criteria

Food handlers who are engaged in food preparation, serving, and Cleaning

Exclusion criteria

Food handlers who have skin irritation, eczema, and inflammation

Sample size determination

Sample size (n) was determined using a formula to estimate single population proportion. Taking 50% prevalence of bacterial hand contamination (p=0.5), 95%

$$n=\frac{(z\propto/2)^{2}*P(1-P)}{d^{2}}=\frac{(1.96)^{2}*(0.5)^{2}}{(0.05)^{2}}\approx 384,$$

where:

P- Bacterial hand contamination rate

z - z-statistics value that corresponds to 97.5 percentile cut-off point in the standard normal distribution

d - Margin of error

Since the total number of the source population was 500, correction formula was used to adjust the sample size to the population size and the sample size was calculated further as

$$\frac{n}{1+\frac{n}{N}}=\frac{384}{1+\frac{384}{500}}\approx 218$$

Finally by considering a 10% (22 subjects) non response rate, the final sample size was determined as:

N+ 22 ≈ 240

Sampling technique

Simple random sampling technique was employed. Study participants were selected by lottery method from the roster lists of food handlers which was obtained from students' cafeteria offices of Jimma University main campus.

Variables of the study

Dependent variables

Bacterial hand contamination

Types of bacterial hand contaminants

Independent variables

- Sociodemographic factors
- Hand washing habit
- Fingernail status
- Presence of jewelers on fingers
- Regular medical checkup
- Hygiene training
- Outer protective coat, and Hair cover
- Cleanness of outer garments

Data and specimen collection

Data related to socio-demographic characteristics, and personal hygiene practices of food handlers was collected by face to face interview method using structured questionnaire, and observational checklist. The tool was first prepared in English and then translated into the national language. Three sanitarians and two medical laboratory professionals were recruited for data collection and microbiological analysis. The data collectors were trained for two days by the principal investigator on data, and specimen collection procedures. After interviewing participants were asked to give hand rinse samples in sterile plastic bag (Stomacher@400 Classic; Seward, Worthing, UK) for microbiological analysis.

Before starting any meal preparation activity including hand washing (if any), participant's hands were sampled for microbial testing. Notification was not given in advance, and extra hand hygiene was not allowed during the hand rinse sample collection. A sterile polyethylene plastic bag technique was employed to collect the hand rinse samples. Participants were asked to dip their hands into sterile polyethylene plastic bag containing 100 milliliter of buffered peptone water (0.1% BPW) (Difco/Becton Dickinson, Franklin Lakes, and NJ). The bag was grasped tightly around the participant's wrist and the Peptone buffer was massaged through the wall of the bag by the investigator for one 1 minute, over all surfaces of the participant's hand, particularly around the nails and palm. The bag was immediately sealed and transported to Jimma University medical microbiology laboratory for examination [27,28].

Isolation and identification of potential food borne bacterial pathogens

All media used in this study were from Oxoid Ltd. and were prepared according to the manufacturer's instructions. The hand rinse samples were vortexed for one minute prior to microbiological examination. A loop full of each sample was separately spread-plated onto MacConkey (for detection of enteric bacteria), MSA (for detection of staphylococci), and XLD (for detection of Salmonella, and Shigella). Rappaport vassiliadis (RV) was used as a primary enrichment for the identification of Salmonella and Shigella. The bacterial colonies grown on the agar media were presumptively identified by colonial morphology and gram staining and a battery of biochemical tests like reaction on oxidase, catalase, simmon citrate, indole production, urease, motility, coagulase, methyl red-voges proskaeur (MR-VP), LDC, KIA, gas and Hydrogen Sulfide (H2S) production [29,30] (Figure 1).

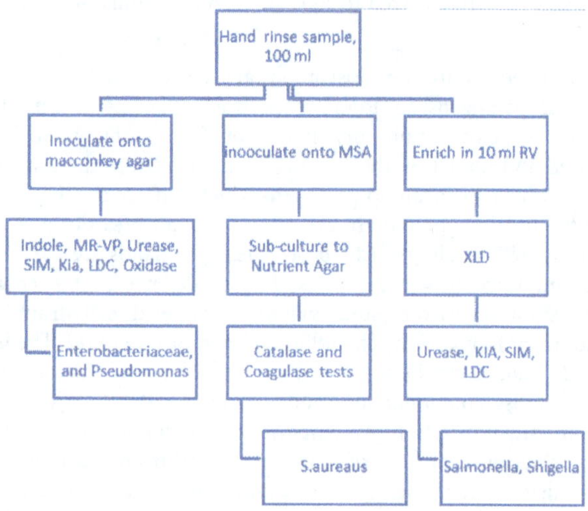

Figure 1: Simplified laboratory flow chart for identification of potential food borne bacterial hand contaminants.

Quality control

To manage the quality of the work SOP was strictly followed during processing of each sample. All the instruments used for sample processing were checked for proper functioning as far quality control strains of *S. aureus* (ATCC 6538) and *E. coli* (ATCC 25922) were used. Data consistency and completeness were made all the way during data collection, data entry and analysis. Culture Medias were prepared based on the manufactures instruction. Then the sterility of culture media was checked by incubating 5% of the batch at 35 - 37oc overnight and observed for bacterial growth. Those Media which shows growth was discarded.

Data processing and analysis

All components of data were entered and cleaned, coded and analyzed using SPSS version 16.0, computer software. Data was organized, summarized, and presented in simple descriptive Statistical methods. Chi-square test was used for checking any possible association between various categorical variables, and p-value<0.05

considered as significant. The findings of the study were compared to other studies.

Ethical Consideration

The study was conducted after obtaining ethical clearance from Jimma University College of public health and Medical Sciences Ethical review Board. Permission letter was obtained from Jimma University Students' Service Dean Office to students' cafeteria office. Informed consent was obtained from participants after explanation of the purpose of the study and procedure of sample collection. In addition, participation in the study was made by willingness of study participants. All personal information about the study participants were kept confidential.

Dissemination of the findings

The finding of the study was disseminated to college of medical sciences and public health, Jimma University as a requirement for partial fulfillment of graduate study. The copy of the thesis results was provided to Student Cafeteria Offices of JU main campus. Furthermore a copy of the study will be submitted to health science library and Department of Medical Laboratory Sciences and Pathology. Finally, study results will be sent to the respective scientific journals requesting for publication.

Operational definition

Bacterial hand contamination: presence of one or more potential food borne bacterial hand contaminants

Food borne diseases - intoxication, infection, or illness contracted by the consumption of contaminated food

Food handler - a person who is engaged in the process of food preparing, serving, cleaning, and etc.

Potential food borne bacterial contaminants – bacterial pathogens that can cause food contamination or spoilage

Personal hygiene - refers to those protection measures primarily with the responsibility of the individual, which promote and limit the spread of infectious disease, like hand washing using soap and water, keep body clean etc.

Risk factor: - a factor whose presence is associated with an increased probability of bacterial hand contamination

Result

Two hundred thirty food handlers were participated in this study making a response rate of 95.83%. From these 194(84.3%) of participants were females while 36(7.7%) were males. The mean and median age of the study subjects were 28.65(SD=8.09), and 26 respectively, whereas the minimum and maximum ages were 18 and 55 years respectively.

About half of the food handlers 119(51.7%) were single, while 86(37%) of were married. The educational background is found as no formal education 28(12.2%), elementary school 115(50%), secondary school 72(31.3%), high school and above 15(6.5%). Regarding their job position 73(31.7%) were Cookers, 99(41.3%) were servers and 58(25.2%) were cleaners. Concerning service years, majority 185 (63%) of food handlers have served for a period of less than five years in the student cafeterias of JU (Table 1).

Variables categories		Frequency	Percent (%)
Sex	Male	36	15.7
	Female	194	84.3
Age	≤20 years	33	14.4
	21-30 years	124	53.9
	31-40 years	47	20.4
	41	26	11.3
Marital-status	Single	119	51.7
	Married	86	37.4
	Divorced	25	10.9
Ethnicity	Oromo	89	38.7
	Amhara	56	24.3
	Gurage	18	7.8
	Dawuro	32	13.9
	Kafa	16	7.0
	Others	19	8.3
Religion	Orthodox	118	51.3
	Muslim	60	26.1
	Protestant	52	22.6
Education	Illiterate	28	12.2
	Elementary	115	50.0
	Secondary	72	31.3
	High-school & above	15	6.5
Job-position	Cook	73	31.7
	Waiter	99	43.1
	Cleaner	58	25.2
Service years	<2	58	25.2
	2-4	87	37.8
	5-7	40	17.4
	8-10	25	10.9
	>10	19	8.7
Income	420	160	69.6
	470	70	30.4

Table 1: Distribution of socio-demographic characteristics of food handlers working in the student cafeterias of JU main campus, May 2012-Aprill 2013.

Personal hygiene practices of food handlers

In the present study out of the total participants 164 (71.3%) have worn outer protective Coat, 93(40.4%) have worn appropriate hair cover, 120 (52.2%) have kept their outer garments clean. Out of the total participants 160 (69.6%) have got informal food hygiene training, 131(57%) have got regular medical checkups, 185(80.4%) have trimmed fingernails, and 58(25.2%) have worn rings. Out of the total participants hand washing habit using soap and water is reported by 177 (77%) after toilet, 132 (57.4%) after touching dirty materials, and 201(57%) before food handling (Table 2).

Variables	Categories	Frequency	Percent (%)
Protective outer garment	Observed	164	71.3
	Not observed	66	28.7
Hair cover	Observed	93	40.4
	Not observed	137	59.6
Hand washing habit after toilet	With soap and water	177	77.0
	With water only	53	23.0
Hand washing habit after touching dirty materials	With soap and water	132	57.4
	With water only	98	42.6
Hand washing habit before handling food	With soap and water	201	87.4
	With water only	29	12.6
Finger nail status	Trimmed	185	80.4
	Semi-trimmed	45	19.6
Medical examination	Checked	131	57.0
	Not checked	99	43.0
Presence of rings	Observed	58	25.2
	Not observed	172	74.8
Hygiene training	Trained	160	69.6
	Not trained	70	30.4

Table 2: Personal hygiene practices of food handlers working in the student cafeterias of JU main campus, May 2012 to April 2013.

Types and prevalence of potential food borne bacterial hand contaminants

Bacteriological investigation of 230 hand rinse samples was performed out of which 114(49.6%) tested positive for one or more potential food borne bacterial hand contaminants, and 73(31.7%) were tested positive for Enteric pathogens. A total of 171 bacteria were isolated from which 109 (63.7%) cases belong to the family of Enterobacteriaceae. In this study the following bacteria's were isolated with the corresponding prevalence rate: *Staphylococcus aureus* 54(23.5%), *Klebsiella spp.* 37(16.1%), *E. coli* 25(10.9%), and *Enterobacter spp.* 21(9.1%), *Citrobacter spp.* 10(4.3%), *Pseudomonas aeruginosa* 8(3.5%), *Serratia marcescens* 6(2.6%), *Proteus spp.* 5(2.2%), *Providencia rettegri* 3(1.3%), and *salmonella species* 2(0.9%). While no *shigella species* was isolated (Table 3).

Bacteria isolated	Frequency	Percent (%)
Staphylococcus aureus	54	23.5
E. coli	25	10.9
Klebsiella spp.	37	16.1
Enterobacter spp.	21	9.1
Citrobacter spp.	10	4.3
Proteus spp.	5	2.2
Serratia marcescens	6	2.6
Providencia rettegri	3	1.3
Pseudomonas aeruginosa	8	3.5
Salmonella spp.	2	0.9

Table 3: Type and prevalence of potential food borne bacterial hand contaminants among food-handlers working in the student cafeterias of JU main campus, May 2012 to April 2013.

Factors associated with bacterial hand contamination

In the present study, no statistical association was found between bacterial hand contamination rate, and gender, educational background, job position, medical check-up, food hygiene training, hand washing habit, and fingernail status. However, bacterial hand contamination rate have significant association with service years, age, and cleanness of outer garments.

The isolation rate of potential food borne bacterial hand contaminants was much higher 25(75.8%) among food-handlers of ≤20 years age group, and lower 10(38.5%) among those ≥41 years age group. There is significant difference in isolation rate of potential food borne bacterial hand contaminants by age groups (Chi-square=11.308, DF=3, P=0.01) (Figure 2).

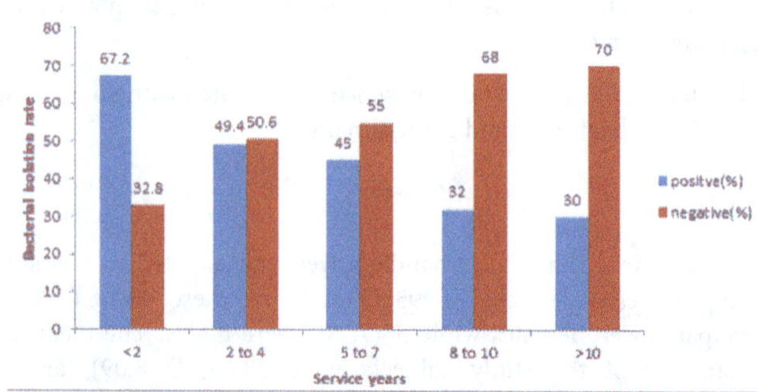

Figure 2: Isolation rate of potential food borne bacterial pathogens among food-handlers working in the student cafeterias of JU main campus in accordance to their service years, May 2012 to April 2013.

Bacterial hand contamination rate have significant association with service years of participants (χ^2=13.732, DF=4, P=0.008). The isolation rate of potential food borne bacterial hand contaminants was relatively higher 39(67.2%) among food handlers served for a period of less than two years, and lower 6(30%) among those served for a period of greater than 10 years.

The isolation rate of bacterial hand contaminants was lower 49 (40.8%) among participants with clean outer garments, compared to 65 (59.1%) with unclean outer garments. There is significant association between bacterial hand contamination rate and cleanness of outer garments (χ^2=7.653, P=0.006) (Table 4).

Gender	Hand rinse culture result		Total (%)	
	Positive (%)	Negative (%)		χ2=0.448, DF=1 Pvalue= 0.503
Female	98(50.5)	96 (49.5)	194 (84.3)	
Male	16(44.4)	20 (55.6)	36 (15.7)	
Total	114	116	230 (100)	

Table 4: Bacterial hand contamination rate and associated factors among food handlers working in the student cafeterias of JU main campus, May 2012 to April 2013.

Discussion

Food handlers are an important vehicle for microorganisms, and improper handling practices may cause food contamination and consequently food borne diseases, which pose a potential risk to public health [31]. This study is taken to assess bacterial hand contamination among food handlers working in the student cafeterias of Jimma University main campus.

In this study 49.6% participants' hands were contaminated with one or more potentially food borne bacterial contaminants. Staphylococcus aureus 23.5%, *Klebsiella species* 16.1%, *E. coli* 0.9%, *Enterobacter species* 9.1%, *Citrobacter species* 4.3%, are among the most commonly isolated bacterial hand contaminants. The overall hand contamination rate of enteric bacterial contaminants was 31.7% among the participants. Similar types of bacterial contaminants were identified in Gondar [32], Nigeria [33], Egypt [34], Iran [35], Brazil [36] and Turkey [37].

Toxin-producing strains of Staphylococcus aureus are the leading cause of gastroenteritis following handling of food by persons who carry this bacterium in their noses and skin [38]. The present study *Staphylococcus aureus* were isolated from 23.5% food handlers' hands. This figure is comparable to 16.5%, 17.5%, and 31% prevalence reported in Gondar, Saudi Arabia, and Egypt respectively [32,34,39]. However, it is higher than 12.6%, and 7.1% incidence reported in Iran [31], and Nigeria [29] respectively. Nevertheless, the finding of the current study is lower than 42%, and 70% prevalence reported in Mexico [40], and Turkey [37] respectively. The discrepancy in socioeconomic status, type of food establishment, and lack of personal hygiene may explain this difference. The Isolation of *Staphylococcus aures*, reflect improper hygiene practices such as pocking fingers into the nose.

Enteric pathogens that are believed to be capable of being transmitted by food workers include, but are not limited to, *E. coli*, *Salmonella spp.*, *Shigella spp.* In addition, pathogens such as *Proteus*, and *Klebsiella*, which could originate from raw animal products, can contaminate hands from where they could be transferred to foods, equipment and other workers [15].

Enteric pathogens are among the transient hand flora that can be easily removed by hand washing. Isolation of these organisms includes a *faeces*-to-hand spread and indicating a poor hygiene practices of the food handlers [41]. Their presence indicates fecal contamination and poor hygiene practices food handlers are not taking enough care of hand hygiene [42]. In the present study' Enterobacteriaceae were identified from hands of 31.7% food handlers'. This result is nearly comparable to 38% isolation rate reported in Mexico [40,43], and higher than 6.9% reported in Egypt [39]. However it is lower than 44%, and 55.6% reported in South Africa [20], and Brazil [31,34] respectively. This could be resulted due to difference in source population, and type of food establishment. Isolation of *Enterobacteriaceae* from hands reflects contamination with fecal matter, and inadequate and poor hand washing habit which may pose potential risk of food borne outbreaks.

E. coli is naturally found in the human intestine and although most strains are harmless, some serotypes 0157:H7 can cause serious illness [44]. *E. coli* is normally absent from hands and the presence of *E. coli* gives a better indication of recent fecal contamination with enteric pathogens [20]. *E. coli* was detected on the hands of 10.9% of food handlers' in the current study, which is in line with 7.8%, and 6.8% carriage reported in Turkey, and Brazil respectively [36,37]. However, it is lower than 22% carriage reported in Iran [36]. Nevertheless, this figure is higher than 3.9%, 3.1%, 2.5%, and 1.8% isolation rate reported in Turkey [25], Gondar [32], Saudi Arabia [34], and Nigeria [33] respectively. The difference between our results and the previous studies may be attributed to sampling techniques.

In our study, no significant association was found for bacterial hand contamination by sex, educational background, medical check-up, training status, hand washing habit, and fingernail status of food handlers. However, there was significant association between bacterial hand contamination rate and service years (Chi-square=13.732, DF=4, P<0.05). This result indicated that food handlers more work experience have less risk of bacterial hand contamination. This could be explained as food handlers with more work experience have better personal hygienic practices than inexperienced food handlers. There is a significant difference in bacterial hand contamination rate among different age groups (χ^2=11.308, DFP=3, P=0.010). This can be explained as younger food handlers have poor hygienic practices. The bacterial hand contamination rate has significant association Cleanness of outer garments (χ^2=7.653, DF=1, P=0.006). Undoubtedly, in-depth training about personal hygienic practices of new employees, inexperienced, and young food handlers could minimize the effect of service on bacterial hand contamination rates

Persons working in food services have to go through periodic medical examination. The interview result of our study showed that only 56.7% of food handlers had taken medical checkup. This figure is comparable to 63.2% reported in Mekele University [45]. However, it is much higher than 22.7% reported in Mekele [46], and the result reported in Bahirdar in which none of the participants come across regular medical examinations [47,48]. The difference with respect to medical checkup can be explained by better provision and enforcement in Jimma University.

It is known that improper handling is one of the main causes of food borne disease and that inappropriate hand hygiene is an important risk factor for food contamination [31]. Food handlers should always wash their hands when their level of cleanliness may affect food quality; for example: just before food handling, after any interruption, after touching contaminated material, after using the bathroom and whenever else needed. They should not smoke, sneeze, spit, cough, eat, handle money or engage in any act that could contaminate the food during the performance of their activities [23].

Hygienic assessment of the food handlers revealed that 77% of food handlers have a habit of hand washing with soap and water after toilet, while others used only water. This figure is nearly similar to 70.4%, and 89% reported in Mekele, and Gondar respectively [32,38]. However, it was lower than 90.6%a reported in Bahirdar [44]. In the present study only 57% of food handlers have hand washing habit after touching dirty materials, and different body parts such as nose. This result shows food handlers negligence, and lack of awareness on sources of food contamination.

Food handlers should receive training before starting work in any food establishment, with a periodic refreshing training [47]. In this study 68.7 % food handlers have got short course of training on food hygiene. This figure is much higher than 14%, and 12.3% reported in Bahirdar, and Mekele respectively [44,48]. This gap can be due to both studies enumerated only certified trainings. However, in the current study food handlers have got only short course of food safety training organized by the student cafeteria office. None of the food handlers were certified by formal training. Effective training of food handlers, may lead to an improvement in hygienic practices.

Food handlers should cover hair and wear appropriate protective covering , cut their fingernails short and during handling they should remove jewelry from their hands[47]. In the present study, 164 (71.3%) food handlers were observed wearing outer working Coat, while only 40.4% had worn hair net. This result is in line with the report a cross-sectional study in mekele in which 72.6% of the food handlers were found wearing outer working garments, and 39% had worn hair net [38]. Nevertheless, it is higher than the figure reported in Ambo in which only 28% of food handlers' worn outer garment and hair covers [48]. This gap might be due to differences in socio-economic condition.

Moreover, in our study 80.4% of food handlers' fingernails were trimmed. This figure is by far comparable to 76.2%, and 88.4% reported in Mekele town [42], and Mekele University [44] respectively. However, it is higher than 70% reported in Ambo [49]. Even though it had no association with the isolation rate of potential bacterial pathogens in this study, fingernails can serve as a vehicle for transport of microorganisms from their source to the foods or/and directly into the body. Beside this, 25.2% food handlers have worn finger ornaments. This figure is similar to 27.1% reported in Ambo [28], and lower than 35.7% reported in Mekele [38].

Limitation of the Study

As far as the study design is cross sectional, it simply provides information about relationship between the dependent and independent variables. Beside this Total Plate Count and Colliform count were not done because of resource and time constraint. Serological identification of *Salmonella* species was not carried out. Antimicrobial susceptibility test for potential food borne bacterial contaminants was not done. Moreover, there is a scarcity of studies focused on isolation of bacteria from hands. This fact makes difficult the comparison of our results with that found by other researchers especially from developing countries.

Conclusion and Recommendations

In conclusion, our findings showed 114 (49.6%) carriage of potential food borne bacterial hand contaminants and 73(31.7%) were tested positive for enteric bacterial hand contaminants. The following food borne bacterial hand contaminants were isolated with the corresponding prevalence rate: S. aureus 54(23.5%), *Klebsiella spp.* 37(16.1%), *E. coli* 25(10.9%), *Enterobacter spp.* 21(9.1%), *Citrobacter spp.* 10(4.3%), *Serratia marcescens* 6 (2.6%), *Pseudomonas aeruginosa* 8(3.5%), *Proteus spp.* 5(2.2%), *Providencia rettegri* 3(1.3), and *salmonella spp.*2 (0.9%). These findings emphasized the importance of food handlers hand as potential vector of food borne bacterial pathogens that could constitute a potential risk of food borne disease outbreaks. Bacterial hand contamination rate have significant association with service years (Chi-square=13.732, DF=4, P=0.008), age (χ^2=11.308, P=0.010) and cleanness of outer garments (χ^2=7.653, P=0.006). Despite short course of informal food hygiene training none of the participants has been certified by formal training.

Based on the findings of the study the following recommendations are made:

As a responsible body to Jimma University:

Instruction regarding proper methods of hand washing should become a part of new employees, as well as young and inexperienced food handlers' orientation, education.

Food handlers should be well trained about personal hygienic practices pointing out on importance of hand hygiene and cleanness of outer garments

Close follow up, and regular supervision of personal hygienic practices of food handlers should be used as controlling strategies

Future studies should focus on enumeration of bacterial hand contaminants, and assessing sanitary facilities of the working environment.

References

1. WHO (2002) WHO global strategy for food safety: safer food for better health. Geneva, Switzerland.
2. http://www.afro.who.int/index.php?option=com_docman&task=doc.
3. WHO Consultation (2006) World Health Organization (WHO) Consultation to Develop a Strategy to Estimate the Global Burden of Food borne Diseases.
4. Centers for Disease control and Prevention (2005) Foodborne Illness. International Food Safety Consultancy.
5. World Health Organization (2007) Food Safety and Foodborne Illness-Fact sheet No. 237.
6. Centers for Disease control and Prevention (CDC) (2005) Foodborne Illness. International Food Safety Consultancy.
7. CDC (2011) Estimates. CDC Estimates of Foodborne Illness in the United States. National Center for Emerging & Zoonotic Infectious Diseases Division of Foodborne, Waterborne, and Environmental Diseases.
8. World Health Organization (2000) Food borne Disease: A focus for Health Education. Geneva.
9. FAO Food and Nutrition (2003) Joint FAO/WHO Publication Assuring Food Safety and Quality: Guidelines For Strengthening National Food Control Systems. Paper 76.

10. Brundtland GH. Food Chain 2001 - "Food Safety a World-wide Challenge. WHO, Uppsala, Sweden, updated.
11. Ministry of Health (2011) Planning and Programming Department. Health and Health Related Indicators.
12. WHO (2004) World Health Organization global strategy for food safety: safer food for better health.
13. Käferstein FK (2003) Food safety: the fourth pillar in the strategy to prevent infant diarrhoea Bull World Health Organ 81: 842-843.
14. Zain MM, Naing NN (2002) Sociodemographic characteristics of food handlers and their knowledge, attitude and practice towards food sanitation: a preliminary report. Southeast Asian J Trop Med Public Health 33: 410-417.
15. Michaels B, Keller C, Blevins M, Paoli G (2004) Prevention of food worker transmission of foodborne pathogens: risk assessment and evaluation of effective hygiene intervention strategies. Food Service Technology.
16. Guzevich J, Ross M (1999) Evaluation of risks related to microbiological contamination of ready-to-eat food by food preparation workers and the effectiveness of interventions to minimize those risks.
17. Gun W, Satu S (2007) Microbial contaminants & Contamination routes in food industry: 1st open seminar arranged by SAFOODNET in food safety and hygiene networking within new member states and associated candidate Countries.
18. Mohan V (2001) An evaluation of health status of food handlers of eating establishments in various educational and health institutions in Amritsar City. Indian Journal of Community Medicine 26(2): 80-84.
19. Bloomfield SF, Nath KJ (2009) Use of ash and mud for hand washing in low income communities. An IFH expert review.
20. Pickering AJ, Boehm AB, Mwanjali M, Davis J (2010) Efficacy of waterless hand hygiene compared with handwashing with soap: a field study in Dar es Salaam, Tanzania. Am J Trop Med Hyg 82: 270-278.
21. Murat B, Azmi SE, Gokhan K (2006) The evaluation of food hygiene knowledge, attitude, and practice of food handlers in food businesses in Turkey. Food Control 17: 317-322.
22. Lues JFR, Tonder IV (2007) The occurrence of indicator bacteria on hands and aprons of food handlers in the delicatessen sections of a retail group. Food Control 18(4): 326-332.
23. Snyder OP (2010) A "Safe Hands" Hand wash program for retail food operations. Hospitality Institute of Technology and Management.
24. Codex Alimentarius (2003) Recommended international code of practice general principles of food hygiene. CAC/RCP 1-1969.
25. Harrison WA, Griffith CJ, Ayers T, Michaels B (2003) Bacterial transfer and cross-contamination potential associated with paper-towel dispensing. Am J Infect Control 31: 387-391.
26. Acikel CH, Ogur R, Yaren H, Gocgeldi E (2008) The hygiene training of food handlers at a Teaching Hospital. Food Control.
27. Fagernes M, Lingaas E (2011) Factors interfering with the microflora on hands: a regression analysis of samples from 465 healthcare workers. J Adv Nurs 67: 297-307.
28. Josie L, Traub-Dargatz, J, Weese S, Rousseau JD (2006) Pilot study to evaluate 3 hygiene protocols on the reduction of bacterial load on the hands of veterinary staff performing routine equine physical examinations. Can Vet J 47: 671-676.
29. Cheesbrough M (2003) Medical Laboratory Technology Manual of Tropical Health. Low Priced Edition.Doddington, Cambridgeshire, England, pp146-215.
30. Buchanan RE and Gribbon NE (1974) Bergeys Manual of Determinative Bacteriology. 8th ed. Williams and Wilkins Co,; Baltimore, U.S.
31. Campos AKC, Cardonha AMS, Pinheiro LBG, Ferreira NR, et al. (2009) Assessment of personal hygiene and practices of food handlers in municipal public schools of Natal, Brazil. Food Control 20(9): 807-810.
32. Andargie G, Kassu A, Moges F, Tiruneh M, Huruy K (2008) Prevalence of bacteria and intestinal parasites among food-handlers in Gondar town, northwest Ethiopia. J Health Popul Nutr 26: 451-455.
33. Ifeadike CO, Ironkwe OC, Adogu PO, Nnebue CC, Emelumadu OF, et al. (2012) Prevalence and pattern of bacteria and intestinal parasites among food handlers in the Federal Capital Territory of Nigeria. Niger Med J 53: 166-171.
34. Fawzi M, Gomaa NF, Bakr WM (2009) Assessment of hand washing facilities, personal hygiene and the bacteriological quality of hand washes in some grocery and dairy shops in alexandria, egypt. J Egypt Public Health Assoc 84: 71-93.
35. Shojaei H, Shooshtaripoor J, Amiri M (2006) Efficacy of simple hand-washing in reduction of microbial hand contamination of Iranian food handlers. Food Research International 39(5): 525-529.
36. Souza PA, Santos DA (2009) Microbiological risk factors associated with food handlers in elementary schools from Brazil. Journal of Food Safety 29(3): 42.
37. Aycicek H, Aydogan H, Kucukkaraaslan A, Baysallar M, et al. (2004) Assessment of the bacterial contamination on hands of hospital food handlers. Food Control 15(4): 253-259.
38. Do Carmo LS, Cummings C, Linardi VR, Dias RS, De Souza JM, et al. (2004) A case study of a massive staphylococcal food poisoning incident. Foodborne Pathog Dis 1: 241-246.
39. Zaglool DA, Khodari YA, Othman RA, Farooq MU (2011) Prevalence of intestinal parasites and bacteria among food handlers in a tertiary care hospital. Niger Med J 52: 266-270.
40. Dharod JM, Stefania Paciello S, BermÃºdez-MillÃ¡n A, Venkitanarayanan K, et al. (2009); Bacterial Contamination of Hands Increases Risk of Crosscontamination among Low-income Puerto Rican Meal Preparers. J Nutr Educ Behav 41(6): 389-397.
41. Jumaa PA (2005) Hand hygiene: simple and complex. Int J Infect Dis 9: 3-14.
42. Zeru K, Kumie A (2007) The sanitary conditions of food establishments in Mekelle Town, Tigray, North Ethiopia. Ethiop. J Health Dev 21(1): 3-11.
43. Abhay BM, Navetta kA, Gargi AM, Ramachandrah CG (2010) Health status and personal hygiene among food handlers working in food establishments around a rural teaching hospital in Wardah district of Maharashtra, India. Global Journal of Health Science 2(2): 198-207.
44. Taulo S, Wetlesen A, Abrahamsen RK, Narvhus JA, et al. (2009) Quantification and variability of Escherichia coli and Staphylococcus aureus cross-contamination during serving and consumption of cooked thick porridge in Lungwena rural households, Malawi. Food Control 20: 1158-1166.
45. Nigusse D and Kumie A (2012) Food hygiene practices and prevalence of intestinal parasites among food handlers working in Mekelle University students cafeteria, Mekelle. GARJSS 1(4): 065-071.
46. Abera B, Biadegelgen F, Bezabih B. (2010) Prevalence of Salmonella typhi and intestinal parasites among food handlers in Bahir Dar Town, Northwest Ethiopia. Ethiop J Health Dev. 24: 46-50.
47. http://www.afro.who.int/index.php?option=com_docman&task=doc.
48. Gudeta D (2007) Sanitary Survey of Food and Drinking Establishments in Ambo Town West Showa Zone Oromia Region. MSc. Thesis, Addis Ababa University, Faculty of Medicine.
49. Fadel HM, Ismail J (2009) Prevalence and Significance of Staphylococcus aureus and Enterohacteriaceae species in Selected Dairy Products and Handlers. International Journal of Dairy Science 4 (3): 100-108.

A Randomized Open Comparative Clinical Trial on the Effectiveness, Safety and Tolerability of a Homeopathic Medicinal Product for the Treatment of Painful Teething in Children

Miek C Jong[1,2,3,*], Cynthia Verwer[1], Lucy van de Vijver[1], Petra Klement[4], Julia Burkart[4] and Erik Baars[1,5]

[1]*Department Nutrition & Health, Louis Bolk Institute, Driebergen, The Netherlands*

[2]*Department of Health Sciences, Mid Sweden University, Sundsvall, Sweden*

[3]*National Information and Knowledge Center on Integrative Medicine (NIKIM), Amsterdam, The Netherlands*

[4]*Deutsche Homöopathie-Union, DHU-Arzneimittel GmbH & Co. KG, Karlsruhe, Germany*

[5]*Department of Care, Professorship Anthroposophic Healthcare, University of Applied Sciences, Leiden, The Netherlands*

[*]**Corresponding author**: Miek C Jong, Louis Bolk Institute, Department Nutrition & Health, Hoofdstraat 24 and 3972 LA Driebergen, The Netherlands, E -mail: m.jong@louisbolk.nl

Abstract

Background: Homeopathic products are sold over the counter and are often used for treatment of self-limiting complaints in children such as painful teething.

Objective: To investigate the effectiveness, safety and tolerability of the homeopathic product ChamBell-5-02, in the treatment of children with painful teething in comparison to another homeopathic product.

Design: A multicenter, randomized, open, comparative clinical trial with two parallel treatment groups at three outpatient pediatric clinics in Russia.

Methods: Children aged ≤ six years with painful teething were enrolled from March-July 2009 in the study and randomized to receive either ChamBell-5-02 tablets (Dentokind®; intervention group) or homeopathic suppositories (Viburcol®; control group). Exclusion criteria were: fever of ≥38°C and severe comorbidity. Primary effectiveness endpoints were change of total severity scores of subjective complaints (TSSC) and clinical signs (TSCS) rated by investigators after seven days of treatment. Treatment satisfaction and safety (via number of adverse events (AEs)) were assessed.

Results: A total of 200 children (100 per group) were included and analyzed. TSSC/ TSCS decreased after the 7-day treatment period from median 7.0 to 1.0/6.0 to 1.0 points in the intervention group and from median 5.0 to 1.0/5.5 to 1.0 points in the control group. Compared to the control group children receiving ChamBell-5-02 had about five/2.5 time higher odds of showing improvement (TSSC/TSCS: odds ratio resulting from proportional odds model was 5.1 (95%-CI: 2.7-9.4, p<0.0001) / 2.5 (95%-CI: 1.5-4.4, p=0.0011). Furthermore the intervention group showed a more favorable outcome regarding treatment satisfaction (ratings very satisfied: intervention group: n=94; control group: n=58). No AEs were recorded in the intervention group. In the control group three mild to moderate, non-serious AEs occurred.

Conclusions: Overall it can be concluded that in this study ChamBell-5-02 tablets showed to be effective, safe and well tolerated.

Keywords: Homeopathy; Randomized clinical trial; Children; Dentition; Teething; Dentokind; Viburcol

Introduction

Teething is known as a natural process by which the first teeth appear in children. The first period of teething takes about two and a half years, with the first tooth erupting between four and ten months and all other teeth before the age of three years. Around the age of six, children begin to lose their primary teeth and the first permanent teeth erupt [1]. A variety of symptoms has been shown to accompany teething [2]. This includes irritated and painful gums, crying, irritability, drooling, sleep disturbances and loss of appetite. Teething symptoms in children can create much distress in parents [3,4]. Often, parents consult family or friends for advice on effective treatments as to alleviate their child's discomfort and pain [5]. It has been reported that the majority of parents (63-88%) manage teething symptoms using some form of over-the-counter (OTC) medication [3,6,7]. The most commonly used medications for painful teething in children are paracetamol and analgesic and anesthetic gels, containing choline salicylate, lidocaine hydrochloride or benzocaine [3,6,7]. However, use of these OTC medications might be associated with unwanted side-effects and for some topical teething gels cases of potential life-threatening risks have been reported [8-10]. There is growing interest among parents for safe and effective medicinal products. Some Complementary and Alternative Medicine (CAM) may offer these medicinal products.

As defined by the National Center for Complementary and Alternative Medicine (NCCAM), CAM covers a broad variety of therapy approaches that are not generally considered part of conventional medicine. A recently published review reported that prevalence rates for overall CAM use in children ranged from 10.9–87.6% for lifetime use and from 8–48.5% for current use [11]. Homeopathy is listed in many studies among the most popular CAM modalities for children [12-16]. A population-based cohort study in the South-West of England showed that 11.8% of children up to 8.5 years of age had used a homeopathic product, most common for self-limiting infantile conditions such as colic, cuts and bruises, and teething [17]. The predominant reason why parents choose homeopathy is that they want safe treatment options for their children. Parents have reported to fear side effects associated with conventional medication and to seek effective and safe alternatives [18,19].

The investigational homeopathic preparation (Dentokind®, ChamBell-5-02) is sold over the counter since 1984 in the Netherlands and up to now also in 18 other countries for self-care of painful teething in children. ChamBell-5-02 is a complex homeopathic product containing five individual homeopathic substances. It was developed by homeopathic physicians through careful selection of individual remedies based on their clinical experience and with the goal of addressing the most common acute symptoms associated with teething. The present study was proposed as a randomized controlled study to obtain data on the clinical use, safety and effectiveness of ChamBell-5-02 for regulatory purposes as required for marketing authorization in Russian Federation. A comparative design with another homeopathic product (Viburcol®, VIB), which was already on the market in the Russian Federation for treatment of painful teething, was requested by the Russian regulatory authorities.

Material and Methods

Study design and approval

A prospective, multicenter, randomized, open-label, comparative, controlled clinical trial with two parallel groups was conducted in Moscow, Russia. The study was approved by the Independent Ethics Committee of the Russian Federation (Protocol No. 23, December 10, 2008) and by the Ethics Committee of the Russian State Medical University of the Federal Agency for Healthcare and Social Developments (Protocol No. 86, January 19, 2009). The study was conducted in accordance with the Russian Federation National Standards of Good Clinical Practice.

Study population

Children were recruited at three outpatient pediatric clinics in Moscow, Russia (The State Educational Institution for Higher Professional Education "Russian State Medical University" and the State Healthcare Institution of Moscow City "Children City Clinical Hospital No. 13" and "Children City Policlinic No. 55"). Eligible children were those of either gender, aged up to six years, with one or several symptoms accompanying teething. Exclusion criteria were hyperthermia of over 38.0°C, severe concomitant diseases (renal failure, heart anomalies, circulatory failure, cardiomyopathy, decompensated kidney and liver, immunosuppressive conditions, oncological diseases), known or suspected hypersensitivity to any component of the study medication, participation in clinical studies within the past six months before the start of the study or use of any other medicinal products used for the treatment of symptoms accompanying teething within the last seven days. Informed consent was obtained from the parents for participation of their child in the study. The first child was included in March 2009 and the last child completed the study in July 2009.

Intervention

Children who fulfilled all eligibility criteria were randomly allocated either to the intervention group (n=100) or to the control group (n=100). ChamBell-5-02 tablets; the treatment of the intervention group, is a complex homeopathic product containing five homeopathic substances: Belladonna D6, Chamomilla D6, Ferrum phosphoricum D6, Hepar sulfuris D12 and Pulsatilla D6 and was administered orally for seven days. Children aged up to one year received ChamBell-5-02 tablets with a dosage regime of one tablet every hour up to six tablets per day (acute symptoms). After symptoms reduced one tablet three times a day was administered. Children aged 1-6 years received two tablets every hour up to a maximum of twelve tablets per day (acute symptoms). After symptoms reduction the dosage was two tablets three times per day.

The control group received VIB suppository, which is a complex homeopathic medicinal product with six homeopathic ingredients: Chamomilla recutita D1, Atropa bella-donna D2, Solanum dulcamara D4, Plantago major D3, Pulsatilla pratensis D2, Calcium carbonicum Hahnemanni D8. It was administered rectally for a period of seven days. For children aged up to six months the maximum daily dose was two suppositories a day. Children older than six months of age received a maximum of four suppositories (at a body temperature of ≥ 37.5°C) a day. When body temperature normalized one suppository was used for further 3-4 days 1-2 times per day (with preventive purpose).

Study procedure

The study involved three clinic visits. At baseline visit (Day 0), children were randomly allocated to the intervention or control group, baseline values of subjective complaints and clinical signs were assessed, study medication was handed out and treatment started. Randomization lists were generated by the Laboratory of Biostatistics State Research Center for Preventative Medicine (Moscow, Russia) with a random block size of four in order to guarantee a balanced allocation. According to the randomization list, 50% of the children were allocated to the intervention group and 50% to the control group. At each center, children were assigned a study number in ascending order based on entry in the trial. For each study number, the investigator received a sealed envelope containing the name of the study medication to be given to the child according to the randomization list. The envelope was opened after the children's parents had provided signed informed consent. The second visit (Day 3-5) was a follow up visit at which subjective complaints, clinical signs and possible adverse events (AEs) were evaluated. The third visit (Day 7) was the termination visit and end of the study with final assessment of subjective complaints and clinical signs, evaluation of study medication's effectiveness and tolerability, as well as evaluation of overall satisfaction with the treatment. Duration of individual observation was eight days. There was no run-in or post-treatment period.

Objectives

The purpose of this study was to assess the effectiveness, safety and tolerability of ChamBell-5-02 compared with another homeopathic medicinal product in the treatment of children with painful symptoms of teething. Primary endpoints were changes in total severity scores of subjective complaints (TSSC; unmotivated anxiety, gingival tenderness and appetite disorder - each of the above with maximum two points, otalgy, stool softening, sleep-onset insomnia and frequent awakenings - each of the above with maximum one point; maximum total score: ten points) and changes in total severity scores of clinical signs (TSCS; skin pallor, gingiva condition: hyperemia, gingiva condition: swelling, gingiva condition: hematoma and hyperemia around the mouth - each of the above with maximum one point, drooling and hyperthermia - each of the above with maximum two points, maximum total score: nine points) after treatment with study medication for 3-5 and seven days. Complaints and clinical signs were evaluated and scored by the investigator at the respective center. Secondary endpoints regarding effectiveness were changes in the severities of individual complaints, changes in the severities of individual signs, effectiveness assessments by investigators and children/parents using the 4-point rating Integrative Medicine Outcome Scale (IMOS [20]), treatment satisfaction assessment by children/parents using the 4-point rating Integrative Medicine Patient Satisfaction Scale (IMPSS [20]) and time taken for all subjective complaints and for all clinical signs to disappear. Secondary endpoints regarding safety were tolerability of study medication assessed by investigators and children/parents and incidence of AEs and adverse drug reactions (ADRs).

Sample size

Calculation of sample size was carried out based on power estimation assuming a scenario if 100 children per group are recruited. The primary outcome refers to the difference on a 10-point and 9-point scale respectively. As a measurement of the minimal relevant effect in case of questionnaires the minimal important clinically relevant difference can be regarded. It is usually set as 10% of the range (here: about one point). The standard deviation of the scale is about two. At a level of significance of α=0.05 and n=100 per group power of β=0.94 would be achieved to potentially distinguish a difference of greater than one point between the effectiveness of the study medications.

Statistical analyses

The statistical analysis was based on the full analysis data set (FAS), including all children who were randomized and who received the study medication at least once and had at least one measured post baseline effectiveness response. In case of premature withdrawal of children, the LOCF (last observation carried forward) method was used to replace missing observations regarding primary effectiveness variables. In order to assess the impact of drop-outs on effectiveness results, a subset of observed cases (OC) was evaluated. Safety analysis included all randomized children who received at least one dose of study medication. The homogeneity of the two treatment groups was assessed by comparison of demographic data and data obtained at the baseline visit (Day 0). Baseline values of primary variables were included as covariates in the respective models. Continuously or quasi-continuously scaled variables were investigated whether prerequisites for parametric approach were fulfilled. In case of categorically scaled variables, counts and percentages were reported, and ordinal logistic regression (proportional odds model (POM)), χ^2-Test as well as Armitage Trend Test were applied for comparisons. A rejection-criterion of 0.05 was set for all statistical tests. If tests allowed, the statistics were two-tailed.

Results

Baseline characteristics

A flow diagram of children included and excluded in the study is shown in Figure 1. A total of 200 children were randomized, 100 in each group. Recruitment took place from March-June 2009. Study follow-up was performed from March-July 2009. The trial ended because the planned number of participants was reached. The FAS population consisted of 200 children (100 in each group) and 198 children were included in the OC analysis. In Table 1, demographic and clinical characteristics are shown.

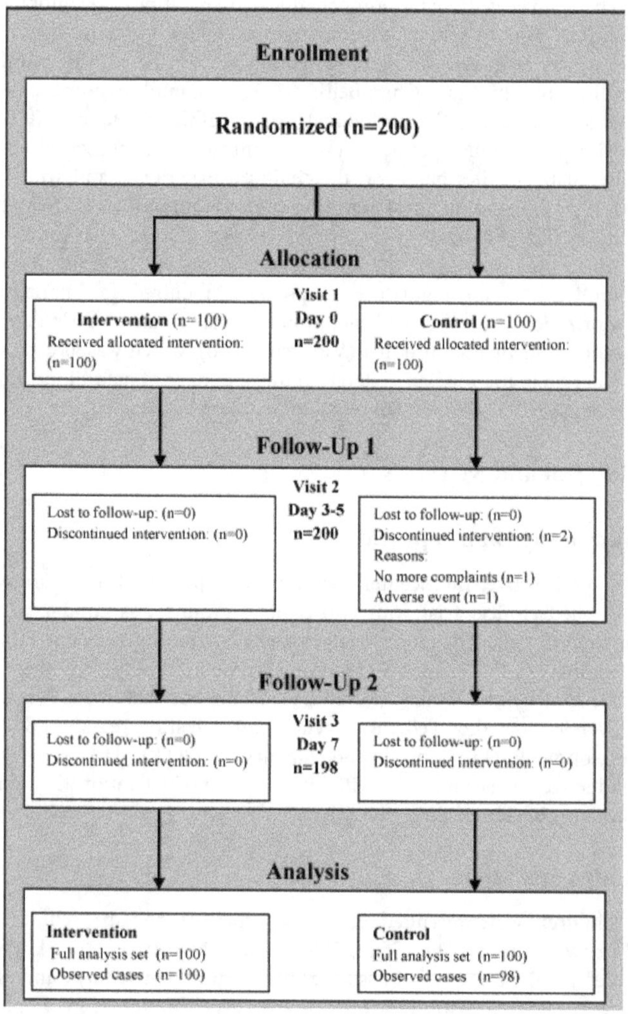

Figure 1: Flow diagram of participants.

Characteristics	Intervention group (n=100)	Control group (n=100)
Age [months] (median [P25, P75]		
Infants <12 months Toddlers/ children ≥ 12 months	7.5 [6.5, 9.0] 19.5 [14.0, 33.5]	6.0 [4.0, 8.0] 18.0 [14.0, 26.0]
Sex (n boys/n girls)	47/53	48/52
Duration of painful teething prior to study start (n)		
1 day 2 days 3-4 days More than 4 days	16 34 23 26*	25 44 18 13
Concomitant diseases (n)	32	29
Concomitant medication (n)	6	6
n- refers to number of children * - for one child duration of painful symptoms prior to study start was unknown		

Table 1: Demographic and clinical characteristics, FAS analysis.

Primary and secondary effectiveness endpoints

Primary effectiveness endpoints: In the intervention group the TSSC reduced from baseline median value 7.0 points over 3.0 points (Day 3-5) to 1.0 point after seven days of treatment. The TSSC assessed in the control group decreased from median 5.0 points (baseline) to 3.0 points (Day 3-5) to 1.0 point after seven days (Figure 2).

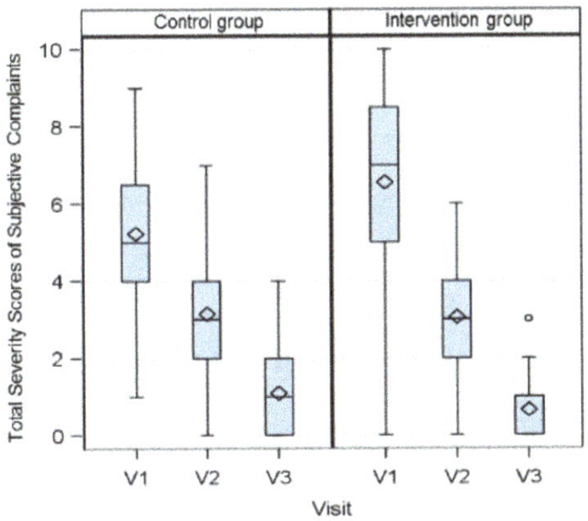

Figure 2: Total Severity Scores of Subjective Complaints (TSSC) at baseline visit (V1, Day 0), follow-up visit (V2, Day 3-5) and termination visit (V3, Day 7), FAS analysis. Note: Boxwhiskerplot showing mean, SD, median, minimum, P25%, P75% and maximum.

In a baseline adjusted POM those children receiving ChamBell-5-02 had five times higher odds of showing improvement after seven days of treatment than children in the control group (odds ratio resulting from baseline adjusted POM: 5.1 (95%-CI: 2.7-9.4, p<0.0001; FAS). After 3-5 days of treatment odds ratio resulting from baseline adjusted POM was 4.5 (95%-CI: 2.4-8.2, p<0.0001; FAS).

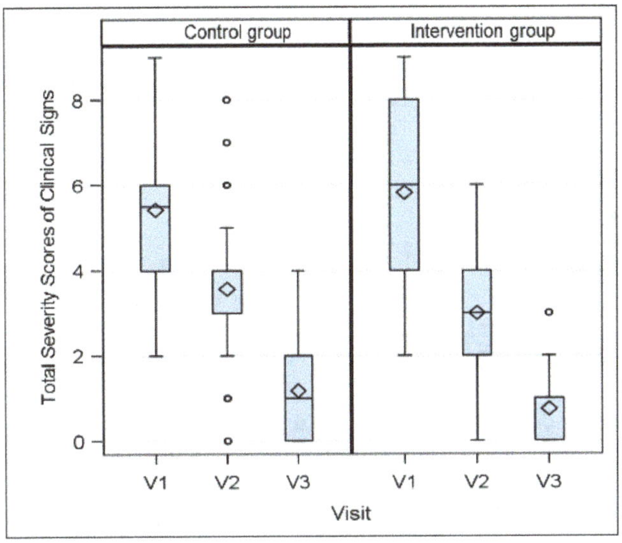

Figure 3: Total Severity Scores of Clinical Signs (TSCS) at baseline visit (V1, Day 0), follow-up visit (V2, Day 3-5) and termination visit (V3, Day 7), FAS analysis. Note: Boxwhiskerplot showing mean, SD, median, minimum, P25%, P75% and maximum.

TSCS assessed in the intervention group at each visit day (Day 0, Day 3-5, Day 7) decreased from median 6.0 points over 3.0 points to 1.0 point. In the control group a reduction from baseline median value 5.5 points to 4.0 points to 1.0 point was recorded (Figure 3). An odds ratio of 2.5 (95%-CI: 1.5-4.4) was found, indicating that children of the intervention group had 2.5 times higher odds of showing improvement after seven days of treatment compared to the children of the control group (baseline adjusted POM: p=0.0011; FAS). The odds ratio resulting from baseline adjusted POM at Day 3-5 was 4.8 (95%-CI: 2.7-8.5, p<0.0001; FAS). The OC analysis confirmed the findings for the primary effectiveness criteria of the FAS analysis (data not shown).

Secondary effectiveness endpoints: Improvement of individual complaints after seven days of treatment was seen in the following number of children of the intervention/control group (out of 100 children each): unmotivated anxiety– 88%/79%, gingival tenderness – 73%/55%, appetite disorder– 83%/66%, otalgy– 56%/18%, stool softening- 75%/36%, sleep-onset insomnia- 57%/54% and frequent awakenings- 74%/59%. With the exception of the complaint sleep-onset insomnia with a recorded deterioration in 3%/2% of children in the intervention and control group respectively, no change in the severity of respective complaint was recorded for the remaining number of children after seven days of treatment (most of these children didn't show the complaint at baseline at all).
Compared to the control group improvement of two out of seven individual complaints (gingival tenderness: Armitage Trend Test: p=0.0130, appetite disorder: Armitage Trend Test: p=0.0107; FAS) was observed in significantly more children of the intervention group.

Individual signs improved after seven days of treatment in following numbers of children of the intervention/control group (out of 100 children each): skin pallor 33%/30%, gingival hyperemia 91%/75%, gingival swelling 59%/41%, drooling 86%/83%, hyperemia around the mouth 51%/37%, hyperthermia 82%/86%. For the remaining number of children no change in the severity of respective sign was recorded after seven days of treatment (many of the children didn't show the sign at baseline at all). Comparing the two groups the signs gingival hyperemia (Armitage Trend Test: p=0.0057; FAS) and gingival swelling (Armitage Trend Test: p=0.0157; FAS) improved in significantly more children of the intervention group than in children of the control group. For all other categories no significant differences were observed. For the sign gingival hematoma no valid results were obtained for the comparison between the groups as strong baseline differences existed (only eight children of the control group and 24 children of the intervention group showed the sign at baseline at all).

After seven days of treatment with ChamBell-5-02 almost all children/parents and investigator (n=99 out of 100 each) of the intervention group rated "no complaints" or "major improvement" (final effectiveness assessments by investigators and children/parents by means of IMOS). In comparison to the other homeopathic preparation the overall outcome in the intervention group was significantly better (Armitage Trend Test: p<0.0001; FAS) (Table 2). Furthermore almost all children/parents (n=99 out of 100) in the intervention group were 'very satisfied' or 'satisfied' with the ChamBell-5-02 treatment (assessment by means of IMPSS). Compared to the assessment of children/parents in the control group the outcome in the intervention group was more favorable (Armitage Trend Test: p<0.0001; FAS) (Table 3).

Assessment	Investigator		Children/Parents	
	Control group (n=100)	Intervention group (n=100)	Control group (n=100)	Intervention group (n=100)
No complaints	28	47	36	62
Major Improvement	52	52	54	37
Improvement	20	1	9	1
No change	0	0	1	0
Deterioration	0	0	0	0
Result (Armitage Trend Test)	p<0.0001		p<0.0001	

Table 2: IMOS: Final effectiveness assessments by investigators and children/parents at termination visit (Day 7), FAS analysis. Note: Analyzed by means of descriptive statistics (counts) for the different categories of the IMOS.

Regarding the time taken for all subjective complaints and clinical signs to disappear (TSSC/TSCS = 0) in few children of the intervention group (complaints: n=8 children, signs: n=1 child) and the control group (complaints: n=7 children, signs: n=2 children) first clinical effects were seen after three to five days. At the end of treatment duration, subjective complaints and clinical signs disappeared completely in 47%/45% out of 100 children of the intervention group and in 33%/39% out of 100 children of the control group. Between the treatment groups no significant differences were noted with respect to time for complete disappearance of signs (Armitage trend test: p=0.5008; FAS). With respect to the time for disappearance of complaints a tendency for shorter durations was seen for the intervention group (Armitage trend test: p=0.0829; FAS).

Assessment	Control group (n=100)	Intervention group (n=99*)
Very satisfied	58	94
Satisfied	38	5
Neutral	3	0

Dissatisfied	1	0
Very dissatisfied	0	0
Result (Armitage Trend Test)	p<0.0001	
* For one patient assessment was unknown.		

Table 3: IMPSS: Treatment satisfaction evaluation by children/parents at termination visit (Day 7), FAS analysis. Note: Analyzed by descriptive statistics (counts) for the different categories of the IMPSS.

Safety and tolerability

During the 7-day treatment period children of the intervention group took on average 78 ChamBell-5-02 tablets (median: 78, P25%: 51, P75%: 88). Children of the control group received on average 23 suppositories (median: 24, P25%: 23, P75%: 24).

During the whole treatment period three out of 200 (1.5%) children experienced AEs. Serious AEs were not reported. The recorded AEs (allergic dermatitis (probably related), erythema (likely related) and anorectal discomfort (unlikely related) occurred in three children of the control group (3.0% out of 100 children) and were all of mild to moderate intensity. One of these children discontinued treatment and withdrew from the study due to the AE. In the intervention group no AEs were reported. Results of final treatment tolerability evaluated by investigators and children/parents are shown in Table 4.

Assessment	**Investigator**		**Children / Parents**	
	Control group (n=100)	Intervention group (n=99)*	Control group (n=100)	Intervention group (n=99)*
Very good	57	95	56	97
Good	41	4	43	2
Satisfactory	1	0	1	0
Poor	1	0	0	0
Result (Armitage Trend Test)	p<0.0001		p<0.0001	
*For one patient assessment was unknown				

Table 4: Final tolerability evaluation by investigators and children/parents at termination visit (Day 7), FAS analysis. Note: Analyzed by descriptive statistics (counts) for the different categories.

Almost all children/parents and investigators rated the tolerability of ChamBell-5-02 as 'very good' or 'good'. In comparison to the homeopathic suppositories the outcome in the intervention group was significantly better (Armitage Trend Test: p<0.0001; FAS).

Discussion

The present study demonstrated that both homeopathic study medications reduced total severity scores of subjective complaints, including individual symptoms such as unmotivated anxiety, gingival tenderness, appetite disorders and otalgy in teething children after seven days of treatment. Total severity scores of clinical signs, as associated with individual signs such as drooling, hyperemia and hyperthermia, also lowered after seven days of treatment in the homeopathic treatment groups. ChamBell-5-02 tablets appeared to be slightly more effective than the homeopathic suppositories in reducing teething complaints and clinical signs. The observed reductions in total severity scores of subjective complaints and clinical signs were also reflected by the effectiveness assessments of investigators and children/parents, as either a major improvement or total recovery from painful teething was observed for almost all children (99%) in the intervention group and 80-90% of the children in the control group.

To our best knowledge, this study is the first randomized controlled trial on effectiveness of homeopathic medications for painful teething. A number of studies have demonstrated the effectiveness of homeopathy for other (self-limiting) conditions in children. A study by Haidvogl et al. [21] in children with acute respiratory tract infections and ear complaints, showed significant rapid improvements upon homeopathic medications compared to conventional treatment. The rate of symptom improvement in children with acute otitis media was also faster upon treatment with homeopathic ear drops compared to standard therapy only [22]. Another randomized-controlled study on acute otitis media reported that children who received homeopathic treatment improved faster than those conventionally treated [23]. Furthermore, children treated with homeopathy did not require any additional antibiotic treatment [23].

Despite these positive finding, the effectiveness of homeopathy is still heavily debated [24]. Based on the perceived implausibility of any conceivable mechanism of action for homeopathy, specifically the highly diluted medications, all (placebo)-controlled studies and other available evidence on homeopathy is rejected [25] or regarded as placebo effects [26]. Regrettably, the rejection of homeopathy within conventional medicine is in sharp contrast to the beliefs and behaviors of patients and parents. Many patients and parents accept and use homeopathic medicines for themselves or their children, either prescribed by (homeopathic) physicians or through self-care [12,27,28]. The observation that personal use of CAM (including homeopathy) is relatively high among conventional healthcare professions [29,30], could indicate that attitudes shift when conventional healthcare professions become patients or parents themselves. Although the scientific critique on homeopathy is expected to continue, recent studies on cost-effectiveness of homeopathy may bring another viewpoint into the debate. Studies by Kooreman and Baars [31,32] reported that patients whose general practitioner has additional CAM training (including homeopathy) had lower health costs. Furthermore, homeopathic treatment of children with rhinopharyngitis was associated with lower direct medical costs and less sick leave time for their parents compared to standard antibiotic treatment [33]. Because of the rapidly growing health care cost in Western societies, cost-effective treatment options such as homeopathy may gain new (politic) interest.

Another important advantage of the use of homeopathy in children is its apparent excellent safety profile. In the present study, both homeopathic medications were very well tolerated in children. Only three mild, non-serious adverse reactions (1.5% of total study population) were reported in the control group. Conventional OTC medications for painful teething, such as teething gels, have failed to demonstrate any specific benefits and have the potential to be harmful in overdose [34]. Unintentional parent-caused overdose in the form of frequent use of teething gels over several months has led to potential lethal risks as children were hospitalized due to salicylate intoxication [9] or methemoglobinemia [10]. Common side effects such as reduced gag reflex and irritated oral sensation have also been reported for teething gels [35]. Altogether, these findings suggest that the presently investigated homeopathic product ChamBell-5-02 may be a better alternative for children with painful symptoms of teething, with lower risks than conventional OTC treatment options like teething gels.

The present study was specifically designed for regulatory purposes. It also had its limitations. First of all, the study had an open label design. Both investigators and children/parents knew that the study was undertaken to investigate whether ChamBell-5-02 was comparable with the other homeopathic product in symptom relief of teething. Even though the primary effectiveness endpoints were partly based on objective clinical signs such as skin pallor, gingiva condition, drooling, hyperemia and hyperthermia, it cannot be excluded with certainty that in particular the subjective complaints measured in the intervention group may have been overestimated relative to the control group. Secondly, ChamBell-5-02 was administered orally and compared to a homeopathic medicinal product as control that was administered rectally. To specifically investigate comparable effectiveness, it would have been better if the homeopathic medicinal products under investigation were administered in a similar manner. Another limitation was that the current study design did not control for the natural course of the disease and regression to the mean. Teething symptoms such as drooling, ear rubbing, irritability, hyperthermia and loss of appetite have been reported specifically within an eight-day time frame of teething [36]. This covers a four day period before the tooth emerges, the day itself, and up to three days after tooth eruption. As children in the present study already exhibited teething symptoms for some days prior to start of the study, the observed reduction in total severity scores of subjective complaints and clinical signs may have reflected the natural decline of teething symptoms, rather than a direct effect of the homeopathic study medication itself. Teeth often emerge in clusters, meaning that successive non-first teeth emerge on the same day as another tooth, or teeth emerge within five days of another tooth [36]. Thus teething symptoms can be exhibited over a longer period of time, dependent on the number of teeth erupting. The number of erupting teeth however, was not recorded in the present study. Other studies in children have shown that homeopathic medications achieve symptom relieve specifically within the first week after treatment, more so than standard, conventional therapy [21-23]. Based on these findings, it can be hypothesized that ChamBell-5-02 may have reduced symptoms more rapidly than the natural course of teething. Further research is warranted to confirm this hypothesis. As recommended in the roadmap for future CAM research [37], further research on ChamBell-5-02 may include comparative effectiveness research in a real world setting comparing ChamBell-5-02 to conventional treatment strategies. Despite these limitations, the present study served its purpose as a large randomized controlled study demonstrating the clinical use of ChamBell-5-02 in children, its excellent safety profile and treatment satisfaction of parents/children with ChamBell-5-02.

As nowadays healthcare costs are escalating, the attention for managing one's own health and self-care is growing [38]. It is expected that the use of OTC medications for symptom management in children will further increase [39]. Since in the present study, ChamBell-5-02 was shown to be safe, excellently tolerated and to reduce symptoms of teething, ChamBell-5-02 could be advised in the support of self-management of teething in children. It is known that the use of OTC medications may increase the risk that self-treatment is undertaken when medical care should have been sought [40]. Therefore, it remains important that parents are always alert that some symptoms in their children could not be attributed to teething and may have a more serious underlying cause. This would require the physicians' attention and conventional treatment if necessary.

In conclusion, the findings in the present study suggest that the OTC homeopathic medicine ChamBell-5-02 may offer a pragmatic treatment alternative to conventional OTC teething gels for symptom relieve of painful teething in children.

Acknowledgement

The study was sponsored by the Deutsche Homöopathie-Union, DHU-Arzneimittel GmbH & Co. KG, Karlsruhe, Germany.

We thank all investigators and children with their parents who participated in this study and T Keller (Leipzig) for his assistance in the statistical analysis and the preparation of the publication manuscript.

Additonal Declaration of Former Publication

Information about the study has been published on the website of Federal Service for Surveillance in the Sphere of Healthcare and Social Development of Ministry of Health of Russian Federation at:

http://www.roszdravnadzor.ru/medicines/control_for_doklin_i_klin_issl/info?year=2009

Study registration number: 567

Parts of the results of this study have been published earlier by Ilyenko LI, Kholodova IN, Syrieva TN, Il'ina ID, and Kholodov DI, in the Russian language in the Journal Pediatriya, 2010. 89 (4): 106-110©. For the present study all data were newly entered, validated and analysed according to ICH-GCP guidelines. Permission to publish the newly analyzed data was obtained from the Pediatriya Journal on November 9, 2013 by the Deputy editor-in-chief of the Journal Pediatriya" (n.a. G.N. Speransky), Prof. T.V. Kazyukova, PhD, MD.

Conflict of Interest

M. Jong was an employee of VSM Geneesmiddelen bv (sister-company of Deutsche Homöopathie Union) from 2001 till 2008.

P. Klement and J. Burkart are employees of Deutsche Homöopathie-Union, DHU-Arzneimittel GmbH & Co. KG, Karlsruhe, Germany.

References

1. Buckler JMH (1974) A Reference Manual of Growth and Development. (2nd edn) Blackwell Science Oxford.
2. McIntyre GT, McIntyre GM (2002) Teething troubles? Br Dent J 192: 251-255.
3. Wake M, Hesketh K, Allen M (1999) Parent beliefs about infant teething: a survey of Australian parents. Journal of Pediatrics and Child Health 35: 446–449.
4. Owais AI, Zawaideh F, Bataineh O (2010) Challenging parents' myths regarding their children's teething. International Journal of Dental Hygiene 8: 28–34.
5. Trajanovska M, Manias E, Cranswick N, Johnston L (2010) Parental management of childhood complaints: over-the-counter medicine use and advice-seeking behaviours. J Clin Nurs 19: 2065-2075.
6. Kakatkar G, Nagarajappa R, Bhat N, Prasad V, Sharda A, et al. (2012) Parental beliefs about children's teething in Udaipur, India: a preliminary study. Braz Oral Res 26: 151-157.
7. Plutzer K, Spencer AJ, Keirse MJNC (2012) How first-time mothers perceive and deal with teething symptoms: a randomized controlled trial. Child: Care, Health and Development 38: 292–299.
8. Curtis LA, Dolan TS, Seibert HE (2009) Are one or two dangerous? Lidocaine and topical anesthetic exposures in children. J Emerg Med 37: 32-39.
9. Williams GD, Kirk EP, Wilson CJ (2011) Salicylate intoxication from teething gel in infancy. The Medical Journal 194: 146-148.
10. Balicer RD, Kitai E (2004) Methemoglobinemia caused by topical teething preparation: a case report. Scientific World Journal 4: 517-520.
11. Italia S, Wolfenstetter SB, Teuner CM (2014) Patterns of Complementary and Alternative Medicine (CAM) use in children: a systematic review. Eur J Pediatr 173: 1413-1428.
12. Gottschling S, Gronwald B, Schmitt S, Schmitt C, Längler A, et al. (2013) Use of complementary and alternative medicine in healthy children and children with chronic medical conditions in Germany. Complement Ther Med 21: 61-69
13. Jean D, Cyr C (2007) Use of complementary and alternative medicine in a general pediatric clinic. Pediatrics 120: 138–141.
14. Robinson N, Blair M, Lorenc A, Gully N, Fox P, et al. (2008) Complementary medicine use in multi-ethnic paediatric outpatients. Complement Ther Clin Pract 14: 17–24.
15. Vlieger AM, van de Putte EM, Hoeksma H (2006) The use of complementary and alternative medicine in children at a general paediatric clinic and parental reasons for use. Ned Tijdschr Geneeskd 150: 625–630
16. Zutavern A, Schaaf B, von Berg A, Borte M, Herbarth O, et al. (2007) Inanspruchnahme von Homöopathie und Konsultation von Heilpraktikern - Ergebnisse einer deutschen Geburtskohortenstudie (LISA) im Alter von 2 Jahren [Use of homeopathy and consultation with alternative medicine practitioners: Results of a German birth cohort study (LISA) at the age of 2 years]. Monatsschrift Kinderheilkunde 5: 439–445
17. Thompson EA, Bishop JL, Northstone K (2010) The use of homeopathic products in childhood: data generated over 8.5 years from the Avon Longitudinal Study of Parents and Children (ALSPAC). J Altern Complement Med 16: 69-79.
18. Steinsbekk A, Bentzen N, Brien S (2006) Why do parents take their children to homeopaths? -- an exploratory qualitative study. Forsch Komplementmed. 13: 88-93.
19. Thompson EA, Dahr J, Susan M, Barron S (2007) Setting standards in homeopathic practice--a pre-audit exploring motivation and expectation for patients attending the Bristol Homeopathic Hospital. Homeopathy 96: 243-246.
20. Steinsbekk A (1999) Data collection in homeopathic practice – A proposal for an international standard. HomInt R&D NewsLetter 2: 14-15
21. Haidvogl M, Riley DS, Heger M, Brien S, Jong M, et al. (2007) Homeopathic and conventional treatment for acute respiratory and ear complaints: a comparative study on outcome in the primary care setting. BMC Complement. Altern Med 7: 7.
22. Taylor JA, Jacobs J (2011) Homeopathic ear drops as an adjunct to standard therapy in children with acute otitis media. Homeopathy 100: 109-115.
23. Sinha MN, Siddiqui VA, Nayak C, Sing V, Dixit R, et al. (2012) Randomized controlled pilot study to compare homeopathy and conventional therapy in acute otitis media. Homeopathy 101: 5-12.
24. Rutten L, Mathie RT, Fisher P, Goossens M, van Wassenhoven M (2013) Plausibility and evidence: the case of homeopathy. Med Health Care Philos. 16: 525-532.
25. Smith K (2012) Against homeopathy--a utilitarian perspective. Bioethics. 26: 398-409.
26. Shang A, Huwiler-Muntener K, Nartey L, Jüni P, Dörig S, et al. (2005) Are the clinical effects of homoeopathy placebo effects? Comparative study of placebo-controlled trials of homoeopathy and allopathy. Lancet. 366: 726-732.
27. Lert F, Grimaldi-Bensouda L, Rouillon F, Massol J, Guillemot D, et al. (2014) Characteristics of patients consulting their regular primary care physician according to their prescribing preferences for homeopathy and complementary medicine. Homeopathy 103: 51-57.
28. van Wassenhoven M, Ives G (2004) An observational study of patients receiving homeopathic treatment. Homeopathy 93: 3-11.
29. Vlieger AM, van Vliet M, Jong MC (2011) Attitudes toward Complementary and Alternative Medicine: A National Survey among Paediatricians in the Netherlands. European Journal of Pediatrics. 170: 619-624.
30. Jong MC, van Vliet M, Huttenhuis S, van der Veer D, van den Heijkant S (2012) Attitudes toward integrative paediatrics: a national survey among youth health and physicians in The Netherlands. BMC Complement Altern Med 12: 4.
31. Kooreman P, Baars EW (2012) Patients whose GP knows complementary medicine tend to have lower costs and live longer. Eur. J. Health Econ 13: 769-776.
32. Baars EW, Kooreman P (2014) A 6-year comparative economic evaluation of healthcare costs and mortality rates of Dutch patients from conventional and CAM GPs. BMJ Open. 27: 4.
33. Trichard M, Chaufferin G, Nicoloyannis N (2005) Pharmacoeconomic comparison between homeopathic and antibiotic treatment strategies in recurrent acute rhinopharyngitis in children. Homeopathy 94: 3-9.
34. Cranswick N, McGillivray G (2001) Over-the-counter medication in children: friend or foe? Australian Prescriber 24: 149–151.
35. Nield LS, Stegner JP, Kamat D (2008) Common pediatric dental dilemmas. Clinical Pediatrics 47: 99–105.

36. Macknin ML, Piedmonte M, Jacobs J, Skibinski C (2000) Symptoms associated with infant teething: a prospective study. Pediatrics 105: 747–752.

37. Fischer FH, Lewith G, Witt CM, Linde K, von Ammon K, et al. (2014) High prevalence but limited evidence in complementary and alternative medicine: guidelines for future research. BMC Complement Altern Med. 14: 46.

38. Hemwall EL (2010) Increasing access to nonprescription medicines: a global public health challenge and opportunity. Clin Pharmacol Ther. 87: 267-269.

39. Allotey P, Reidpath D, Elisha D (2004) "Social Medication" and the Control of Children: A Qualitative Study of Over-the-Counter Medication Among Australian Children. Pediatrics 114: 378-383.

40. Bradley CP, Bond C (1995) Increasing the number of drugs available over the counter: arguments for and against. Br J Gen Pract. 45: 553-556.

28

The Accuracy of Plant Identification in a Longitudinal Ethno Botanical Project in Coastal Ecuador

David S. Kiefer[1*], **Lauren Moscoe**[2], **Jack Buchanan**[3] **and Catherine Woodward**[4]

[1]*Department of Family Medicine, School of Medicine and Public Health, University of Wisconsin-Madison, USA*

[2]*Department of Botany, University of Wisconsin-Madison, USA*

[3]*Nelson Institute for Environmental Studies, University of Wisconsin-Madison, USA*

[4]*Ceiba Foundation for Tropical Conservation, USA*

[*]**Corresponding author**: Kiefer DS, Clinical Assistant Professor, Department of Family Medicine, School of Medicine and Public Health, University of Wisconsin-Madison, USA, E-mail: david.kiefer@fammed.wisc.edu

Abstract

Background: Preserving traditional environmental knowledge about herbal medicine in the face of rapid environmental, economic and cultural change depends in part on the identification of traditionally used medicinal plants to their Latin binomial. When financial, legal, and/or time constraints prevent the collection of voucher specimens or the use of advanced molecular technologies, arguably the "gold standards" for plant identification, alternative methods such as photography and morphological descriptions may still be able to assist identification. There are unknowns about the relative accuracies of these different techniques. This paper compares the efficacy of several methods to correctly identify plants across five separate site visits in the province of Manabí, Ecuador.

Methods: Plants that were identified to genus-, and species-level accuracy during each of the five site visits were totaled, and the type of data (expert consultation, written, photographic, and morphological) leading to the identification noted. Percentage accuracy was calculated as the number of unambiguous identifications to Latin binomial divided by the total number of common plant names recorded for each site visit.

Results: Ninety-six common plant names were recorded across the five site visits, while each individual visit yielded information about 26-54 plants, reflecting significant overlap. In addition to interview data, site visit 4 uniquely collected additional photographic (34 plants) and morphological data (12 plants). Photographs were more effective in aiding identification to both genus (12) and species (4) than morphological data (4 genus and 0 species identifications). Percentage accuracy for the first four site visits ranged from 27-36%; site visit 5 yielded 91% accuracy, but only when considering a limited subset of the plants.

Conclusions: Photographic, and morphological data can aid identification of medicinal plant species to Latin binomial when time, money and/or collection permits are lacking, but should not be considered reliable substitutes for plant voucher specimens or advanced molecular technologies.

Keywords Traditional environmental knowledge (TEK); Latin binomial; Morphology; Plant identification

Introduction

The race is on to catalog plant use before the associated knowledge and natural resources disappear. The literature contains compelling evidence that traditional environmental knowledge (TEK) may be threatened by rapid changes in cultural [1], economic [2], and environmental conditions [3], and associated disruptions in the transmission of such knowledge across generations [4]. One type of TEK is that pertaining to herbal medicine (referred to hereafter as TEK-HM).

Efforts to catalog and preserve TEK-HM exist in numerous forms and involve a variety of community members and researchers, the latter from such diverse fields as anthropology [5,6], linguistics [7], pharmacy [8-10], health care [7-11], botany [12-14], chemistry [15], ecology [3], geography [16] and public health [7]. Some of these research efforts are community-based and are either directed by or actively involve "cultural insiders." [17].

One challenging, yet important, step of TEK-HM projects is the identification of plant specimens to their Latin binomial. Although valuable information is contained in plant common names, Latin binomials are additionally important for TEK-HM research. A reliance on common names may lead to confusion if more than one taxon is referred to by a single common name (homonymy) or if a single taxon is referred to by many different common names (synonymy) [18]. Ambiguities and inconsistencies in common names may occur within a community, among common-language communities, or among language groups [19]. Latin binomials, however, allow for unambiguous communication, which is important for clinical applications [20], informed consumption [21], and accurate communication about TEK-HM [7].

Furthermore, Latin binomials contain information about evolutionary relationships that may offer insight into ecology, biochemistry, and morphology. Plant identification in TEK-HM projects is especially difficult because researchers often encounter specimens removed from their ecological context (e.g., in markets) or as isolated plant parts (e.g., only the leaves, roots, flowers, or fruits). However, as best as possible, researchers attempt to elaborate complete voucher specimens and deposit them in local herbaria to provide tangible evidence of the research undertaken [22]. Plant identification often requires researchers to use a dichotomous key and to then confirm identification by matching the voucher specimen with others already present in herbaria. Accurately done, this approach can provide an exact match for plants collected in the field. Although generally more expensive, if sufficient material is not available to identify the plant using a key, plant identification can be carried out through laboratory-based techniques such as DNA barcoding [23] or spectrometric methods [24]. When applied correctly, the accuracy of employing a dichotomous key using voucher specimens and these laboratory methods for plant identification make them the "gold standards" or the ideal to which ethnobotanical research projects strive.

The above-mentioned techniques and methodologies can be difficult to successfully execute, especially in a community far removed from research centers and associated herbaria. One pressing challenge is the difficulty in obtaining permits to collect plant material. Although some government institutions are actively working to simplify permit procedures, the steps to obtain permits are often ambiguous, and the frustrating process may take months or years (Tulio Medina, Ministry of the Environment, Peru, and pers. comm.). In addition, complex legal frameworks have decreased the ease of accessing specimens from ex situ collections, partially because curators are afraid of disobeying laws they may not understand [25]. To circumvent this challenge, past research efforts have used numerous approaches to improve on the possibility of correct plant identification on-site. For example, some have employed digital, high-resolution photography [26].

This article discusses one community-based, multi-year project, in which the ultimate goal was to accurately identify all plants mentioned by study participants, some of which were incorporated in a community medicinal garden (described below). This project included multiple site visits by researchers with different backgrounds, each of whom employed slightly different methodologies.

Throughout the process, we explored the efficiency and effectiveness of different methodological approaches to plant identification. In this paper, we investigate the hypotheses that 1) repeated site visits, regardless of the researchers' techniques or experience, would eventually lead to accurate plant identification, and 2) detailed morphological descriptions and high-quality photographs could assist in accurate plant identification above and beyond qualitative ethnographic research techniques.

Methods

Study site

Five separate visits by researchers of different backgrounds and levels of training took place over a four-year time period to the county of Jama, Ecuador (Table 1). The coastal county of Jama, in the province of Manabí, Ecuador, has a population of approximately 25,000, who live in rural villages and small towns. The largest urban setting is the town of Jama. Latitudinal and climatic gradients create a mixture of vegetation types, including semi-deciduous tropical forest and humid montane forest embedded within a largely agricultural landscape. We conducted this TEK-HM project in the community of Tabuga (population approximately 750) near the Lalo Loor Dry Forest Reserve, a biological station operated by the Ceiba Foundation for Tropical Conservation. The Ceiba Foundation is an advocate for sustainable community development, habitat protection, and ecological research, and, as per the community of Tabuga's request, is working to create a living collection of local medicinal plants at the reserve's nature center, accompanied by a written document. Their well-established relationships with people in the area and the application of our research interests to an expressed community need were important factors in our decision to pursue this research at this site [27].

Site Visit	Time period	Level of training	Discipline
1	April-May, 2011	Undergraduate	Ecology
2	January, 2013	MD, and PhD student	Medical, Botany
3	July, 2013	Undergraduates	Pharmacy
4	January, 2014	PhD student	Agroecology
5	April-May, 2014	Undergraduate	Ecology

Table 1: Personnel characteristics of the five Manabí site visits.

Site Visits

There was some variation in the research goals and techniques for the five site visits, though all collected information about common names of plants and uses of those plants, and all cross-checked this information with available printed information. None of the five projects had official collecting permits that would allow corroboration of voucher specimens with herbarium specimens, partly due to logistics and partly due to an evolution in the goals of the projects, where early priorities did not include a taxonomic focus. Details about each of the five site visits are below.

The project began with Site Visit 1 (SV1), the efforts of an undergraduate intern of the Ceiba Foundation in conjunction with community members in Tabuga. SV1 involved the location of willing community participants with knowledge of herbal medicine, and ad hoc collection of information about any and all plants described as having medicinal properties and local availability. The intern recorded common names, medicinal uses, and plant preparation. Ceiba Foundation scientists assisted in the identification of plants to Latin binomials using available taxonomic keys, ecological and herbal texts, and professional experience with the local flora.

Knowing that the preliminary work was started during SV1, Site Visit 2 (SV2) was designed to extend those findings, with the understanding that even more follow-up work would be necessary. The goals of SV2 were to begin the process of documentation of TEK-HM, to comprehensively survey the herbal medicines being used in the community, and to provide educational herbal medicine resources for the community. Semi-structured interviews were conducted with ten key informants identified by Ceiba employees who lived in the community. Informants were asked to name plants they used medicinally and describe their uses and preparations.

Living specimens were photographed when possible, and detailed taxonomic notes were taken. Interviews were audio-recorded and transcribed.

The intention of Site Visit 3 (SV3) was to corroborate accuracy of previously collected data by revisiting the informants from SV2 with the transcribed and summarized information. Of the ten original informants, seven were located and the community herbal information was reviewed and corrected; either the corrected information was reviewed orally (n=4) or as a written, corrected document (n=3).

In addition, a local herbal medicine expert in the town closest to the field site was interviewed about the common names, use, and preparation of 20 medicinal plants. Photographs were taken of specimens during this interview. Site Visit 4 (SV4) aimed to improve botanical accuracy of data from previous site visits through interviews, photographs, and morphological data collection.

Most individuals (n=9) interviewed during SV2 were re-interviewed using a semi-directed interview method. When possible, detailed photographs of the plants were taken. Detailed morphological characteristics, including flower and fruit characteristics, were recorded for plants perceived as more obscure or difficult to identify.

Site Visit 5 (SV5), as with SV1, involved a Ceiba Foundation intern working in conjunction with community members. SV5's primary goal was to create signage, with corresponding common names and Latin binomial names, for the plants in the medicinal plant garden at the Lalo Loor Dry Forest reserve. As such, a limited subset of plants was the focus of this effort. Plant uses and Latin binomial names were corroborated from past site visits through the involvement of community contacts and Ceiba Foundation biologists.

Plant identification

From December 2013, through September 2014, the plant lists resulting from each of the site visits were then analyzed by the authors of this paper in order to identify plants to a likely family, genus, or Latin binomial. This analysis used a variety of methods, including cross-referencing the common plant name with published literature on TEK-HM for Ecuador or surrounding regions, comparing likely Latin binomial with internet sources and images, and consulting other scientists with experience in tropical botany. A plant was given a Latin binomial identification only if there was no ambiguity about the Latin binomial name corresponding to its common name. In this analysis, no ambiguity resulted in three ways. First, there was no ambiguity if a plant with a given common name had no alternative identification, such as with ajo (garlic), which could distinctly only be Allium sativum. The second method for achieving a definitive identification to Latin binomial occurred when the detailed documentation of morphological characteristics with photographic and/or written description was considered adequate and unambiguous. Third, we considered there to be no ambiguity if all cross-referencing for a given common name only yielded one Latin binomial that could then be corroborated by tropical botanists familiar with the local flora.

From this analysis, a simple percentage accuracy was calculated (number of unambiguous identifications to Latin binomial divided by the total number of common names in that plant list). In some cases, there were numerous species for a given plant genus, or there was a lack of plant characteristics necessary to identify a plant beyond the plant family. These plants were recorded as identified to "genus" and "Family", respectively. Finally, for some plants, there was a lack of information to allow any accurate identification. In such cases, it was not possible to come up with a scientific name of any type.

Results

Information for 96 plants resulted from the five site visits (Table 2), though an individual site visit only yielded information for 26-54 plants (Tables 2 and 3). There was some overlap and some uniqueness between the five site visits with respect to the plants documented (Table 2). For some of these site visits, the overlap was predictable. For example, 18 plants documented in SV3 were also documented in SV2; ten of these overlapping plants occurred because a 10-plant booklet prepared from SV2 was used to guide discussions during follow-up interviews during SV3.

	SV1			SV2			SV3			SV4			SV5		
Common name	*	G	S	*	G	S	*	G	S	*	G	S	*	G	S
Agua del carmen										*					
Ajenjo										*			*		X
Ají													*		X
Ajo				*		X	*		X				*		X
Albahaca	*		X				*						*		X
Albahaca de mentha	*	X											*	X	
Altamara				*											
Altamisa				*		X	*								
Amanza toro										*			*		X
Ardor				*											
Ayahuasca										*		X	*		X
Badeilla										*	X				
Begonia	*	X													
Berro	*		X	*											
Biblia				*						*					
Café													*		X
Calaguala							*								
Campana										*	X				
Caña agria										*					
Cedrón				*	X										
Chala	*			*						*					
Chanca piedra				*		X									
Chilinche										*					
Cigarillo				*		X									
Congona	*									*	X		*		X
Cordoncillo	*	X		*		X									

Corrimiento	*	X							*			*		X
Doña Juana									*					
Dulcamara									*	X		*		X
Emori	*	X												
Escancel	*		X	*			*			*		X	*		X
Espanto	*			*						*	X		*	X	
Geranio				*	X					*			*	X	
Gualanga	*									*	X				
Guayaba							*	X		*	X		*		X
Hierba buena				*		X							*		X
Hierba chivo				*		X	*		X	*		X	*		X
Hierba luisa	*		X	*		X	*		X	*		X	*		X
Hierba mora										*	X		*		X
Higo				*											
Huaco	*	X													
Jengibre	*	X		*	X					*	X		*	X	
Jorra	*									*	X				
Lechuga				*		X									
Limón	*	X		*		X				*		X	*		X
Limoncillo				*		X									
Llanten				*	X		*	X		*	X		*	X	
Malacapa				*						*					
Mango				*		X									
Manzanilla				*		X	*		X	*		X			
Mate	*		X	*						*		X			
Matico				*		X									
Menta silvestre	*	X								*					
Milton							*								
Monte	*	X													
Muyuyu	*		X							*		X	*		X
Nacerera										*					
Noni	*		X							*		X			
Oreganita	*		X												
Oregano	*			*		X				*			*		X
Oreganón	*		X	*	X		*	X		*	X		*		X

Ortiga				*		X				*	X				
Paico	*		X	*		X	*		X	*		X	*		X
Palo santo													*		X
Papaya				*		X							*		X
Pegador										*					
Pestaña				*											
Piña de monte	*	X													
Piñuella	*	X													
Piñon				*						*		X			
Plátano													*		X
Poleo				*											
Pomón										*	X				
Rábano										*		X			
Romedillo							*								
Ruda castilla	*	X		*		X	*		X	*		X	*		X
Ruda clavellina										*			*		X
Ruda de gallinaso	*			*			*			*			*	X	
Ruda de muerto							*								
Sábila	*		X	*	X		*	X					*		X
San Juanito	*														
Santa María				*									*		X*
Santa Maria del bosque	*		X							*	X				
Suelda consuelda				*											
Tamarindo										*		X			
Tiatina	*		X				*			*		X	*		X
Tilo				*		X	*		X	*		X	*		X
Tres puntas							*								
Uña de gato										*	X				
Uvilla				*	X										
Valeriana	*	X		*	X					*	X		*		X
Verbena	*	X		*			*			*					
Verde laya															
Zapallo										*					

Zaragoza	*		X	*			*			*					
Zorrilla	*						*			*					

Table 2: Compilation of plants, alphabetical by most accepted common name spelling, from five site visits (SV1-SV5), and identifications to genus (G) and species (S). The symbol * indicates the plant was documented during that site visit.

Table 3 lists, for each site visit, the number of plants documented and respective identifications. The percent accuracy, calculated by dividing the number of plants identified to species by the total number of plants documented during that site visit, is also listed. The percent accuracy varied slightly between SV1-SV4. Site visit 5 had a much higher accuracy (91%), although, as analyzed in the discussion, this research effort was conducted on a limited subset of plants, namely those that were planted in the Ceiba Foundation medicinal plant garden and ones for which Latin binomial names were likely known.

Site visit #	# Plants	Type of data1	# Only identified to Genus	# Identified to species	Accuracy of Latin Binomial(%)
1	39	Expert	15	14	36
2	47	Expert;Written	9	16	34
3	26	Expert	3	7	27
4	54	Expert; Written;Morph	17	16	29
5	34	Expert; Written	6	31	91
Overall	96	Expert; Written;Morph	21	51	53

Table 3: Plants documented and respective identifications for each site visit and for the project as a whole, with percent accuracy of identification to *Genus species*

1. Types of data used to identify plants:

Expert: Consultation with tropical botanists familiar with the local Ecuadorian flora

Written: Reputable primary or secondary sources of local plants, including internet sources

Morph: Detailed documentation of morphological characteristics with photographic and/or written description considered adequate by taxonomists

Site visit 4 used methods unique from the others: detailed documentation of morphological characteristics (plant form, leaf and/or flower characteristics) with photographic (macro photographs of flowers, when possible) or written descriptions. In this case, there were photographs for 34 plants and morphological descriptions for 12 plants.

Table 4 shows the tendency of the photographs or morphological descriptions to have aided in identification to Latin binomial. Detailed photography aided in the identification of 12 plants to genus and four plants to species, whereas the morphological details aided in the identification of four plants to genus and zero to species.

Method	Total plants on which the method was used	Of total plants, number unambiguously identified through other methods	Of total plants, number whose identification to genus was aided by the given method	Of total plants, number whose identification to species was aided by the given method
Detailed photographs. Including floral macro-photographs when possible	34	7	12	4
Detailed morphological descriptions	12	2	4	0

Table 4: The effectiveness of detailed photographic or morphological details in leading to an accurate identification in Site Visit 4 (SV4).

Overall, gleaning information from Table 2, of the 96 plants listed by common name during the five site visits, 51 (53%) of the plants were identified to their Latin binomial (Table 3). An additional 21 plants were identified to Genus when the five site visits were analyzed as a whole (Table 3).

Discussion

The results of our research did not support our initial hypotheses that 1) repeated site visits, regardless of the researchers' techniques or experience, would eventually lead to accurate plant identification, and 2) written morphological descriptions and high-quality photographs could assist in accurate plant identification above and beyond qualitative ethnographic research techniques.

In addition, a "hidden agenda" of sorts was the hope that there was some taxonomic alternative to the two "gold standards", voucher specimens (labor intensive, requiring permits), or DNA barcoding (expensive, requiring a laboratory). We can simply summarize our findings by stating that repeated site visits without collection permits or consistent access to full plant specimens did not lead to an evolution toward great accuracy, nor did one attempt at using photography or a morphological description of a subset of the plants. All site visits, regardless of methodology or researcher training hovered around 30-40% accuracy, minus the spuriously high percentage of the SV5 (a calculation based on a limited subset of the plants).

Overall, the five TEK-HM site visits had varying levels of success in identifying the plants species from common names to Latin binomial (Table 3). Even SV5, arguably the culmination of the four years of fieldwork, only led to the definitive identification of 31 plant species. Although this was 91% of the 34 plants detailed in the sign-making project for the medicinal plant garden, it was still just 32% (31/96 plants) in the context of the combined plant list from all five site visits. Predictably, given the pleas from taxonomists, a TEK-HM project that is not grounded in voucher specimens and corresponding herbaria identification, or, more recently, DNA barcoding or spectrophotometry, is unlikely to yield a high percentage of plants unequivocally identified to Latin binomial, even with the cross-referencing, photography, and morphological description approaches of this investigation.

It is interesting to view the results from this project as a whole in comparison to the gold standard methods alluded to above. If we assume that exact plant matches were to occur with the correct application of herbarium-matched voucher plant specimens or laboratory methods, then the overall 53% accuracy using mixed methodology (expert consultation, written cross referencing, photography, morphological descriptions) falls far short of the ideal.

Our results, in retrospect, should come as no surprise. Researchers in the fields of botany and ethno botany have long emphasized the importance of voucher specimens for optimal scientific rigor [7,22,28]. Clearly, as our results show, there are no shortcuts to accurate plant identification: not with repeated site visits, nor with a diverse researcher team. It goes without saying that a focused, taxonomically-oriented research agenda, allowing ample time to procure collecting permits, the deposition of plant specimens in a local herbarium, and support for follow up identification efforts, would have significantly improved the rate of successful identification of the plants in this project [25,27]. The difficulties in establishing such a comprehensive project are worth enduring, as exemplified by the alternative (these results). The community of Tabuga and the Ceiba Foundation are on board with a future goal of obtaining appropriate permits to enable collection of voucher specimens and confirmation of identity in a local herbarium.

Some lessons from this project may have applicability for future TEK-HM work. The relative ineffectiveness in retroactively using morphological characteristics for plant identification speaks to the complexity of plant dichotomous keys and the difficulty in predicting, without a key in hand, which characteristics will turn out to be the crucial details at branch points. Having the relevant keys in the field would certainly be a step in the right direction, although transporting such texts (even in electronic form) is not always a viable option. Photographs were slightly more useful than morphological descriptions because they allowed for the possibility to cross reference and compare with abundant internet resources and scientific papers including high-quality photographs.

With an eye toward a broader view of herbal medicine use, these results parallel challenges with plant identification in clinical medicine [20]. Some TEK-HM studies have attempted to definitively identify plants, realizing the clinical importance of traditional plant use in the context of pharmaceutical co-use or other medical interventions [29,30]. The dynamic nature of plant use only increases the challenge of and need for more accurate communication about plants and plant names. For example, when immigrants arrive in new places with their plants, their plant use may change and it may or may not be communicated with their health care provider [30-32]. The accurate identification of plants and then a substantive discussion about their use in the clinical environment would do much to foster the safe and effective application of herbal medicines and the continuance of TEK-HM.

Acknowledgements

The work presented here was partly carried out while Dr. Kiefer was Research Fellow supported by a National Research Service Award (T32AT006956) from the National Center for Complementary and Alternative Medicine (NCCAM) at the National Institutes of Health (NIH) to the University Of Wisconsin Department Of Family Medicine (UWDFM). Dr. Kiefer also received financial support from a Wisconsin Alumni Research Foundation (WARF) Discovery Challenge award. The authors of this paper wish to thank the many community members of Tabuga for their generous donation of time, sharing their knowledge and experience, and the student researchers (Dena Goldberg, Heather Hresko, Rebecca Grupe, and Ryan Swanson) for all of their efforts in data collection.

References

1. Benz BF, Cevallos EJ, Santana MF, Rosales AJ, Graf MS (2000) Losing knowledge about plant use in the Sierra de Manantlan Biosphere Reserve, Mexico. Economic Botany 54(2): 183-191.
2. Reyes-García V, Vadez V, Huanca T, Leonard WR, McDade T (2006) Economic development and local ecological knowledge: a deadlock? quantitative research from a native Amazonian society. Human Ecology 35(3): 371-377.
3. Salick J, Fang Z, Byg A (2009) Eastern Himalayan alpine plant ecology, Tibetan ethnobotany, and climate change. Global Environmental Change 19(2): 147-155.
4. Turner NJ, Ignace MB, Ignace R (2000) Traditional ecological knowledge and wisdom of aboriginal peoples in British Columbia. Ecological Applications 10(5): 1275-1287.
5. Girón LM, Freire V, Alonzo A, Cáceres A (1991) Ethnobotanical survey of the medicinal flora used by the Caribs of Guatemala. Journal of Ethnopharmacology, 34(2-3): 173-187.
6. Merlin MD (2003) Archaeological evidence for the tradition of psychoactive plant use in the old world. Economic Botany 57(3): 295-323.
7. Balick MJ, Cox PA. (1996) Plants, people, and culture: the science of ethnobotany. Scientific American Library, New York.
8. Michel J, Duarte RE, Bolton JL, Huang Y, Caceres A, et al. (2007) Medical potential of plants used by the Q'eqchi Maya of Livingston, Guatemala for the treatment of women's health complaints. Journal of Ethnopharmacology 114(1): 92-101.
9. Andrade-Cetto A (2009) Ethnobotanical study of the medicinal plants from Tlanchinol, Hidalgo, México. Journal of Ethnopharmacology 122(1): 163-171.
10. De la Cruz de MG, Malpartida SB, Santiago HB, Jullian V, Bourdy G (2014) Hot and cold: medicinal plant uses in Quechua speaking communities in the high Andes (Callejón de Huaylas, Ancash, Perú). Journal of Ethnopharmacology 155(2): 1093-117.
11. Cáceres A, López B, González S, Berger I, Tada I, Maki J (1998) Plants used in Guatemala for the treatment of protozoal infections. I. Screening of activity to bacteria, fungi and American trypanosomes of 13 native plants. Journal of Ethnopharmacology 62(3): 195-202.
12. Schultes RE (1969) Hallucinogens of plant origin. Science 163(3864): 245-254.
13. Meyer RS, Bamshad M, Fuller DQ, Litt A. (2014). Comparing medicinal uses of eggplant and related Solanaceae in China, India, and the Philippines suggests the independent development of uses, cultural diffusion, and recent species substitutions. Economic Botany 68(2): 137–152.
14. Vandebroek I, Balick MJ. (2014). Lime for chest congestion, bitter orange for diabetes: foods as medicines in the Dominican community in New York City. Economic Botany, 68(2): 177–189.
15. Heitzman ME, Neto CC, Winiarz E, Vaisberg AJ, Hammond GB (2005) Ethnobotany, phytochemistry and pharmacology of Uncaria (Rubiaceae). Phytochemistry 66(1): 5-29.
16. Corlett JL, Dean EA, Grivetti LE (2003) Hmong gardens: botanical diversity in an urban setting. Economic Botany 57(3): 365-379.
17. McClatchey W (2007) Two Ethnobotanists. Ethnobotany Research & Applications 5: 95-96.
18. Soleri D, Worthington M, Aragón-Cuevas F, Smith SE, Gepts P (2013) Farmers' varietal identification in a reference sample of local Phaseolus species in the Sierra Juárez, Oaxaca, Mexico. Economic Botany 67(4): 283-298.

19. Emshwiller E (2006) Evolution and conservation of clonally propagated crops. In TJ Motley, N Zerega, HB Cross [eds.] Darwin's harvest: new approaches to the origins, evolution, and conservation of crops, 308–332. Columbia University Press New York.
20. Kiefer D, Tellez-Girón P, Bradbury J (2014) A pilot study of herbal medicine use in a Midwest Latino population. Wisconsin Medical Journal 113(2): 64-71.
21. Cimino M (2010) Ensuring the specific identity and quality of herbal products by the power of DNA. HerbalGram 86: 50-57.
22. Nguyen MLT (2005) Cultivated plant collections from market places. Ethnobotany Research & Applications 3: 5-16.
23. Chase MW, Fay MF (2009) Barcoding of plants and fungi. Science 325(5941): 682-683.
24. Durgante FVM, Higuchi N, Almeida A, Vicentini A (2013) Species spectral signature: discriminating closely related plant species in the Amazon with near-infrared leaf-spectroscopy. Forest Ecology and Management 291(C): 240-248.
25. Galluzzi G, López Noriega I (2014) Conservation and use of genetic resources of underutilized crops in the Americas: a continental analysis. Sustainability 6: 980-1017.
26. Thomas E, Vandebroek I, Van Damme P (2007) What works in the field? A comparison of different interviewing methods in ethnobotany with special reference to the use of photographs. Economic Botany 61(4): 376-384.
27. Engels JMM, Dempewolf H, Henson-Apollonio V (2010) Ethical considerations in agro-biodiversity research, collecting, and use. Journal of Agricultural and Environmental Ethics 24(2): 107-126.
28. Bye RA, Linares E (1983) The role of plants found in Mexican markets and their importance in ethnobotanical studies. Journal of Ethnobiology 3(1): 1-13.
29. Ceuterick M, Vandebroek I, Torry B, Pieroni A (2008) Cross-cultural adaptation in urban ethnobotany: the Colombian folk pharmacopoeia in London. Journal of Ethnopharmacology 120: 342-359.
30. Vandebroek I, Balick MJ, Ososki A (2010) The importance of botellas and other plant mixtures in Dominican traditional medicine. Journal of Ethnopharmacoly 128(1): 20-41.
31. Mehta DH, Gardiner PM, Phillips RS, McCarthy EP (2008) Herbal and dietary supplement disclosure to health care providers by individuals with chronic conditions. Journal of Alternative and Complementary Medicine 14: 1263-1269.
32. Kuo GM, Hawley ST, Weiss LT, Balkrishnan R, Volk RJ (2004) Factors associated with herbal use among urban multiethnic primary care patients: a cross-sectional survey. BMC Comp Alt Med 2(4): 18.

Traditional Bone-Setters and Fracture Care in Ekiti State, Nigeria

Owoseni Joseph Sina[1,*] **and Ibikunle Ayodele M**[2]

[1]*College of Medicine and Health Sciences (Medical Sociology), Afe Babalola University, Ado-Ekiti, Nigeria*

[2]*Department of Sociology, Ekiti State University Ado Ekiti, Nigeria*

***Corresponding author**: Owoseni Joseph Sina, College of Medicine and Health Sciences (Medical Sociology), Afe Babalola University, Ado-Ekiti, Nigeria, E-mail: owoshynah@yahoo.com

Abstract

In Nigeria, the practice of traditional bone setting (TBS) is extensive as in other developing nations. Traditional bonesetters play an imperative role in fracture care. Though, the outcome of the intervention of TBS treatment is usually poor with profound effects on the patient in the future. This study seeks to examine the activities of traditional bone setters on fracture care in Ekiti State, Nigeria.

Survey method was applied in the study. 250 questionnaires were administered to owners of traditional bone centres and their clients respectively. Ten (10) of such centres were selected for the study in Ekiti.

The findings indicated that majority of the bone setters had little or no formal education. Many of them acquired the schema used through ancestral/supernatural power. The TBS lack basic knowledge of investigations and wound care while most of their clients patronized them because of poverty, ignorance and superstitious beliefs.

Provision of adequate basic equipment in health institutions may reduce the rate at which people utilize Traditional bone centres against medical advice.

Keywords: Traditional bone setters; Fracture; Care; Nigeria

Introduction

In Nigeria, with high level of accidents recorded every day, the traditional care givers still remain popular despite the high level of education and the existence of modern health care facilities [1]. In Nigeria, there are traditional medical practitioners - herbalists, bone-setters and religious practitioners. In the main, traditional healers and bonesetters were practicing long before orthodox medicine was introduced to the developing world Hoff, 1997.

Contemporarily, both orthodox and traditional medicines are coexisting side by side and both are patronized by patients [2]. Basically, in Nigeria, the traditional bone setters enjoy more confidence and patronage from people than any other group of traditional care-givers [3].

On the whole, the traditional bonesetter's practice is a highly specialized form of traditional medicine. It is usually passed from father to son but some outsiders also receive their training through apprenticeship [4]. Traditional bone setting is an old practice found almost in all communities of Nigeria especially in the rural communities of Ekiti State. Traditional Bone setting (TBS) is popular in Africa because its practitioners lay claims to supernatural influences [5].

World Health Organization (2002) describes traditional bone-setting as that health practices, approaches, knowledge and beliefs incorporating plant, animal and mineral based medicines, spiritual therapies, manual techniques and exercises, applied singularly or in combination to diagnose and treat fracture in human body.

In a further explanation, Ekere [6] reiterates that; traditional medicine is based on the belief that: the natural resources have active therapeutic principles that heal occult supernatural forces, power to change active principles which can be manipulated by those who know how to produce marvelous results. This implies that Africans have belief in using the natural way to treat illnesses than the modern and scientific method that was brought from the western societies [7].

In the main, superstition, ignorance and poverty are the basis for continued patronage despite complications [5]. There are however many complications attributed to the TBS. Indeed, the patrons of this service cuts across every strata of the society including the educated and the rich [3]. Mostly, Africans do believe that diseases and accidents have spiritual components that need to be tackled along with treatment. The major and commonest problems treated by them are fractures and dislocations [3].

Problem

In the main, before the emergence of western invention, every society stipulated methods of doing things even with relation to health. These methods are engrained in the culture and tradition of the people. As it is done in every other aspect, there are traditional means of treating the sick whenever there is the need to do so. African traditional medicine (Alternative medicine) therefore has an important place in the healthcare delivery system among Africans, especially in rural southwest Nigeria. Being widely known as alternative medicine, traditional medicines are utilized informs of treatment and also serves as last resort where other forms of treatment have failed.

According to Omololu, Ogunlade and Gopaldsani [7], traditional medicine has been the first port of call before western or orthodox medicine and a last resort when all orthodox efforts fail. From this assertion, it is indicated that African people firstly put traditional medicine into consideration, whenever they are to undergo any treatment before looking at western method.

On the whole, traditional healers were long practiced before orthodox medicine was introduced into the developing world. The first orthodox hospital was built in Nigeria (Lagos) in 1873. Before this, traditional medicine was the only available form of healthcare, [7]. The art of traditional medicine is so wide that different experts have emerged to have their own area of specialization [8]. There is therefore no disputing the fact that some aspects of trado-medical knowledge system is well structured and organized and has survived through generations to maintain harmony between body, mind and soul within its socio-cultural and religious context. However, different experts have emerged within their ranks including herbalists, bonesetters, psychiatrists, and traditional birth attendants among others [8].

The traditional bone setter is a lay practitioner of joints manipulation. He/she is the unqualified practitioner (in the western training) who takes up the practice of healing without having had any formal training in accepted medical procedures according to Agaja [9].

Functionalism theory

Functionalism sees society as an organic whole, with each of its parts working to maintain the others. This is similar to the way in which parts of the body work to maintain each other and the body as a whole.

To study the function of a social practice or institution is to analyze the contribution which that practices or institution makes to the continuation of the society as a whole. The best way to understand this is through organic analogy; to study a bodily organ, we need to show how it relates to the other part of the body.

Functionalist perspective on health and medicine was formulated largely by Talcott Parsons. He explained that a healthy population is essential to the society. Healthy people can perform the social roles that are necessary to keep the society function optimally. Illness, then, is dysfunctional as it prevents people from performing their social roles, at least temporarily. Thus, the traditional bonesetters play a vital role in the overall functioning of a society by making members who have fractures regain their health. If those who have fractures are not treated, just like the organic analogy as explained by the functionalist, it will hamper the continued existence of the society, as the role they are supposed to play toward the survival of the society were affected.

The practice of traditional bone settings have though existed for centuries, there has however been campaigns against its patronage, especially by the orthodox practitioners. Despite this campaign, it still survives till today. This indicated that the practice of traditional bone setting has an important role that it is playing in the society, to have continued to exist. It would have ceased to be in existence, if it has no role that it is played in the society.

The functionalists explained that the society comprises of structures with each part laying different role toward ensuring the continual survival of the society. They used the organic analogy to explain this whereby organism contains different part, with each part carrying out a particular function toward the sustenance of the organism.

Though the functionalist perspective identified the social institution bone setting as being vital toward the overall functioning of the society by making the members healthy, the failure to recognize that there may be better ways of managing fractures, due to their rigidity and maintaining status quo therefore led to the need to another theory to explain this study

Modernization theory

1. The modernist theorists on the other hand look at how society evolves from tradition to modernity. They explained that societies will join the — developed‖ world when they do away with their traditions and adopt modernity as a way of life.
2. In constructing their accounts of development, they drew on the tradition-modernity distinction of classical sociologists. They placed most emphasis on norms and values that operate in these two types of society. They argued that the transition from the traditional to modernity depended on a prior change in the values, attitudes and norms of people.
3. They called for the total abandoning of the old form of doing things, for the adoption of the western ways.

To synthesize these theories, functionalism and modernization theory, have a common perspective on the importance of ensuring that people who have fractures are treated and continue to contribute their own quota toward having a functional society, they however have point of divergence. While functionalism explain the relevance of the traditional bonesetters toward the continual survival of the society and believes in the maintenance of status quo , modernization theory looks at how the traditional bonesetters have adopted modern form in carrying out treatment among patients. Modernity has made it easier for the traditional bone setters to adopt modern form in the treatment of fracture. This is important as it not only reduce the rate of complication, but also assist in ensuring that proper treatment are received by the patients, which will aid them in their health restoration and optimal functioning in the society.

Both the Traditional bonesetters and the western practitioners are practicing today in Nigeria. Until recently, the relationship that exists between these two kinds of practitioners can best be explained as being that of cat and mouse as the traditional bone setters'method of treatment was regarded as being fetish, primitive and not modern.

Methodology

This study was conducted within Ekiti State. Many communities where traditional bone-setters and their clients could be found were selected for the study.

The communities included in the study were

1. Ado-Ekiti,
2. Ikole-Ekiti,
3. Oye-Ekiti,
4. Ise-Ekiti,
5. Efon-Ekiti,
6. Omuo-Ekiti,
7. Ijero-Ekiti and
8. Ogotun-Ekiti.

Although the number of traditional bone setters that abound in these communities is not well documented due to lack of proper record by the constituted authorities, it is widely accepted that traditional fracture care is utilized in the selected communities.

Thus, the purposive and snowball sampling techniques were used traditional bonesetter practitioners or patients who have fractures. The first bonesetter clinic was identified by the researcher and snowballing technique was used to identify subsequent respondents/interviewees

Although patients were not evenly distributed in the clinics identified, the available number of patients that a clinic can catered for within the period of the study was all selected.

Patients in the clinics range between three and twenty-two. Both quantitative and qualitative methods were used to collect the necessary data. For the quantitative research method, Two hundred and fifty (250) copies of questionnaires were administered among patients in Ten traditional bonesetter's clinics that were identified and visited out of which Two hundred forty-seven (247) copies were retrieved for analysis, while the in-depth interview was conducted with traditional bonesetter practitioners in the Ten clinics and Fifteen patients that were visited.

Quantitative data was analyzed using descriptive statistical tools like tables, percentages, frequency distributions, bar charts and pie-charts, while qualitative data was content analyzed.

Ethical consideration

The anonymity of all respondents was of paramount significance to the researcher. At no point during and after the study was any information given was being used in a manner that would make it feasible to identify the respondent. Participant was given the right to decline from the study at any stage should he/she found it uncomfortable to continue. The study did not cause any harm to the participants in the process of administering questionnaire and in-depth interviews. The participation of the respondents in the study was entirely voluntary.

Findings

This section deals with the analysis and interpretation of data.

Age years	Frequency	Percentage %
Male	166	67.2
Female	81	32.8
Total	247	100
Sex	Frequency	Percentage %
≤ 20	13	5.3
21 – 30	57	23.1
31 – 40	114	46.2
41 – 50	35	14.2
51 yrs and above	28	11.3
Total	247	100
Educational Level	Frequency	Percentage %
No formal schooling	24	9.7
Primary school.	69	27.9
Secondary school	100	40.5
Tertiary school	54	21.9
Total	247	100
Ethnic Group	Frequency	Percentage %
Yoruba	184	74.5
Igbo	4	1.6
Hausa	24	9.7
Others	35	14.2
Total	247	100
Religion	Frequency	Percentage %
Christianity	133	53.8
Muslim	109	44.1
Traditional belief	5	2.0
Total	247	100

Table 1: Distribution of Respondents' Demographic Characteristics.

Table 1 depicts that; out of the total numbers of respondents (247), 166 (66.4%) of them were males. Age ranged between 15 and 72 years (mean ± SEM was 35.44 ± 3.71). 184 (74.5%) participants were Yoruba ethnic group while 63 (25.5%) from other ethic groups. The distribution of participants according to their educational status was varying. The findings showed that few of the respondents were not educated. Education level found to be of no role in the preference of treatment selection. 53.8% of the participants that were Christians still preferred to be treated by TBSs while 44.1% from rural descent preferred to be treated by TBSs

Reasons of preference of TBSs

Figure 1 below indicated that; 38% of the participants from urban community preferred to be treated by TBSs while 48% from rural descent preferred to be treated by TBSs, P=0.021. 192 participants out of 199 responded well to the questionnaire.

The reason for going to TBS was; in 71 participants (37%) was their beliefs, in 27 participants (14.06%) was due to the low cost of TBS, and in 27 participants (14.06%) was due to fear of plaster (Figure 1).

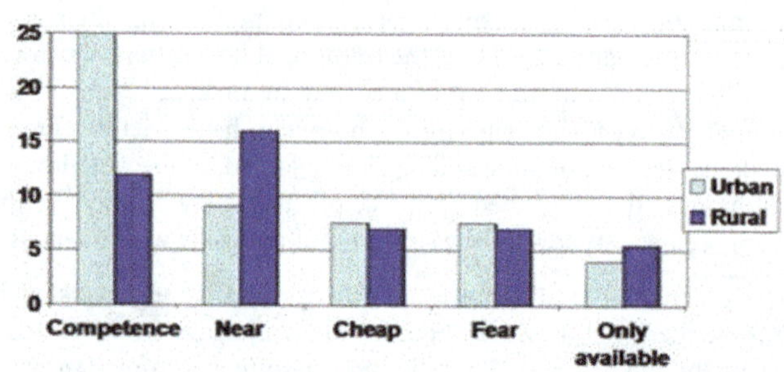

Figure 1: Participants From Urban Community and treatment with TBS's.

TBSs utilization

Examination of the TBSs patronage, 70 (28.3%) of the clients had a past history of treatment by an orthodox practitioner in their previous condition, while 177 (71.7%) were not but the first experience. On the whole, 124 (50.2%) of clients were attended to by bone-setters immediately in their current condition, 123 (49.8%) were not but still kept waiting.

Furthermore, many of those who had been attended to by the orthopaedists in the hospital and still fell back to TBSs indicated various reasons for doing so. The reasons of why do they changed to TBSs were varied. Out of the total respondents, 23 (9.3%) of the clients indicated that, the TBS is the only available nearby service to be utilized, 224 (90.7%) portrayed different medical causes for patronizing TBSs, which ranged from delay in medical services in the hospitals, fear of cast or amputation, occupied wards, less trained doctors, and high cost of hospital treatment (11.2%, 30.8%, 17.7%, 9.1%, 9.7%, respectively), and in 15 (11.5%) because of their beliefs (Figure 2).

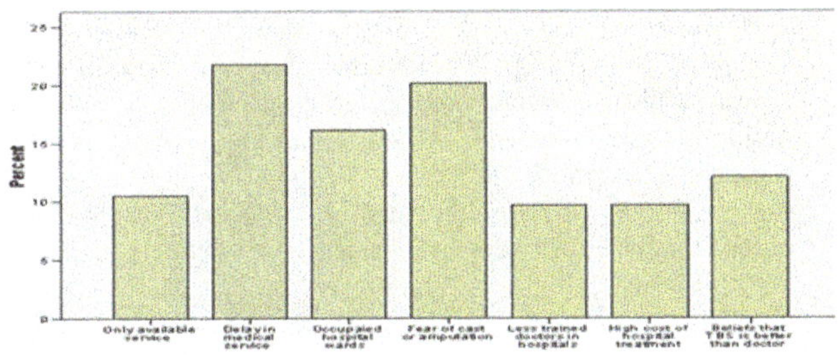

Figure 2: Examination of the TBSs patronage.

This section depicts the end result of the treatment of fracture through TBSs

Out come	Frequency	(%)
Poor	7	(2.8)
Acceptable	33	(13.4)
Good	84	(34.0)
Excellent	123	(49.8)
Total	247	(100.0)

Table 2: Outcome of Treatment Received By the Clients through TBSs.

In the main, investigation about the outcome of their treatment; majority (49.8%) of the respondents indicated that it was excellent and poor in 7 (2.8%) (Table 2). This result really shows the strength of the TBSs in fracture care in Ekiti State, especially the rural communities (Figure 3).

The Figure 3 above is an investigation on the decision maker on utilization of TBSs by the clients. The decision to contact the TBSs was a self-decision in 68 (27.5%), family in 99 (40.1%), relatives in 61 (24.7%), and friend decision in 19 (7.7%).

Source of knowledge of TBSs

An investigation on the source of their knowledge in bone setting, it was revealed that majority of the TBSs interviewed got into the system from self-education, parents or from relatives, and many others indicated that they got into the practice through other different sources.

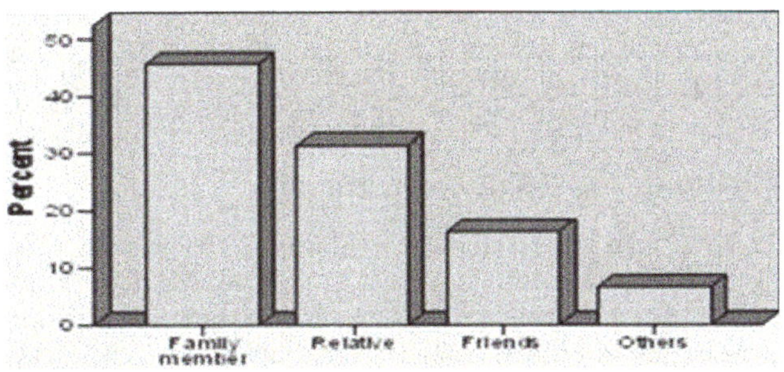

Figure 3: Decision on Service Utilization.

Discussion

The study revealed that males (67.2%) accounted for a large portion of patients seeking TBS treatment and showing that males are predominantly injured. This is no other reason than injuries from accident on "Okada" (Motorcycles). Majority of the unemployed graduates in Ekiti are daily engaging in using motorcycles for commercial purpose in a bid to make ends meet.

Hundred twenty-four (124) of the TBS's clients (50.2%) went to TBS from the start of their injury, this result agrees with Owumi et al. study, where 74.9% of patients were seen initially by TBS [8]. This could be dangerous especially in those that could have sustained concomitant life threatening injuries.

In the main, it is interesting that 49.8% of the patients initially were taken to hospitals before being withdrawn and attended treatment by TBS. This result is comparable to studies by Olorun [10] and Solagberu [11], where the incidences were 50% and 43% respectively. This high percentage requires an audit of our orthodox system in order to correct over inadequacies.

Different kind of fractures and dislocation were managed by the TBS in this study using the splints, herbs, skin lashes, pads and manipulation without consideration for a perfect anatomical reduction and alignment. It is important to raise the level of awareness of our communities about the narrow limit of the TBS in making a diagnosis and proper treatment of orthopaedic and trauma problems and this only can be tackled through a proper health education programs.

The reasons for continued patronage or preference and the attitude of the people and the TBSs are similar in studies conducted in Africa [12].

Patronage as shown in this study is determined by several factors. These factors were found not to be restricted to a particular group of people but involve people from every social strata and academic classes. Findings from the study also indicated that the TBS treatment is also believed to be cheap to the clients.

On the whole, fear of amputation was the reason of patronage in a small percentage of this study (17.7%), this closely agrees with Ogunlusi's [2] study who found that the fear of amputation was in 7%. It is important to educate people and let them know that Modern Orthopaedic Services does primarily save the limbs, and amputation is carried out on limbs that cannot be saved or for dead ones. We revealed that one of the important preference determinant factors included the opinions of family and friends. We found that the decision of seeking treatment at TBS in 68.1% of clients is non-self-decision (family members and friends); this closely agrees with Solagberu and Dada et al, where they found that the initial idea of visiting TBS was from an external person in 75% and 25 of cases respectively [10,11].

Conclusion and Recommendations

In view of the societal confidence, which the TBS enjoy in Nigeria, it is important that efforts be made at regulating their practice including the establishment of a sound referral system and adoption of a standard training curriculum. Though a number of deficiencies of the bone setters have been highlighted in this paper, it is obvious that they can be trained to function at the primary level especially in the rural areas.

1. Although there is a number of qualified orthopaedic surgeons and well-equipped hospitals in Nigeria at the moment, treatment is still obtained from traditional bonesetters by a large number of our population.
2. In spite of the complications, TBS continue to have patronage from both the highly educated and the illiterate. Possible reasons for this include culture and beliefs, ignorance and third-party advice, and also overcrowding of hospitals with trauma cases.
3. More collaborative effort is needed to raise awareness of complications that may arise from seeking management in TBS.
4. To achieve that, an extensive study of the current status of TBS including the obstacles and motivations for change is mandatory.

References

1. Orjioke CJG (2005) Does traditional medicine have a place in Primary Health Care? Orient J of Medicine.
2. Ogunlusi DO, Ikem IC, Oginni (2007) Why Patients Patronize Traditional Bone Setters. The Internet Journal of Orthopedic Surgery 4: 2.
3. Thanni LO (2000) Factors influencing patronage of traditional bone setters. West Afr J Med 19: 220-224.
4. Oyebola DD (1980) Yoruba traditional bonesetters: the practice of orthopaedics in a primitive setting in Nigeria. J Trauma 20: 312-322.
5. Udosen AM, Etiuma AU, Ugare GA (2005) Femoral Artery Aneurysm, a Complication of Traditional Bonesetting, (A case report). NigJSurg.
6. Ekere AU (2003) The scope of extremity amputations in a private hospital in the south-south region of Nigeria. Niger J Med 12: 225-228.
7. Omololu AB, Ogunlade SO, Gopaldasani VK (2008) The practice of traditional bonesetting: training algorithm. Clin Orthop Relat Res 466: 2392-2398.
8. Owumi BE, Jerome T (2012) Yoruba traditional bonesetters: the practice of orthopaedics in a primitive setting in Nigeria. J trauma 20: 312–322.
9. Agaja SB (2000) Prevalence of limb amputation and role of TBS in Nigeria. Nig J surgery 7: 79.
10. OlaOlorun DA, Oladiran IO, Adeniran A (2001) Complications of fracture treatment by traditional bonesetters in southwest Nigeria. Fam Pract 18: 635-637.
11. Solagberu BA (2005) Long bone fractures treated by traditional bonesetters: a study of patients' behaviour. Trop Doct 35: 106-108.
12. Ikpeme IA, Udosen AM, Okereke-Okpa I (2007) Patients' perception of traditional bone setting in Calabar. Port Harcourt medical Journal 1: 104-108.

Efficacy and Safety of Sansoninto in Insomnia with Psychiatric Disorder: An Open-Label Study

Tsuyoshi Miyaoka*, **Kiminori Kawano, Motohide Furuya, Rei Wake, Sadayuki Hashioka, Kristian Liaury, Erlyn Limoa, Keiko Tsuchie, Michiyo Fukushima, Tomoko Araki and Jun Horiguchi**

Department of Psychiatry, Shimane University School of Medicine, Izumo, Japan

***Corresponding author**: Tsuyoshi Miyaoka, Department of Psychiatry, Shimane University School of Medicine, 89-1 Enyacho, Izumo 693-8501, Japan, E-mail: miyanyan@med.shimane-u.ac.jp

Abstract

Background: Prior research confirms that insomnia is highly prevalent in patients with psychiatric disorders. Benzodiazepine hypnotics, causing serious disadvantages, have been widely used in psychiatry for a long time. Sansoninto (SNT), Japanese herbal medicine, is used for patients with weakness and fatigue, annoyance, insomnia, amnesia, and neurotic symptoms.

Objective: The efficacy and safety of SNT was examined in adult psychiatric disorder patients with insomnia symptoms.

Methods: Eighty-one adults with sleep disturbance meeting DSM-IV-TR diagnostic criteria for psychiatric disorders (schizophrenia: 17; monopolar depression: 20; bipolar depression: 10; adjustment disorder: 12; anxiety disorder: 5; others: 17) were treated openly for four weeks with SNT (2.5-7.5 g) at bedtime. Patients maintained sleep throughout the study. Efficacy was analyzed using a repeated measures methodology. The primary outcome was the Pittsburgh Sleep Quality Index (PSQI). The secondary outcomes were the Insomnia Severity Index (ISI), Athens Insomnia Scale (AIS), Clinical Global Impression-Improvement (CGI-I), and change of dosage of benzodiazepine hypnotics (diazepam equivalent).

Results: After 4 weeks of SNT therapy, significant symptom reduction was observed on all parameters (PSQI: 10.22 ± 3.23 vs. 3.11 ± 3.52; ISI: 20.63 ± 4.86 vs. 3.38 ± 5.10; AIS: 17.41 ± 4.69 vs. 2.85 ± 4.23; dosage of benzodiazepine hypnotics [diazepam equivalent, mg]:10.5 ± 4.71 vs. 2.98 ± 3.37). No withdrawal involved treatment-related adverse events.

Conclusion: Data from this 4-week open-label study suggests SNT was an effective and generally well tolerated treatment for insomnia symptoms in this sample of adult patients with psychiatric disorders.

Keywords: Psychiatric disorder; Sunsoninto (SNT); Insomnia; Japanese Herbal Medicine

Introduction

Sleep disturbances are common in individuals with psychiatric disorders [1]. For example, sleep problems are present in approximately 80% of patients with a major depressive disorder (MDD) [2], in 30% to 80% of patients with schizophrenia [3], and in at least 55% of individuals with active substance abuse [4]. Although these sleep disturbances often are secondary to the psychiatric illness, recent observations strongly suggest that sleep disorders should be actively treated parallel to psychiatric disorders. The few studies regarding this matter indicate that separate treatment of comorbid sleep disturbances exerts positive effects on the course of the psychiatric disorder and may prevent relapse [5]. Sleep disturbance is not only one of the most common symptoms of psychiatric disorders, but also one of the major determinants relating to quality of life (QOL) for patients with psychiatric disorders [6-8].

Benzodiazepines quickly gained acceptance as the preferred treatment for insomnia after appearing on the pharmaceutical market in 1960. Despite clinical guidelines recommending their use [9], there are still claims that the benefits of this older generation of hypnotics are outweighed by serious disadvantages including daytime sedation, dependence, rebound insomnia, slurred speech, staggering gait, poor judgment, and slow uncertain reflexes. Not surprisingly, many patients with sleep difficulty have turned to Japanese herbal medicine (kampo medicine) to manage their sleep problems and improve their QOL.

Kampo medicines use natural substances that generally have low toxicity and few side effects, treats disease as unique to the individual, and balance homeostasis and increasing immunity to diseases. Among traditional prescriptions used to treat sleep disorders, sansoninto (SNT; *suazaoretang*), a well-known traditional sedative, is used for patients with weakness and fatigue, annoyance, insomnia, amnesia, and neurotic symptoms [10]. In the classical literature, SNT is said to 'nourish the blood' and calm the nerves to eventually bring on a tranquilizing sensation and reduce the effect of sleep disturbance. SNT is a combination of five medicinal herbs: Jujube seed (*Zizyphi Semen*),

Poria sclerotium (*Poria*), Cnidium rhizome (*Cnidii Rhizoma*), Anemarrhena rhizome (*Anemarrhenae Rhizoma*) and Glycyrrhiza (*Glycyrrhizae Radix*) [11] (Table 1).

In experimental studies, SNT showed the hypnotic effect on sleep enhancement and its underlying mechanisms may be mediated through the activation of serotonergic system in additional to the activation of gamma-amino butyric acid A (GABAA) receptors in rat [12,13]. At the global metabolomics levels, SNT can increase sleep activity and exhibit binding affinity for serotonaergic receptors in a model of insomnia drosophilia [14]. Jujube seed, as the principal drug in the SNT, has exhibited the central nervous system tranqualizing effect. Spinosin has been proposed as the active component in Jujube seed [15]. In addition, the hypnotic effect of Jujube seed may be mediated by the anticholinergic and antihistamine action of betulic acid, an active compound of Jujube seed [16,17].

SNT is also available in the United States, but as an over-the-counter dietary supplement. Despite its popularity, no scientific evidence to back up claims of efficacy or safety in clinical use of SNT. Pharmaceutical companies are generally reluctant to conduct any randomized controlled trial for SNT, which is already on the market and approved by regulatory bodies. However, it is unethical not to conduct clinical trials to outline the safety profile of SNT; clinical trials will also provide basic knowledge to reveal possible mechanisms of SNT's effectiveness. An observation period of four weeks can start to expose any unknown side effects and may verify an ancient tradition that SNT is effective in improving sleep quality, sleep latency, sleep disturbance, sleep efficiency, and daytime function in patients with psychiatric disorders.

The objective of this four-week open study in a naturalistic setting was to evaluate the efficacy and safety of SNT in patients with psychiatric disorders.

Method

Herbal formula

The SNT formula used in this study is an herbal extract powder produced according to the good manufacturing procedures (GMP) of the certified company Tsumura Pharmaceutical Co., Ltd. (Japan), for the purpose of meeting international market standards of quality and uniformity. Apart from providing SNT, Tsumura Pharmaceutical was not involved in any other sponsorship, study design, or monitoring of the participants. In Japan, SNT has been approved by the Ministry of Health, Labour and Welfare, and is covered by the National Health Insurance plan. The compounds were classified on the basis of the constituent herbs of SNT on a chromatogram (Table 1).

Constituent of SNT	Compounds
JP Juijube seed (Zizyphi Semen)	Sanjoinine A
JP Poria sclerotium (Poria)	Dehydropachymic acid
JP Conidium rhizome (Chidii Rhizoma)	Geissoschizine methyl ether, hirsuterine, hirsutine
JP Anemarrhena rhizome (Anemarrhenae Rhizom)	Anemarsaponin AIII, Anemarsaponin C
JP Glycyrrhiza (Glycyrrhizae Radix)	Formononetin, formononetin-7-O-glucoside Liquiritigenin, liquiritin, liquiritin apioside, glycyrrhizin, glycyroside, isoliquiritin apioside, isoliquiritin, isoliquiritigenin, glycylcoumarin

Table 1: Classification of compounds identified in the three-dimensional chromatogram.

Preparation of herbs

All herbal components of SNT were prepared in large computer-controlled boiler which collected volatile oils and herbal broth, pumped into a vacuum drying condenser, and sprayed onto a base material. These granulated compounds were then vacuum-dried at low temperatures before being siphoned into a separate sterile-room, where they were packaged, labelled, and sealed. Granules were packed in aluminium foil packages and are administered orally at a dose of 2.5-7.5 g once per day. For quality assurance of the active ingredients in SNT, HPLC (high performance liquid chromatography) fingerprinting was employed to identify substances in the final product (Figure 1). No animal products, endangered species, or restricted herbal ingredients were used in this study. Each batch of SNT was also tested for E. coli, Salmonella (bacteria count), and heavy metals.

Figure 1

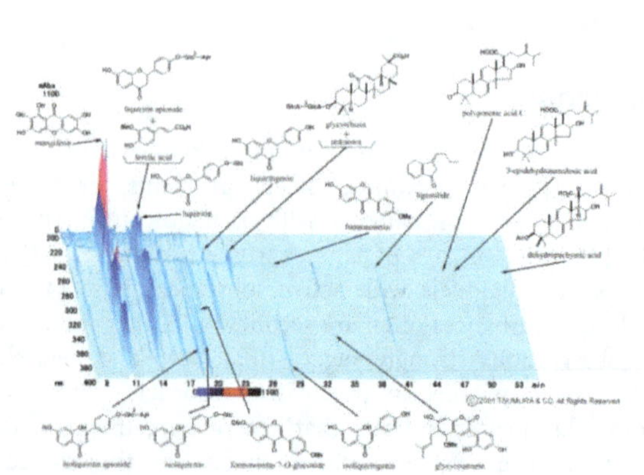

Figure 1: High performance liquid chromatography.

Recruitment of subjects

Patients of the Department of Psychiatry of the Shimane University Hospital were enrolled in the study. The study obtained approval from the Shimane University Hospital Institutional Review Board (No. 1067). Participants were recruited between April 2011 and April 2012. All participants understood the nature of the trial and willingly signed the informed consent form.

Eligibility criteria

The subjects enrolled in the study were patients with psychiatric disorders meeting DSM-IV-TR criteria [18], ranging from 27-80 years of age, with a Pittsburgh sleep quality index (PSQI) of greater than six. These patients spent 45 minutes or more falling asleep, slept less than six hours, and had struggled with this issue continuously for at least one month.

Ineligibility criteria

Patients with psychiatric disorders were ineligible to participate in the study if (1) they had had a major incident within three months of the study, (2) were working the nightshift, (3) lacked time or had timing conflicts, (4) had confounding disease such as obstructive sleep apnea-hypopnea, restless legs syndrome, cardiac arrthythmia, acute myocardial infarction, high blood pressure, diabetes, or cancer, (5) were currently taking pharmaceuticals that affect melatonin, acetylcholine, adenosine or prostaglandins, (6) were unable to read and fill out the forms for the study, or (7) had any evidence of renal or liver dysfunction as defined by a level of at least 1.5 times of the upper reference limit (serum creatinine: 1.3 mg/dL, blood urea nitrogen: 22 mg/dL, serum aspartate-aminotransferase (AST): 25 IU, alanine-aminotransferase (ALT): 29 IU/L).

Study design and procedure

Psychiatrists, physicians, and nurses were briefed on important points prior to the start of the study and attended a training session to ensure their duties were conducted in accordance with good clinical practice guidelines. Participants underwent an initial screening phase of two visits. On the first visit, they were interviewed to obtain information about their medical history and were later subjected to a clinical examination. The second visit determined the baseline data on symptoms and included a basic health assessment that consisted of complete blood counts and biochemical function tests. These tests were performed to ensure the eligibility of each patients and to identify respondents with potential poor compliance. At the end of the second visit, each eligible patient was provided with sufficient SNT for a treatment dose of 2.5-7.5 g once daily (at bed-time) to take until the next visit. No other herbs were allowed during the study period.

Follow-up visits were scheduled for the first and fourth weeks of the study. Physical examinations, basic health assessments, and biochemical function tests for each patient were carried out the end of the study. At the end of the trial, the participants received a further physical examination, including blood tests. Patients were contacted by telephone one to two days prior to each visit to encourage their continued participation. Throughout the study, leftover packages were counted to monitor each patient's compliance. The occurrence of adverse effects (AEs) was recorded on every visit.

Efficacy

The primary outcome parameter evaluated prior to and following the four week intervention was the PSQI. The PSQI is a multidimensional, self-administered, health status measure that probes clinically important, patient-relevant symptoms in the areas of sleep quality and quantity. The PSQI comprises a 19-item questionnaire with seven sub-scales (subjective sleep quality, sleep latency, sleep duration, habitual sleep disturbances, sleep efficiency, use of sleep medication, and daytime dysfunction) [18]. Each subscale is rated 0-3 with the higher scores reflecting more severe sleep complaints. The sum of the scores indicates the patient's overall sleep experience. The lower the overall score, the better the person sleeps. The tool possesses adequate internal reliability, validity, and consistency for clinical and community samples of psychiatric patients [19], However, the questions are heavily based on memory over the past month. Therefore, the study included four secondary outcome parameters: the Insomnia Severity Index (ISI) [20], Athens Insomnia Scale (AIS) [15], Clinical Global Impression-Improvement (CGI-I) [21], and dosage of benzodiazepine hypnotics (diazepam equivalent) [22].

Safety assessment

To set up an active safety surveillance system, we first surveyed the traditional medicine practitioners currently using SNT in the treatment of sleep difficulty to ascertain any AEs these practitioners had noticed. They reported that such medication occasionally resulted in gastrointestinal discomfort such as acid regulation, heartburn, and abdominal discomfort when SNT was administered orally at a dose of 2.5-7 g, once per day. We included these on our list for surveillance. We also included the AEs most frequently reported by the National Reporting System: abdominal fullness, diarrhoea, vomiting, nausea, urticaria, itching, purpura, jaundice, skin vesicles (or local reddish swelling), edema, hypotension, bradycardia, dyspnoea, fever, muscle cramps, and sleepiness on our surveillance list. Other possible AEs were enquired about as the 21st item. All subjects were required to take objective laboratory tests to detect any abnormal liver, blood, or kidney findings at the baseline and after four weeks of SNT therapy.

Statistical analysis

Our analysis focused mainly on changes in the seven-domain constructs of the PSQI assessment. The study described the treatment effects as changes in mean differences among the participants between the baseline scores and those measured at visits on weeks one and four. Separate linear regression models were constructed for the response variables of differentiated scores on subjective sleep quality, sleep latency, sleep duration, habitual sleep disturbances, use of sleep medication, and daytime dysfunction subscales. The explanatory variables in the final regression model were age, marital status, educational level, and baseline severity of psychiatric symptoms. To examine improvement across the month, two indicator variables for visits at weeks one and four were also included in the regression model. The coefficients of the two indicator variables represent the differences between the average values of measured scores for the visits at weeks one and four versus those at baseline. We assumed correlated error terms among the repeated measurements for each participant. Finally, each single PSQI score item was also examined separately to identify any PSQI items sensitive to treatment by SNT. All of the above analyses were performed using the SAS (9.2 edition) software package. On the basis of data from previous reports, we calculated the required sample size to be 75 [5].

Results

Study population

Of 99 sample patients, 18 were deemed to be ineligible. The principal reasons for ineligibility were a disinterest in participation (n=12), medical conditions and medications (n=3), failure to show up for further study (n=2), and lack of evidence of severe sleep difficulty (n=1). In all, 81 of the initial participants intending to treat (ITT) completed the 4-week study without any major protocol violation. For safety analysis, full analysis set testing was performed.

Table 2 summarizes the baseline demographics and clinical characteristics of the study. The patients in the study had a mean age of 44.5 ± 8.4. All subjects were diagnosed with insomnia associated with psychiatric disorder according to International Classification of Sleep Disorders Second Edition (ICSD-2) [23], and classified as: schizophrenia, 17; monopolar depression, 20; bipolar type I, 4; bipolar type II, 6; adjustment disorder, 12; anxiety disorder, 5; and others, 17. At the start of SNT administration, all subjects were receiving BZD hypnotics (one kind of drug, 44; two or more kind of drugs, 37).

Clinical Characteristics	
Sex, n (male/female)	35/46
Age, mean ± SD, year	44.5 ± 8.4
Diagnosis	
Schizophrenia	17
Monopolar depression	20
Bipolar affective disorder	
Type I	4
Type II	6
Adjustment disorder	12
Anxiety disorder	5
Others	17
Hypnotics	
Diazepam equivalent (mg)	10.5 ± 4.7
One drug	44
Two or more drugs	37

Table 2: Demographic and clinical characteristics of 81 patients completing a 4-week trial of SNT.

Efficacy

After four weeks of treatment, there were significant improvements in each of the PSQI subscales. The magnitudes of improvement in the PSQI subscales were 30% for subjective sleep quality, 22% for sleep latency, 27% for sleep duration, 9.3% for habitual sleep disturbances, and 27% for daytime dysfunction (Table 3). The mean amount of time to fall asleep per day was reduced from 60.6 ± 46.0 minutes at the baseline to 31.0 ± 20.0 minutes at the end of the study. The mean sleep duration per day was prolonged from 4.7 ± 1.0 hours at the baseline to 6.5 ± 1.1 hours after four weeks treatment. In other secondary outcomes, ISI, AIS, and CGI, significant improvement of symptoms was observed. The mean dosage of benzodiazepine hypnotics was reduced significantly after 4-week treatment by SNT (Table 3).

	Baseline	**After 4 weeks of TJ-103 therapy**	**P-value**
	(mean ± SD)	**(mean ± SD)**	
Pittsburg Sleep Quality Index	10.22 ± 3.23	3.11 ± 3.52	<0.0001
Subjective sleep quality	2.56 ± 0.57	0.78 ± 0.85	<0.0001
Sleep latency	2.64 ± 0.58	0.58 ± 0.74	<0.0001
Sleep duration	2.33 ± 0.92	0.64 ± 0.73	<0.0001
Habitual sleep efficacy	2.14 ± 1.12	0.20 ± 0.49	<0.0001
Sleep disturbance	1.15 ± 0.48	0.33 ± 0.50	<0.0001
Daytime dysfunction	2.68 ± 0.54	0.58 ± 0.89	<0.0001
Insomnia Severity Index	20.63 ± 4.86	3.38 ± 5.10	<0.0001
Athens Insomnia Scale	17.41 ± 4.69	2.85 ± 4.23	<0.0001
Hypnotics			
Diazepam equivalent (mg)	10.5 ± 4.71	2.98 ± 3.37	<0.0001
Tablets	1.46 ± 0.95	0.59 ± 0.45	<0.0001

Table 3: Major variables of baseline and week 4 measurements summarized as mean difference.

Among those ITT, psychiatric symptom scores of one of 81 patients had increased at the end of the study. Ten of these patients reported sleep quality at the same level as their baseline, one reported sleep quality worse than her baseline, and the remaining nine perceived better sleep quality by week four.

Safety and adverse effects

No tested biomarker demonstrated significant changes after the 4-week SNT intervention. No participant withdrew from the study due to AEs. Intolerable side effects resulting in withdrawal included two events of stomach ache and nausea. We carried out periodic evaluation of any unexpected symptom during the treatment period and found the perception of gastrointestinal discomfort two days after SNT consumption, but it was dramatically relieved after SNT discontinuance. We were unable to rule out the possibility that ingesting SNT will cause the deterioration of pre-existing gastrointestinal symptoms.

Discussion

To the best of our knowledge, this study is the first to investigate the potential efficacy and safety of SNT in improving sleep quality in psychiatric disorders with sleep difficulty as measured by PSQI. Our results demonstrated a significant improvement in sleep quality of patients with psychiatric disorders after four weeks of SNT treatment.

Although we used self-comparison to rule out potential confounding effects of BMI, smoking, exercise, and socioeconomic status, the possibility of placebo effect might still exist.

The present data showed that one week of SNT treatment had no effect, but there was significant improvement in sleep quality after a four-week treatment at a dose of 2.5-7.5 g once daily (Figure 2). From a physiologically based pharmacokinetic point of view, it takes more than one week to demonstrate the symptom-relief effect of the active ingredients in SNT, which appears to resemble a slow-acting drug, and it may not be appropriate to compare its action head-to-head with conventional medications of rapid action, such BZD hypnotics. The outcome of the evaluation study provides valuable evidence to avoid a direct comparison of the SNT formula with rapid action medications in future randomized controlled trials.

Figure 2

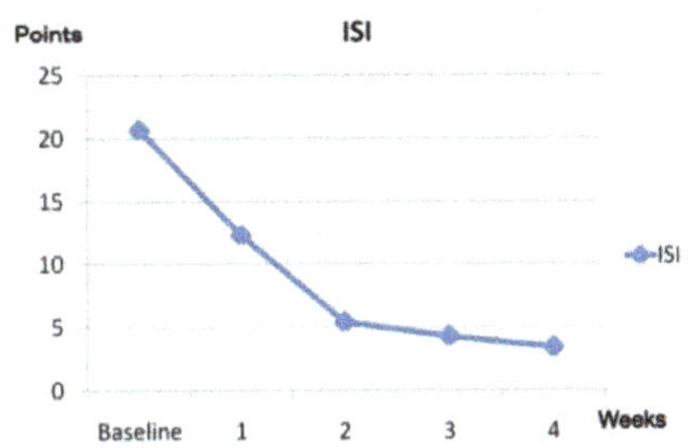

Figure 2: SNT treatment.

The dose of BZD hypnotics was reduced at almost the same time as improvement of the score, and the dose was further reduced with an improvement in the score. At week 4, the dose of BZD hypnotics had been reduced to about one third of that used at baseline. During the observation period, reducing the dose of BZD hypnotics did not cause any adverse events that may pose serious problems in medical practice, such as inter dose rebound insomnia.

Although an immediate effect of SNT cannot be expected due to its characteristics, the effect was observed after four weeks in the 34 subjects who switched to exclusive-use, and especially at week 2, 31 of the 34 subjects had been able to switch to SNT alone. This result suggests that continuous administration at least for one month would be ideal in order to reduce the dose of co-administered BZD hypnotics.

Generally, if the duration of administration of BZD hypnotics exceeds six months to one year, about 80% of patients experience withdrawal symptoms [24]. Therefore, as a method for gradual reduction of BZD hypnotics, reducing the daily dose about 25% every two to four weeks is recommended [25]. Most subjects in this study had taken BZD hypnotics for more than one year, and the speed of reduction was faster than recommended. However, because of the small number of subjects and the lack of evaluation of the effect of concomitant psychotropic drugs, it is difficult to assert that SNT has potential to prevent withdrawal symptoms.

With regard to the basic research examining the treatment of insomnia, current pharmacologic approaches have largely focused on the activity of γ-amino butyric acid A (GABAA), one of the inhibitory neurotransmitters in the central nervous system. In an experimental mouse model, it had been suggested that SNT has an activity different from that of synthetic hypnotics such as BZD. This is because SNT had no effect on pentobarbital (PB)-induced sleep in unstressed mice, and it reverses the stress-induced decrease and/or increase in PB sleep by improving stress-induced functional changes in the central nervous system rather than by acting like a synthetic hypnotic on GABAA receptors [26]. Yang et al. reported that SNT increases sleep activity and exhibits binding affinity for serotonin receptors. These results implicate the hypnotic effect of SNT, and its effects may be mediated through serotonergic activation. It provided strong evidence that the hypnotic effect of SNT occurred at the level of global metabolomics. By using a metabolomic approach, this study also demonstrates that metabolomics could provide a very promising way to elucidate the therapeutic mechanisms of Japanese herbal medicines [27].

Clinical trials have never explored the SNT dosage used in this study (2.5-7.5 g once daily). Without the present data, TM practitioners in Japan will continue to prescribe SNT to patients in their everyday practice based on documentation from a thousand years ago. The results of this study show (about IIb level) [15] that to participants had to withdraw from the study due to AEs, and that the two leading adverse drug reactions included stomach ache and nausea. The AEs discovered by this study, though not serious enough to prohibit the use of this formula clinically, show that TM practitioners must be alert to the possibility that prescribing SNT can cause severe adverse gastrointestinal effects. Further research to clarify the safety of SNT use is necessary [28].

The present study recruited psychiatric patients with poor sleep and used self-comparison to rule out the potential confounders of BMI, age exercise, and socioeconomic status. This type of study presents particular advantages. Limited subject numbers allow simple and comprehensive data analysis that can be used to identify possible trends, which a larger sample size could prove significant. Participants do not have to spend the extended amount of time necessary for a crossover design, an alternate method for dealing with a limited number of subjects. Additionally, this type of study avoids the ethical dilemma regarding giving a placebo to symptomatic participants who could be receiving valid treatment.

A major limitation of our study is its observational nature or lack of a randomized placebo group. Therefore, our claim of efficacy associated with SNT might not be as strict as that from a randomized clinical trial (RCT). No matter how common the use of SNT is in Japan, no RCT has been conducted yet. The evidence we obtained from the present study can provide important data on the safety profile of SNT and direct evaluation of its effectiveness, and meanwhile this study can serve as prior data for the design of RCTs. Another limitation of this study is that since participants were psychiatric patients with sleep problems in Japan, caution in generalizing these findings to patients in other nations is necessary.

Limitation

Given the design characteristics of this trial, the present findings should be taken cautiously. Study limitations include its open design and its small sample size. In an open-label study, both placebo effects and the effects of medication previously prescribed cannot be ruled out as explanations for the observed improvements.

Conclusion

Excluding psychiatric patients with a past history of stomach ache, diarrhoea, and dizziness, the dosage form and prescription pattern of the SNT preparation appears to be well tolerated and valuable as a short-term alterative therapeutic option for improving daytime dysfunction in psychiatric patients with poor sleep quality during their psychiatric phase. A placebo effect, natural fluctuation, insufficient follow-up time, and/or other unobserved factors could confound the results of the current study. A prospective randomized, double-blind, controlled trial to further evaluate the efficacy of SNT on psychiatric patients with sleep difficulty is warranted in the future.

Authors Contributions

T. Miyaoka created the study design and coordination, patient recruitment, conceived the study, and helped draft the manuscript. M. Furuya conducted paper preparation and submission. R. Wake, S. Hashioka, K. Kawano, K. Liaury, E. Limoa, K. Tsuchie, M. Fukushima, and Jun Horiguchi were responsible for data acquisition and obtained the funding for the study. T. Araki and M. Fukushima performed all statistical analyses and interpretation of the data. All authors have read and approved the paper.

Acknowledgments

Part of this work was supported by Grant-in-Aid for Scientific Research on Priority Areas No. 13770544 and 50284047 from the Ministry of Education, Science, Sports and Culture and 012 from the Ministry of Health Labour Sciences Research Grant of Japan.

References

1. Abad VC, Guilleminault C (2005) Sleep and psychiatry. Dialogues Clin Neurosci 7: 291-303.
2. Tsuno N, Besset A, Ritchie K (2005) Sleep and depression. J Clin Psychiatry 66: 1254-1269.
3. Cohrs S (2008) Sleep disturbances in patients with schizophrenia : impact and effect of antipsychotics. CNS Drugs 22: 939-962.
4. Mahfoud Y, Talih F, Streem D, Budur K (2009) Sleep disorders in substance abusers: how common are they? Psychiatry (Edgmont) 6: 38-42.
5. Smith MT, Huang MI, Manber R (2005) Cognitive behavior therapy for chronic insomnia occurring within the context of medical and psychiatric disorders. Clin Psychol Rev 25: 559-592.
6. Zammit GK, Weiner J, Damato N, Sillup GP, McMillan CA (1999) Quality of life in people with insomnia. Sleep 22 Suppl 2: S379-385.
7. Bélanger L, Morin CM, Langlois F, Ladouceur R (2004) Insomnia and generalized anxiety disorder: effects of cognitive behavior therapy for gad on insomnia symptoms. J Anxiety Disord 18: 561-571.
8. Riedel BW, Lichstein KL (2000) Insomnia and daytime functioning. Sleep Med Rev 4: 277-298.
9. National Institutes of Health (2005) National Institutes of Health State of the Science Conference statement on Manifestations and Management of Chronic Insomnia in Adults, June 13-15, 2005. Sleep 28: 1049-1057.
10. www.consensus.nih.gov/2005/2005InsomniaSoS026html.htm
11. Wang YC (1983) Hand book of Commonly Used Chinese Herbal Prescriptions, Oriental Healing Arts Institute, Long Beach CA
12. Ministry of Health (2006) Labour and Welfare, "The Japanese Pharmacopeia, Fifteenth Edition (15th edn)
13. Yi PL, Tsai CH, Chen YC, Chang FC (2007) Gamma-aminobutyric acid (GABA) receptor mediates suanzaorentang, a traditional Chinese herb remedy, -induced sleep alteration. J Biomed Sci 14: 285-297.
14. Yi PL, Lin CP, Tsai CH, Lin JG, Chang FC (2007) The involvement of serotonin receptors in suanzaorentang-induced sleep alteration. J Biomed Sci 14: 829-840.
15. Yang B, Zhang A, Sun H, Dong W, Yan G, et al. (2012) Metabolomic study of insomnia and intervention effects of suanzaoren decoction using ultra-performance liquid-chromatography/electrospray-ionization synapt high-definition mass spectrometry. J Pharm Biomed Anal 58: 113-124.
16. Li Y, Liang X, Xiao H, Bi K (2003) Determination of spinosin in rat plasma by reversed-phase high-performance chromatography after oral administration of Suanzaoren decoction. J Chromatogr B Analyt Technol Biomed Life Sci 787: 421-425.
17. Chen CY, Chen YF, Tsai HY (2008) What is the effective component in suanzaoren decoction for curing insomnia? Discovery by virtual screening and molecular dynamic simulation. J Biomol Struct Dyn 26: 57-64.
18. American Psychiatric Association (2000) Diagnostic and Statistical Manual of Mental Disorders, revision (DSM-IV-TR) (4thedn), American Psychiatric Association, Washington DC
19. Buysse DJ, Reynolds CF 3rd, Monk TH, Berman SR, Kupfer DJ (1989) The Pittsburgh Sleep Quality Index: a new instrument for psychiatric practice and research. Psychiatry Res 28: 193-213.
20. Bastien CH, Vallières A, Morin CM (2001) Validation of the Insomnia Severity Index as an outcome measure for insomnia research. Sleep Med 2: 297-307.
21. Soldatos CR, Dikeos DG, Paparrigopoulos TJ (2000) Athens Insomnia Scale: validation of an instrument based on ICD-10 criteria. J Psychosom Res 48: 555-560.
22. Guy W (1976) National Institute of Mental Health. CGI, Clinical Global Impression In ECDEU Assessment Manual for Psychopharmacology. revised Rockville MD: 534-537.
23. Inagaki A, Inada T (2006) Dose equivalence of psychiatric drugs. Jpn J Clin Psychopharmacol 9: 1443-1447.
24. American Academy of Sleep Medicine (2005) International Classification of Sleep Disorders (2nd edn) Diagnostic and Coding Manual. American Academy of Sleep Medicine Westchester IL
25. Rickels K, Case WG, Schweizer EE, Swenson C, Fridman RB (1986) Low-dose dependence in chronic benzodiazepine users: a preliminary report on 119 patients. Psychopharmacol Bull 22: 407-415.
26. Catena-Dell'Osso M, Marazziti D, Rotella F, Bellantuono C (2012) Emerging targets for the pharmacological treatment of depression: focus on melatonergic system. Curr Med Chem 19: 428-437.
27. Saito K, Umeda S, Kawashima K, Kano Y (2000) Pharmacological properties of traditional medicines. XXVI. Effects of Sansohnin-to on pentobarbital sleep in stressed mice. Biol Pharm Bull 23: 76-79.
28. WHO (2000) General guidelines for methodologies on research and evaluation of traditional medicines. Document: WHO/EDM/TRM/ 2000.1 Geneva, Switzerland.

Permissions

All chapters in this book were first published in A&IM, by OMICS International; hereby published with permission under the Creative Commons Attribution License or equivalent. Every chapter published in this book has been scrutinized by our experts. Their significance has been extensively debated. The topics covered herein carry significant findings which will fuel the growth of the discipline. They may even be implemented as practical applications or may be referred to as a beginning point for another development.

The contributors of this book come from diverse backgrounds, making this book a truly international effort. This book will bring forth new frontiers with its revolutionizing research information and detailed analysis of the nascent developments around the world.

We would like to thank all the contributing authors for lending their expertise to make the book truly unique. They have played a crucial role in the development of this book. Without their invaluable contributions this book wouldn't have been possible. They have made vital efforts to compile up to date information on the varied aspects of this subject to make this book a valuable addition to the collection of many professionals and students.

This book was conceptualized with the vision of imparting up-to-date information and advanced data in this field. To ensure the same, a matchless editorial board was set up. Every individual on the board went through rigorous rounds of assessment to prove their worth. After which they invested a large part of their time researching and compiling the most relevant data for our readers.

The editorial board has been involved in producing this book since its inception. They have spent rigorous hours researching and exploring the diverse topics which have resulted in the successful publishing of this book. They have passed on their knowledge of decades through this book. To expedite this challenging task, the publisher supported the team at every step. A small team of assistant editors was also appointed to further simplify the editing procedure and attain best results for the readers.

Apart from the editorial board, the designing team has also invested a significant amount of their time in understanding the subject and creating the most relevant covers. They scrutinized every image to scout for the most suitable representation of the subject and create an appropriate cover for the book.

The publishing team has been an ardent support to the editorial, designing and production team. Their endless efforts to recruit the best for this project, has resulted in the accomplishment of this book. They are a veteran in the field of academics and their pool of knowledge is as vast as their experience in printing. Their expertise and guidance has proved useful at every step. Their uncompromising quality standards have made this book an exceptional effort. Their encouragement from time to time has been an inspiration for everyone.

The publisher and the editorial board hope that this book will prove to be a valuable piece of knowledge for researchers, students, practitioners and scholars across the globe.

List of Contributors

Tenaw Gualu Melesse, Girma Alem Getie, Haymanot Zeleke Mitiku and Girmay Tsegaye
Department of Nursing, College of Health Sciences, Debremarkos University, Debremarkos, Ethiopia

Yohannes Ayalew
Departments of Nursing and Midwifery, School of Allied Health Sciences, College of Health Science, Addis Ababa University, Addis Ababa, Ethiopia

Ghosh AK
The Jagaddal Noapara Homoeopathic Medical Association, West Bengal, India

Richa Gupta and Suman Bala Sharma
Department of Biochemistry, University College of Medical Sciences, University of Delhi, India

Usha Rani Singh
Department of Pathology, University College of Medical Sciences, University of Delhi, India

Mukesh C. Sharma
Drug Research Laboratory, School of Pharmacy, Devi Ahilya University, Takshila Campus, Khandwa Road, Indore, M.P, India

Erica B. Oberg, Ryan Bradley, Kieran Cooley, Heidi Fritz, Joshua Z. Goldenberg, Dugald Seely, Jane D. Saxton and Carlo Calabrese
Pacific Pearl La Jolla, San Diego, CA 92037, USA

Mahendra Kumar Trivedi, Shrikant Patil and Harish Shettigar
Trivedi Global Inc., 10624 S Eastern Avenue Suite A-969, Henderson, NV 89052, USA

Mayank Gangwar and Snehasis Jana
Trivedi Science Research Laboratory Pvt. Ltd, Madhya Pradesh, India

Seung-Mo Kim and Min-Ah Kwak
Department of Internal Medicine, College of Korean Medicine, Daegu Haany University, Daegu, Korea

Ae Ryun Choi
Department of Sasang Constitutional Medicine, College of Korean Medicine, Daegu Haany University, Daegu, Korea

Im Hee Shin
Department of Medical Statistics, School of Medicine, Catholic University of Daegu, Daegu, Korea

Byung Seok Kim and Chang Hyeong Lee
Department of Internal Medicine, School of Medicine, Catholic University of Daegu, Daegu, Korea

Paul C. Chikezie
Department of Biochemistry, Imo State University, Owerri, Nigeria

Okey A. Ojiako
Department of Biochemistry, Federal University of Technology, Owerri, Nigeria

Xiangping Kang, Guoqin Jin, Xueli Zhang, Zhangbin Gong and Yanwu Xu
Department of Biochemistry, Institute of Basic Medicine, Shanghai University of Traditional Chinese Medicine (TCM), Shanghai 201203, China

Chao Liang
Experiment in TCM, Department, Institute of Basic Medicine, Shanghai University of Traditional Chinese Medicine (TCM), Shanghai 201203, China

Zhifen Han
Experiment Center for Teaching & Learning, Shanghai University of Traditional Chinese Medicine (TCM), Shanghai 201203, China

Jie-Jun Li, Jin-Feng Jiang, Ying Jiang and Xiao-Jing Wu
Key Laboratory of Acupuncture Combined with Medication, The Second Clinical Medical College, Nanjing University of Traditional Chinese Medicine, Nanjing 210046, China

Keck T
Department of ENT Medicine, Head and Neck Surgery, Krankenhaus, Elisabethinen GmbH Graz, Austria

Strobl A
Department of ENT Medicine, Head and Neck Surgery, Krankenhaus der Barmherzigen Schwestern Linz Betriebsgesellschaft m.b.H, Linz, Austria

Stracke B
Department of Clinical Research, Dr. Willmar Schwabe GmbH & Co. KG, Karlsruhe, Germany

Richard Pearlman and Jonathan Wolfe
School of Medicine, University of South Alabama, Mobile, Alabama, USA

John E. Kovaleski
Department of Health, Physical Education, University of South Alabama, Mobile, Alabama, USA

Wei Liu
Edward Via College of Osteopathic Medicine Auburn, Auburn, Alabama, USA

Satyendra Kumar and Arun Gupta
Medical Affairs and Clinical Research Division, Dabur Research and Development Centre, Dabur India Limited, Uttar Pradesh, India

Raman Ghungralekar
Department of Kayachikitsa, R A Podar Medical (Ayurvedic) College and M A Podar hospital, Mumbai, Maharashtra, India

Vaishali Shailesh Deshpande
Department of Kayachikitsa, Sumatibhai Shah Ayurved Mahavidyalya, Malwadi, Mumbai Pune, Maharashtra, India

Mohamed M Elseweidy
Faculty of Pharmacy, Zagazig University, Zagazig, Egypt

Aswathy Rajan and Ramanibai Ravichandran
Department of Zoology, University of Madras, Chennai, India

Upma Bagai
Department of Zoology, Panjab University, Chandigarh, India

A Timucin Atayoglu
Medipol University, Department of Family Medicine, Istanbul, Turkey
Holistic and Integrative Medicine Association, Istanbul, Turkey

Ayten Guner-Atayoglu, Gulcin Kuran-Cetinkale and M Ali Cetinkale
Holistic and Integrative Medicine Association, Istanbul, Turkey

Elena Mejías Gil
University of Extremadura, Avda de Elvas S/N, 06006 Badajoz, España, Spain

María Victoria González López-Arza
Medicine and Surgery Department, University of Extremadura, Spain

Radosław Kujawski, Magdalena Borowska, Katarzyna Manikowska, Joanna Liberska, Michał Szulc and Piotr Ruszkowski
Department of Pharmacology, Poznan University of Medical Sciences, Poland

Justyna Baraniak, Malgorzata Kania and Agnieszka Gryszczyńska
Department of Pharmacology and Phytochemistry, Institute of Natural Fibers and Medicinal Plants, Poland

Marcin Ożarowski
Department of Pharmacology and Phytochemistry, Institute of Natural Fibers and Medicinal Plants, Poland
Department of Pharmaceutical Botany and Plant Biotechnology, Poznan University of Medical Sciences, Poland

Małgorzata Kujawska
Department of Toxicology, Poznan University of Medical Sciences, Poland

Joanna Bartkowiak-Wieczorek
Department of Clinical Pharmacy and Biopharmacy, Poznan University of Medical Sciences, Poland

Agnieszka Sobczak
Department of Pharmaceutical Chemistry, Poznan University of Medical Sciences, Poland

Joanna Cichocka
Wielkopolska Centre for Advanced Technologies (WCAT), Adam Mickiewicz University in Poznan, Poland

Oroma B Nwanodi
Department of Obstetrics and Gynecology, Locum Tenens, Salinas CA, USA

Aiman Abbas Jafri, Suman Bala Sharma, Mohit Mehndiratta and Nikhil Khurana
Department of Biochemistry, University College of Medical Sciences (University of Delhi), Dilshad Garden, Delhi, India

Kalpana Luthra
Department of Biochemistry, All India institute of Medical Sciences, Ansari Nagar, Delhi, India

Usha Rani Singh
Department of Pathology, University College of Medical Sciences (University of Delhi), Dilshad Garden, Delhi, India

Hsien-Tsung Yao
Department of Nutrition, China Medical University, 91, Hsueh-Shih Road, Taichung, 404, Taiwan

Lorenzo Freti, Vincenzo Condemi, Massimo Gestro and Umberto Solimene
Department of Biomedical Sciences for Health-State University of Milan; Via Mangiagalli 31, Milan, Italy

Marianna Mazza, Marco Di Nicola and Luigi Janiri
Institute of Psychiatry and Clinical Psychology, Catholic University of Sacred Heart, Largo A. Gemelli 8, Rome, Italy

Andrea Antonietti
Fondazione Don Gnocchi Onlus, IRCCS Santa Maria Nascente Centre; Via Alfonso Capecelatro 66, Milan, Italy

Hoorieh Mohammadi Kenari and Maryam Taqavi Shirazi
Research Institute for Islamic and Complementary Medicine, Iran University of Medical Sciences, Tehran, Iran

Rozita Jafari
School of Health Management and Information Sciences, Iran University of Medical Sciences, Tehran, Iran

Maryam Moghimi
Persian Medicine Offices of Ministry of Health and Medical Education, Tehran, Iran

Ahmed T. El-Olemy
Department of Public Health and Community Medicine, Faculty of Medicine, Tanta University, Egypt
Department of Academic Affairs and Training Unit, National Center for Complementary and Alternative Medicine, Ministry of Health, Riyadh, Saudi Arabia

Fawehinmi AB
Nigeria Natural Medicine Development Agency Lagos, Nigeria

Oyedeji FO
Department of Chemistry, University of Ibadan, Nigeria

Tsegaye Assefa, Haymanot Tasew and Jemal Beker
Department of Medical Laboratory Sciences and Pathology College of Public Health and Medical Sciences, Jimma University, Ethiopia

Beyene Wondafrash
Department of Nursing, College of Public Health and Medical Sciences, Jimma University, Ethiopia

Cynthia Verwer and Lucy van de Vijver
Department Nutrition & Health, Louis Bolk Institute, Driebergen, The Netherlands

Miek C Jong
Department Nutrition & Health, Louis Bolk Institute, Driebergen, The Netherlands
Department of Health Sciences, Mid Sweden University, Sundsvall, Sweden
National Information and Knowledge Center on Integrative Medicine (NIKIM), Amsterdam, The Netherlands

Petra Klement and Julia Burkart
Deutsche Homöopathie-Union, DHU-Arzneimittel GmbH & Co. KG, Karlsruhe, Germany

Erik Baars
Department Nutrition & Health, Louis Bolk Institute, Driebergen, The Netherlands
Department of Care, Professorship Anthroposophic Healthcare, University of Applied Sciences, Leiden, The Netherlands

David S. Kiefer
Department of Family Medicine, School of Medicine and Public Health, University of Wisconsin Madison, USA

Lauren Moscoe
Department of Botany, University of Wisconsin-Madison, USA

Jack Buchanan
Nelson Institute for Environmental Studies, University of Wisconsin-Madison, USA

Catherine Woodward
Ceiba Foundation for Tropical Conservation, USA

Owoseni Joseph Sina
College of Medicine and Health Sciences (Medical Sociology), Afe Babalola University, Ado-Ekiti, Nigeria

Ibikunle Ayodele M
Department of Sociology, Ekiti State University Ado Ekiti, Nigeria

Tsuyoshi Miyaoka, Kiminori Kawano, Motohide Furuya, Rei Wake, Sadayuki Hashioka, Kristian Liaury, Erlyn Limoa, Keiko Tsuchie, Michiyo Fukushima, Tomoko Araki and Jun Horiguchi
Department of Psychiatry, Shimane University School of Medicine, Izumo, Japan

Index